MTP International Review of Science

Physiology
Series One

Consultant Editor
A. C. Guyton

Publisher's Note

The MTP International Review of Science is an important new venture in scientific publishing, which is presented by Butterworths in association with MTP Medical and Technical Publishing Co. Ltd. and University Park Press, Baltimore. The basic concept of the Review is to provide regular authoritative reviews of entire disciplines. Chemistry was taken first as the problems of literature survey are probably more acute in this subject than in any other. Biochemistry and Physiology followed naturally. As a matter of policy, the authorship of the MTP Review of Science is international and distinguished, the subject coverage is extensive, systematic and critical, and most important of all, it is intended that new issues of the Review will be published at regular intervals.

In the MTP Review of Chemistry (Series One), Inorganic, Physical and Organic Chemistry are comprehensively reviewed in 33 text volumes and 3 index volumes. Physiology (Series One) consists of 8 volumes and Biochemistry (Series One) 12 volumes, each volume individually indexed. Details follow. In general, the Chemistry (Series One) reviews cover the period 1967 to 1971, and Physiology and Biochemistry (Series One) reviews up to 1972. It is planned to start in 1974 the MTP International Review of Science (Series Two), consisting of a similar set of volumes covering developments in a two year period.

The MTP International Review of Science has been conceived within a carefully organised editorial framework. The overall plan was drawn up, and the volume editors appointed by seven consultant editors. In turn, each volume editor planned the coverage of his field and appointed authors to write on subjects which were within the area of their own research experience. No geographical restriction was imposed. Hence the 500 or so contributions to the MTP Review of Science come from many countries of the world and provide an authoritative account of progress.

Butterworth & Co. (Publishers) Ltd.

INORGANIC CHEMISTRY SERIES ONE

Consultant Editor
H. J. Eméleus, F.R.S.
*Department of Chemistry
University of Cambridge*

Volume titles and Editors

1 **MAIN GROUP ELEMENTS—HYDROGEN AND GROUPS I–IV**
Professor M. F. Lappert,
University of Sussex

2 **MAIN GROUP ELEMENTS—GROUPS V AND VI**
Professor C. C. Addison,
F.R.S. and Dr. D. B.
Sowerby, *University of Nottingham*

3 **MAIN GROUP ELEMENTS—GROUP VII AND NOBLE GASES**
Professor Viktor Gutmann,
Technical University of Vienna

4 **ORGANOMETALLIC DERIVATIVES OF THE MAIN GROUP ELEMENTS**
Dr. B. J. Aylett, *Westfield College, University of London*

5 **TRANSITION METALS— PART 1**
Professor D. W. A. Sharp,
University of Glasgow

6 **TRANSITION METALS— PART 2**
Dr. M. J. Mays, *University of Cambridge*

7 **LANTHANIDES AND ACTINIDES**
Professor K. W. Bagnall,
University of Manchester

8 **RADIOCHEMISTRY**
Dr. A. G. Maddock,
University of Cambridge

9 **REACTION MECHANISMS IN INORGANIC CHEMISTRY**
Professor M. L. Tobe,
*University College,
University of London*

10 **SOLID STATE CHEMISTRY**
Dr. L. E. J. Roberts, *Atomic Energy Research Establishment, Harwell*

INDEX VOLUME

PHYSICAL CHEMISTRY SERIES ONE

Consultant Editor
A. D. Buckingham
*Department of Chemistry
University of Cambridge*

Volume titles and Editors

1 **THEORETICAL CHEMISTRY**
Professor W. Byers Brown,
University of Manchester

2 **MOLECULAR STRUCTURE AND PROPERTIES**
Professor G. Allen,
University of Manchester

3 **SPECTROSCOPY**
Dr. D. A. Ramsay, F.R.S.C.,
National Research Council of Canada

4 **MAGNETIC RESONANCE**
Professor C. A. McDowell.
F.R.S.C., *University of British Columbia*

5 **MASS SPECTROMETRY**
Professor A. Maccoll,
*University College,
University of London*

6 **ELECTROCHEMISTRY**
Professor J. O'M Bockris,
University of Pennsylvania

7 **SURFACE CHEMISTRY AND COLLOIDS**
Professor M. Kerker,
Clarkson College of Technology, New York

8 **MACROMOLECULAR SCIENCE**
Professor C. E. H. Bawn,
F.R.S., *University of Liverpool*

9 **CHEMICAL KINETICS**
Professor J. C. Polanyi, F.R.S.,
University of Toronto

10 **THERMOCHEMISTRY AND THERMO-DYNAMICS**
Dr. H. A. Skinner, *University of Manchester*

11 **CHEMICAL CRYSTALLOGRAPHY**
Professor J. Monteath
Robertson, F.R.S., *University of Glasgow*

12 **ANALYTICAL CHEMISTRY —PART 1**
Professor T. S. West,
Imperial College, University of London

13 **ANALYTICAL CHEMISTRY —PART 2**
Professor T. S. West,
Imperial College, University of London

INDEX VOLUME

ORGANIC CHEMISTRY SERIES ONE

Consultant Editor
D. H. Hey, F.R.S.,
*Department of Chemistry
King's College, University of London*

Volume titles and Editors

1 **STRUCTURE DETERMINATION IN ORGANIC CHEMISTRY**
Professor W. D. Ollis, F.R.S.,
University of Sheffield

2 **ALIPHATIC COMPOUNDS**
Professor N. B. Chapman,
Hull University

3 **AROMATIC COMPOUNDS**
Professor H. Zollinger, *Swiss Federal Institute of Technology*

4 **HETEROCYCLIC COMPOUNDS**
Dr. K. Schofield, *University of Exeter*

5 **ALICYCLIC COMPOUNDS**
Professor W. Parker,
University of Stirling

6 **AMINO ACIDS, PEPTIDES AND RELATED COMPOUNDS**
Professor D. H. Hey, F.R.S.,
and Dr. D. I. John, *King's College, University of London*

7 **CARBOHYDRATES**
Professor G. O. Aspinall,
Trent University, Ontario

8 **STEROIDS**
Dr. W. F. Johns, *G. D. Searle & Co., Chicago*

9 **ALKALOIDS**
Professor K. Wiesner, F.R.S.,
University of New Brunswick

10 **FREE RADICAL REACTIONS**
Professor W. A. Waters,
F.R.S., *University of Oxford*

INDEX VOLUME

PHYSIOLOGY
SERIES ONE

Consultant Editors
A. C. Guyton,
Department of Physiology and Biophysics, University of Mississippi Medical Center and
D. F. Horrobin,
Department of Physiology, University of Newcastle upon Tyne

Volume titles and Editors

1 **CARDIOVASCULAR PHYSIOLOGY**
Professor A. C. Guyton and Dr. C. E. Jones, *University of Mississippi Medical Center*

2 **RESPIRATORY PHYSIOLOGY**
Professor J. G. Widdicombe, *St. George's Hospital, London*

3 **NEUROPHYSIOLOGY**
Professor C. C. Hunt, *Washington University School of Medicine, St. Louis*

4 **GASTROINTESTINAL PHYSIOLOGY**
Professor E. D. Jacobson and Dr. L. L. Shanbour, *University of Texas Medical School*

5 **ENDOCRINE PHYSIOLOGY**
Professor S. M. McCann, *University of Texas*

6 **KIDNEY AND URINARY TRACT PHYSIOLOGY**
Professor K. Thurau, *University of Munich*

7 **ENVIRONMENTAL PHYSIOLOGY**
Professor D. Robertshaw, *University of Nairobi*

8 **REPRODUCTIVE PHYSIOLOGY**
Professor R. O. Greep, *Harvard Medical School*

BIOCHEMISTRY
SERIES ONE

Consultant Editors
H. L. Kornberg, F.R.S.
Department of Biochemistry University of Leicester and
D. C. Phillips, F.R.S., *Department of Zoology, University of Oxford*

Volume titles and Editors

1 **CHEMISTRY OF MACRO-MOLECULES**
Professor H. Gutfreund, *University of Bristol*

2 **BIOCHEMISTRY OF CELL WALLS AND MEMBRANES**
Dr. C. F. Fox, *University of California, Los Angeles*

3 **ENERGY TRANSDUCING MECHANISMS**
Professor E. Racker, *Cornell University, New York*

4 **BIOCHEMISTRY OF LIPIDS**
Professor T. W. Goodwin, F.R.S., *University of Liverpool*

5 **BIOCHEMISTRY OF CARBO-HYDRATES**
Professor W. J. Whelan, *University of Miami*

6 **BIOCHEMISTRY OF NUCLEIC ACIDS**
Professor K. Burton, F.R.S., *University of Newcastle upon Tyne*

7 **SYNTHESIS OF AMINO ACIDS AND PROTEINS**
Professor H. R. V. Arnstein, *King's College, University of London*

8 **BIOCHEMISTRY OF HORMONES**
Professor H. V. Rickenberg, *National Jewish Hospital & Research Center, Colorado*

9 **BIOCHEMISTRY OF CELL DIFFER-ENTIATION**
Professor J. Paul, *The Beatson Institute for Cancer Research, Glasgow*

10 **DEFENCE AND RECOGNITION**
Professor R. R. Porter, F.R.S., *University of Oxford*

11 **PLANT BIOCHEMISTRY**
Professor D. H. Northcote, F.R.S., *University of Cambridge*

12 **PHYSIOLOGICAL AND PHARMACO-LOGICAL BIOCHEMISTRY**
Dr. H. K. F. Blaschko, F.R.S., *University of Oxford*

MTP International Review of Science

series:

Physiology
Series One

Volume 3
Neurophysiology

Edited by **C. C. Hunt**
Washington University School of Medicine

Butterworths · London
University Park Press · Baltimore

THE BUTTERWORTH GROUP

ENGLAND
Butterworth & Co (Publishers) Ltd
London: 88 Kingsway, WC2B 6AB

AUSTRALIA
Butterworths Pty Ltd
Sydney: 586 Pacific Highway 2067
Melbourne: 343 Little Collins Street, 3000
Brisbane: 240 Queen Street, 4000

NEW ZEALAND
Butterworths of New Zealand Ltd
Wellington: 26–28 Waring Taylor Street, 1

SOUTH AFRICA
Butterworth & Co (South Africa) (Pty) Ltd
Durban: 152–154 Gale Street

ISBN 0 408 70483 7

UNIVERSITY PARK PRESS

U.S.A. and CANADA
University Park Press
Chamber of Commerce Building
Baltimore, Maryland, 21202

Library of Congress Cataloging in Publication Data

Hunt, Carlton C., 1918–
  Neurophysiology.

  (Physiology, series one, v. 3) (MTP International
review of science)
  1. Neurophysiology. I Title. II. Series.
III. Series: MTP international review of science.
[DNLM: 1. Neurophysiology. W1PH951D/
WL102 N497] QP1.P62 vol. 3 [QP355.2] 599'.01'08s
[599'.01'88]
ISBN 0–8391–1052–9   74–13476

First Published 1975 and © 1975

BUTTERWORTH & CO (PUBLISHERS) LTD

Typeset, printed and bound in Great Britain by
REDWOOD BURN LIMITED
Trowbridge & Esher

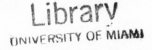
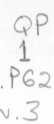

Consultant Editor's Note

The International Review of Physiology, a review with a new format, is hopefully also new in concept. But before discussing the new concept, those of us who are joined in making this review a success must admit that we asked ourselves at the outset: Why should we promote a new review of physiology? Not that there is a paucity of reviews already, and not that the present reviews fail to fill important roles, because they do. Therefore, what could be the role of an additional review?

The International Review of Physiology has the same goals as all other reviews for accuracy, timeliness, and completeness, but it has new policies that we hope and believe will engender still other important qualities that are often elusive in reviews, the qualities of critical evaluation and instructiveness. The first decision toward achieving these goals was to design the new format, one that will allow publication of approximately 2500 pages per edition, divided into eight different sub-speciality volumes, each organised by experts in their respective fields. It is clear that this extensiveness of coverage will allow consideration of each subject in far greater depth than has been possible in the past. To make this review as timely as possible, a new edition of all eight volumes will be published every two years giving a cycle time that will keep the articles current. And in addition to the short cycle time, the publishers have arranged to produce each volume within only a few months after the articles themselves have been completed, thus further enhancing the immediate value of each author's contribution.

Yet, perhaps the greatest hope that this new review will achieve its goals of critical evaluation and instructiveness lies in its editorial policies. A simple but firm request has been made to each author that he utilise his expertise and his judgement to sift from the mass of biennial publications those new facts and concepts that are important to the progress of physiology; that he make a conscientious effort not to write a review consisting of annotated lists of references; and that the important material he does choose be presented in thoughtful and logical exposition, complete enough to convey full understanding and also woven into context with previously established physiological principles. Hopefully, these processes will bring to the reader each two years a treatise that he will use not merely as a reference in his own personal field but also as an exercise in refreshing and modernising his whole body of physiological knowledge.

Mississippi

A. C. Guyton

Preface

In inviting contributions to this volume the aim has been to provide the reader with a view of the current state of knowledge in a number of areas of neurophysiology. Topics have been selected to sample representative areas of the peripheral and central nervous system. The coverage in this volume is not comprehensive but over the course of several volumes it is hoped that representation will become more complete.

The selection also reflects the editor's view that the study of the structure and function of individual neurons, the characteristics of their synaptic interactions and the way such neurons are interconnected is a very productive approach to the understanding of nervous system function. In this regard the application of knowledge gained from study of the peripheral nervous system has been especially important to an understanding of mechanisms involved in the central nervous system.

The nervous system provides a good example of the artificiality of dividing biology into molecular, cellular and systemic compartments. In understanding functions of the nervous system one frequently must consider mechanisms at all these levels.

St. Louis,   Carlton C. Hunt
Missouri

Contents

Identifiable neurones and invertebrate behaviour   1
S. B. Kater, C. B. Heyer and C. R. S. Kaneko, *University of Iowa*

Synaptic transmission   53
A. R. Martin, *University of Colorado Medical Center, Denver*

Vestibular system   81
W. Precht, *Max-Planck Institute for Brain Research, Frankfurt*

The neurophysiology of movement performance   151
R. Porter, *Monash University, Clayton, Victoria*

**Superior colliculus: structure, physiology and possible
functions**   185
B. Gordon, *University of Oregon*

Aspects of the recovery process in nerve   231
P. De Weer, *Washington University School of Medicine, St. Louis,
Missouri*

The physiology of skeletal muscle   279
A. J. Buller, *University of Bristol*

Neural substrates of somatic sensation   303
E. R. Perl, *University of North Carolina School of Medicine,*
and J. G. Boivie, *Karolinska Institute, Stockholm*

Index   411

1
Identifiable Neurones and Invertebrate Behaviour

S. B. KATER, C. B. HEYER and C. R. S. KANEKO
University of Iowa

1.1   INTRODUCTION   2

1.2   APPROACHES TO NEURAL IDENTITY   3
      1.2.1   *The population approach*   3
      1.2.2   *The hunt-and-poke approach*   4
      1.2.3   *The identifiable neurone approach*   4

1.3   IDENTIFIABLE NEURONES OF INVERTEBRATES   5
      1.3.1   *Criteria*   5
      1.3.2   *A portrait of a neurone*   8
      1.3.3   *A limitation of the identifiable-neurone approach*   8

1.4   INVERTEBRATE BEHAVIOUR   10
      1.4.1   *Contributions of cellular approaches to invertebrate behaviour:*
              simple reflexes   11
      1.4.2   *Contributions of cellular approaches to invertebrate*
              behaviour: fixed action patterns   11
              1.4.2.1   *Central programmes*   12
              1.4.2.2   *Command elements*   12
      1.4.3   *Higher-order control*   13
              1.4.3.1   *Plasticity*   14

1.5   ANALYSIS OF NEURAL SYSTEMS MEDIATING DISCRETE BEHAVIOURS   16
      1.5.1   *Reflexes*   16
              1.5.1.1   *The leech reflex shortening*   16
              1.5.1.2   *The crayfish tail flip*   18

1.5.2   *Central programmes*   21
        1.5.2.1   *The cardiac ganglia*   22
        1.5.2.2   *The stomatogastric ganglion: pyloric cycle*   24
        1.5.2.3   *The stomatogastric ganglion: gastric mill cycle*   25
1.5.3   *Sensory modulation of central programmes*   28
1.5.4   *Plasticity*   31
        1.5.4.1   *The crayfish tail flip*   31
        1.5.4.2   *The* Aplysia *gill-withdrawal response*   32
1.5.5   *Arousal*   36

1.6   ADDITIONAL DIRECTIONS   37
1.6.1   *Developmental studies*   38
1.6.2   *Genetic studies*   39

1.7   CONCLUSIONS   42

      ACKNOWLEDGEMENTS   42

1.1   INTRODUCTION

This chapter is aimed at providing neurobehavioural scientists with a view of a field that has become a primary focus of research during the last decade, namely, work on the integrative neuronal processes that contribute to the generation of specific behaviours in invertebrates. Research in this area forms a continuum ranging from primarily behavioural to primarily physiological studies, depending upon the suitability of the experimental animal for each kind of approach. One extreme is exemplified by research on molluscs where information on identifiable neurones abounds but behaviourally relevant information is far more difficult to obtain. The majority of arthropod investigations, on the other hand, have yielded a wealth of information on the neuromuscular control of specific acts, but only recently have we obtained data on the integrative cellular processes underlying these well-defined behaviours. No single organism is suited uniquely for the broad analyses required for understanding how cellular processes mediate behavioural responses; investigations are carried out on a wide variety of species with the specific attributes of each being emphasised and directed towards a common goal.

The pioneering ideas of many investigators are fused into what is now a basic approach in this area, but the work of one individual, C. A. G. Wiersma, seems to us to mark the beginning of this approach. The demonstration by Wiersma and his colleagues[1], that individual routinely-identifiable neural elements could be activated to evoke precisely-defined behavioural acts, lit the imaginations of investigators the world over. If we can 'command' a behaviour with a single neurone, might we be able to identify neurones co-ordinating behavioural outputs, or neurones acting in decision making processes, or even neurones with sufficient plasticity to alter a preprogrammed response as a result of past experience? It is the products of this sort of creative inquiry that provide the basis of this chapter.

The volume of literature generated by neurobehavioural research on invertebrates far exceeds the scope of this chapter. We will restrict ourselves to an examination of a variety of invertebrate systems which can provide, by virtue of their identifiable nerve cells, insights into how neural networks mediate behavioural processes at different levels. We have chosen our examples to demonstrate particular points rather than attempting a comprehensive treatment of this entire area. The reader requiring detailed information is directed to the more comprehensive review treatments of the individual facets of our topic: invertebrate behaviour[2-4], neuroanatomy[5-8], and neurophysiology[5,6,9,10,239].

As we progress through this chapter it should become clear to the reader that the use of invertebrates may be considered as one of many possible tools for the study of how neural interactions mediate behavioural outputs. The reason for employing this particular tool is primarily the smaller number of neurones involved and the added reproducibility afforded experimental design. Perhaps as we explore the use of this tool the essential message will be that pointed out by Donald Maynard[11] before his untimely death early this year: 'The more powerful the conceptual tools, the greater the intrinsic complexity of the "simple systems" can be.'

1.2 APPROACHES TO NEURAL IDENTITY

A single opportunity to record from a given neurone cannot provide the amount of information required for an intracellular analysis of neural elements underlying the generation of discrete behavioural acts. Given this limitation, several alternative and complementary approaches to the characterisation of the role of individual neurones have been developed. Three of the more common approaches are: (a) population, (b) 'hunt and-poke' and (c) identifiable neurones.

1.2.1 The population approach

When investigating the properties of a morphologically homogeneous population of neurones, a composite or average picture of individual neurones often emerges. This *population approach* is best illustrated by our concept of 'the vertebrate spinal motoneurone'. The name in itself implies a knowledge of a well-studied single nerve cell, but in fact, we have amalgamated anatomical and physiological data from thousands of 'similar' motoneurones to construct a model with characteristic attributes. A large number of spinal motoneurones may lack one or more features of such a model and likewise many less frequently observed characteristics can be absent from the model. Where the population approach must be relied on, it is recognised that greater acuity of anatomical and physiological investigations often reveals subdivisions in any given class of nerve cells. The value of the population approach for the study of large numbers of 'homogenous' cells is clearly demonstrated by our detailed knowledge of the several vertebrate cell types. The shortcomings of the method are, however, equally obvious. What does one conclude when only one or a few neurones display an unusual and interesting characteristic rarely observed in the population? Are there simply few neurones in this class that display this characteristic, or do all neurones in the population display this feature on rare occasion? With large populations it is difficult to conceive of penetrating the 'same' neurone in any two preparations; if, indeed, 'same' has any meaning for such situations.

1.2.2 The hunt-and-poke approach

At the extreme from the population approach is the philosophy that even rarely observed neural phenomena are valuable additions to our growing dictionary of the neural vocabulary. Such a theme is the basis of the *hunt-and-poke* approach. The search for the neural mechanisms underlying oscillatory motor outputs is a good example of this methodology. Two alternative hypotheses are considered: oscillatory motor outputs could arise from the properties of single oscillating neurones, or such outputs could be the result of specific neural networks. The failure to detect single oscillating neurones led some to favour the latter hypothesis (e.g. Page and Wilson[12]), but persistent investigation by Mendelson[13] revealed individual oscillating neurones in both crabs and lobsters whose properties suggest that they could fulfil the criteria for the drivers of stereotyped motor output. Mendelson reports that such neurones were difficult to locate and to hold with microelectrodes but asserts that his localisation 'encourages the belief that such neurones are present elsewhere'[13]. Our inability to locate routinely and record from neurones like Mendelson's oscillators severely limits the kinds of investigations we can perform. Finding unique neurones in the central nervous systems throughout the animal kingdom has often revealed exciting information and whetted our appetite for more detailed data. All too often, however, we are frustrated by the technical difficulties encountered in attempts to localise such neurones routinely.

1.2.3 The identifiable neurone approach

Systems with *identifiable neurones* offer a viable alternative to the population and hunt-and-poke approaches cited above. The depth of our knowledge of the Mauthner neurone, the best-known, identifiable, vertebrate neurone, demonstrates the value of being able to locate a specific neurone routinely. The rationale for employing identifiable neurones is, in some ways, similar to that for tissue culture: having a large supply of equivalent cells. Understanding the role of any cell and the mechanisms by which its function is fulfilled usually requires a series of complementary experiments. Even though such experiments may be performed and replicated over a period of months or even years, we must analyse and inter-relate data as if they were all obtained from the same cell. In fact, we can never study the 'same' neurone in two different animals, but by working with identifiable nerve cells we can examine corresponding neurones, which, based on specific criteria, are equivalent in all representatives of the species. In making such assumptions of equivalence, however, we must take into account the previous developmental histories and potentially disparate genetic backgrounds of each individual we examine.

1.3 IDENTIFIABLE NEURONES OF INVERTEBRATES

1.3.1 Criteria

Both morphological and physiological criteria can be employed to establish neuronal identity. In the central nervous system (CNS) of many invertebrates, neuronal somata are predominantly arranged as a cortex around a central neuropilar region and can often be identified by their relative location on the surfaces of the ganglia. For instance, in the leech, *Hirudo medicinalis*, darkfield illumination of the living ganglia allows one to observe the somata of a large percentage of the constituent neurones with a low-power dissection microscope. These neurones appear to be arranged in a highly stereotyped fashion from animal to animal, and the division of each segmental ganglion into six discrete packets greatly facilitates identification of individual cell bodies[14]. In some animals (e.g. arthropods in general), a connective tissue sheath surrounding the ganglia obscures direct visualisation of nerve cell bodies. Such sheaths can be removed mechanically (e.g. Otsuka et al.[15]) to allow mapping of the somata (e.g. lobster ganglia (Otsuka et al.[15], Davis[16])). While desheathing is required to see the neurones of some animals, it may not be of general applicability. In insects, for example, the sheath provides an ionic barrier from the haemolymph[17-24], and its removal appears detrimental to neural function (e.g. Hoyle[9], Murphey, personal communication). On the basis of visual criteria alone, the most readily identifiable neurones are those of certain gastropod molluscs. Recognition of this situation led Arvanataki and Chalazonitis[25] and Tauc[26] to begin electrophysiological investigations of what has become a classical preparation in this area, the sea hare, *Aplysia*. Large size (up to 1 mm in diameter) and contrasting pigmentation provide a nearly flawless index for identification of some gastropod neurones. Variations in the hue of cytoplasmic pigmentation of several gastropod species[27] can be employed to distinguish particular neurones reliably. To the indices of colour and size can be added location. While the absolute location of particular cells may vary over the surface of a ganglion, the relative positions of neurones to one another and to various nerve trunks is rather constant (e.g. Kerkut and Meech[28]). In the buccal ganglia of the fresh-water snail, *Helisoma*, one can reliably identify and record from cells 9 through 14[29], even though each is only *ca.* 10 μm in diameter, because of the fixed association of these cell bodies in a stereotyped anatomical pattern designated the aster complex. It is our experience, however, that definitive specification of a particular neurone usually requires not only a series of morphological cues but also complementary physiological data.

Many nerve cells fall into the category of identifiable neurones even though they cannot be impaled by a microelectrode under visual control. While such neurones are not as routinely accessible as their visually identifiable counterparts, physiological indices can be sufficient for identification. A widely employed approach with arthropods (see reviews by Atwood[30] and Usherwood[31]) is to record extracellularly from motor roots and identify, by spike height, the particular elements innervating individual muscle fibres. Such an approach has a limited value for studying the integrative processes governing the output of the neurone under study, and as stated at the outset of this paper, we will restrict our discussion to the situation where information processing at the intracellular level is available. In crustacea the approach has developed from purely extracellular analysis to analysis of intracellular information by taking two directions. Takeda and Kennedy[32] visually identified somata in desheathed abdominal ganglia of crayfish and used physiological criteria to identify them as specific motoneurones. A variety of physiological criteria (see a review by Kennedy[33]), have now been applied to the kind of soma maps of crustacean ganglia produced by Otsuka et al.[15]. The second approach is that of recording directly from neuronal processes located in the neuropil since these structures are closer to the actual sites of synaptic inputs than the soma proper. This approach is exemplified by Sandeman's work on motoneurones controlling rapid eye withdrawal in the crab, Carcinus. Conventional histological reconstructions of the brain and optic tract revealed a single large diameter axon and its major process within the brain which were, on intracellular analysis, confirmed as motoneurones involved in eye withdrawal[34]. While this neurone could not be penetrated under visual control, it could be penetrated routinely in the brain because of its consistent morphology. Intracellular analysis of the various regions of this neurone allowed Sandeman[35] to construct a map correlating the structural and functional properties of this neurone. Using a similar approach many, usually large, neurones whose morphology can be recognised histologically, are being investigated by intracellular techniques in the context of their roles in mediating behavioural processes (e.g. Murphey[36]).

There has been a significant increase in both the breadth and depth of our knowledge of identifiable neurones as a consequence of intracellular staining techniques as advanced by the introduction of the dye, Procion yellow, by Stretton and Kravitz[37]. One need only compare the morphological and physiological pictures developed by Sandeman (see earlier) before[34,35] and after[38] his injection of Procion yellow into the eye withdrawal motoneurone to understand how intracellular staining can increase the depth of our understanding of specific identifiable neurones. Not only was he able to locate and describe a specific integrating segment of this neurone and suggest the location of synaptic inputs, but he was also able to identify the soma which previous conventional histology had failed to define. Intracellular staining also will allow us to increase enormously the number of neurones which can be considered identifiable. Neurones previously impaled blindly and characterised by physiological criteria can now gain a morphological identity. Perhaps most significant, however, is the fact that units identified solely by extracellular analysis of nerve trunks can now be identified within the central nervous system as specific nerve cells, and they are thus potentially available for intracellular analysis as identifiable neurones. This is readily accomplished by employing the axonal iontophoretic technique of Iles and Mulloney[39] or one of its later modifications[40,41]. In its simplest form, the cut end of a nerve trunk is immersed in a pool of cobalt chloride[42], allowed to incubate for a specified period, developed with ammonium sulphide, and then treated by conventional histological procedures (for alternative methods and details, see Kater and Nicholson[8]). By implementing this procedure one can obtain details of the morphology of neurones whose axons course down any specified nerve trunk. Once the morphology within the CNS of particular neurones is known, one can readily move to standard intracellular recording and polarisation procedures to complete specific identification of particular cells. These methods are not only of value on preparations where cells cannot be impaled under visual control but also on preparations where visual criteria have usually played a key role in identification. Many neurones whose morphology was previously known only in terms of their somata are now characterised more completely in terms of axons, branch patterns and dendritic morphology (e.g. Selverston and Kennedy[43], Baylor and Nichols[44] and Kater and Kaneko[45]). Therefore, while intracellular staining is not, in these cases, a basis for identification, it can provide additional data on the structure–function relationships within and between neurones and groups of neurones involved in the generation of specific behaviours.

In many cases, a demonstration of neural identity requires all three of the criteria cited above: visualisation within living ganglia, physiological data and neuronal geometry as revealed by intracellular staining. The insect case illustrates this point. Since it is impractical to remove the surrounding sheath from insect ganglia (see earlier), one cannot observe individual cell bodies for directed microelectrode impalement. Hoyle and Burrows[46] and Hoyle[9] penetrating blindly into the cortex of locust ganglia first identified particular neurones on the basis of physiological indices and then filled these cells with Procion yellow. Examination of histological sections revealed that recordings were made from the somata of specific cells that could then be more routinely penetrated by cuing on physical landmarks (e.g. tracheae) on the external surface of ganglia. Such a combined approach allows one to: (a) penetrate routinely particular neurones, (b) define precisely the physiological inputs to and outputs from these cells which are part of particular circuits, and (c) examine the morphological correlations of neural connections forming functional circuits. Furthermore, the resolution of such morphological interactions need not be limited to the level of the light microscope. Pitman et al.[47] found cobalt to be a promising intracellular stain specifically because of its electron opacity. More recently, Purves and McMahan[48] have taken a well-identified and physiologically characterised motoneurone in the leech[49,50] and characterised its fine structure and the morphology of synapses impinging on it by adapting ultrastructural procedures to the study of Procion-filled neurones. This demonstrates our potential for elucidating the fine structure of nearly any neurone that can be penetrated by a microelectrode.

In addition to the facility with which we can explore both anatomy and physiology by employing identifiable nerve cells, we have the opportunity to examine, at the level of single cells, biochemical phenomena supporting and perhaps directing specific neural functions. Large numbers of functionally equivalent neurones can be harvested from many animals to allow analysis of neurotransmitters (e.g. Otsuka[15]; Rude et al.[51]) and related enzymes (e.g. Hall et al.[52] and Coggeshall et al.[53]) as well as details of RNA and protein metabolism (e.g. Wilson and Berry[54] and Wilson[55]). The results of these studies indicate that specific biochemical characteristics might themselves act as additional criteria for the identification of specified neurones (e.g. Gainer[56-58]).

1.3.2   A portrait of a neurone

We now have the armaments to provide an in-depth portrait of any identifiable neurone if it warrants detailed understanding. The best example of such an analysis is the 'Parabolic Burster' of certain gastropod molluscs. This neurone was first characterised in *Aplysia* (cell 3 of Strumwasser[59]; Br of Arvanataki and Chalazonitis[25]; R15 of Frazier *et al.*[60]) on the basis of its unique pattern of spontaneously generated action potentials. Similar neurones (see discussion on neuronal homology, Sakharov[61] and Kater and Kaneko[45]) now have been located in *Tritonia*[62], *Helix*[63], *Otala*[56-58] and *Helisoma*[45]. Of continued interest is the question of the mechanisms underlying the burst shown to be endogenous to these single cells (e.g. Strumwasser[64]) and persisting even in a relatively intact animal[45]. In addition to standard intracellular recording techniques, Parabolic Bursters have been analysed in terms of current–voltage relationships by employing current (e.g. Chalazonitis and Arvanataki[65] and Gainer[57]) and voltage clamp techniques (e.g. Wachtel and Wilson[66] and Faber and Klee[67]) as well as by employing specific agents like tetrodotoxin and ouabain[68]. Synaptic inputs to these neurones have been examined electrophysiologically, pharmacologically[69] and in terms of behaviourally relevant stimuli[45,70-72]. Recordings have been obtained for periods in excess of 24 h and reveal a modulation of its activity in a circadian rhythm[58,73]. Strumwasser[59] has vigorously pursued the basis of this phenomenon and, as a result of studies on RNA synthesis, has pointed out the possibility that circadian activity of metabolic processes might mediate the circadian electrical events. A direct complement to our information on circadian properties of this neurone was provided by Gainer's comparison[56,57] of electrical and metabolic properties of the Parabolic Burster in *Otala* in normal and diapausing animals. His findings that the incorporation of radio-labelled amino acid was inversely proportional to spontaneous electrical activity and that an entire class of polypeptides was absent from diapausing electrically-silent neurones, suggests a most promising avenue of establishing cause–effect relationships between biochemical and electrical phenomena in individual neurones. To all of these data on Parabolic Bursters can be added our ability to analyse the morphology of these neurones (e.g. by intracellular staining techniques[45]) even, should we require it, to the ultrastructural level.

1.3.3   A limitation of the identifiable neurone approach

Having detailed many of the assets of the identifiable-neurone approach, we should point out here that, as with the population approach, the picture developed for a given neurone is indeed a composite; in this case of data collected from many animals. Care must be taken on this point because there is some degree of variability for nearly any trait one might measure. We can illustrate this point with examples of morphological variability. By employing one of the many intracellular staining techniques now available[8] it is possible to ask questions about the reproducibility of neuronal geometry and assess directly the equivalence of identified neurones in different animals. At present there are insufficient data to make broad, general statements on the constancy of neuronal geometry in animals of the same species. However, this question has been approached by Stretton and Kravitz[74] and their results are consistent with those of less detailed studies. The intracellular stain Procion yellow was used to reveal the morphology of an identified motoneuron (I_2) in the abdominal ganglia of six different lobsters. Figure 1.1 shows the similarity of the coarse features of these neurones, but closer inspection reveals dissimilarities. For instance, the point of origin of branches B and C is quite different in one of the six cases (displaced by *ca.* 150 µm). Another obvious difference is in the origin of the branches designated as 'A'. A similar observation on the reproducibility of neuronal branching patterns has been reported for an endogenously bursting gastropod neurone[45]. As pointed out by Stretton and Kravitz[74], the significance of differences such as those in Figure 1.1 is not readily assessed and it would be of considerable interest to determine whether compensatory changes in the shapes of other neurones is associated with these variations. Variability such as that shown in Figure 1.1 appears to be attributable to two factors: differing genetic backgrounds and disparate developmental processes. Recently, Macagno *et al.*[75] examined the neuronal morphology of an identified neurone at the ultrastructural level in an isogenic, similarly reared, population of the small crustacean, *Daphnia magna*. They found that

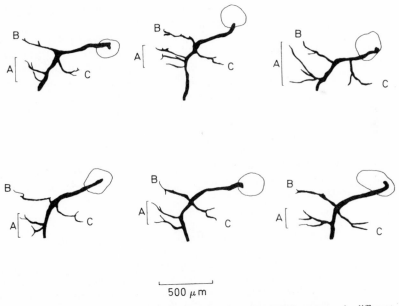

500 µm

Figure 1.1 Variability of the neuronal geometry of identified neurones in different animals. Motoneurone I_2 in the second abdominal ganglion of the lobster was intrasomatically injected with Procion yellow. The simplified and reduced horizontal projections shown from six different animals demonstrates the degree of variability of neuronal geometry (i.e., branching pattern) encountered. (From A. O. W. Stretton and E. A. Kravitz, Figure 6 in Chapter 2 of *Intracellular Staining in Neurobiology*, S. B. Kater and C. Nicholson (editors), Springer-Verlag, N.Y., by courtesy of Springer-Verlag.)

the gross features of a particular neurone were reproduced quite well within animals of a single clone, but that the finer details (at the level of terminals) was highly variable. Another interesting finding along this line is derived from comparative studies on various species of leech[76]. The morphology of the somata and neural processes of the Retzius' cells in four different genera of leech were shown to be quite constant. This demonstration suggests that there has been an evolutionary conservation of coding for specific neuronal morphology. Comparative analyses of this type may well provide an understanding of the functional significance of particular neuronal structures. The data presently at hand serves as sufficient warning against considering identifiable neurones as totally equivalent throughout all representatives of a given species. If one must assume the equivalence of particular neurones for a given experimental design, animals might be selected with greater awareness of genetic background, previous environmental conditions and age of each animal than has usually been the case in the past.

1.4 INVERTEBRATE BEHAVIOUR

Since the vast majority of the literature on the study of behaviour concerns vertebrate behaviour, nearly all the organising principles of behaviour theory are vertebrate orientated. Questions arise as to how applicable such principles might be to the study of animal behaviour in general, and invertebrate behaviour in particular and what contributions studies utilising invertebrate subjects might have in shaping general behaviour theory. It appears that ethological and/or physiological descriptions of invertebrate behaviour have been limited by a vertebrate behaviour oriented vocabulary. One example of such descriptive limitation is manifested in the prevalent assumption that phenotypic similarity (i.e. analogous behaviour) is a sufficient criterion for the classification of patterns of invertebrate behaviour in vertebrate-derived terms.* Certainly the use of the same term for phenomena demonstrable in single-celled protozoa and phenomena shown in vertebrates is misleading at the organismic level and incorrect at a mechanistic level. Before such general terms can be accurately applied to representatives of different phyla, the nearly impossible standard of proving homology of the behaviours must be attained or mechanistically orientated classifications must be adopted.

---

* This assumption might be consistent if one restricts ones inquiry to the level of the organismic black box while maintaining a clear view of the procedures which comprise the operationally defined term of interest. For instance, Corning and Lahue[2] have constructed a table of examples of habituation as demonstrated in various invertebrate phyla. They include ten criteria for habituation, taken largely from the criteria of Thompson and Spencer[77], and indicate which of the criteria are met in each example they cite (see also Eisenstein and Peretz[78]). It is fairly clear that, as defined by the procedures they outline, each example is consistent with a general profile which may be termed habituation. However, as Corning and Lahue point out, if one extends the level of inquiry to the cellular black box and attempts to delimit the mechanisms which underlie the behaviour in terms of cellular interactions or even subcellular events, habituation becomes a general term for a number of different processes. There are a number of other examples which may be cited: fixed action patterns, various conditioning paradigms, etc.

1.4.1 Contributions of cellular approaches to invertebrate behaviour: simple reflexes

Paradoxically, the comparison of cellular mechanisms mediating types of behaviours which demonstrate the shortcomings of broad descriptive schemes also point up the areas in which the comparative approach to behaviour is most useful. It has been argued that a mechanistic analysis of behaviour is often impossible in vertebrates while it is much more approachable in representatives of the various invertebrate phyla. Such analyses can be quite free of confusing terminology while contributing a good deal to the library of mechanisms of behaviour which might be employed throughout the animal kingdom. In fact, however, cellular analyses of behaviour of various invertebrates has added little in the way of general statements at the level of simple reflexively organised behaviours. The type of interactions of agonistic and antagonistic elements and the contribution of various peripheral receptor inputs are already well-known for spinal behaviours of mammals (for Refs. see Granit[79]). The type of interactions originally described in mammals have even served as models for similar interactions which have been, and are now being, elucidated in the control of behaviour of various invertebrate species. There are, of course, differences in the interactions of, for instance, proprioceptors and muscle tension in mammals and arthropods[80] correlated with anatomical differences (i.e. endoskeleton v. exoskeleton). The point here is that detailed mechanisms will have to be worked out for each phylum (and possibly each class) and that the analyses of reflexes in the class Vertebrata are at a more advanced state than for the various other classes and phyla.

1.4.2 Contributions of cellular approaches to invertebrate behaviour: fixed action patterns

Analyses of chained reflexes or fixed-action patterns (FAPs) have received considerable attention at the behavioural level as a result of the efforts of psychologists and ethologists. At the cellular, mechanistic level there is a contrasting dearth of information. This is somewhat surprising since the behavioural analysis suggests that such behaviour should be easily evoked and quite stereotyped given the correct set of environmental stimuli. In the vertebrates, the dearth of information has been due, in part, to the reluctance of ethologists to 'interfere' with behaviours and, in part, to the technical difficulties inherent in such an analysis. A number of neurobiologists have begun the analysis of FAPs in invertebrate preparations for two reasons: (a) the percentage of an organism's total behaviour which is made up of FAPs apparently increases as one descends the phylogenetic scale and (b) FAPs which are indistinguishable from normally occurring FAPs can be easily evoked in animals which have been rendered suitable for cellular analyses. For example, Willows and his colleagues have demonstrated the stereotyped nature of the swimming response of *Tritonia* (Figure 1.2), the extremely fixed nature of the FAP[81] and are currently working out the neural circuitry which underlies the FAP[82-85]. Although the bases for various FAPs seem to have been more thoroughly described for this case and a number of other invertebrate cases (e.g. insect flight[86]) than in any vertebrate example, it appears that

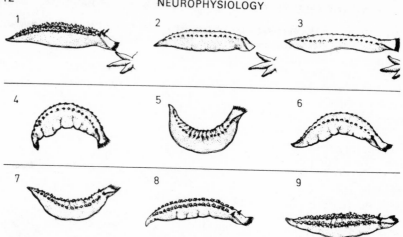

Figure 1.2 The Fixed Action Pattern (FAP) swimming escape response of the gastropod mollusc, *Tritonia*. The animal comes in contact with an aversive stimulus such as a starfish (1). It first pulls in extended parts of its body (2). Next there is an elongation and enlargement of the head and tail regions into paddle-like structures (3). The animal then begins a series of ventral (4) and dorsal (5) flexions causing vigorous, poorly directed swimming movements. The response ends with a series of gradually weakening upward bends (6–9) with short intervals of relaxations between them. (From A. O. D. Willows, 1971, 'Giant Brain Cells in Mollusks'. *Scientific American*, 224 : 68–75.)

the mechanisms of the various FAPs will have to be worked out for each example as was the case for simple reflexes. On the other hand, the cellular analysis of the FAP of locust flight, as well as succeeding demonstrations in other invertebrates (see later), has served to frame and emphasise a concept that appears to have relevance to organisation of behaviour across phyla. This is the concept of a central programme.

1.4.2.1 Central programmes

Wilson[87], working on the flight system of the desert locust, and Bullock[88], in a theoretical paper, proposed that patterned behaviour could be sustained completely independently of afferent input. In such instances, the neuronal circuitry which determines phasing of antagonistic sets of muscles to give the oscillatory behaviour is complete, and afferent information serves only to maintain a general level of 'excitability' within the circuit[86]. Such centrally programmed behaviours have been demonstrated in other phyla (e.g. molluscs[85,89]). The relevance of the concept of centrally programmed behaviour is that it identifies one end of a theoretical continuum ranging from completely reflexive to completely centrally programmed behaviours. Behaviours might thus be categorised as to their relative position along such a continuum.

1.4.2.2 Command elements

Another concept derived from cellular analyses of an invertebrate FAP is that already mentioned above, the command element. This idea, pioneered and christened by C. A. G. Wiersma, was derived from his work on decapod crustaceans. In its strictest usage it applies only to arthropod locomotion and is defined by its experimentally derived properties as described most recently by Davis and Kennedy[90-92]. From the properties of this particular class of individual interneurones, however, it is possible to extract a concept which has general applicability as a possible mechanism for organising behaviours. This seems valid even though the exact nature of the connectivity which mediates the effects observed when command interneurones are stimulated, is unknown for even arthropod systems and will most likely be different in other phyla. The extraction might be formulated as follows. There are neural elements which may be stimulated in a non-patterned manner to give well organised behavioural outputs indistinguishable from those occurring naturally in the freely moving animal. Stated in this form, behaviour evoked by stimulation of diffuse neuroanatomical areas or behaviour which is inconsistent or fragmentary in form would not be considered under the control of command elements (e.g. the majority of behaviours which may be evoked by brain stimulation in vertebrates). Nevertheless, the concept of command elements is readily applied to behaviour in phyla other than the arthropods. Among the chordates stimulation of a single Mauthner cell in certain teleosts and larval anurans results in a stereotyped complex of responses[93]. In addition, Shik et al.[94] have shown that non-patterned stimulation of a well localised mid-brain area evokes locomotor behaviour in mesencephalic cats. In molluscs, Willows[95] has demonstrated evoked swimming in response to stimulation of a particular group of neurones. It may be that commonly used stereotyped behaviours are built into all animals and controlled through command elements.

1.4.3 Higher-order control

The above concepts, derived from reductionistic invertebrate behavioural analyses, have provided generalisations applicable to the study of behaviour across phyla and might, with further confirmations, attain the status of tenets in a general behaviour theory. It is the delineation of such mechanisms, which come under the realm of higher-order control, that should prove the real strength of the comparative approach to the cellular analysis of behaviour. The success of the above mentioned research programmes in providing descriptions of general mechanisms in the organisation of behaviour has prompted a considerable thrust of research aimed specifically at the cellular delineation of such higher-order control aspects of behaviour as behavioural choice and plasticity of behaviour. A number of laboratories are beginning to establish hierarchies of behaviour for molluscan preparations (e.g. Davis and Mpitsos[96], Kater and Kaneko, unpublished observations) in which the ease of determining cellular interactions is the forté of the preparation. The faith is that the establishment of such hierarchies coupled with the neuronal analysis of the control of the individual behaviours will allow one to study the interaction of the control elements for pairs of behaviours. Such neuronal interactions can then be compared with the behavioural interactions in order to establish the mechanisms which mediate choice between behaviours. The assumption of this approach is that the organisation of the various behaviours to be studied will be similar to those already studied. That is, the behaviours will be organised such that the control elements will be routinely identifiable and relatively few in number (e.g. Kater and Rowell[89]) thereby allowing analyses of control elements' interaction. Although as yet unsubstantiated, this assumption is not unreasonable. Moreover, the possibility of approaching such interactions in any system opens up a level of behavioural control which has been as yet unexplored at the mechanistic level in any phylum.

1.4.3.1 Plasticity

The investigation of plasticity of behaviour has taken two approaches. The first has been to adopt behavioural paradigms such as classical conditioning to use with single neural elements. By defining stimulation of one nerve and its consequent action on an individual neurone as the conditioned stimulus and doing likewise for an unconditioned stimulus, Kandel and Tauc[97] were able to demonstrate both sensitisation and learning at the single cell level. They showed an increased efficacy of evoking a conditioned response similar to the unconditioned response, following repeated pairings of the two stimuli. Unfortunately, classical conditioning was demonstrated for unidentified cells only. Sensitisation, which they term heterosynaptic facilitation, has been further investigated in the readily-identified neurone R2 (nomenclature of Frazier, et al.[60]) of Aplysia (e.g. Haigler and von Baumgarten[98]). Such studies have given us some insight into cellular sensitisation mechanisms but the relationship such mechanisms have to whole-animal sensitisation or behaviour is as yet uncertain.

A second approach to behavioural plasticity has been to employ whole-animal preparations. Following a demonstration of such behavioural phenomena as habituation, classical conditioning or operant conditioning, there is an attempt to work out the neuronal basis of these phenomena. Of the three phenomena mentioned, only habituation has yielded to neurophysiological analysis. Examples of such analyses will be discussed below. Although classical conditioning has been demonstrated in both arthropods and molluscs[2], attempts to dissect such conditioning have been lacking. One example where this type of analysis is in progress employs the gastropod mollusc, Pleurobranchia. The behavioural demonstration of a classical conditioned feeding response has been completed[99] (Figure 1.3) and the analysis of the feeding response is underway (e.g. Davis et al.[100]). Such work should soon give us some notion of the kinds of changes that take place at the cellular level which underlie classical conditioning.

Similarly, examples of the neuronal description of operant conditioning are in progress. Horridge[101] demonstrated that an insect (cockroach or locust) learns to hold his leg elevated as a result of application of an aversive stimulus, electric shock, when the leg is lowered. Hoyle has extented the neuronal analysis of this problem in the desert locust. He has applied Horridge's operant conditioning-yolked control paradigm to an adductor muscle in the locust leg. This muscle is likely, although not conclusively proven to be, involved in the conditioned positional response[102,103]. Since the muscle is

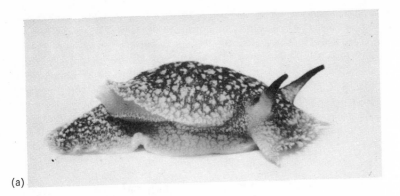

(a)

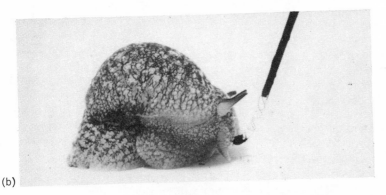

(b)

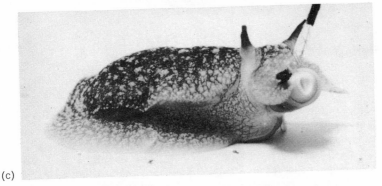

(c)

Figure 1.3 A classically conditioned feeding response in the marine gastropod mollusc, *Pleurobranchea californica*. (a) The resting animal. (b) The response of a naïve animal to presentation of the tactile conditioning stimulus (CS). The tactile stimulus is a touch with a hand-held glass rod (wrapped with wire for visualisation in the photograph). The CS normally evokes a withdrawal response. Following a series of trials in which food is placed on the end of the glass rod to act as the unconditioned stimulus (US), the presentation of the glass rod *alone* evokes the conditioned feeding response (c). (From G. Mpitsos and W. J. Davis, *Science.*, in press. By courtesy of the American Association for the Advancement of Science.)

innervated by a single excitatory axon, the rate of firing of the neurone can be substituted in the original paradigm for lowering of the leg, i.e. if the average frequency of discharge of the axon falls below some arbitrary criterion a shock is delivered to the whole leg. The results are strikingly similar to those obtained in the whole-animal preparation[104]. In addition, the soma of this neurone has been identified recently[46] and the analysis of interneurones which might influence its response begun[105].

1.5 ANALYSIS OF NEURAL SYSTEMS MEDIATING DISCRETE BEHAVIOURS

In this section we want to look at a few of the preparations with identifiable neurones that are currently being used in neurophysiological investigations of the circuitry underlying behaviour in invertebrates. The list is not meant to be exhaustive, but rather representative of the types of approaches being employed currently. Examples have also been selected for the contributions they have made to our general understanding of neural mechanisms of behaviour. Finally, we will examine some of the more recent variations on the general approach which show promise as future resources. As was pointed out at the beginning of this chapter, investigations are being performed on a variety of animals since no single organism provides the optimal situation for every type of analysis. We will examine some preparations which have, thus far, provided key information about reflexively controlled behaviours, others which provide information primarily about central programmes and yet other animals which show how sensory information can be integrated into central programmes. Finally, this section will provide examples of the neural analysis of behavioural plasticity.

1.5.1 Reflexes

1.5.1.1 The leech reflex shortening

The relatively simple nervous system of the leech, composed of a chain of 21 nearly identical ganglia, each containing *ca.* 300–400 neurones, combined with the relatively limited behavioural repertoire of the animal, makes the preparation seem particularly suitable for the study of mechanisms underlying simple reflex behaviours. Progress has been made in this direction, primarily using an isolated ganglion and attached body wall preparation. Three components of the cutaneous sensory system have been characterised[14]. Intracellular recordings have been made from neuronal somata identified on the basis of a number of criteria. Three types of mechanoreceptors have been studied. In each hemiganglion, there are three cells responding to light touch applied to the skin (T-cells), two to pressure (P-cells), and two to noxious mechanical stimulation (N-cells). The receptive field of each neurone has been mapped and found to be remarkably similar from segment to segment and animal to animal. Many of the central connections formed among these sensory neurones have also been mapped and found to be remarkably similar from segment to segment and animal to animal[44]. For example, P-cells inhibit T-cells, although the effect is probably not monosynaptic. Synaptic interactions among the T-cells are extensive. Each T-cell is coupled electrotonically with eleven other T-cells in three ganglia. In addition, activity in one T-cell evokes IPSPs in the other T-cells with which it is coupled. These IPSPs are synchronous in T-cells within each hemiganglion, but are not coordinated between two sides of the same ganglion nor among T-cells in adjacent ganglia. The electrical coupling of the T-cells is rather unique in being doubly rectifying. That is, depolarisation can pass in both directions but hyperpolarisation cannot pass in either direction. In addition, soma recordings during hyperpolarisation of one neurone reflect a decrease in the apparent size of the electrotonic EPSP from the second T-cell, and depolarisation of the soma appears to increase the effectiveness of the coupling.

The segmental motor system of the leech[49,106] is also relatively simple. The musculature of the body wall can be divided into three layers: longitudinal, circular and two sets of oblique fibres. In addition, there are muscles for dorsoventral flattening and erection of the annuli into ridges. Each ganglion contains six excitatory motoneurones to the longitudinal muscle fibres. One large motoneurone (L-cell) innervates the entire half of the body wall; two divide the field into dorsal and ventral halves, each innervating one half; and the three remaining each innervate one-third of the field. The two L-cells within a ganglion are strongly coupled electrotonically. In addition, there are two inhibitory motoneurones, one each to the dorsal and ventral halves of the body wall. There are four excitatory motoneurones for the circular muscles, one each for the two oblique layers, one for the dorsal–ventral fibres, and one for erecting the annuli into ridges. There is an additional inhibitory motoneurone to the dorsoventral fibres. Because of the relative simplicity of the system, it should be possible to specify which motoneurones are active during a limited repertoire of movements.

Connections between sensory neurones and the L-cell have been mapped[50,107]. These include chemical excitation of the L-cell by N-cells chemical excitation and electrical coupling from the P-cells and rectifying electrical synapses allowing depolarisation of the L-cells by T-cells.

Records have been made during simple reflex activation of the L-motoneurone by light tactile stimulation of the skin resulting in discrete activation of individual, identified T-cells. A single EPSP from a T-cell, in the absence of background activity, is never enough to evoke an action potential in the L-cell in the ganglion-body wall preparation, but repetitive touches can evoke marked shortening of the segment mediated by the firing of the two coupled L-cells. Although such a reflex appears to be very simple, the connectivity involved is rather complex. For example, three distinct kinds of electrical coupling are involved. The two L-cells are coupled with a strong, non-rectifying synapse. This assures synchrony of firing and therefore bilateral shortening of the whole segment. The significance of characteristics of the other two types is not clear. The T-cell–L-cell coupling is via a rectifying electrical synapse. The significance of an electrical rather than a chemical synapse at this point has not been clarified. It does not appear to involve synchrony and, since more than one impulse in the T-cell is required to produce an L-cell response, it does not seem that the short latency of the electrical synapse is significant.

Unlike P-cell and N-cell synapses on the L-cell, the T-cell synapse does not fatigue, and since many normal activities of the leech should activate T-cells, they may function to produce maintained synaptic drive on the L-cell[107]. Finally, T-cells are coupled by a doubly rectifying electrical synapse, the significance of which has not been established, although it may be related to the apparent effect of membrane potential on the strength of coupling mentioned earlier. Activation of both P-cell and N-cells can elicit the shortening reflex described, but the inevitable concurrent activation of T-cells precludes a study of reflexes initiated by these cells.

Although the study of such a simple reflex has not yet added much to our general understanding of reflexive behaviours (other than to emphasise the actual complexity of the interactions involved) the system would appear to be potentially quite useful in future studies on factors affecting integration in simple behavioural systems. For example, increased concentrations of extra-cellular potassium produced by neural activity in the leech has been studied[108], and this system might be used to investigate the effects of such non-synaptic signalling on integration. The role of after-effects (e.g. hyperpolarisation following one or more spikes) on integration of a simple behaviourally signi-ficant circuit might be considered[109]. For example, it has been shown that a brief large hyperpolarisation of the soma of P-cells or N-cells can increase transmitter release for > 20 s without apparently altering the size of the action potential of the presynaptic terminal (at least in the case of the P-cell to L-cell synapse[107]). The effects of afterhyperpolaristion on integration might explain the existence of rectification of the T–T and T–L cells in the reflex just dis-cussed. In Gunther Stent's laboratory one of the primary goals for the leech as a useful experimental animal is now being realised with the development of a more intact preparation for a direct analysis of behaviours.

1.5.1.2 The crayfish tail flip

The neural basis of much more complex behaviours has been studied in inver-tebrates. Perhaps one of the most complete analyses to date is concerned with the tail flip escape response of crayfish. We will consider part of the circuitry as an example of what a more complex, reflexly evoked, motor output may tell us about the organisation involved in the production of such behaviours.

The total behaviour (a FAP) involves a number of components (turning the eyestalks inward, the antennae and all legs forwards, and the swimmerets upwards, as well as the tail flip[1]). In 1938, Wiersma[110] reported that even single shocks to the ventral nerve cord could elicit the complex behaviour including activation of motoneurones to the fast flexor muscles of the abdomen by the giant axons present in the cord. There are four such axons. Two of these, the medial giants, are single cells with unbranched axons in the ventral nerve cord and somata and dendritic fields only in the brain. The lateral giants, however, are not in fact axons, but electrotonically coupled sections of axons from cells with somata and dendritic fields in each segment. It has been shown recently[111], that the tail flips mediated by lateral or medial giant stimulation are not identical. The medial giants result in a backward, horizontal propulsion. while the lateral giants cause a more vertical backward thrust. Further, the two responses are not elicited in the same way. Stimulation of the head region usualy elicits responses mediated by the medial giant, while tactile stimullation to the abdomen causes lateral giant firing[112]. The circuitry underlying one component of this system, the input–output relations of the tail flip mediated by the lateral giant in the isolated crayfish abdomen, has been most extensively studied, and we will confine our discussion to this aspect of the behaviour. A summary of the results is provided in Figure 1.4. The analysis has provided insights into the roles of individual neurones as well as the organisation of the neurones in a more complex behaviour than that involving

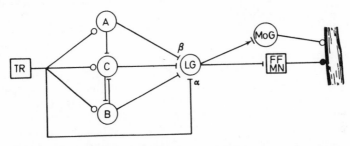

Figure 1.4 A schematic diagram of the excitatory connections involved in the tail-flip response of the isolated crayfish abdomen. Stimulation of tactile receptors can cause activity in several inter-neurones and finally activation of motoneurones to the phasic flexor muscles of the abdomen. For simplicity, synapses are shown on the soma, although morphological data indicates that they occur on branches of the cells. Populations of elements are indicated by squares; single neurones are represented by circles, electrical synapses are represented by bars (the one to the motor giant is rectifying); antifacilitating chemical synapses are designated by open circles; and facilitating chemical synapses are represented by filled circles. TR, tactile receptors; A, a unisegmental tactile interneurone; B and C, multisegmental tactile inter-neurones; LG, lateral giant neurone; MoG, motor giant motoneurone; FF MN, fast flexor motoneurones innervating phasic flexor muscles. (From R. S. Zucker, *J. Neurophysiol.* 35, p. 616, Fig. 22.)

a sensory to motoneurone pathway, and thus may suggest models for the production of other more complex reflex behaviours.

Rapid flexion of the crayfish abdomen mediated by the lateral giant can be elicited primarily by tactile stimulation. Intracellular recordings from the lateral giant show a large complex EPSP on stimulation of carapace tactile receptors. The response is especially strong to stimulation of receptors on the segment from which the recording is being made, but responses to stimulation of any abdominal segment can be recorded. The waveform of the EPSP is very complex. The first component of the EPSP is relatively constant and of short latency; it is the result of direct electrical synapses from the tactile afferents to the lateral giant[113,114]. The later components are much more variable[113]. Zucker[114] reasoned that if tactile pathways were the ones exciting the lateral giant, then abdominal tactile interneurones would be expected to mediate these later components. He studied the behaviour of three such inter-neurones during tactile excitation of the lateral giant, as well as the effects of direct stimulation of the interneurones. One (interneurone A) is a unisegmental tactile interneurone receiving input from a single segment[115]; the other two (interneurones B and C) are multisegmental, receiving information from the ipsilateral second through fourth segments and the entire abdomen, respectively[114]. The result suggests that the three interneurones are typically activated monosynaptically, by means of chemical synapses from primary tactile afferents. Antifacilitation is usually seen at synapses onto multisegmental interneurones while those to interneurone A frequently show facilitation at moderate frequencies. Other less common forms of input to these interneurones are also seen[114]. Further, interneurone A electrically excites interneurone C, and interneurones B and C are reciprocally electrically coupled. The lateral giant is excited by electrical synapses from all three interneurones.

Rapid flexion of the crayfish tail is mediated by the fast flexor muscles. These are innervated by ten fast flexor motoneurones: nine excitatory and one inhibitory[116]. One of the excitatory motoneurones, the motor giant, is excited by the lateral giant via a rectifying, electrotonic junction[117]. Morphological data, based on patterns of branching revealed by Procion yellow dye injections, suggest that the other motoneurones should be activated by one, two, three or four of the giants[33,116]. Penetration of branches of these motoneurones near the site of activation by the lateral giant confirms that there is an electrical synapse from one or both lateral giants at this point (as predicted by the morphology). The analysis further reveals that the activation of the motoneurone axon by the synapses requires the initiation of a dendritic spike which then propagates to encounter a region of low safety factor where dentrites and the neurite from the soma join the main axon. This organisation accounts for a lability of the lateral giant–motoneurone synapse, a feature normally associated with chemical transmission[118]. The inhibitory motoneurone receives a longer latency hyperpolarising PSP during activation of the lateral giant. Since the morphology of the inhibitory motoneurone is similar to that of the excitatory motoneurones, the delay is probably due to chemical synaptic transmission[116].

The activation of the fast flexor muscles by these motoneurones reveals that the neuromuscular junction of the motor giant fatigues rapidly even at low rates of stimulation[119], whereas the jucntion potentials produced by the remaining eight fast flexor motoneurones are facilitating. Thus repetitive activation of the lateral giant should produce repetitive flexions of the abdomen, first primarily through the motor giant and subsequently by other remaining fast flexor motoneurones.

The circuitry summarised in Figure 1.2 does not define completely the connectivity involved in the escape behaviour mediated by the lateral giant. It does not include movements of cephalothorax appendages nor does it account for the apparent differential effects of the lateral giant in various abdominal segments[111,120]. Even with a given segment, it does not include alternate methods of activating the interneurones shown nor other interneurones which are undoubtedly involved, and does not provide mechanisms for such observed properties as recurrent inhibition[121]. Yet the circuitry outlined together with information about the functioning of the neurones and their connections, does account for many of the characteristics of the system.

The significance of using identified cells of known morphology is emphasised at several points in this analysis. The main branching patterns of the motoneurones[116] and the lateral giant are remarkably constant, facilitating penetration of cells at several places, such as near the site of synaptic inputs. As discussed, this was necessary to clarify the electrical nature of the lateral giant–motoneurone synapse. In addition, knowledge of morphology provides for reasonable speculation about the organisation of inputs to the lateral giant. Recordings within the lateral giant indicate a high firing threshold from the site of synaptic input whereas the smaller interneurones have relatively low thresholds for firing. As Zucker[114] points out, chemical EPSPs can excite low threshold cells, but cannot summate linearly if they are very large. (Indeed the reversal potential of 40 mV for tactile afferent EPSPs in the interneurone studied is below the threshold for activation of the lateral giant.) Thus, firing the lateral giant appears to be dependent on inputs showing both convergence and electrical transmission.

The organisation of the circuit supports the concept of hierarchically ordered neurones[115,122]. There are five levels of cells represented by the crayfish tail flip. First are the primary tactile afferents, each responding to the deformation of a single hair of the carapace. Kennedy[115] considers segmental interneurones as next in the hierarchy. For example, interneurone A integrates only excitatory information from a single class of receptors in a single segment. Then come the multisegmental interneurones, which receive inputs of more than one modality from several segments as well as inputs from lower order interneurones. In the crayfish the next step is the highest order interneurone, the lateral giant. Again, it integrates information coming directly or indirectly from the levels below it. Finally, of course, are the effectors of the system, the motoneurones. The information flow is unidirectional; communication is among cells in the same level or to higher-order cells, never to cells lower on the hierarchy. It will be interesting to see how well this pattern holds for other systems and the nature of exceptions when they occur.

1.5.2 Central programmes

The controversy over the possible existence of central programmes was eliminated by Wilson's demonstration of behaviourally relevant patterned output in the absence of patterned input[87,123]. However, the behaviour, locust flight, has proved difficult to analyse electrophysiologically. The mapping of motoneurones involved and characterisation of certain aspects of their morphology[124], as well as recording during flight of semi-intact preparations[125], has not added much to the consideration of the mechanisms involved. A number of models of neural interactions have been proposed to explain the patterned output[123], but sufficient data to implicate a single model has not been presented. The system is still under study and more information should be forthcoming.

Another approach to mechanisms underlying centrally patterned output has been to study interactions in the very small autonomic ganglia of arthropods. Of these ganglia, the cardiac, controlling the neurogenic activity of heart muscle, and the stomatogastric, controlling various foregut movements, have been studied extensively. Three systems will be considered here in some detail. Each demonstrates principles of organisation which may be basic to other systems using centrally patterned output.

1.5.2.1 The cardiac ganglia

The heart beat of most and possibly all arthropods is neurogenic. Each beat is initiated by a small group of neurones (varying from nine to several hundred in number) contained in a cardiac ganglion. These cells are capable of producing a patterned output which is generally unaltered by isolation from the animal. Control is also exerted over the ganglion by inhibiting and accelerating fibres coming from the central nervous system. Although the details of neural characteristics and connectivity vary among the many preparations studied, there are certain similarities of organisation underlying this rhythmic output in all systems. We will consider first the pattern producing interaction within the ganglion and then some aspects of this control by the CNS. Much early work has been reviewed by Hagiwara[126].

Cardiac ganglia are neural networks specialised for production of synchronous bursts of activity in motoneurones to the heart muscle. The muscle fibre membrane frequently shows little or no regenerative capability[127-129]; thus bursts of spikes in the motoneurone are required to produce the sustained contraction necessary for ejection of the blood. Polyneuronal innervation[128] and the small size of individual junction potentials recorded from muscle fibres[127,129] further suggest that synchronous output through all motoneurones involved would be required to produce adequate contraction of the heart as a whole.

The somata of these neurones are electrically inexcitable but the electrotonic decay of action potentials and synaptic potentials can be recorded from the soma. Two functional types of neurones have been identified electrophysiologically in the cardiac ganglion. In the lobster, for example, there are five large anterior cells which send axons to the muscle and are apparently motoneurones[130]. There are four additional small cells in the posterior part of the ganglion which do not send axons out of the ganglion. These are assumed to be pacemaker neurones controlling the frequency of output[126]. Although such a system of nine cells would appear to be relatively simple, it has been difficult to characterise all of the connections and interactions. This is primarily due to the poor visibility of small cells in decapods, the most extensively studied group. Still, a general picture can be made by comparing work on several related preparations.

There is little data on the cells designated as 'pacemakers' in decapods. At least one cell of this group usually fires before the motoneurones in the lobster[130], and there is some evidence for electrotonic coupling among them[126], but there is no intracellular data on the mechanisms underlying this firing. In some crabs, one of the posterior cells is large. Early intracellular recordings showed pacemaker potentials and no discernible EPSPs preceding spikes[131], but more recent observations in the crab *Eriocher japonicus* reveal the presence of small synaptic potentials (probably produced by the small pacemaker cells) and weak electrotonic coupling between motoneurones and the large cell[132]. In this animal, synchronous EPSPs in the motoneurone and the posterior large cell preceding each burst still suggest that activity in the small cells initiates the burst. Only in *Limulus*[133] and the stomatopod *Squilla*[134] have good intracellular records from pacemaker cells been made, and only in the latter system can these be considered 'identifiable cells'. The cardiac ganglion of *Squilla* consists of 14–16 cells, all of which can be visualised and studied intracellularly. Records from somata of cells initiating the first output reveals the presence of slow depolarising potentials which do not depend on the presence of spikes but which appear to underly the burst of spikes (initiated in the axon) when spikes are present[134,135]. In this system, the synchrony of pacemaker cell output is assured in several ways. The cells are closely electrotonically coupled at the soma-dendrites allowing spread of the slow potential between cells. In addition, there is both morphological and physiological evidence for the electrotonic coupling of axons. Since action potentials can initiate slow waves, this provides an additional mechanism for assuring synchrony[135].

Motoneurones have generally been classified as followers[126], but in many systems are capable of producing slow potentials and burst output in the absence of the input of the pacemaker cells[132,136]. The persistence of slow waves in the presence of tetrodotoxin demonstrates that they do not require the presence of spikes anywhere in the system and that motoneurones may also be classified as endogenous pacemaker cells[137]. The large cells are electrotonically coupled in decapod crustacea. The attenuation factor is very small (e.g. 1.5) for long current pulses passed between the soma of adjacent cells, but much larger for short pulses the duration of action potentials[126,132], indicating that the coupling takes place between dendrites and lower somata but not axons[132].

Two points can be made about the mechanisms underlying rhythmic output in the system. First, there is extensive electrotonic coupling between pacemaker cells[134], motoneurones[126,138] and pacemaker and motoneurones[126,132]. It would appear that such coupling would insure synchronous output. The second point is the role of slow potentials initiating bursts of spikes in the neurones. Production of the slow potential controls the frequency of bursts[134], at least in *Squilla* and *Limulus*[133] and probably in the decapods also, but they have additional functions. It is the slow depolarisation of non-spike potentials which accounts for the coupling and therefore at least some of the synchronous firing in motoneurones. Further, at least in the crab, the EPSPs produced by the pacemaker cells trigger production of the slow potential in motoneurones. In this case it is the ability of the soma-dendritic membrane of the motoneurone to generate a sustained depolarisation which is responsible for the sustained burst of spikes required for adequate muscle contraction.

There are generally three pairs of extrinsic nerves (two accelerators, one inhibitor) which must normally regulate the output of the ganglion *in vivo*[126]. The effects of these fibres on the whole rhythm have been studied (see Hagiwara[126], for a review) but the mechanism of action has been difficult to assess in decapods. Although some direct input to motoneurones can be recorded, the major effects appear to be dependent on input to the pacemaker cells, but no intracellular records are available. The effects of extrinsic nerve firing on the pacemaker cells of *Squilla* have been reported. Stimulation of the inhibitory fibre results in monosynaptic, chemically mediated IPSPs. The magnitude of the conductance change and ease with which chloride or current injection into the soma alters the size of the IPSP, suggests that the synapses occur on or near the soma. The effects generally do not outlast the stimulation of the nerve[139]. In contrast, stimulation of either accelerator nerve produces no measurable EPSP or soma conductance change, but even a single shock can markedly alter the rate of rise of the pacemaker potential between spikes and the effects can greatly outlast the duration of nerve stimulation. Blocking of the effect by high magnesium or low calcium suggests that it is chemically mediated. It has been suggested that the transmitter may act directly on the membrane producing the pacemaker potential[140]. The significance of these differences has not been pursued nor has the generality for other cardiac ganglia been established. However, the results are consistent with observations by Rao[141] on the sensitivity of burst frequency to the pattern of inhibitory input and suggest the mechanism for the blocking of accelerator input by stimulation of inhibitory fibres[126].

1.5.2.2   *The stomatogastric ganglion: pyloric cycle*

The cardiac ganglia offer information on the type of organisation involving slow potentials and electrotonic coupling whereby a system of neurones can produce a patterned output. Although numerous interactions may be involved, the output itself is quite simple. The stomatogastric ganglia of larger decapod crustacea offer two additional models for the central control of patterned output. The ganglia, located within the lumen of the aorta and anterior of the dorsal region of the cardiac stomach, contain 30–35 neurones, at least 24 of which are motoneurones[11]. Although the soma position is not as consistent as in many central nervous systems' ganglia, motoneurones can be identified on the basis of general position and neuromorphology and confirmed by recording from roots innervating specific muscles. Identification of interneurones is more difficult. The somata are generally electrically inexcitable, but decrementally conducted spikes and synaptic potentials can be recorded by intrasomatic electrodes.

Two cycles of output can be recorded from intact and semi-isolated preparations. One involves 14 neurones driving the muscles of the pyloric filters and related structures. The second involves two subsystems containing a total of *ca.* 12 neurones, which control the musculature of the gastric mill. In contrast to the simple synchronous output of the cardiac ganglia, each cycle in the stomatogastric ganglia requires the sequential firing of neurones or sets of neurones controlling synergistic and antagonistic muscles. We will consider interactions among the components of the two systems separately, and then discuss some data on extrinsic control of the ganglion.

The pyloric cycle occurs in isolated ganglia essentially unchanged from that which can be recorded in intact animals[11,142]. There appear to be essentially three functional groups of neurones and the basic pattern of the cycle involves sequential activity in these three groups. Four neurones (three identified as motoneurones with specific muscles) initiate the cycle, firing for 100–300 ms. This is followed by a 50–200 ms pause and a brief (100 ms) discharge in the second group involving two motoneurones. The third group of eight motoneurones begins firing before the second group ceases and fires repetitively for 200–400 ms. Hence, the total cycle lasts less than 1 s[11,143]. A variety of interactions among these 14 cells has been mapped by simultaneous recording and/or stimulation of two cells either intra- or extracellularly. There are some individual variations of synapses among cells of any group or between groups, but the basic pattern of electrotonic coupling of cells firing synchronously (i.e. the four neurones of the first group and the eight neurones of the second group) and the reciprocal inhibition between the three groups (i.e. between neurones firing out of phase) can be observed. Because the recording site is far from the synaptic site in many instances, it is difficult to determine unequivocally that these represent monosynaptic interactions. However, this appears to be the case for many if not all pyloric cycle interactions thus far studied. Changes in the rhythm produced by the intracellular depolarisation or hyperpolarisation of group I neurones and the observation of maintained bursting activity in these neurones in the absence of firing in other cells, suggest that all or part of the group I neurones may form an intrinsic pacemaker and therefore be responsible for the frequency of the patterned output. When they are silent, the regular rhythmicity of the other two groups is lost and they fire with irregular alternations[11]. The pause between group I and group II firings then appears to be the result of neurones recovering from group I inhibition, with group II recovering first and then being inhibited by the firing of recovered group III neurones[11].

The basic pattern proposed involves a pacemaker determining the rhythmicity, electrotonic coupling of synchronous units, and reciprocal inhibition between alternating units. However, many of the details remain to be worked out. For example, there is no evidence on the source of rhythmicity in group I neurones: i.e. whether rhythmicity results from properties inherent in each neurone, in one or two neurones of the group, or in some characteristic of their coupling. Further, the significance of apparently different forms of inhibition and strengths of electrotonic coupling must be investigated before the functioning of the system is completely understood.

1.5.2.3 The stomatogastric ganglion: gastric mill cycle

Neurones controlling muscles of the gastric mill do not consistently show regularly patterned output in the intact animal in the absence of food[142] nor in the isolated preparation. However, patterned output can be recorded from neurones controlling muscles in the two functional subsystems of the gastric mill (i.e. those controlling the medial tooth and the lateral teeth) either separately or in co-ordinated activity on numerous occasions even if these patterns cannot be elicited at will. Further, interactions between neurones can be mapped as in the pyloric system.

Each subsystem consists of synergistic and antagonistic muscles controlled by motoneurones in the ganglia and motoneurones of the same muscle or the synergistic muscles tend to fire synchronously and to alternate with the firing of motoneurones to antagonists[11] (Selverston and Mulloney, unpublished results). The patterns of connectivity among neurones are much more complex than those encountered in the cardiac ganglion or the pyloric cycle of the stomatogastric ganglia. They involve not only ten motoneurones but one and probably two interneurones as well. In general, there is electrotonic coupling between synchronously firing neurones. However, in the case of motoneurones which control muscles to the lateral teeth there is also some type of reciprocal inhibition between two such electrically coupled neurones (LGN and MGN of Figure 1.5). The precise nature of this interaction has not been specified.

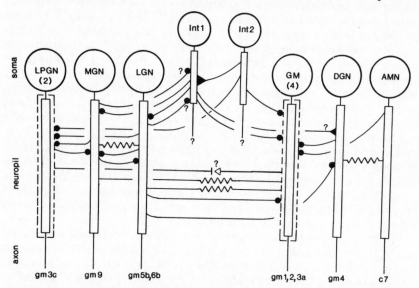

Figure 1.5 A diagram of neurones in the lobster stomatogastric ganglion involved in producing the gastric mill cycle. The sites of synapses and electrotonic coupling are schematic and not meant to represent actual morphology. Question marks indicate connections not as well established as most and the lack of information on the destination of axons of interneurones one and two. ◀, excitatory chemical synapses; ● inhibitory synapses; ⋀⋀ excitatory electronic coupling; ▷ ⊢ rectifying excitatory electrotonic coupling. Numbers at the end of the axons refer to the muscles innervated by each cell. (By courtesy of Brian Mulloney and Allen I. Selverston.)

In this system, a second group of two neurones is coupled electrotonically (LPGN of Figure 1.5) and the two antagonistic groups are reciprocally inhibitory. In addition there is a neurone, identified as an interneurone (that is, no muscle innervation has been found), which inhibits and is inhibited by one or both of the first two neurones. Finally, there appears to be a second interneurone (whose soma has not yet been found) which excites interneurone one and inhibits the LPGNs. There is no clear indication of pacemaker activity in any of the neurones involved in the subsystem, yet stable rhythmic output involving alteration of the two antagonistic sets of moto neurones is often recorded. It has been suggested that the pattern is generated by the reciprocal inhibitory connections between interneurone one and LGN and MGN (Selverston and Mulloney, unpublished results). Interneurone one would therefore act as a switch for the alternate firing of antagonists.

Connections within the second subsystem controlling the median tooth again include electrotonic coupling among two sets of neurones controlling the same or synergistic muscles. In this set of neurones however, there is not reciprocal, but rather one way inhibition of one group (DGN and MGN) onto the antagonistic motoneurone group (GM of Figure 1.5). In addition, interneurones one and two inhibit the second group of motoneurones (GM). Again, none of the neurones involved show pacemaker activity. Alteration of the antagonist is presumed due to alternating activity in interneurone one, as driven by connections in the first subsystems. In addition there are connections between the two subsystems (see Figure 1.5).

A number of problems must be clarified before the system can be understood. For example, the precise nature of many presumed synapses needs to be specified before the role of such interactions in the pattern generation becomes clear. In particular, the interactions of LGN and MGN with interneurone one need to be studied, since it is proposed that these produce the entire pattern of alternating firing in gastric mill neurones. It is not clear why the firing rates in LGN and MGN should slow, allowing interneurone one to fire and inhibit them, nor is it obvious why the reverse, allowing the resumption of activity in LGN and MGN, occurs. Even more difficult to explain is rhythmic output from the second subsystem in the absence of activity in the first. None of the patterns of connectivity thus far elucidated suggest a mechanism for such output. The system of neurones controlling the activity of gastric mill muscles may therefore provide a model of a system in which the generation of patterned output is not dependent on endogenous pacemaker activity of one or a few neurones, but on the patterns of connectivity and such parameters as fatigability of the neurones involved. Before this can be proven, however, further study is needed.

The presence of extrinsic control of at least some aspects of ganglion activity is suggested by observations on pattern variation recorded in intact animals. Here the patterned output may be altered by the presentation of food, even before it reaches the stomach[142]. One such system for control has been studied[144]. Two fibres innervating the stomatogastric ganglion were stimulated. They appeared to directly excite the pacemaker neurones of the pyloric cycle and perhaps also directly inhibit their antagonists. Low frequency firing (2 Hz), of the two fibres (whose effects were individually similar and additive) tended to increase the cycle frequency, although higher rates of firing disrupted the pattern and finally (20 Hz) halted most activity. High firing rates in the fibres also tended to inhibit the GM motoneurones of the gastric mill cycle. Neither the precise mechanism by which these fibres exert their effects, nor the function of such innervation in the intact animal is known.

Although many details remain to be studied, the autonomic ganglia of arthropods suggest three patterns of interactions which may produce the rhythmic output of centrally controlled programmes. Cycle frequency may be determined by pacemaker activities endogenous to specific neurones or by patterns of connectivity among non-pacemaker neurones. Synchrony of firing is often attained by synchrony of input and/or electrotonic coupling of elements and the alternation or sequencing of output is frequently the result of inhibitory interactions. The applicability of these models to other systems remains to be demonstrated. For example, the neurones involved in pattern formation in the stomatogastric ganglion are motoneurones. Reciprocal inhibitory coupling can be shown among motoneurones for some dipteran flight systems[145], but the patterns of output are so different from that of locusts, for example, as to suggest that they are probably produced by different mechanisms[146]. In the latter system, there is no evidence for sufficient coupling of motoneurones to produce patterned output[46,122,125]. In such systems, if reciprocal coupling is involved, it might be among interneurones driving motoneurones[123]. Pattern formation by pacemakers was demonstrated in two of the small ganglia discussed. The presence of apparent pacemaker neurones has been reported for crustacean central ganglia[13]; these may be involved in producing the motor rhythm of ventilation.

1.5.3 Sensory modulation of central programmes

We turn now to consideration of several systems in which the interaction of peripheral sensory input and a central programme have been examined in relation to specific invertebrate behaviours. The bulk of the literature on this subject is concerned with various arthropod preparations. Among the crustacea, metachronal swimmeret beating has received the most attention[90,92,147-151]. In insects, ventilation (for a review see Miller[152]; Farley and Case[153] and Mill[154]), walking (e.g. Pearson[155]), stridulation (e.g. Bentley[156,157]), and flight (for a review see Wilson[86,158]) have all been approached from this point of view. The basis of these analyses is a behaviour which is very well defined. In the case of locust flight, the mechanics and aerodynamics have been characterised and quantified[86]. The motor units which control the behaviours have also been rigorously characterised (e.g. the muscles and motoneurone axons which control roll, pitch, and yaw in locust flight and walking in the cockroach[159]). The effect of various afferent inputs on the output of the system is also easily monitored. For example, it has been shown that thoracic stretch receptors[160,161], companiform sensilla on the wing vein[162], sensory hairs on the head[163-165] and the visual input of the eyes[166] contribute to the maintenance of various aspects of locust flight through the tonic modulation of the central programme.

The major limitation of such work is that, although general effects of sensory input may be characterised and the central programme component of the behaviour demonstrated through deafferentation, neither the specific action of the various inputs nor the neuronal network underlying the central programme have been worked out for any arthropod behaviour. Amongst the molluscs, the technical difficulties of recording central synaptic events are significantly less than in arthropods and, therefore, the opportunity to monitor the elements of the central programme as well as the effect of input is correspondingly enhanced. The problems encountered in the characterisation of the various peripheral motor and sensory apparatuses (see earlier) may also be avoided by choosing a behaviour which does not involve peripheral nerve nets. The most frequently studied molluscan behaviour is that of feeding. The analyses of the buccal ganglia (which control feeding behaviour) of marine gastropods such as *Aplysia*[167-171], *Navanax*[172-174], *Archidoris*[175], and *Anisidoris*[176,177] have emphasised the neuronal properties of the system as opposed to the analysis of the behaviour. Davis, Seigler and

Mpitsos[100] working on *Pleurobranchia* and Murray[178] and Woollacott[179] working independently on *Navanax* have begun behaviour oriented work on these marine gastropods, but this work is as yet preliminary. Although further investigation of the feeding behaviour in these various marine gastropods might reveal an interplay of the centrally programmed and sensory elements, no conclusions may be made at this time. In the pulmonates, feeding behaviour has been shown to be built upon a central programme which is a function of the connectivity of the several motoneurones and few interneurones located in the buccal ganglia[29]. Berry[180,181] has concentrated on the electrotonically coupled 'trigger' network in *Planorbis*. Kater (unpublished observations) has shown that the feeding of *Planorbis* is reliant upon a central programme similar to the one Kater and Rowell described for *Helisoma*[29]. In the latter preparation, it has been demonstrated that stretch receptors in the muscles of the buccal mass evoke EPSPs in the retractor and IPSPs in the protractor motoneurones. The output of the receptors is proportional to the drag on the system imposed by the substratum on which the snail feeds. This

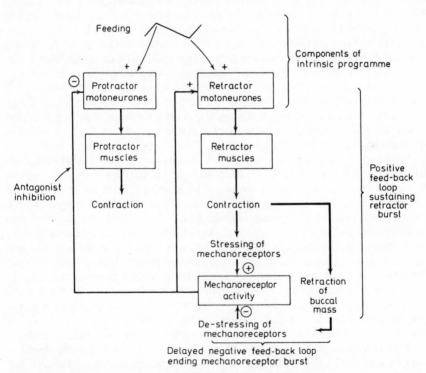

Figure 1.6 Diagrammatic representation of the modulation by sensory feed-back of the central programme which controls feeding behaviour in the fresh water snail, *Helisoma trivolvis*. The central programme is the result of the intrinsic properties of, and interconnections between, the motoneurones and interneurones of the buccal ganglia. The intrinsically programmed motoneurone output is modulated by feed-back of mechanoreceptors. (From S. B. Kater and C. H. F. Rowell (1973). *J. Neurophysiol.*, **36,** 142)

type of sensory modulation of a centrally programmed behaviour can adapt the behaviour to variability of the environment allowing compensation for load variation.

The analyses of the interaction of sensory input and central programmes point up two factors which correlate well with the presence of central programmes and with the relative importance of the central programme in the overall mediation of the behaviour. The first is the frequency of occurrence of the behaviour, those behaviours which occur more frequently tend to be mediated by central programmes. The second point is the degree of independence of the central programme machinery from effects of sensory input is a function of the variations in load inherent in the behaviour which the machinery mediates[155]. The examples cited above are entirely consistent with these notions. Behaviours such as the heartbeat of various decapod crustaceans persist continually throughout the life of the animal and should be relatively independent of changes in load. This behaviour is mediated by a relatively independent central programme. Progressively lower frequency of occurrence and higher variability in load are seen in stomatogastric activity, stridulation, insect flight, ventilation in insects, insect walking and gastropod feeding. Pearson[155] points out that, in his studies of cockroach walking, he has noticed a progressive independence of the central programme from sensory input as the rate of locomotion increases. This rate increase and increased autonomy of the central programme occurs only on smooth surfaces where load variations are at a minimum. Pearson (personal communication) has pointed out two additional generalities which he has derived from a consideration of both vertebrate and invertebrate literature. There is a positive correlation of central programme mediation and rhythmic, complex movements. There is also a negative correlation between sensory modulation and rapidity of movement of centrally programmed behaviours.

Conclusions on the organisation of centrally programmed behaviours are severely limited by our lack of knowledge of cellular events which comprise the programming machinery. However, it appears that those behaviours in which the effectors serve multiple functions (e.g. appendages in locomotion, support, etc.) are organised such that the final common path motoneurones do not participate directly in the programming circuit. Conversely, in behaviours mediated by fixed function effectors (e.g. decapod cardiac motoneurones and muscles, and motoneurones and muscles of pulmonate feeding apparatuses), the motoneurones also constitute part of the centrally programmed circuit. This is not surprising but it does necessitate the placement of the central programme circuit at least one level upstream from the motoneurones in the former case. Such a situation allows for direct sensory input at the level of the motoneurone or the interneurones in either a phasic or tonic manner.

The correlations pointed out above might have been derived from a consideration of vertebrate neurophysiological literature. Saccadic eye movements and ventilation are behaviours of common occurrence and relatively constant load, and appear to be mediated by central programmes relatively independent of sensory feed-back. Vertebrate locomotion is subject to a greater variation in load and is less frequent in occurrence than ventilation or eye movement and has a proportionally reduced centrally programmed component (i.e. higher degree of sensory modulation). One possible reason for the de-emphasis of the concept of central programmes in the vertebrate literature might be that the proportion of vertebrate behaviour which is non-rhythmic, unique and highly variable is very high as compared to that in invertebrates. Another possibility is the success of the analysis of reflex vertebrate behaviours. Nevertheless, a number of vertebrate neurobiologists have proposed modes of nervous system function similar to the concept of central programming[182,184]. The comparative approach provides the neurophysiologist with examples of non-modulated centrally programmed behaviours. The utilisation of the identifiable neurone approach will facilitate the detailed analysis of such systems, and their interaction with sensory input, at a cellular level.

1.5.4 Plasticity

As discussed earlier, the problem of plasticity in invertebrates has been approached in several ways, but only habituation has yet proven amenable to investigation on both behavioural and single cell neurophysiological levels. We will consider two such studies of habituation: the crayfish tail flip described earlier and the gill withdrawal response of the sea hare, *Aplysia*.

1.5.4.1 The crayfish tail flip

A number of recordings from intact animals indicate that the medial and lateral giant axons do not mediate all tail-flip responses in the crayfish. They are involved almost exclusively in the initiation of escape responses to sudden stimuli and do not fire, for example, during sustained cycles of swimming[112,185] The lability of the behaviour elicited by lateral giant firing has been studied[186]. Electrophysiological studies show that repetitive stimulation of the lateral giant can evoke apparently normal tail flips at rates much greater than that seen during habituation of the whole animal[187], whereas input to the lateral giant decreases on repetitive stimulation to tactile afferents or roots containing the processes of these afferents[113]. In a recent, more complete study, Zucker[188] has attempted to define sources of lability in the circuit which can account for the habituation. He has shown that the primary tactile afferents do not show fatigue, that the response decrement cannot be due to properties of adaptation or refractoriness of the tactile interneurones or lateral giant, and confirmed that the lateral giant is capable of initiating tail flips at a rate far in excess of that which is seen in the animal. Response of the tactile interneurones to repeated tactile stimulation parallels the decreased EPSP recorded in the lateral giant, and has a time course very similar to the habituation of the response in the whole animal. Thus, Zucker concludes that the properties of the behaviour can be accounted for by antifacilitation of the chemical synapse between tactile afferents and subsequent interneurones. Although the analysis is indirect, the results of calculations using the probability theory of quantal transmitter release suggest that the cause of the decreased EPSP in the interneurones is a result of decreased transmitter release by presynaptic terminals, rather than postsynaptic mechanisms such as increased inhibition or decreased sensitivity of the postsynaptic membrane. Earlier data showing that picrotoxin (which blocks known inhibitory processes in crustacea) had no effect on habituation of this response, also suggested that inhibitory processes were not involved[189].

Although study of the crayfish has allowed determination of the site of habituation in one behaviourally relevant neural circuit, the response lacks many of the properties of habituation found in other systems (as summarised by Thompson and Spencer[77]). The time parameters for the change are quite short; there is no interganglionic generalisation, and no dishabituating stimulus has been found. Whether these will prove a serious drawback to the general applicability of this model remains to be seen.

1.5.4.2 The Aplysia *gill withdrawal response*

The second response which we will consider, habituation of gill withdrawal in *Aplysia*, does demonstrate more features of habituation. We will look at the neural control of gill movements in *Aplysia*, then describe some properties of habituation and dishabituation of the withdrawal response, and finally consider whether the mechanisms underlying the behaviour might have general applicability to other systems.

The gill of *Aplysia* is a large external respiratory organ composed of *ca*. 16 individual pinnules. It can be withdrawn with the siphon into the mantle cavity and covered by the mantle shelf. The posterior edge of the mantle shelf forms the siphon and the anterior mantle shelf contains the purple gland[190,191]. Weak tactile stimulation of the gill produces a small local contraction of the stimulated pinnule[192], whereas strong tactile stimulation of the gill or weak stimulation of the siphon or mantle shelf produces complete withdrawal of the gill into the mantle cavity and contraction of the mantle shelf and siphon[190]. The pinnule response can be elicited in an isolated gill and is therefore undoubtedly mediated by peripheral neurones[192]. Total gill withdrawal, however, requires that connections between the abdominal ganglion and the gill remain intact[190]. The latter response has been studied in a number of preparations of varying degrees of intactness, from the isolated abdominal ganglion with or without the siphon and gill, to the intact, unrestrained animal[193]. The gill is also under control of central commands as part of a movement resulting in the aeration of the gill and mantle cavity[194].

Although the complete neural circuitry for control of gill movements has not been worked out, several elements are known. Ten neurones causing contractions of various parts of the gill, siphon and mantle shelf have been identified[195]. Of these, five produce movements of the gill, four produce movements of the siphon and one (L7) produces movements of the gill, siphon and mantle shelf. Not all responses of the gill are similar. For example, stimulation of neurone L7 produces a contraction like that seen during the gill withdrawal reflex, while the combined stimulation of two other neurones (LDG$_1$ and LDG$_2$) produce patterns which appear similar to centrally commanded gill movements[195]. Results of simultaneous intracellular recordings from muscle fibres in the gill and neural somata in the abdominal ganglion indicate that at least three neurones (L7, LDG$_1$ and LDG$_2$) synapse directly on the muscle without intervention of peripheral interneurones[190, 196]. Cell bodies of presumed primary mechanoreceptor neurones have been identified in the abdominal ganglion and some of their receptive fields mapped[195]. Siphon sensory cells can produce large apparently monosynaptic EPSPs in L7 and other gill motoneurones, as well as polysynaptic input[191, 195]. While gill withdrawal requires synchronous activation of motoneurones, the centrally commanded movement requires sequential activation of two groups of motoneurones. This appears to be accomplished by input producing simultaneous excitation of one group and inhibition followed by rebound firing in the second group[195]. Tentative circuits for these behaviours are presented in Figure 1.7. The study of habituation and dishabituation of the centrally-mediated response is based on the circuit proposed in Figure 1.7(c).

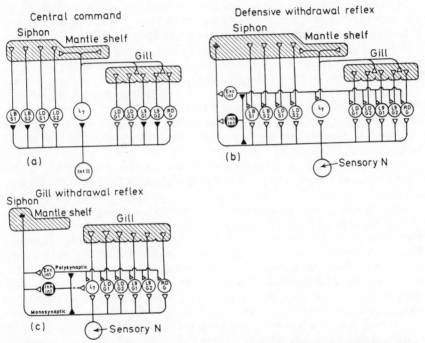

Figure 1.7 A diagram of the neural circuitry underlying gill movements in *Aplysia*. The sites of synapses are schematic and not meant to represent actual morphology. Filled triangles represent inhibition; open triangles indicate excitation. (a) Circuit for the centrally commanded control of gill movement. Interneurone II probably represents several closely coupled neurones. These excite some motoneurones and inhibit other to produce a sequentially patterned motor output. (b) Circuit for the total defensive withdrawal reflex including siphon, mantle, and gill components. The motoneurones and inhibitory interneurones are identified cells, while the sensory neurones and excitatory interneurones represent classes of cells. (c) Circuit for the components of the gill withdrawal reflex receiving the most detailed study (see text for discussion). As in (b), the sensory neurones and excitatory interneurones are classes of cells, while the inhibitory interneurones and motoneurones are identified cells. The relative strength of muscular contractions produced by various motoneurones is indicated by the size of the triangle representing neuromuscular synapses. The sensory input is mediated both directly and via interneurones. (From E. R. Kandel, 1973. The *Neurosciences*. F. O. Schmitt, editor, MIT Press, in the press.)

Habituation studies have dealt with the withdrawal of the gill[190,191,197] the pinnule response[192] and withdrawal of the siphon with and without connections to the abdominal ganglion[193,198]. Of these, only short-term habituation of gill withdrawal elicited by stimulation of the purple gland or the siphon has been studied at the single neurone level. Habituation of the response in the restrained animal has been reported[197]. Simultaneous recording from motoneurones (especially L7) during habituation reveals a parallel decrease in amplitude of the EPSP produced by tactile stimulation[199]. Similar habituation by stimulation of the root containing sensory information as well as records from root and sensory somata during habituation demonstrated that the decrement is not due to receptor fatigue[191,200]. No change in motor response of the gill either to motoneurone stimulation or during centrally-commanded movements is recorded[190,200], suggesting that decrement in neuromuscular transmission does not normally play a part in habituation of the response. Because tactile stimulation may activate motoneurones by more than one path, the total habituation response undoubtedly involves many synapses. However, it has been modelled by considering a single siphon sensory cell synapse onto L7. The time course of habituation in the restrained animal is closely paralleled by size changes in the EPSP at this synapse, making it a likely model for the whole process underlying the behaviour[191,200]. Much indirect evidence suggests that the decrement is due to decreased transmitter release rather than postsynaptic mechanisms[191,195], but the distance between the motoneurone soma and the synaptic site precludes proof at this time.

Once the response has been habituated, two processes can lead to its recovery. Spontaneous recovery involves a rapid phase of 10–20 min, accounting for about three-quarters of the recovery, followed by a slower, more variable return which may last many hours[197]. Alternatively, a sufficiently strong stimulus to any area of the body results in immediate recovery (dishabituation). This latter process has been studied in the restrained animal and correlated activity has been recorded from the neurones involved. The behavioural data shows much more variation than do the neural recordings[191,197,199].

A study was undertaken to define the nature of disinhibition. Since early work by Pavlov, habituation has frequently been ascribed to an inhibitory process and dishabituation has been attributed to removal of the habituation. However, work on some vertebrate systems suggests that habituation is due to a decreased excitatory drive rather than increased inhibition. It is further proposed that dishabituation is a special case of sensitisation and is independent of the mechanism for habituation[201]. The gill withdrawal reflex of *Aplysia* offers a good system in which to test this hypothesis. In most instances habituation of withdrawal to simulation of the purple gland does not interact with habituation to stimulation of the siphon[191]. After habituation of one pathway (e.g. to siphon stimulation) the dishabituating stimulus is applied and responses of the previously habituated and non-habituated pathways (i.e. stimulation of the siphon and purple gland) were tested. If dishabituation is simply the removal of habituation, the dishabituatory stimulus should increase the efficacy of siphon stimulation but have no effect on the response to purple gland stimulation. If dishabituation is only a special case of sensitisation, then the response to both paths should be facilitated. Although the results on the restrained animal are somewhat variable, responses to purple gland stimulation were often facilitated during disinhibition of the habituated response to siphon stimulation[191], confirming the latter hypothesis. Records from a primary motoneurone involved (L7) showed a corresponding lack of interaction between decreases in the EPSPs evoked by repeated stimulation of the siphon and purple gland or stimulation of the nerves containing their afferents. Further, the dishabituating stimulus increased EPSPs in both decremented and non-decremented pathways, paralleling the behavioural observations. Further analysis involved recording from the somata of siphon sensory neurones and L7 during the habituation–dishabituation paradigm. Whether the recorded sensory neurone was in the habituated or non-habituated pathway, the dishabituating stimulus increased the size of its EPSP onto L7. During the dishabituating stimulus, the sensory neurone did not fire but was in fact, hyperpolarised[191]. Thus, facilitation of the EPSP could not be attributed to one known mechanism of plasticity in single synapses, post-tetanic potentiation. This confirmed earlier work which suggested that hetero-synaptic facilitation in another network of *Aplysia* cells was not due to post-tetanic potentiation[202].

Results of these studies on the gill withdrawal reflex and *Aplysia* are consistent with the suggestions from vertebrate work[201] and Zucker's[188] analysis of the crayfish, that habituation is due to decreased excitatory drive. In addition, they lend support to the concept of the separateness of the paths involved in habituation and dishabituation, suggesting that dishabituation is indeed only a special case of sensitisation[191,201]. Although no mechanism for dishabituation can be proposed at this time, it is interesting to note that the dishabituating stimulus produced a hyperpolarisation in the sensory neurone. Habituation at another molluscan synapse (the giant synapse of the squid stellate ganglion) is abolished by hyperpolarisation of the presynaptic terminal[203], and we have mentioned that large, short hyperpolarisation of somata of some leech neurones can facilitate transmission for at least 20 s following the pulse[107].

Habituation of the gill withdrawal reflex in *Aplysia* demonstrates many but not all of the features of habituation summarised by Thompson and Spencer[77]. Generalisation between siphon and purple gland stimulation was not generally seen, but this does not mean that the reflex cannot generalise to stimuli more closely spaced within the receptive field[191]. However, the habituation response studied also does not show increased rate of decrement with repeated habituation series. It has been suggested that the latter may be a serious drawback to the use of this system as a model for long-term learning[204]. The problem is emphasised by the work of Schwartz et al.[205] on the isolated abdominal ganglion of *Aplysia*. The changes in synaptic efficacy associated with habituation and dishabituation of the gill withdrawal reflex were not altered by a 95% inhibition of protein synthesis by one of several antibiotics over a 6 h period. Although new protein synthesis may not be involved in short-term learning, the evidence suggests that it is involved in long-term learning[206,207]. Recently, work has been begun on habituation of the siphon and gill withdrawal reflex in unrestrained animals. In this case, a response decrement to repeated habituation series can be seen, suggesting that this system might also contribute to understanding mechanisms of long-term neural changes[195].

1.5.5 Arousal

Preceding examples illustrate the extent to which we can analyse the mechanisms by which specified neuronal circuitry can mediate particular behavioural acts. As our knowledge of any behaviourally relevant neural circuit approaches completion, however, we become increasingly aware of the existence of higher-order neuronal machinery that can bias the output of such circuits. From behavioural studies we know that such amorphous phenomena as motivation and arousal play significant roles in determining the probability of activation of the majority of acts in an animal's behavioural repertoire. As demonstrated by the studies of Moruzzi and Magoun[208] on the reticular formation of the vertebrate brain, neurobiologists can examine biasing phenomena such as arousal. In the remainder of this section we will look at an example of how such questions can be approached in invertebrates with identifiable neurones and note particularly how recent technological advances have increased our facility for exploring such questions.

A good example of the approach to higher-order biasing systems in invertebrates is a series of investigations on a single sensory interneurone, the descending contralateral movement detector (DCMD) of orthopteran insects. The DCMD, a visual interneurone approximately four synapses removed from primary photoreceptors in the compound eye, produces no observable change in the locust's behaviour when activated to fire by intracellular depolarisation[209]. Rather than driving a particular behaviour, this neurone exerts a biasing effect on follower cells.

The DCMD is one of the best characterised sensory interneurones in the animal kingdom[210]. Its response characteristics have been extensively described in terms of its extracellularly recorded responses[211,212] (see also a review by Rowell[210]). It is quite responsive to small movements, with the most effective stimulus being a contrasting object moving through the visual field. Among the more interesting properties of the DCMD are its incremental and decremental response properties[210,213-215]. There is habituation of the response to repeated stimulation of a given area of the eye, but the response can be renewed by stimulus presentations to a slightly different receptive field. The quantitative characteristics (e.g. time course) of the DCMDs habituatory responses make this neurone most sensitive to novel stimuli and led Rowell[209] to suggest that: 'This would be an appropriate property for a neurone conveying warning information.' In summarising a series of experiments implicating the DCMD as part of an arousal system Rowell pointed out[209] that: 'Almost any sensory stimulus strong enough to "catch the animal's attention" would dishabituate the visual unit's response once.'

Many interesting characteristics of the DCMD were, until quite recently, refractory to analysis due to inability to record routinely the intracellular activity of the DCMD and potential follower cells. Rowell and O'Shea took the first step in overcoming these problems by precisely defining the morphology of the DCMD through the use of the axonal iontophoretic technique of Iles and Mulloney[39] (see also Kater and Nicholson[4]). A series of preparations, stained in this way, revealed that the location of the DCMD soma was quite constant in different animals and therefore amenable to penetration by stereotactically positioned microelectrodes. Furthermore, the staining revealed that the majority of the DCMDs terminals were in the metathoracic ganglion: the location of the motoneurones controlling the locust's jump. The most significant findings to date is the recent demonstration that the DCMD actually biases, but does not drive, follower neurones. (Burrows and Rowell, personal communication.)

The results of the most recent experiments on the DCMD seem to confirm Rowell's long-stated hypothesis that the DCMD mediates some aspect of arousal. In the locust, a high priority response to aversive stimuli is to initiate a jump by extension of the large, specialised hind legs on the metathorax. Burrows and Rowell (personal communication) have shown that the output of the DCMD on either side of the animal produces subthreshold EPSPs in the fast extensor motoneurones to this leg and also apparently mediates inhibition to antagonist motoneurones. While the DCMD activity does not result in the generation of action potentials in extensor motoneurones, it raises their level of excitability and thus positively biases these cells for firing as a result of direct activation of the jump mechanism. Thus, the DCMD has receptive properties which make it responsive primarily to novel stimuli and output characteristics which produce a positive biasing of an avoidance response. Taken together, these features demonstrate a role for the DCMD as part of an arousal network which if examined on purely behavioural criteria would seem far more diffuse than the actual neuronal machinery underlying this process.

1.6 ADDITIONAL DIRECTIONS

The examples cited above demonstrate the major trend of research on identifiable neurones and invertebrate behaviour: description of neuronal circuitry underlying discrete behaviours. This sort of investigation has contributed to our rudimentary understanding of neurobehavioural strategies, but the development of general theories of neurobehavioural organisation requires considerably more data over a variety of behaviours and across the breadth of the animal kingdom. At present, our information is too limited to even speculate on the homology, analogy and convergent evolution of neurobehavioural mechanisms. Even the very appealing concepts of central programmes and command interneurones must be subjected to the scrutiny of the comparative approach before they can be elevated to the level of theorems of neurobehavioural organisation. Thus, a most important avenue for future research is the continued dissection of behaviourally relevant circuits over a wide variety of organisms. This may well yield information on the frequency of usage of particular integrative mechanisms and might also indicate the breadth over which there has been an evolutionary conservation of neuronal machinery.

Outside of the mainstream of investigations, several additional avenues of research make use of the feature of invertebrate neural organisation and promise to make significant contributions to neurobehavioural theories. Perhaps foremost among these is an area of inquiry which asks what specifies the organisation of neural elements into functional networks underlying a particular act. Several investigators have begun to study the development of invertebrate nervous systems and the genetic specification of neuronal organ-isation. Such approaches will yield data on how neural networks become organised and might also expedite our understanding of the 'finally' organised adult nervous system.

1.6.1 Developmental studies

A series of investigations on flight and song production in crickets is an excellent example of a systematic multidisciplinary approach to a neuro-behavioural problem. There are 12 stages in the life cycle of the cricket and none of these wing-dependent behaviours occur until after the final imag-inal moult when newly formed wings are present. Flight and song production are the result of highly stereotyped motor outputs which are readily quantified by electromyographic analysis of the relevant musculature. By employing such an analysis Bentley and Hoy[216] have demonstrated that: (a) pattern generating neuronal circuitry is not functional at hatching, (b) there is an increase in the ability to generate patterns which arises in an orderly fashion over the last four moults, and (c) functional outputs can be generated before the final moult (i.e. to the adult, winged stage). This system offers an oppor-tunity to examine, in detail, the development of centrally programmed motor output connections. Bentley[217] has begun such an analysis by examining neuronal geometry of relevant neurones in the meso- and metathoracic ganglia (the location of wing motoneurones). Staining specific neurones (by the axonal iontophoretic technique[39]) can provide data (to the ultrastructural levels) on the changes in neuronal architecture associated with the onset of functional circuitry. Bentley[217] has already found that: (a) key neuronal somata are present at very early stages, (b) neurones in very young animals appear to have rather restricted branching patterns (especially at the tertiary and quater-nary levels) when compared with their adult counterparts (i.e. animals with functional circuitry), and (c) to the level of resolution of the light microscope, the essential features of the architecture of relevant neurones are achieved somewhat before the stage of first pattern generation. This study defines a critical period during which the major morphological features of the system are present, but the motor output cannot be evoked. This time might represent a period of synaptogenesis and certainly warrants detailed investigation.

Another example of developmental neurobehavioural investigations in-volves measuring the precision of re-specification of neurones in regenerating systems. Young[218] using physiological, morphological and behavioural techniques has demonstrated the presence of serially homologous motoneu-rone somata in the meso- and metathoracic ganglia of the cockroach. He has transplanted metathoracic legs to the mesothoracic segment and found that the leg musculature becomes specifically innervated by the appropriate homologous neurones of the new segmental ganglion. Furthermore, when regeneration occurs, transplanted legs function normally during walking. Pearson and Bradley[219], in another regeneration experiment on cockroach leg motoneurones, demonstrated an apparently normal motor output from a re-innervated system. These investigations on the specificity of regeneration of motor systems are complemented by studies on regeneration of connections between sensory cells and interneurones. For example, the anal cerci of crickets bear displacement sensitive hairs innervated by sensory neurones at their bases. These peripheral sense cells send processes into the CNS and synapse on elements of the giant fibre systems. Edwards and Sahots[220] obtained evidence for a remarkable degree of specificity of these connections by transplanting cerci onto the stumps of mesothoracic legs. The cerci were thus fully half the length of the animal away from their normal location, but still relatively close to the giant fibres which pass through the mesothoracic ganglion. These authors obtained both electrophysiological and morphological evidence that the cercal sensory cells formed functional synapses with the giant fibres at this new location. While the precise nature of the specification is as yet unclear (since there are several giant fibres) these results led the authors to suggest that perhaps there were mechanisms for whole cell recognition as opposed to specification to particular synaptic areas. Investigations of this system are continuing with a major effort towards increasing the level of resolution of particular cellular interactions (e.g. Edwards and Palka[221] and Murphey[36]).

The leech preparation (see above) recently has been employed to examine the specificity of regenerated connections between neurones in the CNS. Severing the connective between two segmental ganglia interrupts connections between sensory and motor cells in these ganglia. Baylor and Nichols[222] and Jansen and Nichols[223], examined, by intracellular microelectrode recordings, the nature of the interactions between neurones (known to be interconnected in unoperated animals) in leeches whose connectives had been cut 5–27 weeks earlier. The pattern of connections between sensory and motor cells was like that of intact animals and suggests a great degree of specificity for the regeneration process. A most interesting and unexplained result of the experimental treatment was that the sign of the net synaptic potential could be reversed. That is, in some of the connections (e.g. posterior sensory cell to anterior motor cell) where a presynaptic action potential normally evoked a small inhibitory and much larger excitatory PSP in the motoneurone, the predominant response of these cells in regenerated animals was primarily inhibitory. Further studies demonstrated that connections were altered not only between ganglia whose connective had been severed, but also throughout the animal. It was also shown that more extensive isolation of ganglia from their normal inputs could result in substantial modification of connections even within a single ganglion. There are still several questions about the precise nature of some of the connections examined in these studies, many of which might be resolved by studies of neuronal geometry using intracellular staining.

1.6.2 Genetic studies

Genetic variability between animals of the same species might result in sufficient phenotypic variability to significantly confound experimental results if one assumes equivalence of identified neurones among the individuals of the species (see Sections 1.2.3 and 1.3.3). However, such genetic variability might be employed as a valuable resource for the dissection of neural circuitry underlying behaviours. The establishment of isogenic lines (e.g. by inbreeding) of experimental animals might be used to reduce undesirable phenotypic variability. This technique could also be employed to provide a series of lines which, by virtue of their genetic differences, displayed behavioural differences. The neural bases of these behavioural differences could then be elucidated to add to our understanding of the necessary and sufficient characteristics of neural circuits for particular behaviours.

Genetic analysis of invertebrate behaviour patterns is already being employed on systems with identifiable neurones. We can again draw our example from work on cricket sound production. There are several specific and precisely defined songs in the repertoire of crickets; among these is the calling song which is used by males in attracting receptive females. Bentley[224] and Bentley and Hoy[225], have studied the calling song which can be divided into 'phrases' that can be sub-divided into 'chirps', 'trills' and individual sound pulses. In all, 18 parameters of the song were available for analysis either as sound output or as muscle activity recorded electromyographically. In the first study, Bentley[224], demonstrated that specific characteristics of the song were under direct genetic control and that this specification could resolve as little as a single action potential in the pattern of motor output of homologous motoneurones of differing genotypes. These studies made use of differences in song patterns of two species of cricket which will interbreed when brought together. Bentley and Hoy[225], asked: '(a) can hybridisation be used to reveal the basic features of the genetic system controlling song pattern? (b) can manipulation of the genotype be used to test hypotheses about the structure of the neuronal pattern generating network? Their results suggest a strong affirmation on both counts. For example, two hypotheses were consistent with the available data on the mechanism of generation of the B_1-type chirping song of $Gryllus$ $campestris$: two separate neuronal oscillators controlling phrase and patterns within the phrase or a single oscillator with an accumulating refractoriness for both. Their data strongly supported the two oscillator hypothesis and provided information of the sort not previously available. The cricket sound production system with its demonstrated feasibility for genetic and developmental as well as behavioural and neurophysiological analysis, is clearly among the outstanding preparations presently available.

The cricket sound production system has been shown to be polygenic and multichromosomal. Finer resolution, that is in terms of single genes and specific neural elements, should also be possible. Ideally, we would like to examine the effects of genetic modifications at the membrane level. A model system for this approach has been developed amongst a group of invertebrates often referred to as aneural organisms, the protozoa. Eckert and his co-workers have examined the unicellular organism, $Paramecium$, in terms of specific behaviours, sensory processes and specific effectors[226-228]. A $Paramecium$ swimming, by ciliary action, in the anterior direction can be induced to increase its rate by stimulation of its posterior surfaces and, likewise, its direction of ciliary beating and swimming can be reversed by stimulation of its anterior surfaces. Forward ciliary beating is governed by non-regenerative potassium currents. The rate of beating is a function of the degree of hyperpolarisation induced by the potassium efflux[227]. Ciliary reversal, on the other hand, is brought about by inward calcium currents which can produce regenerative all-or-none action potentials[229].

As pointed out by Kung and Eckert[230], attempts to increase our understanding of membrane phenomena like regenerative ion activation have not taken advantage of one of the most useful approaches for determining mechanisms of biological function, such as modification or deletion of single molecules that contribute to the organisation of complex functions. A genetic analysis of *Paramecium*[231] has provided the basic information for a series of studies on a fundamental problem in neurobiology, electrical excitability. By screening pure clones of various genetic backgrounds Kung[231] was able to isolate a single gene mutation, 'Pawn', which failed to swim backwards in response to depolarisation of its cell membrane. Subsequently, Kung and Eckert[230] were able to demonstrate that the Pawn mutation was apparently due to a blockage of the normal calcium activation mechanism and that other behavioural and membrane characteristics of mutant animals were identical with normal animal (see also Kung and Naitoh[232]). This study gains special significance when one considers the resolution of the genetically coded information. Alteration of a single gene, and thereby the specific product(s) regulated by this gene, completely disabled the diagnostic feature of an excitable system: regenerative ion activation.

Single gene effects on both the behaviour and nervous system of more complex invertebrates have also been reported. Benzer and his co-workers are examining problems of genetics and neural function in the fruit fly, *Drosophila*. The forté of this approach has been an imaginative consolidation of available techniques, from a variety of areas, into analytical methods specifically applicable to neurobehavioural problems. One of these, a countercurrent distribution method, provides a screen for kinetic and tropic behavioural mutations which can then be examined with respect to the mechanisms underlying these aberrant behaviours[233]. Another highly successful tool is the production of gynandromorphs; composite animals which are a mosaic of male and female characteristics. Thus, by appropriate markers and screening techniques, flies can be obtained in which particular regions are male and others female. Specific mutations associated with the male genotype then can be located in restricted regions of the animal. By using this approach, Hotta and Benzer[234] have been able to specify anatomical regions associated with behavioural differences arising from single gene mutations. They have used the technique to demonstrate, for example, that certain mutations showing behavioural abnormalities have their effect completely within the eye. The gynandromorph technique allowed these authors to rule out possible abnormalities in other locations such as visual integrating centres within the brain. This technique is quite valuable since it can be used to determine the level of organisation effected by specific genetic coding. *Drosophila* is also being used for genetic analysis of events recorded intracellularly from single neurones. Ikeda and Kaplan[235] have masterfully overcome the technical problems of intracellular recording from this tiny animal. They have taken their analysis of a behavioural mutant showing abnormal leg shaking to the level of events occurring intracellularly in two types of neurones in the CNS. In mutant flies specific motoneurones display aberrant, rhythmic bursting patterns of action potentials. Ikeda and Kaplan then made use of the gynandromorph approach to demonstrate that aberrant motor activity can be expressed in as little as one half of the thoracic ganglion[236]. With further elucidation of levels of genetic control, work on *Drosophila* could provide fundamental information for neurobiologists.

1.7 CONCLUSIONS

We have shown that systems with identifiable neurones offer a set of unique advantages for neurobehaviourists and suggested that a comparative approach is required for obtaining a more complete understanding of neurobehavioural problems. At our present level of knowledge and technical competence, we can begin to ask about the limits to, and significance of, variability at the cellular and subcellular levels and their relevance to behavioural output. Investigations on the development, genetics and evolution of behaviourally relevant processes are being carried to the neuronal and molecular level and thus allow us to begin replacing somewhat amorphous behavioural concepts with cellular mechanisms.

Acknowledgements

We are grateful to Drs. R. K. Murphey and C. Nicholson for their comments on this manuscript. The authors were partially supported by the following grants during the course of writing this paper: PHS grant 1 R01 NS09696 (S.B.K.), NSF predoctoral fellowships (C.B.H.), NSF predoctoral traineeship (C.R.S.K.).

References

1. Wiersma, C. A. G. (1952). Neurons of arthropods. *Cold Spring Harbor Symp. Quant. Biol.*, **17**, 155
2. Corning, W. C., Dyal, J. and Willows, A. O. D. (1973). *Invertebrate Learning.* (New York: Plenum Press)
3. Special Issue. (1972). Invertebrate behaviour. *Amer. Zool.*, **12**, 385
4. Marler, P. R. and Hamilton, W. J. (1967). *Mechanisms of Animal Behavior* (New York: John Wiley and Sons, Inc.)
5. Bullock, T. H. and Horridge, G. A. (1965). *Structure and Function in the Nervous Systems of Invertebrates.* (San Francisco: W. H. Freeman and Company)
6. Kandel, E. R., and Kupfermann, I. (1970). The functional organization of invertebrate ganglia. *Annu. Rev. Physiol.*, **32**, 349
7. Young, J. Z. (1971). *The Anatomy of the Nervous System of Octopus vulgaris.* (Oxford: Clarendon Press)
8. Kater, S. B. and Nicholson (editors). (1973). *Intracellular Staining in Neurobiology* (New York: Springer-Verlag)
9. Hoyle, G. (1970). Cellular mechanisms underlying behavior-neuroethology. *Advan. Insect Physiol.*, **7**, 349
10. Tauc, L. (1967). Transmission in invertebrate and vertebrate ganglia. *Physiol. Rev.*, **47**, 521
11. Maynard, D. M. (1972). Simpler networks. *Annu. N.Y. Acad. Sci.*, **193**, 59
12. Page, C. H. and Wilson, D. M. (1970). Unit responses in the methathoracic ganglion of the flying locust. *Fed. Proc. (Fed. Amer. Soc. Exp. Biol.)*, **29**, 590
13. Mendelson, M. (1971). Oscillator neurons in crustacean ganglia. *Science*, **171**, 1170

14. Nicholls, J. G., and Baylor, D. A. (1968). Specific modalities and receptive fields of sensory neurons in CNS of the leech. *J. Neurophysiol.*, **31**, 740

15. Otsuka, M., Kravitz, E. A. and Potter, D. D. (1967). Physiological and chemical architecture of a lobster ganglion with particular reference to gamma-aminobutyrate and glutamate. *J. Neurophysiol.*, **30**, 725

16. Davis, W. J. (1971). Functional significance of motoneuron size and soma position in swimmeret system of the lobster. *J. Neurophysiol.*, **34**, 274

17. Treherne, J. E. (1961). Sodium and potassium fluxes in the abdominal nerve cord of the cockroach, *Periplaneta americana* L. *J. Exp. Biol.*, **38**, 315

18. Treherne, J. E. (1961). The movements of sodium ions in the isolated abdominal nerve cord of the cockroach, *Periplaneta americana* L. *J. Exp. Biol.*, **38**, 629

19. Treherne, J. E. (1961). Exchanges of sodium ions in the central nervous system of an insect (*Periplaneta americana* L.). *Nature (London)*, **191**, 1223

20. Treherne, J. E. (1961). The efflux of sodium ions from the last abdominal ganglion of the cockroach, *Periplaneta americana* L. *J. Exp. Biol.*, **38**, 729

21. Treherne, J. E. (1961). The kinetics of sodium transfer in the central nervous system of the cockroach, *Periplaneta americana* L. *J. Exp. Biol.*, **38**, 737

22. Weidler, D. J. and Diecke, F. P. J. (1970). The regulation of sodium ions in the central nervous system of the herbivorous insect *Carausius morosus*. *Z. Vergl. Physiol.*, **67**, 160

23. Weidler, D. J. and Diecke, F. P. J. (1970). Hemolymph ionic concentrations and sodium ion regulation by the neural sheath in two stick insect species (*Diapheromera femorata* and *Carausius morosus*). *Z. Vergl. Physiol.*, **69**, 311

24. Weidler, D. J., Myers, G. G., Gardner, P. J., Bennett, A. L. and Earle, A. M. (1971). Defects in the experimental design of radioisotopic studies on the insect nerve cord. *Z. Vergl. Physiol.*, **75**, 352

25. Arvanitaki, A. and Chalazonitis, N. (1955). Les potentiels bioelectriques en docytaires du neurone geant d'*Aplysia* en activite autorhythmique. *C. R. Acad. Sci. Paris*, **240**, 349

26. Tauc, L. (1955). Reponse de le cellule nerveuse du ganglion abdominal d'*Aplysia depilans* a la stimulation directe intracellulaire. *C. R. Acad. Sci. Paris*, **239**, 1537

27. Willows, A. O. D. and Hoyle, G. (1967). Correlation of behavior with the activity of single identifiable neurons in the brain of *Tritonia*. In: *Symposium on Neurobiology of Invertebrates*. (J. Salanki, editor) (New York: Plenum Press)

28. Kerkut, G. A. and Meech, R. W. (1966). The internal chloride concentration of G and D cells in the snail brain. *Comp. Biochem. Physiol.*, **19**, 819

29. Kater, S. B. and Rowell, C. H. F. (1973). Integration of sensory and centrally programmed components in the generation of cyclical feeding activity of *Helisoma trivolvis*. *J. Neurophysiol.*, **36**, 142

30. Atwood, H. L. (1967). Crustacean neuromuscular mechanisms. *Amer. Zool.*, **7**, 527

31. Usherwood, P. N. R. (1967). Insect neuromuscular mechanisms. *Amer. Zool.*, **7**, 553

32. Takeda, K. and Kennedy, D. (1965). The mechanisms of discharge pattern formation in crayfish interneurons. *J. Gen. Physiol.*, **48**, 435

33. Kennedy, D., Selverston, A. I. and Remler, M. P. (1969). Analysis of restricted neural networks. *Science*, **164**, 1488

34. Sandeman, D. C. (1969). The synaptic link between sensory and motoneurones in the eye withdrawal reflex of the crab. *J. Exp. Biol.*, **50**, 87

35. Sandeman, D. C. (1969). The site of synaptic activity and impulse initiation in an identified motoneurone in the crab brain. *J. Exp. Biol.*, **50**, 771

36. Murphey, R. K. (1973). Characterization of an insect neuron which cannot be visualized *in situ*. In: *Intracellular Staining in Neurobiology*. (S. Kater and C. Nicholson, editors) (New York: Springer-Verlag)

37. Stretton, A. O. W. and Kravitz, E. A. (1968). Neuronal geometry: determination with a technique of intracellular dye injection. *Science*, **162**, 132

38. Sandeman, D. C. (1969). Integrative properties of a reflex motoneurone in the brain of the crab *Carcinus maenas*. *Z. Vergl. Physiol.*, **64**, 450

39. Iles, J. F. and Mulloney, B. (1971). Procion yellow staining of cockroach motor neurones without the use of microelectrodes. *Brain Res.*, **30**, 397

40. Mulloney, B. (1973). Microelectrode injection, axonal iontophoresis, and the structure of neurons. In: *Intracellular Staining in Neurobiology* (S. Kater and C. Nicholson, editors) (New York: Springer-Verlag)

41. Kater, S. B., Nicholson, C. and Davis, W. J. (1973). A guide to intracellular staining

techniques. In: *Intracellular Staining in Neurobiology* (S. Kater and C. Nicholson, editors) (New York: Springer-Verlag)

42. Pitman, R. M., Tweedle, C. D. and Cohen, M. J. (1973). The form of nerve cells: Determination by cobalt impregnation. In: *Intracellular Staining in Neurobiology* (S. Kater, and C. Nicholson, editors) (New York: Springer-Verlag)

43. Selverston, A. I. and Kennedy, D. (1969). Structure and function of identified nerve cells in the crayfish. *Endeavour*, **28**, 107

44. Baylor, D. A. and Nicholls, J. G. (1969). Chemical and electrical synaptic connections between cutaneous mechanoreceptor neurones in the central nervous system of the leech. *J. Physiol.* **203**, 591

45. Kater, S. B. and Kaneko, C. R. S. (1972). An endogenously bursting neuron in the gastropod mollusc, *Helisoma trivolvis*: Characterization *in vivo*. *J. Comp. Physiol.*, **79**, 1

46. Hoyle, G. and Burrows, M. (1973). Neural mechanisms underlying behavior in the locust *Schistocerca gregaria*. I. Physiology of identified neurons in the metathoracic ganglion. *J. Neurobiol.*, **4**, 13

47. Pitman, R. M., Tweedle, C. D. and Cohen, M. J. (1972). Branching of central neurons: Intracellular cobalt injection for light and electron microscopy. *Science*, **176**, 412

48. Purves, D. and McMahan, U. J. (1972). The distribution of synapses on a physiologically identified motor neuron in the central nervous system of the leech. *J. Cell Biol.*, **55**, 205

49. Stuart, A. E. (1970). Physiological and morphological properties of motoneurones in the central nervous system of the leech. *J. Physiol.*, **209**, 627

50. Nicholls, J. G. and Purves, D. (1970). Monosynaptic chemical and electrical connexions between sensory and motor cells in the central nervous system of the leech. *J. Physiol.*, **209**, 647

51. Rude, S. R. E., Coggeshall, R. E. and Van Orden, L. S. (1969). Chemical and ultra-structural identification of 5-hydroxytryptamine in an identified neuron. *J. Cell Biol.*, **41**, 832

52. Hall, Z., Bownds, M. D. and Kravitz, E. A. (1970). The metabolism of gamma aminobutyric acid in the lobster nervous system—enzymes in single excitatory and inhibitory axons. *J. Cell Biol.*, **46**, 290

53. Coggeshall, R. E., Dewhurst, S. A., Weinreich, D. and McCaman, R. E. (1972). Aromatic acid decarboxylase and choline acetylase activities in a single identified 5-Ht containing cell of the leech. *J. Neurobiol.*, **3**, 259

54. Wilson, D. L. and Berry, R. W. (1972). The effect of synaptic stimulation on RNA and protein metabolism in the R2 soma of *Aplysia*. *J. Neurobiol.*, **3**, 369

55. Wilson, D. L. (1971). Molecular weight distribution of proteins synthesized in single, identified neurons of *Aplysia*. *J. Gen. Physiol.*, **57**, 26

56. Gainer, H. (1972). Patterns of protein synthesis in individual, identified molluscan neurons. *Brain Res.*, **39**, 369

57. Gainer, H. (1972). Effects of experimentally induced diapause on the electrophysiology and protein synthesis patterns of identified molluscan neurons. *Brain Res.*, **39**, 387

58. Gainer, H. (1972). Electrophysiological behavior of an endogenously active neuro-secretory cell. *Brain Res.*, **39**, 403

59. Strumwasser, F. (1967). Types of information stored in single neurons. In: *Invertebrate Nervous Systems* (C. A. G. Wiersma, editor) (Chicago: University of Chicago Press)

60. Frazier, W. T., Kandel, E. R., Kupfermann, I., Waziri, R. and Coggeshall, R. E. (1967). Morphological and functional properties of identified neurons in the abdominal ganglion of *Aplysia californica*. *J. Neurophysiol.*, **30**, 1288

61. Sakharov, D. A. (1970). Cellular aspects of invertebrate neuropharmacology. *Annu. Rev. Pharmacol.*, **10**, 335

62. Willows, A. O. D. (1968). Behavioral acts elicited by stimulation of single identifiable nerve cells. In: *Physiological and Biochemical Aspects of Nervous Integration* (F. D. Carlson, editor) (New Jersey: Prentice-Hall, Inc.)

63. Sakharov, D. A. and Salanki, J. (1969). Physiological and pharmacological identification of neurons in the central nervous sytem of *Helix pomatia*. *Acta Physiol. Acad. Sci. Hung.*, **35**, 19

64. Strumwasser, F. (1963). A circadian rhythm of activity and its endogenous origin in a neuron. *Fed. Proc. (Fed. Amer. Soc. Exp. Biol.)*, **22**, 220

65. Arvanitaki, A. and Chalazonitis, N. (1967). Electrical properties and temporal organization in oscillatory neurons. In: *Symposium on Neurobiology of Invertebrates* (J. Salanki, editor) (New York: Plenum Press)
66. Wachtel, H. and Wilson, W. A. (1971). *Proc. 25th Intern. Physiol. Congress, Munich,* **9,** 591
67. Faber, D. S. and Klee, M. R. (1972). Membrane characteristics of busting pacemaker neurones in *Aplysia*. *Nature New Biol.,* **240,** 29
68. Strumwasser, F. (1968). Membrane and intracellular mechanisms governing endogenous activity in neurons. In: *Physiological and Biochemical Aspects of Nervous Integration* (F. D. Carlson, editor) (New Jersey: Prentice-Hall, Inc.)
69. Kandel, E. R., Frazier, W. T., Waziri, R. and Coggeshall, R. E. (1967). Direct and common connections among identified neurons in *Aplysia*. *J. Neurophysiol.,* **30,** 1352
70. Stinnakre, J. and Tauc, L. (1966). Effects de l'activation osmotique de l'osphradium sur les neurones de systeme nerveux central de *l'Aplysia*. *J. Physiol. (Paris),* **58,** 266
71. Stinnakre, J. and Tauc, L. (1969). Central neuronal response to the activation of osmoreceptors in the osphradium of *Aplysia*. *J. Exp. Biol.,* **51,** 347
72. Jahan-Parwar, B., Smith, M. and Baumgarten, R. von. (1969). Activation of neurosecretory cells in *Aplysia* by osphradial stimulation. *Amer. J. Physiol.,* **216,** 1246
73. Strumwasser, F. (1965). The demonstration and manipulation of a circadian rhythm in a single neuron. In: *Circadian Clocks* (J. Aschoff, editor) (Amsterdam: North-Holland Publ. Co.)
74. Stretton, A. O. W. and Kravitz, E. A. (1973). Intracellular dye injection: The selection of Procion yellow and its application in preliminary studies of neuronal geometry in the lobster nervous system. In: *Intracellular Staining in Neurobiology* (S. Kater and C. Nicholson, editors) (New York: Springer-Verlag)
75. Macagno, E. R., Lopresti, V. and Levinthal, C. (1973). Structure and development of neuronal connections in isogenic organisms: variations and similarities in the optic system of *Daphnia magna*. *Proc. Nat. Acad. Sci. USA,* **70,** 57
76. Lent, C. M. (1973). Retzius' cells from segmental ganglia of four species of leeches: comparative neuronal geometry. *Comp. Biochem. Physiol.,* **44A,** 35
77. Thompson, R. F. and Spencer, W. A. (1966). Habituation: a model phenomenon for the study of neuronal substrates of behavior. *Psychol. Rev.,* **173,** 16
78. Eisenstein, E. M. and Peretz, B. (1973). Comparative aspects of habituation in invertebrates. In: *Habituation: Behavioral and Electrophysiological Substrates* (H. Peeke and H. Herz, editors) (New York: Academic Press)
79. Granit, R. (1970). *The Basis of Motor Control* (New York: Academic Press)
80. Kennedy, D. (1967). The reflex control of muscle. In: *Invertebrate Nervous Systems* (C. A. G. Wiersma, editor) (Chicago: University of Chicago Press)
81. Abraham, F. D. and Willows, A. O. D. (1971). Plasticity of a fixed action pattern in the sea slug *Tritonia diomedia, Comm. Beh. Biol.,* **6,** 271
82. Willows, A. O. D., Dorsett, D. A. and Hoyle, G. (1973). Neuronal basis of behavior in *Tritonia*. I. Functional organization of the central nervous system. *J. Neurobiol.,* **4,** 207
83. Hoyle, G. and Willows, A. O. D. (1973). Neuronal basis of behavior in *Tritonia*. II. Relationship of muscular contraction to nerve impulse pattern. *J. Neurobiol.,* **4,** 239
84. Willows, A. O. D., Dorsett, D. A. and Hoyle, G. (1973). Neuronal basis of behavior in *Tritonia*. III. Neuronal mechanism of a fixed action pattern. *J. Neurobiol.,* **4,** 255
85. Dorsett, D. A., Willows, A. O. D. and Hoyle, G. (1973). Neuronal basis of behavior in *Tritonia*. IV. The central origin of a fixed action pattern demonstrated in the isolated brain. *J. Neurobiol.,* **4,** 287
86. Wilson, D. M. (1968). The nervous control of insect flight and related behavior. *Advan. Insect Physiol.,* **5,** 289
87. Wilson, D. M. (1961). The central nervous control of flight in a locust. *J. Exp. Biol.,* **38,** 471
88. Bullock, T. H. (1961). The origins of patterned nervous discharge. *Behaviour,* **17,** 48
89. Dorsett, D. A., Willows, A. O. D. and Hoyle, G. (1969). Centrally generated nerve impulse sequences determining swimming behavior in *Tritonia*. *Nature (London),* **224,** 711
90. Davis, W. J. and Kennedy, D. (1972). Command interneurons controlling swimmeret movements in the lobster. I. Types of effects on motoneurons. *J. Neurophysiol.,* **35,** 1

91. Davis, W. J. and Kennedy, D. (1972). Command interneurons controlling swimmeret movements in the lobster. II. Interaction of effects on motoneurons. *J. Neurophysiol.*, **35,** 13

92. Davis, W. J. and Kennedy, D. (1972). Command interneurons controlling swimmeret movements in the lobster. III. Temporal relationships among bursts in different motoneurons. *J. Neurophysiol.*, **35,** 20

93. Diamond, J. (1971). The Mauthner cell. In: *Fish Physiology V: Sensory Systems and Electric Organs* (W. S. Hoar and D. J. Randall, editors) (New York: Academic Press)

94. Shik, M. L., Severin, F. V. and Orlovskii, G. N. (1966). Control of walking and running by means of electrical stimulation of the mid-brain. *Biophysics*, **11,** 756

95. Willows, A. O. D. (1967). Behavioral acts elicited by stimulation of single identified nerve cells. *Science*, **157,** 570

96. Davis, W. J. and Mpitsos, G. J. (1971). Behavioral choice and habituation in the marine mollusk *Pleurobranchaea californica* MacFarland (Gastropoda, Opisthobranchia). *Z. Vergl. Physiol.*, **75,** 207

97. Kandel, E. R. and Tauc. L. (1964). Mechanism of prolonged heterosynaptic facilitation. *Nature (London)*, **202,** 145

98. Haigler, H. J. and Baumgarten, R. J. von (1972). Facilitation of excitatory postsynaptic potentials in the giant cell in the left pleural ganglion of *Aplysia californica*. *Comp. Biochem. Physiol.*, **41A,** 7

99. Mpitsos, G. J. and Davis, W. J. (1973). Learning: classical and avoidance condition in the mollusc *Pleurobranchia*. *Science*, **180,** 317

100. Davis, W. J., Siegler, M. V. S. and Mpitsos, G. J. (1973). Distributed neuronal oscillators and efference copy in the feeding system of *Pleurobranchaea*. *J. Neurophysial*, **36,** 238

101. Horridge, G. A. (1962). Learning of leg position by the ventral nerve cord in headless insects. *Proc. Roy. Soc. (London) B*, **157,** 33

102. Horridge, G. A. (1965). The electrophysiological approach to learning in isolatable ganglia. *Anim. Behav.*, **12** (1), 163

103. Hoyle, G. (1965). Neurophysiological studies on "learning" in headless insects. In: *Physiology of the Insect Central Nervous System* (J. W. Beament and J. Treherne, editors) (New York: Academic Press)

104. Hoyle, G. (1973). Neural machinery underlying behavior in insects. In: *The Neurosciences*, in the press (F. O. Schmitt, editor) (Brookline, Mass.: MIT Press)

105. Hoyle, G. and Burrows, M. (1973). Neural mechanisms underlying behavior in the locust *Schistocera gregaria*. II. Integrative activity in metathorasic neurons. *J. Neurobiol.*, **4,** 42

106. Stuart, A. E. (1969). Excitatory and inhibitory motoneurons in the central nervous system of the leech. *Science*, **165,** 817

107. Nicholls, J. G. and Purves, D. (1972). A comparison of chemical and electrical synaptic transmission between single sensory cells and a motoneurone in the central nervous system of the leech. *J. Physiol.*, **225,** 637

108. Baylor, D. A. and Nicholls, J. G. (1969). Changes in extracellular potassium concentration produced by neuronal activity in the central nervous system of the leech. *J. Physiol.*, **203,** 555

109. Baylor, D. A. and Nicholls, J. G. (1969). After-effects of nerve impulses on signalling in the central nervous system of the leech. *J. Physiol.*, **203,** 571

110 Wiersma, C. A. G. (1938). Function of the giant fibers of the central nervous system of the crayfish. *Proc. Soc. Exp. Biol. Med.*, **38,** 661

111. Larimer, J. L., Eggleston, A. C., Masukawa, L. M. and Kennedy, D. (1971). The different connections and motor outputs of lateral and medial giant fibres in the crayfish. *J. Exp. Biol.*, **54,** 391

112. Wine, J. J. and Krasne, F. B. (1972). The organization of escape behavior in the crayfish. *J. Exp. Biol.*, **56,** 1

113. Krasne, F. B. (1969). Excitation and habituation of the crayfish escape reflex: the depolarizing response in lateral giant fibres of the isolated abdomen. *J. Exp. Biol.*, **50,** 29

114. Zucker, R. S. (1972). Crayfish escape behavior and central synapses. I. Neural circuit exciting lateral giant fiber. *J. Neurophysiol.*, **35,** 599

115. Kennedy, D. (1971). Crayfish interneurons. *Physiologist*, **14,** 5

116. Selverston, A. I. and Remler, M. P. (1972). Neural geometry and activation of crayfish fast flexor motoneurons. *J. Neurophysiol.*, **35**, 797
117. Furshpan, E. J. and Potter, D. D. (1959). Transmission at the giant motor synapse of the crayfish. *J. Physiol.*, **145**, 289
118. Zucker, R. S. (1972). Crayfish escape behavior and central synapses. III. Electrical junctions and dendrite spikes in fast flexor motoneurons. *J. Neurophysiol.*, **35**, 638
119. Bruner, J. and Kennedy, D. (1970). Habituation: occurrence at a neuromuscular junction. *Science*, **169**, 92
120. Mittenthal, J. E. and Wine, J. J. (1973). Connectivity patterns of crayfish giant interneurons: visualization of synaptic regions. *Science*, **179**, 182
121. Roberts, A. (1968). Recurrent inhibition in the giant-fibre system of the crayfish and its effect on the excitability of the escape response. *J. Exp. Biol.*, **48**, 545
122. Wilson, D. M. (1970). Neural operations in arthropod ganglia. In: *The Neurosciences, A Second Study Program* (F. O. Schmitt, editor) (New York: Rockefeller University Press)
123. Wilson, D. M. (1966). Central nervous mechanisms for the generation of rhythmic behavior in arthropods. *Symp. Soc. Biol.*, **20**, 199
124. Bentley, D. R. (1970). A topological map of the locust flight system motoneurons. *J. Insect Physiol.*, **16**, 905
125. Kendig, J. J. (1968). Motor neurone coupling in locust flight. *J. Exp. Biol.*, **48**, 389
126. Hagiwara, S. (1961). Nervous activity of the heart in crustacea. *Ergebn. Biol.*, **24**, 287
127. Brown, H. F. (1964). Electrophysiological investigations of the heart of *Squilla mantis*. II. The heart muscle. *J. Exp. Biol.*, **41**, 701
128. Van der Kloot, W. (1970). The electrophysiology of muscle fibers in hearts of decapod crustaceans. *J. Exp. Zool.*, **174**, 367
129. Anderson, M. and Cooke, I. M. (1971). Neural activation of the heart of the lobster *Homarus americanus*. *J. Exp. Biol.*, **55**, 449
130. Hartline, D. K. (1967). Impulse identification and axon mapping of the nine neurons in the cardiac ganglion of the lobster *Homorus americanus*. *J. Exp. Biol.*, **47**, 327
131. Bullock, T. H. and Terzuolo, C. A. (1957). Diverse forms of activity in the somata of spontaneous and integrating ganglion cells. *J. Physiol.*, **138**, 341
132. Tazaki, K. (1972). The burst activity of different cell regions and intercellular coordination in the cardiac ganglion of the crab, *Eriocher japonicus*. *J. Exp. Biol.*, **57**, 713
133. Lang, F. (1971). Intracellular studies on the pacemaker and follower neurons in the cardiac ganglion of *Limulus*. *J. Exp. Biol.*, **54**, 815
134. Watanabe, A., Obara, S., Akiyama, T. and Yumoto, K. (1967). Electrical properties of the pacemaker neurons in the heart ganglion of a stomatopod, *Squilla oratoria*. *J. Gen. Physiol.*, **50**, 813
135. Watanabe, A., Obara, S. and Akiyama, T. (1967). Pacemaker potentials for the periodic burst discharge in the heart ganglion of the stomatopod, *Squilla oratoria*. *J. Gen. Physiol.*, **50**, 839
136. Connor, J. A. (1969). Burst activity and cellular interaction in the pacemaker ganglion of the lobster heart. *J. Exp. Biol.*, **50**, 275
137. Tazaki, K. (1971). The effects of tetrodotoxin on the slow potential and spikes in the cardiac ganglion of a crab *Eriocher japonicus*. *Jap. J. Physiol.*, **21**, 529
138. Tazaki, K. (1972). Electrical interaction among large cells in the cardiac ganglion of the lobster, *Panulirus japonicus*. *J. Exp. Zool.*, **180**, 85
139. Watanabe, A., Obara, S. and Akiyama, T. (1968). Inhibitory synapses on pacemaker neuron: in the heart ganglion of a stomatopod, *Squilla oratoria*. *J. Gen. Physiol.*, **52**, 908
140. Watanabe, A., Obara, S. and Akiyama, T. (1969). Acceleratory synapses on pacemaker neurons in the heart ganglion of a stomatopod, *Squilla oratoria*. *J. Gen. Physiol.*, **54**, 211
141. Rao, K. P., Babu, K. S., Ishiko, N. and Bullock, T. H. (1969). Effectiveness of temporal pattern in the input to a ganglion: inhibition in the cardiac ganglion of spiny lobster. *J. Neurobiol.*, **2**, 233
142. Morris, J. and Maynard, D. M. (1970). Recordings from the stomato gastric nervous system in intact lobsters. *Comp. Biochem. Physiol.*, **33**, 969

143. Maynard, D. M. (1969). In: *The Interneuron* 56 (M. A. B. Brazier, editor) (Los Angeles: University California Press)

144. Dando, M. R. and Selverston, A. I. (1972). Command fibers from the supra-oesophageal ganglion to the stomatogastric ganglion in *Panulirus argus. J. Comp. Physiol.*, **78**, 138

145. Mulloney, B. (1969). Organization of flight motoneurons of diptera. *J. Neurophysiol,*. **33**, 86

146. Mulloney, B. (1970). Impulse patterns in the flight motor neurones of *Bombus californicus* and *Oncopeltus fasciatus. J. Exp. Biol.*, **52**, 59

147. Hughes, G. M. and Wiersma, C. A. G. (1960). The co-ordination of swimmeret movements in the crayfish, *Procambarus clarikii* (Girard). *J. Exp. Biol.*, **37**, 657

148. Ikeda, K. and Wiersma, C. A. G. (1964). Autogenic rhythymicity in the abdominal ganglia of the crayfish: the control of swimmeret movements. *Comp. Biochem. Physiol.*, **12**, 107

149. Davis, W. J. (1969). The neural control of swimmeret beating in the lobster. *J. Exp. Biol.*, **50**, 99

150. Davis, W. J. (1969). Reflex organization in the swimmeret system of the lobster I. Intrasegmental reflexes. *J. Exp. Biol.*, **51**, 547

151. Davis, W. J. (1969) Reflex organization in the swimmeret system of the lobster. II. Reflex dynamics. *J. Exp. Biol.*, **51**, 565

152. Miller, P. L. (1966). The regulation of breathing in insects. *Advan. Insect Physiol.*, **3**, 279

153. Farley, R. D. and Case, J. F. (1968). Sensory modulation of ventilative pacemaker output in the cockroach, *Periplaneta americana. J. Insect Physiol.*, **14**, 591

154. Mill, P. J. (1970). Neural patterns associated with ventilatory movements in dragon fly larvae. *J. Exp. Biol.*, **52**, 167

155. Pearson, K. G. (1972). Central programming and reflex control of walking in the cockroach. *J. Exp. Biol.*, **56**, 173

156. Bentley, D. R. (1969). Intracellular activity in cricket neurons during the generation of behaviour patterns. *J. Insect Physiol.*, **15**, 677

157. Bentley, D. R. (1969). Intracellular activity in cricket neurons during generation of song patterns. *Z. Vergl. Physiol.*, **62**, 267

158. Wilson, D. M. (1972). Genetic and sensory mechanisms for locomotion and orientation in animals. *Amer. Sci.*, **60**, 358

159. Pearson, K. G. and Iles, J. F. (1971). Innervation of the coxal depressor muscles of the cockroach, *Periplaneta americana. J. Exp. Biol.*, **54**, 215

160. Gettrup, E. (1962). Thoracic proprioceptors in the flight system of locusts. *Nature (London)*, **193**, 498

161. Gettrup, E. (1963). Phasic stimulation of a thoracic stretch receptor in locusts. *J. Exp. Biol.*, **40**, 323

162. Gettrup, E. and Wilson, D. M. (1964). The lift control reaction of flying locusts. *J. Exp. Biol.*, **41**, 183

163. Camhi, J. M. (1969). Locust wind receptors. I. Transducer mechanics and sensory response. *J. Exp. Biol.*, **50**, 335

164. Camhi, J. M. (1969). Locust wind receptors. II. Interneurons in the cervical connective. *J. Exp. Biol.*, **50**, 349

165. Camhi, J. M. (1969). Locust wind receptors. III. Contributions to flight initiation and lift control. *J. Exp. Biol.*, **50**, 363

166. Goodman, L. J. (1965). The role of certain optomotor reactions in regulating stability in the rolling plane during flight in the desert locust, *Schistocerca gregaria. J. Exp. Biol.*, **42**, 385

167. Strumwasser, F. (1967). Types of information stored in single neurons. In: *Invertebrate Nervous Systems* (C. A. G. Wiersma, editor) (Chicago: University of Chicago Press)

168. Gardner, D. (1969). Symmetry and redundancy of interneural connections in the buccal ganglion of *Aplysia. Physiologist*, **12**, 232

169. Gardner, D. (1971). Bilateral symmetry and interneuronal organization in the buccal ganglia of *Aplysia. Science*, **173**, 550

170. Gardner, D. and Kandel, E. R. (1972). Diphasic postsynaptic potential: a chemical synapse capable of mediating conjoint excitation and inhibition. *Science*, **176**, 675

171. Rose, R. M. (1972). Burst activity of the buccal ganglion of *Aplysia depilans. J. Exp. Biol.*, **56**, 735

172. Levitan, H., Tauc, L. and Segundo, J. P. (1970). Electrical transmission among neurons in the buccal ganglion of a mollusc, *Navanax inermis*. *J. Gen. Physiol.*, **55**, 484
173. Levitan, H. and Tauc, L. (1972). Acetylcholine receptors: topographic distribution and pharmacological properties of two receptor types on a single molluscan neurone. *J. Physiol.*, **222**, 537
174. Spira, M. E. and Bennett, M. V. L. (1972). Synaptic control of electronic coupling between neurons. *Brain Res.*, **37**, 294
175. Rose, R. M. (1971). Patterned activity of the buccal ganglion of the nudibranch mollusc *Archidoris pseudoargus*. *J. Exp. Biol.*, **55**, 185
176. Gorman, A. L. F. and Mirolli, M. (1969). The input–output organization of a pair of giant neurons in the mollusc, *Anisodoris nobilis*. *J. Exp. Biol.*, **51**, 615
177. Gorman, A. L. F. and Mirolli, M. (1970). Axonal localization of an excitatory postsynaptic potential in a molluscan neuron. *J. Exp. Biol.*, **53**, 727
178. Murray, M. J. (1972). The biology of a carniverous mollusc: anatomical, behavioral and electrophysiological observations. *Ph.D. Thesis*, University of California, Berkeley
179. Woollacott, M. H. and Moore, G. P. (1972). Neural correlates of the prey–capture response of *Navanax*. *Physiologist*, **15**, 305
180. Berry, M. S. (1972). A system of electrically coupled small cells in the buccal ganglia of the pond snail *Planorbis corneus*. *J. Exp. Biol.*, **56**, 621
181. Berry, M. S. (1972). Electrotonic coupling between identified large cells in the buccal ganglia of *Planorbis corneus*. *J. Exp. Biol.*, **57**, 173
182. Brown, T. G. (1914). On the nature of the fundamental activity of the nervous centres; together with an analysis of the conditioning of rhythmic activity in progression, and a theory of the evolution of function in the nervous system. *J. Physiol.*, **48**, 18
183. Holst, Erich von. (1937). Vom wesen der ordnung im zentralnervensystem. *Naturwissenschaften*, **25**, 625
184. Weiss, P. (1936). A study of motor coordination and tonus in deafferented limbs of amphibia. *Amer. J. Physiol.*, **115**, 461
185. Schrameck, J. E. (1970). Crayfish swimming: alternating motor output and giant fiber activity. *Science*, **169**, 698
186. Krasne, F. B. and Woodsmall, K. S. (1969). Waning of the crayfish escape response as a result of repeated stimulation. *Anim. Behav.*, **17**, 416
187. Kennedy, D. and Takeda, K. (1965). Reflex control of the abdominal flexor muscles in the crayfish. I. The twitch system. *J. Exp. Biol.*, **43**, 211
188. Zucker, R. S. (1972). Crayfish escape behavior and central synapses. II. Physiological mechanisms underlying behavioral habituation. *J. Neurophysiol.*, **35**, 621
189. Krasne, F. B. and Roberts, A. (1969). Habituation of the crayfish escape response during release from inhibition induced by picrotoxin. *Nature (London)*, **215**, 769
190. Kupfermann, I., Pinsker, H., Castellucci, V. and Kandel, E. R. (1971). Central and peripheral control of gill movements in *Aplysia*. *Science*, **174**, 1252
191. Carew, T. J., Castellucci, V. F. and Kandel, E. R. (1971). An analysis of dishabituation and sensitization of the gill-withdrawal reflex in *Aplysia*. *Int. J. Neuroscience*, **2**, 79
192. Peretz, B. (1970). Habituation and dishabituation in the absence of a central nervous system. *Science*, **169**, 379
193. Carew, T. J., Pinsker, H. M. and Kandel, E. R. (1972). Long-term habituation of a defensive withdrawal reflex in *Aplysia*. *Science*, **175**, 451
194. Kupfermann, I. and Kandel, E. R. (1969). Neural controls of a behavioral response mediated by the abdominal ganglion of *Aplysia*. *Science*, **164**, 847
195. Kandel, E. R. (1973). An invertebrate system for the cellular analysis of simple behaviors and their modifications. In: *The Neurosciences*, in the press (F. O. Schmitt, editor) (Brookline, Mass.: MIT Press)
196. Carew, T. J., Schwartz, J. H. and Kandel, E. R. (1972). Innervation of *Aplysia* gill muscle fibers by two identified excitatory motor neurons using different transmitters. *Physiologist*, **15**, 100
197. Pinsker, H., Kupfermann, I., Castellucci, V. and Kandel, E. (1970). Habituation and dishabituation of the gill-withdrawal reflex in *Aplysia*. *Science*, **167**, 1740
198. Lukowiak, K. and Jacklet, J. W. (1972). Habituation and dishabituation: interactions between peripheral and central nervous systems in *Aplysia*. *Science*, **178**, 1306
199. Kupfermann, I. Castellucci, V., Pinsker, H. and Kandel, E. (1970). Neuronal

correlates of habituation and dishabituation of the gill-withdrawal reflex in *Aplysia*. *Science*, **167**, 1743

200. Castelluci, V., Pinsker, H., Kupfermann, I. and Kandel, E. R. (1970). Neuronal mechanisms of habituation and dishabituation of the gill-withdrawal reflex in *Aplysia*. *Science*, **167**, 1745

201. Groves, P. M. and Thompson, R. F. (1970). Habituation: a dual-process theory. *Psychol. Rev.*, **77**, 419

202. Epstein, R. and Tauc, L. (1970). Heterosynaptic facilitation and post-tetanic potentiation in *Aplysia* nervous system. *J. Physiol.*, **209**, 1

203. Horn, G. and Wright, M. J. (1970). Characteristics of transmission failure in the squid stellate ganglion: a study of a simple habituating system. *J. Exp. Biol.*, **52**, 217

204. Abraham, F. D., Palka, J., Peeke, A. V. S. and Willows, A. O. D. (1972). Model neural systems and strategies for the neurobiology of learning. *Behav. Biol.*, **7**, 1

205. Schwartz, J. H., Castellucci, V. F. and Kandel, E. R. (1971). Functioning of identified neurons and synapses in abdominal ganglion of *Aplysia* in absence of protein synthesis. *J. Neurophysiol.*, **34**, 939

206. Agranoff, B. W. (1967). Agents that block memory. In: *The Neurosciences*. (G. C. Quarton, T. Melnechuk and F. O. Schmitt, editors) (New York: Rockefeller University Press)

207. Barondes, S. H. (1970). Multiple stages in the biology of memory. In: *The Neurosciences A Second Study Program* (F. O. Schmitt, editor) (New York: Rockefeller University Press)

208. Moruzzi, G. and Magoun, H. W. (1949). Brain stem reticular formation and activation of the EEG *Electroenceph. and Clin. Neurophys.*, **1**, 455

209. Rowell, C. H. F. (1973). Boredom and attention in a cell in the locust visual system. In: *Experimental Analysis of Insect Behaviour* (L. Barton Brown, editor) (New York: Springer-Verlag)

210. Rowell, C. H. F. (1971). The orthopteran descending movement detector (DMD) neurones: a characterization and review. *Z. Vergl. Physiol.*, **73**, 167

211. Burtt, E. T. and Catton, W. T. (1954). Visual perception of movement in the locust. *J. Physiol.*, **125**, 566

212. Palka, J. (1965). Diffraction and visual acuity in insects. *Science*, **149**, 551

213. Horn, G and Rowell, C. H. F. (1958). Medium and long-term changes in the behaviour of visual neurones in the tritocerebrum of locusts. *J. Exp. Biol.*, **49**, 143

214. Rowell, C. H. F. and Horn, G. (1968). Dishabituation and arousal in the response of single nerve cells in an insect brain. *J. Exp. Biol.*, **49**, 171

215. Rowell, C. H. F. (1971). Variable responsiveness of a visual interneurone in the free-moving locust, and its relation to behaviour and arousal. *J. Exp. Biol.*, **55**, 727

216. Bentley, D. R. and Hoy, R. R. (1970). Postembryonic development of adult motor patterns in crickets: a neural analysis. *Sciences*, **170**, 1409

217. Bentley, D. R. (1973). Postembryonic development of invertebrate motor systems. In: *Developmental Neurobiology of Arthropods* (D. Young, editor) (Cambridge: Cambridge University Press).

218. Young, D. (1972). Specific re-innervation of limbs transplanted between segments in the cockroach, *Periplaneta americana. J. Exp. Biol.*, **57**, 305

219. Pearson, K. G. and Bradley, A. B. (1972). Specific regeneration of excitatory motoneurons to leg muscles in the cockroach. *Brain Res.*, **47**, 492

220. Edwards, J. S. and Sahota, T. S. (1967). Regeneration of a sensory system: the formation of central connections by normal and transplanted cerci of the house cricket *Acheta domesticus. J. Exp. Zool.*, **166**, 387

221. Edwards, J. S. and Palka, J. (1971). Neural regeneration: delayed formation of central contacts by insect sensory cells. *Science*, **172**, 591

222. Baylor, D. A. and Nicholls, J. G. (1971). Patterns of regeneration between individual nerve cells in the central nervous system of the leech. *Nature* (*London*), **232**, 268

223. Jansen, J. K. S. and Nicholls, J. G. (1972). Regeneration and changes in synaptic connections between individual nerve cells in the central nervous system of the leech. *Proc. Nat. Acad. Sci. USA*, **69**, 636

224. Bentley, D. R. (1971). Genetic control of an insect neuronal network. *Science*, **174**, 1139

225. Bentley, D. R. and Hoy, R. R. (1972). Genetic control of the neuronal network generating cricket (*Teleogryllys gryllus*) song patterns. *Anim. Behav.*, **20,** 478

226. Eckert, R. (1972). Bioelectric control of ciliary activity. *Science*, **176,** 473

227. Eckert, R. and Naitoh, Y. (1972). Bioelectric control of locomotion in ciliates. *J. Protozool.*, **19,** 237

228. Eckert, R., Naitoh, Y. and Friedman, K. (1972). Sensory mechanisms in *Paramecium*. I. Two components of the electric response to mechanical stimulation of the anterior surface. *J. Exp. Biol.*, **56,** 683

229. Naitoh, Y., Eckert, R. and Friedman, K. (1972). A regenerative calcium response in *Paramecium. J. Exp. Biol.*, **56,** 667

230. Kung, C. and Eckert, R. (1972). Genetic modification of electric properties in an excitable membrane. *Proc. Nat. Acad. Sci. USA*, **69,** 93

231. Kung, C. (1971). Genetic mutants with altered system of excitation in *Paramecium aurelia*. I. Phenotypes of the behavioral mutants. *Z. Vergl. Physiol.*, **7,** 142

232. Kung, C. and Naitoh, Y. (1973). Calcium-induced ciliary reversal in the extracted models of 'Pawn', a behavioral mutant of *paramecium*. *Science*, **179,** 195

233. Benzer, S. (1967). Behavioral mutants of *Drosophila* isolated by countercurrent distribution. *Proc. Nat. Acad. Sci. USA*, **58,** 1112

234. Hotta, Y. and Benzer, S. (1970). Genetic dissection of the *Drosophila* nervous system by means of mosaics. *Proc. Nat. Acad. Sci. USA*, **67,** 1156

235. Ikeda, K. and Kaplan, W. D. (1970). Patterned neural activity of a mutant *Drosophila melanogaster*. *Proc. Nat. Acad. Sci. USA*, **66,** 765

236. Ikeda, K. and Kaplan, W. D. (1970). Unilaterally patterned neural activity of gynandromorphs, mosaic for a neurological mutant of *Drosophila melanogaster*. *Proc. Nat. Acad. Sci. USA*, **67,** 1490

237. Galeano, C. (1972). Electrophysiological studies of learning in simplified nervous system preparations. In: *Structure and Function of Nervous Tissue* (G. H. Bourne, editor) (New York: Academic Press)

2
Synaptic Transmission

A. R. MARTIN
University of Colorado Medical Center, Denver

2.1 INTRODUCTION 54

2.2 MEMBRANE PROPERTIES OF EXCITABLE CELLS 54
    2.2.1 *The resting membrane* 54
    2.2.2 *Excitation* 55

2.3 CHEMICAL AND ELECTRICAL SYNAPSES 57
    2.3.1 *Principles of operation* 57
    2.3.2 *Morphological features* 57

2.4 CHEMICAL EXCITATION AND INHIBITION 58
    2.4.1 *Excitatory junctions* 58
    2.4.2 *Inhibitory junctions* 59
    2.4.3 *Presynaptic inhibiton* 60

2.5 RELEASE OF TRANSMITTER FROM NERVE TERMINALS 60
    2.5.1 *The quantal nature of release* 60
    2.5.2 *Evaluation of the quantal parameters,* m, n *and* p 63
    2.5.3 *Spontaneous release* 66
    2.5.4 *Effect of divalent cations* 67
    2.5.5 *Relation between depolarisation and release* 69
    2.5.6 *The vesicle hypothesis* 69

2.6 POST-SYNAPTIC ACTION OF TRANSMITTERS 70
    2.6.1 *Excitatory conductance changes* 70
    2.6.2 *Inhibitory conductance changes* 72
    2.6.3 *Conductance decreases* 72
    2.6.4 *Mixed post-synaptic effects* 72
    2.6.5 *Post-synaptic 'noise'* 73
    2.6.6 *Receptor labelling and density* 74

2.7 CONCLUSION 75
    ACKNOWLEDGEMENT 75

2.1 INTRODUCTION

Synapses are points of functional contact between nerve cells. It is now common to extend this definition to include contact between efferent nerve terminals and muscle cells or cells of other effector organs. The term will be used in this more general sense in the present discussion. Each synapse consists of two basic elements: the presynaptic element is usually a terminal branch of a nerve axon; the post-synaptic element is that part of the post-synaptic cell membrane directly underlying the presynaptic terminal. Between them is a synaptic cleft. A given post-synaptic cell may have upon it only one synapse as, for example, is the case for many skeletal muscle cells, or many hundreds of synapses, as may occur on motor neurones of the spinal cord. At a given synapse, arrival of an action potential in the presynaptic terminal may tend to produce an action potential in the post-synaptic cell or, conversely, may tend to suppress post-synaptic action potential generation. In the former case the synapse is said to be excitatory, in the latter, inhibitory. In general, a cell which is receiving synaptic input on its soma or dendrites cannot communicate this information to its nerve terminals, and hence to the next cells in line, without first generating an action potential. There are only a few known exceptions to this principle; for example, bipolar cells in the retina pass information to higher order cells without action potential generation. In most nerve cells, then, the basic function of the synaptic input is to control or modulate the production of action potentials.

Before dealing directly with synaptic transmission, it will be useful to consider briefly some of the properties of resting and active nerve cell membrane. This will be followed by a brief discussion of some of the general properties of chemical and electrical synapses and then by a discussion of some of the specific characteristics of excitatory and inhibitory synapses. These initial subjects are treated in much more detail in several monographs; the author particularly recommends *Nerve, muscle and synapse* by Katz[1] for those encountering the subject for the first time, and the excellent monograph by Hubbard, Llinàs and Quastel[2] for a still more detailed treatment. The subsequent sections of the present review dealing with release of transmitter from nerve terminals and post-synaptic action of transmitter will deal primarily with the more recent literature to bring the reader up to date on the subject.

2.2 MEMBRANE PROPERTIES OF EXCITABLE CELLS

2.2.1 The resting membrane

One of the characteristics of nerve cells is that they have a 'resting membrane potential'; that is, the membrane is polarised so that the inside of the cell is negative with respect to the outside, usually by 60–90 mV. This potential arises from the distribution of ions across the membrane. Considering only the monovalent ions, the extracellular fluid surrounding neurones contains mainly Na^+ and Cl^-, with only small amounts of K^+. On the other hand, the main internal cation is K^+, and the concentrations of both Na^+ and

Cl^- inside the cell are low. The major counter-ion for K^+ is intracellular protein, which is negatively charged at the internal pH of the cell. The membrane is slightly permeable to all the ionic species mentioned, except the intracellular protein. Permeability is very small indeed to Na^+, but greater by one to two orders of magnitude for K^+ and Cl^-. Recalling that Cl^- is most concentrated outside the cell and K^+ most concentrated inside, it follows that there is a tendency for Cl^- to move into and K^+ to move out of the cell. This tendency for net movement of ions along their concentration gradients is opposed by the membrane potential, the potential gradient being inward for K^+ ions and outward for Cl^-. In many nerve cells the concentration gradient for Cl^- is balanced exactly by the membrane potential and Cl^-, therefore, is in electrochemical equilibrium. In other words, the membrane potential is at the equilibrium potential for Cl^-. K^+, on the other hand, is not quite in equilibrium. Its equilibrium potential (i.e. the potential which would just balance the concentration gradient) is several mV more negative than the resting membrane potential. Since Na^+ is more concentrated outside the cell, it can be seen intuitively that for this ion to be in equilibrium across the cell membrane the inside of the cell would have to be positive rather than negative. Indeed, the equilibrium potential for Na^+ is *ca.* $+50$ mV.

It has already been noted that the cell membrane is permeable to the ions under discussion. Consequently, since neither Na^+ nor K^+ is in equilibrium, there must be a constant leak of Na^+ into and K^+ out of the cell. The internal concentrations are kept constant, however, by an 'active-transport' mechanism which utilises metabolic energy to move Na^+ and K^+ against their electrochemical gradients, thus compensating for the passive leaks. This mechanism is the so-called 'Na^+–K^+ pump'. As mentioned previously, Cl^- is usually at or near equilibrium in most neurones, but recent observations on some cells in the mammalian central nervous system[3] and on *Aplysia* neurones[4] indicate that, in these particular cells, the Cl^- equilibrium potential is more negative than the resting potential and that there is an outwardly-directed Cl^- pump.

The membrane properties outlined above may be summarised by the electrical model shown in Figure 2.1. The fact that there is a charge separation across the cell membrane means that the membrane has the properties of a capacitor. The capacitance per unit area is designated as C_m. The existence of a finite permeability to K^+ is indicated by a conductance channel for this ion (g_K). This channel is in series with a battery with a value, E_K, equal to the K^+ equilibrium potential. Similar conductances and driving potentials are indicated for Cl^- and Na^+. The potentials are related to the concentration gradients for the individual ions and are maintained, as indicated in the previous paragraph, by the appropriate active-transport mechanisms.

2.2.2 Excitation

A small hyperpolarisation impressed on the soma or on a dendrite of a neurone will spread at most only a few mm along its axon. This is because the cell processes are very inefficient as cable conductors. Depolarisations spread with equal inefficiency unless the magnitude of the depolarisation is sufficient to reach the 'threshold potential' for initiation of an action potential. At this point, which is usually 10–20 mV depolarisation, the membrane potential suddenly reverses in the region of excitation, becoming 30–50 mV positive inside, and then returns to normal. This whole process of action-potential generation lasts *ca.* 1 ms. The depolarisation spreads to adjacent regions of the membrane, initiating active responses there and in this way the excitation is propagated along the axon to the nerve terminals.

The action potential arises because the Na$^+$ conductance, indicated in Figure 2.1 by g_{Na}, is dependent on membrane potential. When the cell membrane is depolarised, say by synaptic activity, two things happen. First, because the inside of the membrane is more positive than in the resting

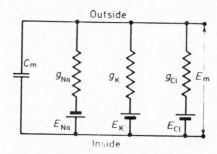

Figure 2.1 Electrical model of a nerve cell membrane. C_m = membrane capacitance; E_{Na}, E_K and E_{Cl} = equilibrium potentials for the respective monovalent ions; g_{Na}, g_K and g_{Cl} = conductance channels in the membrane for the ions. The net membrane potential, E_m, is determined by the three driving potentials and the relative values of the three conductances

steady state, there is a net flux of K$^+$ out of the cell and a net inward movement of Cl$^-$, both of which tend to restore the membrane potential to normal. Secondly, depolarisation results in an increase in g_{Na}, so that there is an increased leak of Na$^+$ into the cell along its electrochemical gradient, tending to depolarise the cell still further. At threshold, these two consequences of depolarisation are in delicate balance. A slight increase in depolarisation results in a further increase in g_{Na}, still more Na$^+$ entry and the depolarisation process becomes explosive. If the Na$^+$ conductance increase persisted the membrane would approach the Na$^+$ equilibrium potential and stay there. However, the increase in g_{Na} is also time dependent and turns off within *ca.* 1 ms. A delayed large increase in g_K then follows, resulting in a rapid efflux of K$^+$ and the consequent repolarisation of the membrane to normal. In summary, then, the ionic events underlying the action potential are a rapid influx of Na$^+$, depolarising the membrane toward E_{Na}, and a subsequent efflux of K$^+$, restoring the membrane to its original resting state.

2.3 CHEMICAL AND ELECTRICAL SYNAPSES

2.3.1 Principles of operation

In general, there are two types of synapses, chemical and electrical. Leaving aside for the moment the question of synaptic inhibition, Figure 2.2 illustrates the principles of operation of electrical and chemical synaptic excitation. In the chemical synapses, the arrival of the nerve impulse in the presynaptic

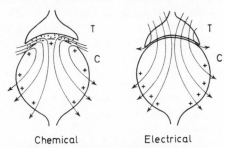

Chemical   Electrical

Figure 2.2 Schematic representation of mode of action of chemical and electrical excitatory synapses. At the chemical synapse an action potential in the presynaptic terminal (T) results in release of transmitter which produces a conductance change in the post-synaptic membrane of the cell (C). This results in a new inward flow of positive current (arrows) and consequent depolarisation of the cell. + signs indicate change in membrane potential from rest. At the electrical synapse, current associated with the presynaptic action potential flows, in part, through the post-synaptic cell, causing depolarisation

terminal results in the release of a transmitter substance which diffuses onto the post-synaptic membrane causing the membrane to become depolarised. The action of the transmitter in producing excitation is to cause net inward movement of positive ions across the membrane and consequent depolarisation of the cell.

At the electrical synapse, depolarisation of the post-synaptic cell is effected by current flow associated with the presynaptic action potential. Some of the current flowing into the presynaptic terminal during the action potential spreads into the post-synaptic cell, as indicated by the arrows, causing depolarisation. In the diagram the plus signs indicate the *change* in membrane potential from the resting state, and the arrows the direction of conventional current flow (i.e. direction of movement of positive ions).

2.3.2 Morphological features

The ultrastructure of chemically-transmitting synapses is rather uniform. The presynaptic and post-synaptic membranes are separated by a cleft *ca.* 250 Å wide with desmasome-like thickenings occurring periodically in the presynaptic membrane. The post-synaptic membrane shows no consistent specialisation; however, at the vertebrate neuromuscular junction it is thrown into deep post-junctional folds. The presynaptic terminal is rich in synaptic vesicles and mitochondria, the former having some tendency to aggregate over the membrane thickenings[5]. There is increasing evidence, which will be discussed in some detail later, that the vesicles are storage particles containing the neurotransmitter. They may be classified into four major types. The most commonly occurring are electron-lucid, circular in profile with a diameter of *ca.* 500 Å, and bounded by a limiting membrane of *ca.* 50 Å. A second type, seen at different synapses, presents a mixture of circular and oval profiles, suggesting that the vesicles are ellipsoidal in shape, rather than spherical. At the crayfish neuromuscular junction, elongated vesicles have been associated with inhibitory synapses and circular ones with excitatory synapses[6]. This relationship has been suggested previously for synapses in general[7] but such a suggestion does not seem to be reasonable. As we shall see later, acetylcholine (ACh) is quite ubiquitous as a transmitter, sometimes being excitatory, sometimes inhibitory, and even having a dual effect on the same post-synaptic cell. It seems unlikely that this, or any other, transmitter is selectively packaged in spherical or ellipsoidal vesicles depending on its ultimate post-synaptic effect. A more logical conclusion would be that certain substances, for example ACh or glutamate, are packaged in spherical vesicles and others, for example γ-aminobutyric acid (GABA), are packaged in ellipsoidal vesicles. A third type of vesicle is seen at adrenergic synapses. This type is electron-dense or 'granular' and is of about the same diameter as other vesicles. These occur in association with electron-lucid vesicles and are depleted by treatments known to deplete the terminals of catecholamines. Finally, there are dense-cored vesicles of larger diameter (*ca.* 1000 Å) whose role in synaptic transmission is unclear.

Electrical synapses are usually characterised by the presence of 'gap junctions' between the pre- and post-synaptic elements. This term is used to describe the close apposition of the pre- and post-synaptic membranes. The synaptic cleft is reduced to the order of a 20–40 Å separation and appears to be bridged by small (*ca.* 10 Å) channels in a periodic array. It is generally assumed that the gap junctions constitute low-resistance pathways between cells, facilitating flow of current from the pre- to the post-synaptic cell. Indeed, there is evidence suggesting that the lattice of 'channels' bridging the gap are true cytoplasmic continuities. The general morphological and physiological characteristics of electrical synapses have been discussed in detail by Bennett[8] and will not be considered further here.

2.4 CHEMICAL EXCITATION AND INHIBITION

2.4.1 Excitatory junctions

Much of our knowledge of excitatory synaptic transmission has been obtained from the vertebrate neuromuscular junction. At this synapse a single action potential in the motor nerve usually results in the generation of a single action potential in each post-synaptic muscle cell. However, transmission may be blocked either by adding a post-synaptic blocking agent (e.g. tubocurarine) to the bathing solution or by adjusting the Mg^{2+} : Ca^{2+} ratio in the bathing solution to reduce transmitter release from the presynaptic terminal. The specific effects of these treatments will be discussed in more detail later. The main point to be made at the moment is illustrated

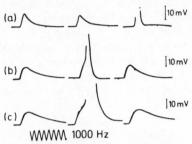

Figure 2.3 Oscilloscope records of end-plate potentials (e.p.p.s) recorded from three different muscle fibres (A, B, C) of cat tenuissimus. Transmission blocked by tubocurarine (A and B) and high Mg (C) so that e.p.p. amplitude is just at threshold for initiation of action potential. In each fibre one out of three trials results in action potential initiation (rapid upward swing of trace). (From Boyd and Martin[9] by courtesy of the Physiological Society)

in Figure 2.3. At a critical level of block one sees an end-plate potential (e.p.p.) in the muscle fibre which, if it reaches threshold, gives rise to an action potential. The records in Figure 2.3 were obtained by inserting a micropipette into the muscle fibre at the point of innervation (the 'end-plate') to record the transmembrane potential, and then stimulating the motor nerve. The resulting e.p.p. rises to a peak in *ca.* 1 ms and then decays with a half time of 1–2 ms. The e.p.p. itself is not propagated but instead decays passively with distance from the end-plate. Its rising phase is associated with a local increase in conductance of the membrane to Na^+ and K^+, caused by the action of ACh released from the presynaptic terminal. The conductance changes are such that the resulting inward movement of Na^+ along its electrochemical gradient is greater than the accompanying outward movement of K^+. Consequently there is a net inward movement of positive ions, resulting in depolarisation. As ACh is removed from the synaptic region by hydrolysis and diffusion the membrane permeability returns to normal and the potential returns to the resting level at a rate determined by the membrane time constant. This overall behaviour is characteristic of excitatory post-synaptic potentials (e.p.s.p.s) in general except, of course, the transmitter substance need not be ACh.

2.4.2 Inhibitory junctions

The process of synaptic inhibition is similar to that just described for excitation, but with one important difference: an increase in Na^+ conductance is never involved. At the crayfish neuromuscular junction, for example, the inhibitory transmitter, GABA, causes an increase in Cl^- conductance in the post-synaptic membrane. A similar increase in Cl^- conductance accompanies inhibition in neurones of the vertebrate central nervous system and in many invertebrate neurones. In some instances the increase in g_{Cl} may be accompanied by an increase in g_K and in some preparations inhibition is associated exclusively with an increase in K^+ conductance. In terms of potential change, an increase in conductance to Cl^- and/or K^+ produces a small hyperpolarisation of the cell or little potential change at all. The main effect is a tendency to hold the membrane at some point below threshold for excitation, thus opposing any depolarising influence from competing excitatory inputs.

2.4.3 Presynaptic inhibition

Excitatory input to a cell may be foiled in yet another way. Inhibitory inputs are known to occur on presynaptic excitatory terminals themselves. The effect of the inhibitory terminal is to reduce the amount of transmitter released from the excitatory terminal and thus the excitatory drive on the post-synaptic cell[10,11]. The underlying ionic events in the excitatory terminal are not known in detail, except at the crayfish neuromuscular junction, where there is good evidence that the membrane permeability to Cl^- is increased[110]. This permeability increase tends to 'short out' the action potential in the terminal and the smaller action potential then releases less transmitter than in the absence of such inhibition. Whether this specific mechanism operates at other sites of presynaptic inhibition is not known.

2.5 RELEASE OF TRANSMITTER FROM NERVE TERMINALS

From the introductory material just presented it can be seen that a discussion of synaptic transmission can be divided conveniently into two separate topics: the mechanism of transmitter release from presynaptic terminals and the effects of the transmitter on the post-synaptic membrane. Details of the release process will be discussed in this section. Most of the information about this process comes from electro-physiological experiments on excitatory synapses in which depolarisation of the post-synaptic cell is used as a measure of transmitter release. In these experiments, then, the post-synaptic membrane is used as a sensitive and rapidly-responding detector of transmitter release. A micropipette is usually placed in the post-synaptic cell near the synapse to record changes in membrane potential as described previously (Figure 2.3). In other experiments, however, recording pipettes are placed extracellularly against the post-synaptic membrane; in this position they become sensitive detectors of current flow into the synaptic region. 'Extracellular e.p.s.p.s' recorded in this way are again a measure of transmitter release.

2.5.1 The quantal nature of release

It has been mentioned previously that the amount of transmitter released from the nerve terminal by an action potential depends on concentrations of Ca^{2+} and Mg^{2+} in the bathing solution. External Ca^{2+} is necessary for release and if its concentration is reduced below normal levels release is attenuated. A similar reduction in release is produced by addition of Mg^{2+} to the bathing solution, Mg^{2+} appearing to displace Ca^{2+} from a membrane site associated with the release process. Consequently, as Ca^{2+} is reduced or Mg^{2+} increased in concentration the amplitude of the synaptic potential becomes progressively smaller. At low levels of release one finds that on successive trials the amplitude of the synaptic potential fluctuates in a stepwise manner, with responses having amplitudes equal to multiples of some irreducible unit size and interspersed with total failures of response. Further reduction in release simply increases the relative number of failures without further reduction in the minimum response. The minimum unit responses are known as 'miniature synaptic potentials' and are also observed in the absence of stimulation, occurring spontaneously at irregular intervals.

These kinds of observations led Fatt and Katz[12] to postulate that the miniature e.p.p., recorded from the frog neuromuscular junction, was the basic 'building block' for the normal response or, in other words, that the normal e.p.p. represented the summed effect of a large number of unit potentials. They proposed further that the miniature e.p.p. was produced by the action of a package, or 'quantum' of acetylcholine molecules. Subsequently del Castillo and Katz[13] formulated the quantum hypothesis of transmitter release to explain the nature of the fluctuations at low release levels. The hypothesis states that there are preformed quanta of transmitter in the nerve terminal and that, on the arrival of a nerve impulse in the terminal, each has a finite probability of being released. If the number of available quanta is n and the average probability of release of a quantum is p then, during a series of successive trials (assuming n is always replenished) the mean number of quanta released (m) will be given by:

$$m = np \qquad (2.1)$$

and the responses should fluctuate in a predictable manner. To use an example, suppose $n=3$ and $p=0.1$ and we have a thousand trials. It is convenient also to define $q=1-p$ ($=0.9$), which is the probability that an individual quantum will not be released. It is clear that the probability of all three quanta being released in a given trial is simply p^3, or 0.001. The probability of two being released is $3p^2q$, or 0.027. The probability of a single release is $3pq^2$ or 0.243, and the probability of no release q^3, or 0.729. Thus in our thousand trials we would expect all three quanta to be released only once, two to be released 27 times, one to be released 243 times and failures to occur 729 times. These expectations are simply the successive terms of the binomial expansion of $(p+q)^3$. In the more general case the expected occurrences of multiple releases are given by the successive terms in the binomial expansion $(p+q)^n$. The probability that x quanta will be released on any given trial (p_x) is given, then, by the appropriate term of the expansion, namely

$$p_x = \frac{n!}{(n-x)!x!} p^x q^{n-x} \qquad (2.2)$$

The immediate difficulty in testing the hypothesis is that n and p are not known. However, del Castillo and Katz made an additional simplifying assumption, namely that when transmission was blocked by low Ca^{2+} or high Mg^{2+} p was very small. In this case, as $p \to 0$ the binomial distribution approaches a limiting form which is identical with the Poisson distribution. The expected distribution of successive quantal releases is then given by the Poisson equation:

$$p_x = \frac{e^{-m} m^x}{x!} \tag{2.3}$$

Since the Poisson equation involves only m, one can simply measure the mean number of quanta released in a series of trials and then predict the expected number of failures, single unit responses, etc. If the hypothesis is correct, the predictions should match the experimentally observed numbers. The success of the predictions at the neuromuscular junction and a wide variety of other synapses is well known[14], and was taken as strong support for the original hypothesis. It was pointed out by Ginsborg[15], however, that although these results were consistent with the hypothesis, they proved only that release was a Poisson process, which in turn implied only that the individual quanta were released independently. In short, neither n nor p is required for a Poisson distribution and Poisson statistics carries no implication at all about their existence. In addition, observations on the crayfish neuromuscular junction[16] and mammalian sympathetic ganglion[17] suggested that Poisson statistics did not hold at all synapses; i.e. the relative numbers of failures and multi-unit responses were not as predicted.

Release at the crayfish neuromuscular junction was re-examined by Johnson and Wernig[18] to determine whether failure to obey Poisson statistics might be an indication that binomial statistics were more appropriate, as implied by the original hypothesis. They recorded synaptic potentials extracellularly from a limited segment of the nerve terminal and kept the preparation at low temperature (2–5 °C) so that individual quanta released from the terminal by nerve stimulation were dispersed in time. In this way, the quantum content of each response was obtained simply by counting the number of miniature potentials occurring after each stimulus.

The point was made earlier that there is no direct way of measuring n and p. However, an indirect measure of p is possible if binomial statistics are assumed. The variance (σ^2) of a binomial distribution is given by

$$\sigma^2 = npq = m(1-p)$$

Consequently,
$$p = 1 - \sigma^2/m \tag{2.4}$$

Experimentally, then, Johnson and Wernig counted the number of quanta released by each of a series of stimuli and calculated the mean number released for the series (m) and the variance (σ^2). Equation (2.4) was used to calculate p, equation (2.1) to calculate n, and the resulting values used in equation (2.2) to predict the expected number of responses in each group (p_x). It should be noted that this is similar to the procedure used previously with Poisson statistics, except that instead of utilising only the mean of the distribution to make the predictions both the mean and variance must now be used. In the experiments, estimates of p ranged between 0.04 and 0.50. With low values of p, both Poisson and binomial predictions were indistinguishable from the experimental results. With high values, the binomial predictions were in extremely good agreement with the experimental observations and the Poisson predictions (using only m) were clearly inappropriate. These experiments, then, provided much more powerful support for the quantum hypothesis than had previously been available.

2.5.2 Evaluation of the quantal parameters, m, n and p

Having established that the characteristics of the transmitter release process are consistent with the binomial hypothesis, it is of obvious interest to have some experimental estimates of all three parameters. One way of doing this has already been mentioned, namely counting quanta released from a limited length of terminal at low temperature and making the appropriate statistical calculations. The method was used previously by Katz and Miledi[19] to determine m, but Poisson statistics was assumed and the analysis carried no further. Estimates of m (and n) for the entire terminal apparatus requires some knowledge of what fraction of the terminal is being sampled by the extracellular micropipette. At the frog neuromuscular junction, this is a few per cent; at the crayfish junction the electrode appears to sample from a single terminal branch, $ca.$ 50 of which arise from each axon.

In experiments using intracellular recording at normal temperatures[9,13], m can be obtained in Mg-blocked preparations by dividing the mean amplitude of a series of evoked responses ($\bar{v}$) by the mean amplitude of the spontaneously occurring unit response ($\bar{v}_1$), i.e.

$$m = \bar{v}/\bar{v}_1 \qquad (2.5)$$

This brings up a point not mentioned previously, namely that at a given synapse the miniature potentials are not constant in size. Their amplitudes vary somewhat, with a standard deviation $ca.$ 30% of the mean. In addition to this straightforward determination, two other methods of obtaining m have been used, both assuming Poisson statistics[2,14]. First, if the mean quantum content is small there will be a significant number of failures. For the Poisson distribution, the fraction of failures, p_0, is given by e^{-m}. Consequently, the number of failures (n_0) observed in N trials should be related to the mean quantum content by

$$m = \ln (N/n_0).$$

The second indirect method makes use of the fact that for the Poisson distribution the coefficient of variation of the quantum content distribution $(CV)_x$ is related to the mean by the equation

$$m = 1/(CV)_x^2.$$

If the unit potentials were all the same size, the coefficient of variation of the amplitude distribution (CV) would be the same as that of the quantum content distribution. In fact, (CV) is larger than $(CV)_x$ by a factor $\sqrt{(1+cv^2)}$, where cv is the coefficient of variation of the unit potentials. Consequently,

$$m = \frac{1+cv^2}{(CV)^2}$$

This calculation is used frequently to determine quantum contents at normal levels of release, particularly at the neuromuscular junction. In such cases the synaptic potential must be reduced below threshold for spike initiation and this is done with a post-synaptic blocking agent such as tubocurarine, with the result that the miniature potentials are reduced below baseline noise levels and no independent measure of unit size is available for use in equation (2.5). Since there are no failures at normal release levels, the coefficient of variation method is the only one available for measuring m. Consequently the method is quite useful; at the same time it must always be regarded with the deepest suspicion. Often corrections must be made for the fact that the unit potentials making up the synaptic potentials do not sum linearly before the method can be used at all and such corrections may not be very accurate. In addition, the estimate itself has an intrinsic coefficient of variation of at least $\pm 10\%$ when two hundred samples are taken, this error increasing linearly as the square root of the number of samples decreases. On top of this, baseline fluctuations may themselves contribute markedly to the measured value of (CV) if recording conditions are not favourable, and finally the method assumes Poisson statistics which may or may not be appropriate for a particular experiment. The corresponding binomial relations for the two indirect methods are

$$m = \frac{-p}{\ln(1-p)} \ln \frac{N}{n_0} \tag{2.6}$$

and

$$m = (1-p)\frac{1+cv^2}{(CV)^2} \tag{2.7}$$

Apart from the statistical method already mentioned, two basic approaches have been used to arrive at an experimental value for p. The first makes use of the observation that at normal release levels the second of two synaptic potentials, separated by, say, 1 s, is usually depressed in amplitude. At the vertebrate neuromuscular junction, for example, the depression is maximal at a separation of ca. 100 ms and the amplitude of the second e.p.p. returns to normal exponentially as the separation is increased, with a time constant of ca. 4 s. If one plots the amplitude of the second response against separation between the two responses and extrapolates the exponential recovery curve to zero separation, a value for 'zero-time depression' may be obtained[14]. This is converted to a value for p if it is assumed that the depression is due entirely to depletion of available quanta (i.e. of n). For example, if the zero-time depression is 25%, then the terminal must have released 25% of its transmitter during the first response or, in other words, p must have been 0.25. Extrapolation of the curve to zero-time is necessary because at short intervals there is a superimposed increase in e.p.p. amplitude (facilitation) which seems to be due to a transient increase in p[20].

A somewhat more complex variation of the depression method, using similar assumptions, consists of measuring the amplitude of successive e.p.p.s during a short, rapid train of impulses[21]. In this case, depression is cumulative and the amplitudes of the responses rapidly approach zero. If we again assume that the depression is due to the terminal running out of transmitter, the sum of the amplitudes of all the responses occurring before zero amplitude is reached must represent the sum total of all the transmitter in the terminal. The ratio of the amplitude of the first response to this sum then must be equal to p. For example, suppose ten responses occur before no more transmitter is released, and their amplitudes total 50 mV. If the first response is 10 mV in amplitude, then it must have been produced by $\frac{1}{5}$ of the total transmitter present and p must have been 0.2. This assumes, of course, a linear relation between transmitter release and depolarisation, but again corrections can be made for non-linearity. In fact, the experiment is somewhat more complicated, since the e.p.p. amplitudes approach a steady state greater than zero and extrapolation to zero is required. The extrapolation may be somewhat hazardous unless one can safely assume that p is constant during the period of rapid decline of the response. In general, this is not a safe assumption[22].

The depression methods both suffer from the same difficulty, namely the assumption that depression is depletion. There is evidence to suggest that this is not completely true. Betz[23] found that depression was not linearly related to the amount of transmitter released. That is, doubling the amount released at a given junction did not double depression. The results were consistent with the idea that during depression both n and p were reduced by approximately equal amounts. The lack of a linear relation between release and depression was subsequently confirmed by Christensen and Martin[22], who introduced a second method of estimating p at the mammalian neuromuscular junction.

The method used by Christensen and Martin makes use of the relation given in equation (2.7) and involves the single assumption that increasing the Ca^{2+} concentration in the bathing solution increases m solely by increasing p, with n remaining constant. The mean amplitude of a series of e.p.p.s and their coefficient of variation were measured in $\frac{3}{4}$ normal Ca^{2+}. The Ca^{2+} concentration was then doubled and the measurements repeated. If we let the subscripts a and b refer to the low and high Ca^{2+} concentrations respectively, we can use equation (2.7) to write:

$$\frac{m_a}{m_b} = \frac{(1-p_a)}{(1-p_b)}\frac{(CV)_b^2}{(CV)_a^2}$$

If the mean response amplitudes, v_a and v_b, are proportional to the mean quantum contents, and if n is unchanged, we can write $m_a/m_b = v_a/v_b$ and $p_b = p_a v_b/v_a$. Substituting these relations into the above equation, we can then solve for p_a in terms of the mean response amplitudes and coefficients of variation at the two Ca^{2+} levels. The method is based on much firmer theoretical grounds than the depression methods, since it has been shown, at least for the crayfish neuromuscular junction[24], that Ca^{2+} does appear to act exclusively on p. It suffers, however, from the difficulties mentioned previously in relation to using the coefficient of variation to measure m and should be regarded with at least equal suspicion. In spite of this, two observations were probably valid:

(a) the values obtained for p were consistently greater than zero, suggesting that binomial statistics were appropriate;

(b) the estimates for p were consistently smaller than those obtained by the depression method at the same junctions.

The second observation is consistent with the idea expressed previously that depression involves a reduction in both n and p and that, consequently, values of p obtained by depression methods are probably overestimates.

Measurements made with the methods just described indicate that the average number of quanta released in a single response ranges from a high of 100–300 at the vertebrate neuromuscular junction[14] to a low of about one at single excitatory and inhibitory synapses on cat spinal motoneurones[25,26]. At the vertebrate neuromuscular junction, estimates of p by depression methods have yielded values ranging from ca. 0.15 to 0.45 (see Ref. 14). Allowing for the intrinsic tendency of the methods to overestimate the release probability, an average value 0.15–0.20 would seem reasonable. The statistical estimates[22] were of this order. As already mentioned, p at the crayfish neuromuscular junction ranged from ca. 0.04 to 0.5[18], and a similar upper limit (0.5) was obtained at inhibitory synapses on spinal motoneurones[26]. The number of available quanta, n, appears to be ca. 1000 at the vertebrate neuromuscular junction[14]. At individual terminals at the crayfish neuro-muscular junction, n ranged from a minimum of 3 to a maximum of ca. 10, and single inhibitory synapses on spinal motoneurones appear to have values of n as low as 4. These low figures raise some difficulties, which will be discussed subsequently, about the interpretation that this parameter represents a population of vesicles.

2.5.3 Spontaneous release

It has already been mentioned that quanta are released spontaneously from nerve terminals. Fatt and Katz[12] measured intervals between successive spontaneous miniature e.p.p.s at the frog neuromuscular junction and showed that they were distributed exponentially, as would be expected if the events occurred randomly in time. Random occurrences, in turn, are consistent with the idea that the successive events occur independently. Since then much effort has been expended to demonstrate with more stringent tests that the quanta are indeed released independently under normal conditions. At invertebrate neuromuscular junctions, spontaneous miniature potentials sometimes occur in a non-random sequence, tending to appear in bursts[27,28]. At the frog neuromuscular junction release becomes non-random in high (15 mM) Ca^{2+} concentrations[29].

Miniature potential amplitudes are usually distributed normally about a mean amplitude which depends on, among other factors, the input impe-dance of the post-synaptic cell. In most cells the mean is between a few tenths of a mV and a few mV. In some preparations, however, either 'giant' or 'subminiature' potentials occur as well. Subminiature populations have been observed at the frog neuromuscular junction during nerve terminal regeneration[30] and after treatment with botulinum toxin[31]. In both cases the spontaneous miniature e.p.p.s had amplitude distributions which, rather than being normal, were skewed into the baseline noise; i.e. there were large numbers of very small potentials. In the regenerating terminals unit potentials evoked by stimulation were, on the contrary, distributed in the usual way around a larger mean, suggesting that the spontaneous potentials and those released by stimulation constituted separate populations. In botulinum-poisoned preparations no release could be evoked, but repetitive stimulation selectively increased the frequency of occurrence of the larger units. In both cases it was considered that the small potentials might possibly arise from the adjacent Schwann cells rather than the nerve terminals. Their nature and significance is not clear. One might suppose, however, that a regenerating or poisoned nerve terminal tends to be generally 'leaky' to quanta so that many would be released spontaneously from positions related more or less unfavourably to post-synaptic receptors. Release from such locations would produce potentials of all amplitudes varying from normal to zero. If evoked, or facilitated, release were still restricted largely to specialised 'release sites' adjacent to the post-synaptic membrane, then quanta released in this way would have the usual amplitude distribution. Thus the disparity between the spontaneous and evoked amplitude distributions would be explained.

There are two distinct types of 'giant' miniature potentials. At the mammalian neuromuscular junction spontaneous potentials of several times the mean amplitude occur infrequently[32]. Their frequency of occurrence is, however, still much greater than would be expected for random coincident release of even two units. They may represent 'fused' multiquantal units, or some other anomalous packaging of ACh either in the nerve terminal or in adjacent Schwann cells. In any case, they do not appear to be released by nerve stimulation[33]. The second type should not be classified as 'giant' since the amplitudes are only two, or occasionally three, times the mean unit amplitude. These are most common in vertebrate autonomic ganglia[34,35]. In the chick ciliary ganglion[35], Martin and Pilar observed that up to 25% of the spontaneous potentials fell outside the normal distribution fitted around the modal amplitude. These appeared to be double releases, but again were too frequent to be the result of random coincidences. The authors suggested that the double releases could be accounted for either by assuming a 'drag' effect (one quantum occasionally pulling another with it) or by assuming that the releases were due to spontaneous activations of single release sites with a very low value of m, so that most such activations produced no release and were unobservable, some produced single quantal releases and a few produced double releases. They were able to account for the tail of the amplitude distribution by assuming a drag effect, but re-examination of the treatment indicates that the test used was totally uncritical in situations where double occurrences constituted $<30\%$ of the total number of spontaneous events. In addition, the drag hypothesis is intrinsically unattractive since it implies that individual quanta would not be released independently in response to stimulation, an implication which is contrary to the available evidence. Taking these considerations into account, the idea that the miniature potentials occur as a result of spontaneous activation of release sites seems much more tenable.

2.5.4 Effect of divalent cations

The two requirements essential for synchronous release of transmitter from presynaptic terminals are depolarisation and external Ca^{2+}. Spontaneous release, of course, occurs in the absence of depolarisation and, as we shall see, is not absolutely dependent on the presence of Ca^{2+} in the external medium. Dodge and Rahamimoff[36] examined carefully the relation between external Ca^{2+} and e.p.p. amplitude at the frog neuromuscular junction. At low Ca^{2+} concentrations the relation was linear on a double logarithmic plot with a slope of almost 4, suggesting that the co-operative action of 4 Ca^{2+} ions was necessary at individual release sites. A simple physical model consistent with this conclusion would be one in which four independent binding sites on a membrane component must be occupied by Ca^{2+} for release to occur. Alternatively, release could depend on the co-operative action of four adjacent membrane components, each requiring one Ca^{2+}. Relations with somewhat smaller slopes have been obtained with other preparations. At the squid giant synapse[37] and the mammalian neuromuscular junction[38], for example, the initial slopes of the double logarithmic plots were *ca.* 2.5, and at the crayfish neuromuscular junction[39,40] about unity.

It is clear that release is associated with Ca^{2+} entry into the nerve terminal. Katz and Miledi[41,42] observed inward currents in the presynaptic terminals of the squid synapse in response to depolarisation, after the Na^+ and K^+ currents normally associated with the action potential were blocked with tetrodotoxin (TTX) and tetraethylammonium (TEA) respectively. The currents were regenerative, showed little inactivation with time and were directly dependent on external Ca^{2+} concentration. The equilibrium potential for Ca^{2+} appeared to be of the order of $+100$ mV. The time-course of the Ca^{2+} current is similar to the later of two phases of Ca^{2+} entry observed in squid axon with the fluorescent indicator aequorin[43]. Aequorin fluorescence has also been observed in the presynaptic terminals themselves during repetitive stimulation[44], again indicating Ca^{2+} entry into the axoplasm. In the superior cervical ganglion of the rat[45], accumulation of $^{45}Ca^{2+}$ by the nerve terminals is markedly accelerated by presynaptic stimulation.

There appear to be two components of spontaneous release, one Ca^{2+}-dependent, one Ca^{2+}-independent. Under otherwise normal circumstances, miniature e.p.p.s continue at a low rate at the vertebrate neuromuscular junction when Ca^{2+} is almost completely absent[46,47]. Their frequency is independent of Ca^{2+} concentration up to *ca.* 10^{-4} M and increases with concentration thereafter[46]. The increase with concentration is approximately linear[48] as opposed to the fourth power relation associated with release in response to depolarisation. Acceleration of spontaneous potential frequency by such treatments as osmotic shock and application of ethanol[49,50] is independent of Ca^{2+}. It was suggested above (p. 67) that spontaneous activity might be the result of spontaneous activation of individual release sites. This suggestion might be applicable to the Ca^{2+}-dependent activity. The Ca^{2+}-independent fraction might then be associated with a more non-specific leak of quanta from the terminals.

Of the other divalent ions, Mg^{2+} is most commonly used as an antagonist of Ca^{2+}. This ion appears to compete directly with Ca^{2+} for membrane binding sites[36,51] and interferes with Ca^{2+} entry into the presynaptic terminal[41,45]. Mn^{2+}[41,52-54] and the trivalent ion La^{3+}[55,56] have antagonistic effects similar to those of Mg^{2+}. Both Sr^{2+} and Ba^{2+} can substitute for Ca^{2+} in the release process[41,52,57-59] but are less effective. In relation to spontaneous release, miniature potential frequency is reduced by Mg^{2+} in normal Ca^{2+} concentrations, but can accelerate spontaneous release in the absence of Ca^{2+}[46,47,59]. La^{2+} produces a marked increase in spontaneous release[54,56,59]. These confusing, and apparently contradictory observations can be given some sense if it is remembered that at least two stages of ionic participation in the release process are involved: entry into the terminal and initiation of release. La^{3+}, for example, competes with Ca^{2+} for membrane sites, blocking Ca^{2+} entry during depolarisation, but does not enter through the Ca^{2+} channels[55]. On the other hand, it apparently accumulates passively in the terminals and is then very effective in accelerating spontaneous release[56,59] either directly, or perhaps by displacing Ca^{2+} from internal binding sites.

2.5.5 Relation between depolarisation and release

It has already been implied that the action potential itself is not essential for synchronous release from presynaptic terminals; artificially imposed depolarisations of the terminal membrane are equally effective. In such experiments[60-64] the Na^+ conductance increase associated with the action potential, and hence the action potential itself, is blocked with TTX. In addition, TEA may be added intracellularly to block the late K^+ current[63]. In the most detailed of the studies on the squid giant synapse[63] brief (1–2 ms) depolarising current pulses in the presynaptic terminal produced no detectable post-synaptic potential until the depolarisation exceeded *ca.* 30 mV (from a resting potential of *ca.* 70 mV). The subsequent relation between e.p.s.p. amplitude and terminal depolarisation was s-shaped, with a maximum slope of a *ca.* tenfold increase in e.p.s.p. amplitude for each 7–10 mV additional depolarisation and saturating when the terminal was depolarised by *ca.* 100 mV. As would be expected, the slope of the 'synaptic transfer curve' was increased by Ca^{2+} and reduced by Mg^{2+}. When pulses of long duration (10–20 ms) were passed, the e.p.s.p. was suppressed and eventually abolished by large depolarisations in the range of 100–200 mV, but appeared as an 'off response' on termination of the depolarisation. These results are consistent with the idea that Ca^{2+} influx is necessary for release; such influx would be suppressed and eventually abolished as the membrane potential approached the Ca^{2+} equilibrium potential. Assuming that the increase in Ca^{2+} conductance produced by depolarisation did not decline immediately at the termination of the pulse, influx at this time would then produce the off response.

2.5.6 The vesicle hypothesis

There is good biochemical evidence that transmitter substances are contained in vesicles. When subcellular particles from cholinergic terminals are separated on sucrose density gradients, the bulk of acetylcholine appears at the same location on the gradient as the vesicle population[65,66]. Similarly, noradrenaline has been shown to occur in association with both small and large dense-cored vesicles[67]. The amount of transmitter contained in each vesicle has not been determined accurately. For cholinergic vesicles, estimates range from *ca.* 10^3 to 10^5[68,69].

At the vertebrate neuromuscular junction, it has now been shown that procedures which produce massive release of ACh from the nerve terminals also result in loss of synaptic vesicles. Such procedures include treatment with La^{3+}[56] or black widow spider venom[70] or prolonged stimulation at low frequency[71,72]. The loss of synaptic vesicles is accompanied by other morphological changes, including swelling and dispersion of mitochondria and appearance of membrane-bound cysternae and 'coated vesicles'. Horseradish peroxidase, which normally does not enter the terminals, is taken up during stimulation, appearing in coated vesicles, cysternae and synaptic vesicles apparently in sequential fashion[72]. The implication of this observation is that vesicles release their content, presumably by fusion with the presynaptic membrane (exocytosis), are recovered as coated vesicles, taking up peroxidase by pinocytosis, move to the internal cysternae, and finally re-form as synaptic vesicles. Uptake of peroxidase into synaptic vesicles has also been observed at the lobster neuromuscular junction[73]. Loss of synaptic vesicles during stimulation and an apparent increase in nerve terminal membrane area, attributed to incorporation of vesicle membranes, has been seen in the superior cervical ganglion[74]. In nerve terminals of the posterior pituitary gland, coated vesicles appear to shed their coats to become synaptic vesicles and both types incorporate peroxidase[75,76].

There is little doubt, then, that the quanta described by Katz and his colleagues[12,13] are represented morphologically by synaptic vesicles. It is still not clear, however, whether or not the number of vesicles is related in any way to the quantal parameter n, the number of quanta available for release. The low values obtained for n in some preparations has already been noted. At the crayfish neuromuscular junction, for example[18,20,24], values of <10 are obtained at a single terminal branch. Furthermore, the parameter appears to be stationary at frequencies up to 20 Hz[20]; i.e. large quantal releases are not followed by small ones and therefore do not appear to deplete the population. The population represented by n, then, appears to be refilled or reactivated rapidly. On the other hand, as noted above, the vesicle population at vertebrate neuromuscular junctions can be depleted by low frequency stimulation. This apparent disparity in behaviour between vesicles and quanta may be attributable to species differences in recovery from depletion. On the other hand, it may be that although the quanta are represented by vesicles the parameter n does not represent the number available for release, but rather the number of release sites on the terminal membrane. The release probability, p, would then represent the average probability of a site interacting with a vesicle and would be dependent on, among other factors, the number and distribution of vesicles in the terminal. This idea is testable if vesicle depletion can be demonstrated at any synapse where binomial statistics are clearly applicable. Such depletion should result in an apparent reduction in p, with little or no change in n.

2.6 POST-SYNAPTIC ACTION OF TRANSMITTERS

2.6.1 Excitatory conductance changes

The post-synaptic conductance changes associated with both excitatory and inhibitory transmission have been discussed in detail by Ginsborg[77]. More recent work on excitatory transmission has been concerned with the dependence on membrane potential of the time course of the post-synaptic conductance changes at the vertebrate neuromuscular junction. Conductance changes are usually measured by 'clamping' the membrane at a fixed potential and measuring the end-plate current (e.p.c.) produced by a single stimulus to the presynaptic nerve. When the membrane is clamped at the Na^+ equilibrium potential there is, of course, no movement of Na^+ in the ionic channels and all the current is due to outward movement of K^+. At the K^+ equilibrium potential, on the other hand, all the current is due to inward movement of Na^+. At some intermediate point (the reversal potential) the inward and outward currents cancel and the net current flow is zero. The reversal potential, in normal conditions, is usually *ca.* −15 mV. At E_{Na}, the half-time decay of the e.p.c. is *ca.* 0.5 ms. This is increased to slightly more than 1.0 ms at the normal resting potential and continues to increase with further hyperpolarisation. This dependence of time course on membrane potential is further exaggerated in the presence of procaine and its analogues, which greatly prolong the e.p.c. at the normal resting potential but have only a slight effect on time course when the membrane is near E_{Na}. These kinds of observations have led to the suggestion that Na^+ and K^+ are carried in separate ionic channels with different characteristic time courses[78,79]. Additional observations on the effects of procaine[80,81] were interpreted as supporting this view and the view that procaine has a selective action on the Na^+ channel. On the other hand, a kinetic model for the effects of xylocaine on ACh receptors has been proposed which does not require separate channels[82,83]. It was pointed out by Kordas[84,85] that the two-channel model implies that near the reversal potential the e.p.c. should be diphasic, a brief phase of outward K^+ current being followed by a more prolonged phase of inward Na^+ current. This type of response was not observed, either in untreated preparations or preparations treated with procaine, where the effect should be more marked. Subsequent experiments by Maeno *et al.*[81] showed diphasic responses in some cases, although perhaps not of the magnitude expected. In any case, the two-channel model fails to account for the continued prolongation of the e.p.c. as the membrane is hyperpolarised beyond the resting potential. This observation leads instead to the hypothesis that the variations in time-course with membrane potential are due to the conductance channels being voltage-dependent. This idea does not, of course, exclude the possibility of separate channels, but separate channels are no longer required.

Magleby and Stevens[86,87] and Kordas[88,89] have shown that the decay of the later portion of the e.p.c. is exponential at all levels of polarisation and Magleby and Stevens have noted, in addition, that the rate constant for the decay process (*a*) is related to the membrane potential (*V*) simply by the expression

$$a = Be^{AV}$$

where A and B are constants. They propose a model in which the binding of ACh to its receptor induces a conformational change responsible for opening end-plate channels. By analogy with the first steps of enzymic catalysis, the binding step is assumed to be rapid and the conformational change rate-limiting. It is postulated that the conformational change is associated with a change in dipole moment of the ACh-receptor complex and hence voltage dependent. The model implies that the decay of the e.p.c. should be largely independent of the dissociation rate constant for the ACh-receptor complex, the rate of diffusion of ACh out of the synaptic cleft and the rate of hydrolysis of ACh by cholinesterase. The anticholinesterase prostigmine, however, prolongs the e.p.c. slightly without affecting voltage dependence; i.e. B is decreased and A unchanged. The authors attribute this effect to an interaction between the drug and the receptor molecules, a conclusion reached previously by Kuba and Tomita[90]. A less detailed model proposed by Kordas[88,89] attributes the rate-limiting step for the decay of the e.p.c. to the dissociation of the ACh receptor complex, with the dissociation rate constant being voltage-dependent. Further experiments are necessary to decide between these possibilities.

2.6.2 Inhibitory conductance changes

At inhibitory synapses of the crayfish neuromuscular junction, where inhibition is normally associated with an increase in g_{Cl}, the relative permeability of the inhibitory conductance channels to other ions has been found to be dependent on the concentration of the transmitter (GABA). Takeuchi and Takeuchi[91] found that at low levels of activation by GABA conductances to NO_3^- and I^- were greater than conductance to Cl^-. When GABA concentrations were increased the conductances to NO_3^- and I^- were lower than to Cl^-. Thus the inhibitory membrane has the remarkable property of varying its anion selectivity with concentration of transmitter. The authors suggest that combination of GABA with the receptors alters the field strength in the membrane and hence its ion-exchange properties.

2.6.3 Conductance decreases

If we refer again to Figure 2.1, it can be seen that the resting potential of the nerve cell membrane is determined by the relative conductances of the membrane to Na^+, K^+ and Cl^-. Given a finite value for g_{Na}, excitation could, in theory be produced by a *decrease* in conductance to K^+. Such excitation has been observed in cells of the sympathetic ganglion of the frog[92]. In this preparation the slow e.p.s.p. is accompanied by an increase in membrane resistance, increases in amplitude with depolarisation and reverses polarity at E_K. The slow e.p.s.p. in the superior cervical ganglion of the rabbit, which is accompanied by a conductance decrease[93] is presumably of similar origin, as are the depolarisations produced by application of ACh to some cortical neurones[94].

2.6.4 Mixed post-synaptic effects

Intensive study of synaptic activation in ganglia of *Aplysia* has revealed an admixture on single neurones of excitatory and inhibitory events having the remarkable property that the events are mediated frequently by the same transmitter and often by the same presynaptic cell. For example, repetitive stimulation of a single neurone can produce first excitation and then inhibition in the follower cell, both responses being mediated by ACh[95]. The excitatory post-synaptic receptor has a low threshold to ACh and becomes desensitised at high stimulation rates; the inhibitory receptor has a higher activation threshold and the inhibitory response is augmented during the stimulus train. Excitation is associated with an increase in g_{Na} and inhibition with an increase in g_{Cl}[96-98]. It is not known whether the post-synaptic receptors can be intermixed or are always associated with separate presynaptic terminal branches of the same neurone. In ganglion cells of the mollusc *Navanax* inhibitory receptors tend to be distributed near the soma and excitatory receptors more distal in the neuropil[98]. In addition to the fast inhibitory response, there is a slower inhibitory potential, also mediated by ACh, which is associated with an increase in K^+ conductance[99]. All three receptors have distinct pharmacological properties: hexamethonium blocks only the e.p.s.p., both the e.p.s.p. and the fast i.p.s.p. are blocked by tubocurarine and the slow i.p.s.p. is blocked selectively by methylxylocholine[97-99]. The same presynaptic neurone can activate all three cholinergic receptors[101]. In addition to the cholinergic receptors, there are also receptors for dopamine (which is the major catecholamine in the mollusc) which mediate both excitatory and inhibitory conductance changes[102]. Inhibition is, in this case, associated with an increase in g_K.

2.6.5 Post-synaptic 'noise'

Application of ACh to the end-plate region of vertebrate muscle has two consequences:
   (a) the end-plate membrane is depolarised;
   (b) this depolarisation is accompanied by an increase in the baseline noise superimposed on the membrane potential recording.
Katz and Miledi[103] have analysed in some detail the relation between depolarisation and increase in noise level on the assumption that the depolarisation may be considered as the summed effect of opening of individual conductance channels and the noise as statistical fluctuations in the average rate of these individual shot effects. If one supposes, for example, that activation of an individual receptor produces an instantaneous depolarisation of amplitude a which then decays exponentially with a time constant τ, it can be shown that the average steady state depolarisation during ACh application (V) is given by

$$V = na\tau,$$

where n is the mean number of elementary events per second. The square of the r.m.s. baseline noise ($\overline{E^2}$) is given by

$$\overline{E^2} = na^2\tau/2$$

It follows that the amplitude of the elementary shot effect is given by

$$a = 2\overline{E^2}/V$$

The factor 2 in this expression depends on the assumption about the shape of the unit shot potential; Katz and Miledi present a convincing argument that the factor is not likely to be >2 nor less than unity. In making experimental measurements allowance was made for the fact that the elementary conductance changes do not sum linearly. Obviously as the depolarisation approaches the reversal potential the contribution of each conductance channel to the developed potential and to the noise will become smaller and smaller. Taking this effect into account, the average value of a at the resting potential was found to be of the order of 0.4 µV. As would be expected if the elementary shot effect represented activation of a single receptor, this value was unaffected by tubocurarine. Although the results were not entirely clear with respect to prostigmine, there was some indication that this drug might affect the receptor in some way to produce a slight increase in a. This would be consistent with the previous suggestion of a direct interaction being responsible for prolongation of the e.p.c.[87]. The frequency distribution of the baseline noise was also examined and was found at 22 °C to be reasonably consistent with the assumptions about the shape of the elementary shot effect, with a value of ca. 10 ms for τ. At lower temperatures there was a loss of higher frequency components, suggesting a possible prolongation of the rising phase of the elementary potential. The frequency spectrum of the current noise recorded extracellularly suggested that the conductance gates were open for ca. 1 ms. In summary, the elementary shot effect produced by ACh appears to involve a channel having a conductance of ca. 3×10^{-11} mho. If one uses a value of 5.5×10^{-8} mho for the conductance change produced by one quantum of ACh[104], this means that one miniature e.p.p. involves the activation of ca. 2000 elementary channels. The authors point out that there is little evidence to suggest that more than one ACh molecule interacts with each receptor, and almost certainly not more than two are involved. This means that a miniature e.p.p. is produced by not more than 4000 molecules of ACh and more probably ca. 2000. This is lower than most estimates of the amount of ACh contained in a quantum by a factor of at least 10.

2.6.6 Receptor labelling and density

The number and density of post-synaptic receptors at vertebrate end-plates has been estimated by binding tritium- or ^{131}I-labelled bungarotoxin to the receptors[105-108]. The binding is irreversible and specific to the end-plate region, and the amount of labelling may be used to calculate the number of receptors occupied in it is assumed that one molecule of bungarotoxin binds to each receptor. Such measurements yield a receptor density of 10^4–10^5 receptors occupied if it is assumed that one molecule of bungarotoxin binds the frog neuromuscular junction[105], may be an overestimate because of the possible presence of extrajunctional receptors[108]. If so, the total number of junctional receptors at the frog end-plate would be of the order of 10^8. If each quantum of ACh activates ca. 2000 receptors, the end-plate could accommodate ca. 50 000 quanta, or ca. 250 times as many as released during a normal e.p.p.

It is of interest to note that the receptor density appears to be identical with the density of cholinesterase sites on the membrane[106]. The receptors are, however, distinct from the cholinesterase molecules since the latter can be removed enzymatically without destroying the sensitivity of the end-plate to ACh[109]. Such removal prolongs both evoked and miniature e.p.p.s without affecting the muscle membrane time constant. Thus it would appear that the e.p.c. is prolonged by removal of cholinesterase. If one accepts the idea that hydrolysis of ACh is not a significant factor in determining the rate constant for decay of the e.p.c.[86-90], it would seem to be necessary to postulate that the end-plate conductance increase is influenced directly by cholinesterase. Prolongation of the e.p.c. by anticholinesterase might then represent some modification of this influence.

2.7 CONCLUSION

The aspects of synaptic transmission considered here have been limited largely to the immediate processes of transmitter release and activation of post-synaptic receptors. With regard to presynaptic events, the major conclusion to be made from the evidence discussed here is that the quantum hypothesis and the associated vesicle hypothesis now seem to be firmly established. One of the remaining problems is the physical significance of the quantal parameter n. It would seem preferable at the moment to assign it to a population of release sites on the presynaptic membrane, but this is a matter for experiment rather than speculation. Post-synaptically, electro-physiological observations have finally been made on the behaviour of individual ACh receptors and measurements of their distribution and density made by radioactive labelling. Further examination of the behaviour of the elementary conductance channels can be expected to provide important information about the intimate processes involved in chemical excitation.

The whole question of longer-term changes in synaptic transmission, including such phenomena as facilitation and post-tetanic potentiation of transmitter release, has not been discussed. Nor was there space to consider the questions of transmitter synthesis and storage or the most important subject of synapse formation during embryogenesis and regeneration. Hopefully the present review will provide readers new to the subject with a basis for further reading about these most fascinating subjects.

Acknowledgement

The author is greatly indebted to Ms. Carole Bucher for assistance in obtaining reference material and preparing the manuscript.

References

1. Katz, B. (1966). *Nerve, Muscle and Synapse* (New York: McGraw-Hill)
2. Hubbard, J. I., Llinàs, R. and Quastel, D. M. J. (1969). *Electrophysiological Analysis of Synaptic Transmission* (Baltimore: Williams and Wilkins)
3. Llinàs, R. and Baker, R. (1972). A chloride-dependent inhibitory post-synaptic potential in cat trochlear motoneurones. *J. Neurophysiol.*, **35**, 484
4. Russell, J. M. and Brown, A. M. (1972). Active transport of chloride by the giant neuron of the *Aplysia* abdominal ganglion. *J. Gen. Physiol.*, **60**, 499
5. Hubbard, J. I. and Kwanbunbumpen, S. (1968). Evidence for the vesicle hypothesis. *J. Physiol.* (*London*), **194**, 407

6. Atwood, H. L., Lang, F. and Morrin, W. A. (1972). Synaptic vesicles: selective depletion in crayfish excitatory and inhibitory axons. *Science*, **176**, 1353

7. Uchizono, K. (1965). Characteristics of excitatory and inhibitory synapses in the central nervous system of the cat. *Nature (London)*, **207**, 642

8. Bennet, M. V. L. (1972). A comparison of electrically and chemically mediated transmission. In *Structure and Function of Synapses* (G. D. Pappas and D. P. Purpura, editors) (New York: Raven Press)

9. Boyd, I. A. and Martin, A. R. (1956). The end-plate potential in mammalian muscle. *J. Physiol. (London)*, **132**, 74

10. Dudel, J. and Kuffler, S. W. (1961). Presynaptic inhibition at the crayfish neuro-muscular junction. *J. Physiol. (London)*, **155**, 543

11. Kuno, M. (1964). Mechanism of facilitation and depression of the excitatory synaptic potential in spinal motoneurones. *J. Physiol. (London)*, **175**, 100

12. Fatt, P. and Katz, B. (1952). Spontaneous subthreshold activity at motor nerve endings. *J. Physiol. (London)*, **117**, 109

13. delCastillo, J. and Katz, B. (1954). Quantal components of the end-plate potential. *J. Physiol. (London)*, **124**, 560

14. Martin, A. R. (1965). Quantal nature of synaptic transmission. *Physiol. Rev.*, **46**, 51

15. Ginsborg, B. L. (1970). The vesicle hypothesis for the release of acetylcholine. In *Excitatory Synaptic Mechanisms, Proceedings of the Fifth International Meeting of Neurobiologists* (P. Anderson and J. K. S. Jansen, editors) (Oslo: Universtet-sforloget.)

16. Bittner, G. D. and Harrison, J. (1970). A reconsideration of the Poisson hypothesis for transmitter release at the crayfish neuromuscular junction. *J. Physiol. (London)*, **206**, 1

17. Blackman, J. G. and Purves, R. D. (1969). Intracellular recording from ganglia of the thoracic sympathetic chain of the guinea pig. *J. Physiol. (London)*, **203**, 173

18. Johnson, E. W. and Wernig, A. (1971). The binomial nature of transmitter release at the crayfish neuromuscular junction. *J. Physiol. (London)*, **218**, 757

19. Katz, B. and Miledi, R. (1965). The effect of temperature on synaptic delay at the neuromuscular junction. *J. Physiol. (London)*, **181**, 656

20. Wernig, A. (1972). Changes in statistical parameters during facilitation at the crayfish neuromuscular junction. *J. Physiol. (London)*, **226**, 751

21. Elmqvist, D. and Quastel, D. M. J. (1965). A quantitative study of end-plate potentials in isolated human muscle. *J. Physiol. (London)*, **178**, 505

22. Christensen, B. N. and Martin, A. R. (1970). Estimates of probability of trans-mitter release at the mammalian neuromuscular junction. *J. Physiol. (London)*, **210**, 933

23. Betz, W. J. (1970). Depression of transmitter release at the neuromuscular junction of the frog. *J. Physiol. (London)*, **206**, 629

24. Wernig, A. (1972). The effects of calcium and magnesium on statistical release parameters at the crayfish neuromuscular junction. *J. Physiol. (London)*, **226**, 761

25. Kuno, M. (1964). Quantal components of excitatory synaptic potentials in spinal motoneurones. *J. Physiol. (London)*, **175**, 81

26. Kuno, M. and Weakly, J. N. (1972). Quantal components of the inhibitory synaptic potential in spinal motoneurones of the cat. *J. Physiol. (London)*, **224**, 287

27. Atwood, H. L. and Parnas, I. (1968). Synaptic transmission in crustacean muscles with dual motor innervation. *Comp. Biochem. Physiol.*, **27**, 381

28. Usherwood, P. N. R. (1972). Transmitter release from insect excitatory motor nerve terminals. *J. Physiol. (London)*, **227**, 527

29. Rotshenker, S. and Rahamimoff, R. (1970). Neuromuscular synapse: stochastic properties of spontaneous release of transmitter. *Science*, **170**, 648

30. Dennis, M. and Miledi, R. (1971). Lack of correspondance between the amplitudes of spontaneous potentials and unit potentials evoked by nerve impulses at regenerating neuromuscular junctions. *Nature New Biol.*, **232**, 126

31. Harris, A. J. and Miledi, R. (1971). The effect of type D botulinum toxin on frog neuromuscular junction. *J. Physiol. (London)*, **217**, 497

32. Liley, A. W. (1957). Spontaneous release of transmitter substance in multiquantal units. *J. Physiol. (London)*, **136**, 595

33. Menrath, R. L. E. and Blackman, J. G. (1970). Observations on the large spontaneous potentials which occur at end-plates of the rat diaphragm. *Proc. Univ. Otago Med. Sch.*, **48**, 72

34. Blackman, J. G., Ginsborg, B. L. and Ray, C. (1963). Spontaneous synaptic activity in sympathetic ganglion cells of the frog. *J. Physiol. (London)*, **167**, 389

35. Martin, A. R. and Pilar, G. (1964). Quantal components of the synaptic potential in the ciliary ganglion of the chick. *J. Physiol. (London)*, **175**, 1

36. Dodge, F. A. and Rahamimoff, R. (1967). Co-operative cation of calcium ions in transmitter release at the neuromuscular junction. *J. Physiol. (London)*, **193**, 419

37. Katz, B. and Miledi, R. (1970). Further study of the role of calcium in synaptic transmission. *J. Physiol. (London)*, **207**, 789

38. Hubbard, J. I., Jones, S. F. and Landau, E. M. (1968). On the mechanism by which calcium and magnesium affect the release of transmitter by nerve impulses. *J. Physiol. (London)*, **196**, 75

39. Bracho, H. and Orkand, R. K. (1970). Effect of calcium on excitatory neuromuscular transmission in the crayfish. *J. Physiol. (London)*, **206**, 61

40. Ortiz, C. L. and Bracho, H. (1972). Effect of reduced calcium on excitatory transmitter release at the crayfish neuromuscular junction. *Comp. Biochem. Physiol.*, **41**, 805

41. Katz, B. and Miledi, R. (1969). Tetrodotoxin-resistant electric activity in presynaptic terminals. *J. Physiol. (London)*, **203**, 459

42. Katz, B. and Miledi, R. (1971). The effect of prolonged depolarisation on synaptic transfer in the stellate ganglion in the squid. *J. Physiol. (London)*, **216**, 503

43. Baker, P. F., Hodgkin, A. L. and Ridgway, E. B. (1971). Depolarization and calcium entry in squid giant axons. *J. Physiol. (London)*, **218**, 709

44. Llinàs, R., Blinks, J. R. and Nicholson, C. (1972). Calcium transient in presynaptic terminals in squid giant synapse: detection with aequorin. *Science*, **176**, 1127

45. Blaustein, M. P. (1971). Preganglionic stimulation increases calcium uptake by sympathetic ganglia. *Science*, **172**, 391

46. Hubbard, J. I., Jones, S. F. and Landau, E. M. (1968). On the mechanism by which calcium and magnesium affect the spontaneous release of transmitter from mammalian motor nerve terminals. *J. Physiol. (London)*, **194**, 355

47. Miledi, R. and Thies, R. (1971). Tetanic and post-tetanic rise in frequency of miniature end-plate potentials in low calcium solutions. *J. Physiol. (London)*, **212**, 245

48. Gage, P. W. and Quastel, D. M. J. (1966). Competition between sodium and calcium ions in transmitter release at a mammalian neuromuscular junction. *J. Physiol. (London)*, **185**, 95

49. Hubbard, J. I., Jones, S. F. and Landau, E. M. (1968). An examination of the effects of osmotic pressure changes upon transmitter release mammalian motor nerve terminals. *J. Physiol. (London)*, **197**, 639

50. Quastel, D. M. J., Hackett, J. T. and Cooke, J. D. (1971). Calcium: is it required for transmitter secretion? *Science*, **172**, 1034

51. Jenkinson, D. H. (1957). The nature of antagonism between calcium and magnesium ions at the neuromuscular junction. *J. Physiol. (London)*, **138**, 434

52. Katz, B. and Miledi, R. (1969). The effect of divalent cations on transmission in the squid giant synapse. *Pubbl. Staz. Zool. Napoli*, **37**, 303

53. Meiri, U. and Rahamimoff, R. (1972). Neuromuscular transmission: inhibition by manganese ions. *Science*, **176**, 308

54. Kajimoto, M. and Kirpekar, S. M. (1972). Effect of manganese and lanthanum on spontaneous release of ACh at frog motor nerve terminals. *Nature New Biol.*, **235**, 29

55. Miledi, R. (1971). Lanthanum ions abolish the calcium response of nerve terminals. *Nature (London)*, **229**, 410

56. Heuser, J. and Miledi, R. (1971). Effect of lanthanum ions on function and structure of frog neuromuscular junctions. *Proc. R. Soc. (London)*, **B179**, 247

57. Dodge, F. A., Miledi, R. and Rahamimoff, R. (1969). Strontium and quanta release of transmitter at the neuromuscular junction. *J. Physiol. (London)*, **200**, 267

58. Meiri, U. and Rahamimoff, R. (1971). Activation of transmitter release by strontium and calcium ions at the neuromuscular junction. *J. Physiol. (London)*, **215**, 709

59. Blioch, Z. L., Glagoleva, I. M., Liberman, E. A. and Nenashev, V. A. (1968). A study of the mechanism of quantal transmitter release at a chemical synapse. *J. Physiol. (London)*, **199**, 11

60. Bloedel, J., Gage, P. W., Llinàs, R. and Quastel, D. M. J. (1966). Transmitter release at the squid giant synapse in the presence of tetrodotoxin. *Nature (London)*, **212**, 49

61. Katz, B. and Miledi, R. (1967). Tetrodotoxin and neuromuscular transmission. *Proc. Roy. Soc. (London)*, **B167**, 8

62. Katz, B. and Miledi, R. (1967). The release of acetylcholine from nerve endings by graded electric pulses. *Proc. Roy. Soc. (London)*, **B167**, 23

63. Katz, B. and Miledi, R. (1967). A study of synaptic transmission in the absence of nerve impulses. *J. Physiol. (London)*, **192**, 407

64. Kusano, K. (1968). Further study of the relationship between pre- and post-synaptic potentials in the squid giant synapse. *J. Gen. Physiol.*, **52**, 326

65. Whittaker, V. P. (1965). The application of subcellular fractionalism techniques to the study of brain function. *Prog. Biophys. Molec. Biol.*, **15**, 39

66. Israël, M., Gautron, J. and Lesbats, B. (1968). Isolement des vésicles synaptiques de l'organe électrique de la torpille et localization de l'acétylcholine à leur niveau. *C.R. Acad. Sci. Paris*, **266**, 273

67. Bisby, M. A. and Fillenz, M. (1971). The storage of endogenous noradrenaline in sympathetic nerve terminals. *J. Physiol. (London)*, **215**, 163

68. Potter, L. T. (1970). Synthesis, storage and release of [^{14}C]acetylcholine in isolated rat diaphragm muscles. *J. Physiol. (London)*, **206**, 145

69. Hubbard, J. I. (1970). Mechanism of transmitter release. *Progr. Biophys. Molec. Biol.*, **21**, 33

70. Clark, A. W., Hurlbut, W. P. and Mauro, A. (1972). Changes in the fine structure of the neuromuscular junction of the frog caused by Black Widow spider venom. *J. Cell Biol.*, **52**, 1

71. Ceccarelli, B., Hurlbut, W. P. and Mauro, A. (1972). Depletion of vesicles from neuromuscular junction by prolonged tetanic stimulation. *J. Cell Biol.*, **54**, 30

72. Heuser, J. E. (1971). Evidence for the recycling of synaptic vesicle membrane during transmitter release at the frog neuromuscular junction. *J. Cell. Biol.*, **57**, 315

73. Holtzmann, E., Freeman, A. R. and Kashner, L. A. (1971). Stimulation-dependent alteration in pyroxidaze uptake at lobster neuromuscular junctions. *Science*, **173**, 733

74. Pysh, J. J. and Wiley, R. G. (1972). Morphologic alterations of synapses at electrically stimulated superior cervical ganglia of the cat. *Science*, **176**, 191

75. Douglas, W. W., Nagasawa, J. and Schultz, R. A. (1971). Coated microvesicles in neurosecretory terminals of posterior pituitary glands shed their coats to become smooth 'synaptic' vesicles. *Nature (London)*, **232**, 340

76. Nagasawa, J., Douglas, W. W. and Schultz, R. A. (1971). Micropinocytotic origin of coated and smooth microvesicles ('synaptic vesicles') in neurosecretory terminals of posterior pituitary glands demonstrated by incorporation of horse radish peroxidase. *Nature (London)*, **232**, 341

77. Ginsborg, B. L. (1967). Ion movements in junctional transmission. *Pharmacol. Rev.*, **19**, 289

78. Maeno, T. (1966). Analysis of sodium and potassium conductances in the procaine end-plate potential. *J. Physiol. (London)*, **183**, 592

79. Gage, P. W. and Armstrong, C. M. (1968). Miniature end-plate currents in voltage clamped muscle fibres. *Nature (London)*, **218**, 363

80. Deguchi, T. and Narahashi, T. (1971). Effects of procaine on ionic conductances of end-plate membranes. *J. Pharmacol. Exp. Ther.*, **176**, 423

81. Maeno, T., Edwards, C. and Hashamura, S. (1971). Difference in effects on end-plate potentials between procaine and lidocaine as revealed by voltage clamp experiments. *J. Neurophysiol.*, **34**, 32

82. Steinbach, A. B. (1968). Alteration by xylocaine (lidocaine) and its derivatives of the time course of the end plate potential. *J. Gen. Physiol.*, **52**, 144

83. Steinbach, A. B. (1968). A kinetic model for the action of xylocaine on receptors for acetylcholine. *J. Gen. Physiol.*, **52**, 162

84. Kordaš, S. (1969). The effect of membrane polarization on the time course of end-plate current in frog sartorius muscle. *J. Physiol. (London)*, **204**, 493

85. Kordaš, M. (1970). Effect of procaine on neuromuscular transmission. *J. Physiol.* (*London*), **209**, 689
86. Magleby, K. L. and Stevens, C. F. (1972). The effect of voltage on the time course of end-plate currents. *J. Physiol.* (*London*), **223**, 151
87. Magleby, K. L. and Stevens, C. F. (1972). A quantitative description of end-plate currents. *J. Physiol.* (*London*), **223**, 173
88. Kordaš, M. (1972). An attempt at an analysis of the factors determining time course of the end-plate current. I. The effects of prostigmine and of the ratio of magnesium to calcium. *J. Physiol.* (*London*), **224**, 317
89. Kordaš, M. (1972). An attempt at an analysis of the factors determining the time course of the end-plate current. II. Temperature. *J. Physiol.* (*London*), **224**, 333
90. Kuba, K. and Tomita, T. (1971). Effect of prostigmine on the time course of the end-plate potential in the rat diaphragm. *J. Physiol.* (*London*), **213**, 533
91. Takeuchi, A. and Takeuchi, N. (1971). Variations in the permeability properties of the inhibitory post-synaptic membrane of the crayfish neuromuscular junction when activated by different concentrations of GABA. *J. Physiol.* (*London*), **217**, 341
92. Weight, F. F. and Votaba, J. (1970). Slow synaptic excitation in sympathetic ganglion cells: Evidence for synaptic inactivation of potassium conductance. *Science*, **170**, 755
93. Kobayashi, H. and Libet, B. (1970). Actions of noradrenaline and acetylcholine on sympathetic ganglion cells. *J. Physiol.* (*London*), **208**, 353
94. Krnjevic, K., Pumain, R. and Renaud, L. (1971). The mechanism of excitation by acetylcholine in the cerebral cortex. *J. Physiol.* (*London*), **215**, 247
95. Wachtel, H. and Kandel, E. R. (1971). Conversion of synaptic excitation to inhibition at a dual chemical synapse. *J. Neurophysiol.*, **34**, 56
96. Blankenship, J. E., Wachtel, H. and Kandel, E. R. (1971). Ionic mechanisms of excitatory, inhibitory and dual synaptic actions mediated by an identified interneuron in abdominal ganglion of *Aplysia*. *J. Neurophysiol.*, **34**, 76
97. Gardener, D. and Kandel, E. R. (1972). Diphasic post-synaptic potential: A chemical synapse capable of mediating conjoint excitation and inhibition. *Science*, **176**, 675
98. Levitan, H. and Tauc, L. (1972). Acetylcholine receptors: topographic distribution and pharmacological properties of two receptor types on a single molluscan neuron. *J. Physiol.* (*London*), **222**, 537
99. Kehoe, J. (1972). Ionic mechanisms of a two-component cholinergic inhibition in *Aplysia* neurones. *J. Physiol.* (*London*), **225**, 85
100. Kehoe, J. (1972). Three acetylcholine receptors in *Aplysia* neurones. *J. Physiol.* (*London*), **225**, 115
101. Kehoe, J. (1972). The physiological role of three acetylcholine receptors in synaptic transmission in *Aplysia*. *J. Physiol.* (*London*), **225**, 147
102. Ascher, P. (1972). Inhibitory and excitatory effects of dopamine on *Aplysia* neurones. *J. Physiol.* (*London*), **225**, 173
103. Katz, B. and Miledi, R. (1972). The statistical nature of the acetylcholine potential and its molecular components. *J. Physiol.* (*London*), **224**, 665
104. Gage, P. W. and McBurney, R. (1972). Miniature end-plate currents and potentials generated by quanta of acetylcholine in glycerol-treated toad sartorius fibres. *J. Physiol.* (*London*), **226**, 79
105. Miledi, R. and Potter, L. T. (1971). Acetylcholine receptors in muscle fibres. *Nature* (*London*), **233**, 599
106. Barnard, E. A., Weickowski, J. and Chiu, T. H. (1971). Cholinergic receptor molecules and cholinesterase molecules at mouse skeletal muscle junctions. (*Nature* (*London*), **234**, 207
107. Fambrough, B. M. and Hartzell, C. H. (1972). Acetylcholine receptors: number and distribution at neuromuscular junctions in rat diaphragm. *Science*, **176**, 189
108. Porter, C. W., Chiu, T. H., Weickowski, J. and Barnard, E. A. (1973). Types and locations of cholinergic receptor-like molecules in muscle fibres. *Nature New Biol.*, **241**, 3

109. Hall, Z. W. and Kelly, R. B. (1971). Enzymatic detachment of end-plate acetyl-cholinesterase from muscle. *Nature New Biol.*, **232**, 62

110. Takeuchi, A. and Takeuchi, N. (1966). On the permeability of the presynaptic terminal of the crayfish neuromuscular junction during synaptic inhibition and the action of 8-aminobutyric acid. *J. Physiol.* (*London*), **183**, 433

3
Vestibular System

W. PRECHT
Max Planck Institute for Brain Research, Frankfurt

3.1   INTRODUCTION   82

3.2   VESTIBULAR RECEPTORS AND PRIMARY NEURONES   82
     3.2.1   *Morphology*   82
     3.2.2   *Physiology*   86
         3.2.2.1   *Receptors*   86
         3.2.2.2   *Canal afferents*   88
         3.2.2.3   *Otolith afferents*   92

3.3   EFFERENT INNERVATION OF VESTIBULAR RECEPTORS   93
     3.3.1   *Morphology of efferent system*   94
     3.2.2   *Physiology and functional importance*   95

3.4   VESTIBULAR NUCLEI: FUNCTIONAL ORGANISATION OF
LABYRINTHINE INPUT   97
     3.4.1   *Field and unitary potentials evoked by stimulation of the
VIIIth nerve*   97
     3.4.2   *Responses to natural stimulation*   100
         3.4.2.1   *Response to stimulation of semicircular canals*   101
             (a)   *Resting discharge*   101
             (b)   *Qualitative aspects*   102
             (c)   *Quantitative aspects*   103
         3.4.2.2   *Stimulation of otolith organs*   107
     3.4.3   *Receptor convergence on vestibular neurones*   110
     3.4.4   *Interaction between the two labyrinths*   111
         3.4.4.1   *Field potentials*   111
         3.4.4.2   *Contralateral excitation of single neurones*   112
         3.4.4.3   *Contralateral inhibition of single neurones*   113
         3.4.4.4   *Functional aspects of crossed inhibition*   113

3.5   VESTIBULO–OCULAR RELATIONS   115
     3.5.1   *Synaptology of vestibulo–ocular reflex*   115
     3.5.2   *Natural stimulation*   118
     3.5.3   *Cerebellar influence on vestibulo–ocular reflex*   120
     3.5.4   *Vestibular nystagmus*   121

3.6   VESTIBULO-CEREBELLAR INTERACTION   124
      3.6.1   *Vestibulo–cerebellar input*   124
      3.6.2   *Cerebello–vestibular projection*   125

3.7   VESTIBULO–SPINAL INTERACTION   127
      3.7.1   *Spino–vestibular input*   128
      3.7.2   *Vestibulo–spinal projection*   129

3.8   VESTIBULAR INTERACTION WITH OTHER SYSTEMS   132
      3.8.1   *Vestibulo–reticular interaction*   132
      3.8.2   *Vestibulo–cortical projection*   133
      3.8.3   *Vestibular effects on autonomic functions*   135

NOTES ADDED IN PROOF   136

3.1 INTRODUCTION

In the past 30 years the knowledge of the vestibular system has been greatly advanced by the application of microphysiological techniques both in primary as well as in higher-order vestibular neurones. During the same time period detailed experimental anatomical studies using modern histological techniques and electron microscopy have added considerable information on the structural organisation of vestibular end organs and central systems. In the account given in this review, emphasis will be placed on these recent developments, and an attempt will be made to correlate physiological and morphological findings. Reference will be made to older studies and/or clinical work if they added significantly to the present-day understanding of the system. Previous reviews will be mentioned in the appropriate sections so that readers interested in the older work may find older references more easily.

3.2 VESTIBULAR RECEPTORS AND PRIMARY NEURONES

In this section a brief account will be given of recent advances in the morphology and physiology of the peripheral vestibular system. Previous reviews on this subject summarising much of the older work are referred to in the appropriate places. The morphology will be described first.

3.2.1 Morphology

A brief description of some recent morphological findings that are of particular interest to physiologists will be given in this section. The vestibular organ, present in all vertebrates, shows some variations of its gross anatomy which are of interest to comparative physiology[1]. In jawless cyclostome fishes (Myxine, Petromycon, Lampetra), only two ampullae are present which are joined by a single semicircular tube. Attached to it is the vestibular sac containing a single macula and the otoliths. In Lampetra both the vestibular sac and the tube show subdivisions which indicate the beginning of the three otolith organs—utriculus, sacculus and lagena—and of anterior and posterior canals. These structures and a third canal—the horizontal or external—are characteristic of true fish, amphibians, reptiles and birds. Finally, in mammals the lagena disappears leaving two otolith organs—utricle and saccula—and three semicircular canals. With the head in the normal position, most of the macula utriculi lies approximately in the horizontal plane, whereas the macula sacculi is orientated roughly in a vertical plane. This geometrical arrangement of the two otolith organs has to be kept in mind when physiological studies of the afferent or central neurones are performed with both receptor organs intact. Thus, it appears that bidirectionality of rolling of the animal about a naso-occipital axis would mainly be monitored by utricular hair cells whereas afferents from the vertical saccular receptors presumably would not detect smaller movements about this axis, and if they did, responses should be independent of the direction of the movement.

The spatial orientation of the semicircular canals is roughly known in most vertebrates but precise measurements are still missing in most cases. Recently, the planar relationship of semicircular canals have been determined in the cat[2]. Angles were calculated between the three ipsilateral canal planes, between pairs of contralateral canal planes, and those formed by stereotaxic planes and canal planes. It was shown that ipsilateral canal planes were orthogonal and that pairs of contralateral synergistically acting canals were nearly co-planar. The most widely used canal in physiological studies—the horizontal canal—forms an angle of 23 degrees with the horizontal stereotaxic plane. In general it may be stated that in most animals the horizontal canal plane is co-planar with the horizontal plane when the head is in the normal position. Even a slight spatial displacement of the canal under study with respect to the plane of rotation may cause endolymph movements in other canals.

Investigations of the biophysical dimensions of the cat labyrinth have been performed, and the data were used for calculating the constants of the fundamental differential equation of the cupula–endolymph system[3–5], and the range of cupula motion occurring during rotations[6]. The calculated values for cupula movements are so small that the original observation of the actual cupula movement in the pike[7] appears to be an artefact. In fact, preliminary observations of the cupula in the frog during motion suggest that the swinging-door model may not be correct, since the cupula is attached to the roof and wall of the ampulla and may, therefore, function rather like an elastic diaphragm[8]. These serious discrepancies between classical and new concepts require further study. The critical dependence of canal response upon its physical dimension has been theoretically treated for a large number of animals of different sizes[9]. It has been shown that changes in certain parameters account for differences in size thus allowing the larger animals to continue to measure angular velocity of head movements. Let us now turn to the structure of the sensory epithelium. Excellent summaries of the morphological features of the sensory region have recently been given[8,10,11] so that only a few major points need to be emphasised in this paper.

The finding that each sensory cell is morphologically polarised due to the relative spatial location of kinocilium and stereocilia is of great functional importance[10,12–14]. In the crista horizontalis all sensory cells have their kinocilia facing the utriculus, whereas in the cristae of the vertical canals the kinocilia are directed towards the lumen of the canal. As will be described in Section 3.2.2, bending of the hair cell tufts toward the kinocilium causes an increase and movement in the opposite direction causes a decrease of resting discharge in primary afferents. On the macula utriculi the sensory cells are polarised toward a curved dividing line running through the middle of the striola, whereas on the saccular maculae they are polarised away from it. Scanning electron micrographs of different receptor regions of the frog show very beautifully the directional orientation of ciliary tufts (Figure 3.1). Note that in the sacculus of the frog the unidirectional orientated kinocilium terminates in a large bulb (Figure 3.1c), making it distinct from the numerous stereocilia. The kinocilia in the utricular hair cells (Figure 3.1b) are about four times as long as the stereocilia. Ultrastructural studies have demonstrated that the mammalian vestibular sense organs contain two types of sensory cells[15,16]. The type I sensory cell is shaped like an amphora. Thick and some medium sized primary vestibular fibres form nerve chalices around these cells. Specific synaptic structures are observed at several places along the extensive chalix–hair cell contact indicating that chemical synaptic transmission takes place from the receptor cell to the afferent nerve terminals. Synaptic boutons of efferent vestibular fibres terminate on the nerve chalices (for details see Section 3.3). The type II sensory cell has an irregular cylindrical shape. The bottom of the cell is in synaptic contact with afferent branches (medium size) of the VIIIth nerve and boutons of efferent vestibular fibres (Figure 3.2e). It is interesting to point out that type II (Figure 3.2e) is the phylogenetically older hair cell type, and is the only cell type found in fish[17,18] and amphibia[14]. Physiological data obtained with primary neurones of mammals do not fall into two categories[19]. This may indicate that the innervation of type I and type II receptors by primary nerve fibres overlaps to some extent, so that a given sensory fibre may not necessarily represent the changes occurring in one or the other receptor group.

A closer inspection of the organisation of the ciliarly tufts (Figure 3.2) shows that the kinocilium protrudes from a notch in the cuticular plate, in contrast with the 60–70 stereocilia which emerge from the cuticle[8,13,14,16,20]. In the frog, the kinociliary bulb of otolith receptors is attached to the otolith membrane[8]. The latter is attached to supporting cells of the epithelium by filament-like structures (Figure 3.1, Figure 3.2e) which cross the submembranous base to become part of the otolith membrane. This submembranous zone is the shearing site for displacement between supporting cells and otolithic membrane. In the canal system, a row of 5–6 stereocilia accompanies the kinocilium across the subcupular space where the kinocilium enters and is embedded in the cupula. The subcupular space is crossed by filaments which anchor the cupula to the supporting cells[21]. In amphibia, there is no doubt that the kinocilia of both the sacculus and utriculus are attached to some of the surrounding stereocilia by filamentous-like structures (Figure 3.2) which bridge the intervening space between the limiting membranes of the cilia[8,14]. At present it is not certain whether similar junctional complexes exist in ciliary tufts of higher vertebrates. The possible functional consequences of the structural arrangement of the cilia will be discussed in Section 3.2.2.

The distal processes of the primary neurones in the vestibular ganglion (ganglion Scarpae) run to the sensory cells. They are myelinated nerve

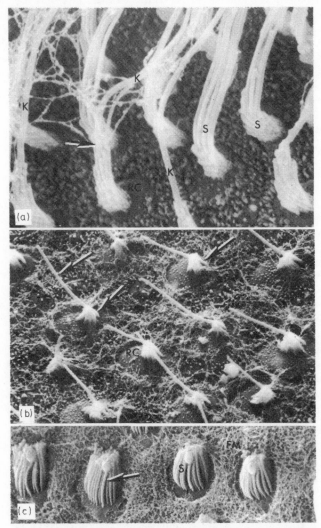

Figure 3.1 Scanning electron micrographs of the three major labyrinthine receptors of the frog. (a) from the crista horizontalis; (b) macula utriculi; and (c) macula sacculi. *Abbreviations:* FM, filamentous material; K, kinocilium; RC, receptor cell; S, stereocilia. Arrows indicate kinocilia. Note the different ratio in length of kinocilia and stereocilia in different receptors. Filamentous material which crosses the subotolithic or subcupular space is seen only over the supporting cells. For more details see text. (By courtesy of Dr. D. Hillman.)

fibres of varying diameter (1–10 μm) which lose their myelin sheath when they pass through the basement membrane into the sensory epithelium[10,11,16,22,23].

The cell bodies of vestibular ganglion cells are devoid of synapses. In mammals they have an approximate diameter of 20–30 μm[22]. Older gross morphological studies of the comparative anatomy of the innervation of the labyrinthine organs are of great value for the experimental physiologist[24]. In amphibia, for example, the main vestibular nerve subdivides into two distinct branches (anterior and posterior) which reach the labyrinthine cavity through two separate holes. Only the anterior branch is entirely vestibular in nature[24] and may be used for selective stimulation and recording.

3.2.2 Physiology

3.2.2.1 Receptors

Vestibular receptors are mechanoreceptors which are excited by shearing of the hair processes or cilia. As shown in Figure 3.2e typical synapses are formed between the hair cell and the primary vestibular neurone. This finding strongly suggests that chemical transmission takes place between receptor cells and afferent nerve terminals. Even when the vestibular apparatus is not stimulated, many afferents tend to show a tonic discharge indicating that some transmitter release occurs in the absence of stimulation. At present the nature of the transmitter substance is not known although some preliminary studies seem to indicate that catecholamines may be likely candidates[25]. As will be shown below, this tonic discharge will increase on bending the cilia in the direction towards the kinocilium, and a decrease in firing occurs on movement in the opposite direction. One may now ask: what mechanism is responsible for increasing or decreasing the amount of transmitter substance released by the sensory cells? In other words, we will have to look for a transducer processes which couples the mechanical force (shearing) to electrical changes in the receptor cell which lead to transmitter release. It is reasonable to assume that the transducer process occurs in the hair cell. In spite of the fact that the mechanism is not known, a few concepts may briefly be mentioned to stimulate further studies in this field (for a review see Ref. 26). The ciliary membrane is covered by potassium salts of acid mucopolysaccharides which are supposed to give the hair processes an electrical (static) surface charge[27–29] thus preventing the cilia from sticking together. Mechanical deformation of the cilia may cause changes in electrical (static) charge and it is assumed that the microphonic potentials that can be recorded in various parts of the inner ear in response to mechanical oscillations are caused by a capacity-governed electrical change across the membrane of the cilia. It is assumed that the microphonic potentials possibly represent a first step in the transducer mechanism, i.e. a kind of receptor potential[26]. As the result of the receptor potential occurring in the apical parts of the receptor (variable capacitor), a generator potential will be produced in the basal part of the receptor cell (variable resistor) by changes of the ionic conductances. This hypothesis implies that the ciliary and apical receptor membrane does not participate in ionic mechanisms of the generator process since these parts are surrounded by endolymph whose sodium and potassium concentration is similar to their intracellular concentration[30]. Thus, it may be assumed that a potassium battery cannot be maintained by those parts of the hair-cell membrane which are surrounded by endolymph,

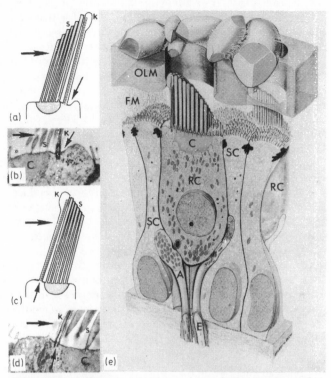

Figure 3.2 Diagrams and electron micrographs showing action of vestibular ciliary apparatus and relationship of vestibular epithelium and otolith membrane: (a, b) show plunging action of kinocilium (arrow) when the hair bundle is moved in the direction of upper arrow; (c, d) cells orientated in opposite direction show that the base of K is raised (arrow); (e) diagram of saccular receptor region constructed on the basis of observations made by scanning and transmission electron microscopy. *Abbreviations:* A, afferent fibre; C, cuticle; E, efferent fibre; FM, filamentous material; K, kinocilium; OLM, otolithic membrane; RC, receptor cell; S, stereocilia; SC, supporting cell. For further description see text. (By courtesy of Dr. D. Hillman.)

but may well be supported by the remainder of the cell which faces normal intercellular fluids (perilymph).

Another hypothesis has recently been suggested solely on the basis of morphological observations of the hair cells[13,14]. Ultrastructural studies of hair cells have shown the existence of an apical attachment of the kinocilium to about five adjacent stereocilia (Figure 3.2). Whereas the stereocilia rest on a rigid cuticular base of the hair-cell membrane, the kinocilium is located over a notch in the cuticle so that, in contrast with the stereocilia, the kinocilary base is in direct contact with the cell cytoplasm (Figure 3.2).

The fact that the kinocilium is attached to adjacent stereocilia implies that shearing motion acting on the whole hair-cell tuft causes a displacement at the kinociliary base whereas the stereocilia will exhibit a sliding action in relation to each other. This plunging-like action of the kinocilium on the surface membrane is illustrated in Figure 3.2a–d for two different positions of the ciliary ensemble: a small dimple of the plasma membrane seen at rest becomes larger as the ciliary tufts are bent towards the kinocilium (Figure 3.2a, b). On the other hand, a withdrawing motion of the kinocilium reduces the distension of the membrane and the surface membrane becomes convex (Figure 3.2c, d). It is possible that the distension of the receptor membrane produces an increase in ionic conductances of the membrane which would cause depolarisation of the hair cell. The resulting increase in transmitter release would explain the increase of activity observed in the vestibular nerve. Conversely, reduction of the distension may decrease the ionic conductance causing hyperpolarisation and decrease in activity in the VIIIth nerve. A similar deformation-sensitive membrane has been demonstrated in pacinian corpuscles in which mechanical forces produce hyper- or depolarisation depending on the direction of the acting force[31]. It should be emphasised that the above hypothesis is entirely based on morphological observations which may or may not be related to the mechanism of the transduction process.

Returning to the experimental side it appears that the d.c. potential changes recorded extracellularly in the sensory epithelium in response to natural stimulation are related to the generator potential[26]. In the horizontal ampulla, negative and positive d.c. potential shifts are generated on utriculopetal and utriculofugal cupula deviation respectively. Conversely, in the vertical ampullae negative and positive d.c. potential changes occur on utriculofugal and utriculopetal endolymph movements, respectively. The differences between horizontal and vertical canals may be explained by the different position of the kinocilium in these two systems (see earlier). Similar d.c. potential changes have been recorded from the maculae of the otolith system[26].

3.2.2.2 Canal afferents

Contrary to the small number of experimental studies performed in the vestibular receptor regions many studies have been devoted to the response characteristics of primary ventibular neurones which are much more readily accessible to physiological investigations. Much of the earlier work has been summarised in previous reviews[32,33] so that the account given in this section will deal mainly with recent studies.

The responses of primary vestibular neurones of the semicircular canals to rotation have been studied extensively in fish[32-35], frog[36, 37], cat[38] and monkey[19,39,40]. A common feature of most primary units recorded from different vertebrates is their resting discharge. In contrast to secondary neurones it is very little affected by anaesthesia[38,41]. Interestingly, the average level of resting discharge appears to be rather low in fish and frog (ca. 10 Hz) and reaches very high average values of 90 Hz in monkeys. The reason for the remarkable differences in resting discharge are not known; possibly they are related to the range of velocities of head and body movements. It is known that the resting discharge of the primary neurones is the most important excitatory input for secondary vestibular neurones and thus is the main source for the vestibular tone of related structures (see Section 3.4). Furthermore, the resting discharge provides the basis for the bidirectional response of canal fibres to rotation and assures the low threshold to natural stimulation. It has been suggested that theoretically a threshold hardly exists at all in spontaneously-active sensory afferents[42]. Indeed, precise determination of threshold acceleration is difficult, because even a slight fluctuation of the resting discharge interferes with the identification of a small response. If so, the regression lines in Figure 3.3 might not be straight in the region close

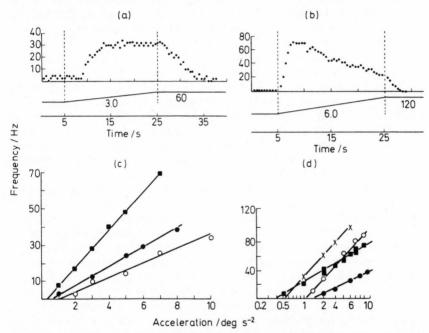

Figure 3.3 Responses of frog vestibular fibres to angular acceleration. Frequency diagrams of discharges of non-adapting (a) and adapting (b) horizontal-canal fibres. Vertical dotted lines indicate beginning and end of acceleration. The line below each frequency diagram indicates velocity of rotation. The left-hand number indicates acceleration, and the right-hand number the velocity of constant rotation (c, d) relation between angular acceleration and maximum frequency increase of afferent fibres. In each diagram, regression lines connect the points obtained from a single fibre by subtracting the resting discharge from average of maximum frequency increase. Note semilogarithmic plot in (d). (From Precht et al.[37] by courtesy of Exp. Brain Res. and Springer Heidelberg.)

to the abscissa, but could extend even to the point of 0 deg s^{-2} in an extreme case. However, with acceleration rates lower than the thresholds determined by this procedure, no significant changes in impulse frequency are observed in most of the neurones. Therefore, this method appears to be a satisfactory one at present. Measurement of threshold for frequency increase to angular acceleration of primary fibres of the frog gave values as low as 0.2 deg s^{-2}. These values are in good agreement with values obtained with secondary vestibular neurones of the cat. It may be added that threshold values for the vestibular nystagmus and perception of angular motion are generally found in a similar range (for a summary see Ref. 43), although values as low as 0.04 deg s^{-2} have been reported for vestibular induced head movements[44]. Horizontal canal neurones respond to ipsilateral acceleration (utriculopetal endolymph movement) with an increase in discharge and to contralateral accelerations (utriculofugal movement) with a decrease in firing. Following cessation of acceleration, i.e. beginning of constant velocity of rotation the discharge frequency returns to resting level. This response pattern is consistent with the polarisation of the sensory hair cells of the horizontal canals (Section 3.2.1). Deviations from this response pattern in some fibres may be attributed to recordings from efferent vestibular fibre (Section 3.3.2). Vertical canal units show opposite responses to rotation due to the different location of the kinocilium.

Following application of acceleration steps of long duration (Figure 3.3) some neurones show no adaptation at all and others are characterised by a significant frequency decline. This is true for all vertebrates studied. In the frog, for example, about two-thirds of the afferents showed adaptation[37]. Adaptation, when present, is usually more marked during the decreasing than during the increasing phase of the responses[39]. It should be pointed out that in theoretical models of vestibular adaptation both a frequency decrease during prolonged acceleration and the presence of secondary responses following velocity steps have been called adaptation[45]. This combination of responses was, in fact, found in primary[39, 46] and secondary vestibular neurones[41]. (Section 3.4.2.1.) Since the occurrence of adaptation has not been considered in the well-known torsion pendulum model (see later) various modifications of the original model have been suggested to account for its presence in the vestibular system of man[45], monkey[39] and frog[37]. At present the precise physiological mechanisms leading to peripheral vestibular adaptation are not known. Since individual primary fibres differ remarkably in their adaptive properties and adaptive behaviour has been observed when polarising currents were applied to the terminal regions, adaptation may not occur in the mechanics of the cupula but rather in the receptors and/or afferent terminals. As pointed out in Section 3.3.2, the efferent vestibular system may contribute to the observed frequency decline.

Units showing no or very little adaptation may serve to test the validity of the torsion pendulum model proposed by Steinhausen[7,47] and developed by others[46,48]. In this model, the cupula endolymph system is treated as an overcritically-damped second-order linear system, the angular displacement of the cupula $\xi(t)$ being related to the input angular acceleration $a(t)$ by the differential equation

$$\Theta\frac{\Delta^2\xi(t)}{\Delta t^2}+\Pi\frac{\Delta\xi(t)}{\Delta t}+\Delta\xi(t)=\Theta a(t) \qquad (3.1)$$

where Θ is the effective moment of inertia of the system, Π the moment of friction at unit angular velocity, and Δ the cupula restoring couple at unit angle. Two time constants determine the behaviour of this system (Π/Δ and

Θ/Π). Studies on single units in fish, frog and monkey have shown that their responses to constant angular acceleration were more or less (see later) consistent with those predicted from equation (3.1). The average time constant Π/Δ in fish[46], frog[37] and monkey primary neurones[39] are in the order of 35, 3 and 6 s, respectively. The differences in the average time constants may be related in part to the physical dimensions of the canals in these species[9]. It should be mentioned that the measurements in fish were obtained in the isolated labyrinth, i.e. in the open-loop situation, whereas closed-loop experiments yielded the data reported in frog and monkey (for time constants of central systems see Section 3.4.2.1). When brief angular accelerations are applied, the response of a given unit is a linear function of acceleration over a wide range of stimulus magnitudes[39]. As accelerations are prolonged, the responses become more and more non-linear[37,39]. Figure 3.3 shows for frog canal units that this statement may be further specified in saying that some units have a linear input–output characteristic even in response to prolonged stimuli, whereas others respond in a non-linear way to the same range of stimulus magnitudes[37]. It should be pointed out that various non-linearities, in particular the asymmetry between excitatory and inhibitory responses, have to be considered in dealing with the overall input–output characteristics of the vestibular system which usually have been described on the basis of linear system theory (for a review see Ref. 49).

The data obtained from experiments employing steps of constant angular acceleration have been complemented by studies of the responses of canal afferents of fish[46] and monkey[40] to sinusoidal stimulation. In general, these studies have demonstrated that the torsion pendulum model, although valid for the motion of cupula and endolymph, may not explain adequately all the response dynamics of the primary canal afferents[40]. Thus, one of the main conclusions made on the basis of the torsion pendulum model was that the peripheral system acts as a faithful velocity transducer since the constant angular force (head acceleration) produces a constant endolymph flow (cupula velocity). As described later, this notion must be modified if one considers the dynamic response characteristics of canal afferents. It has been shown that responses of canal afferents of the monkey[40] were similar to those expected of a linear system when tested with sinusoidal stimuli (0.006–8.0 Hz). The non-linear distortion (ca. 13%) was mainly caused by the asymmetries between the responses obtained in the excitatory and inhibitory direction. Since, for a given frequency, gains and phase lags were relatively independent of stimulus magnitudes the data could be presented as Bode plots and a linear transfer function could be constructed[40]. Two major deviations from the torsion pendulum model were observed in the canal responses. At low frequencies the phase lag with respect to acceleration is less than expected. This effect may be caused by sensory adaptation occurring in these units. At high frequencies there is a gain enhancement and the phase lag with respect to acceleration reaches a maximum and then starts to diminish. The high-frequency lead component may imply that the afferent neurones are not only sensitive to cupula displacement but also to velocity of displacement. It has been suggested that with the aid of velocity sensitivity the peripheral neurones may compensate for the dynamic loads represented by the various vestibular reflexes[40].

Studies of the kind described above are by no means exhaustive. They present, however, a solid basis for further elaboration of the characteristics of the peripheral system. Knowledge of the dynamic characteristics of the primary neurone is of paramount interest since its activity is transferred to higher centres where it is again modified by central mechanisms. Any attempt to analyse the vestibular system on the basis of observation of the final output (nystagmus, sensation of rotation, muscle tension, etc.) must consider the characteristics of primary and higher-order neurones. Unfortunately in the past many observations made in input–output studies have been explained solely on the basis of the cupula-endolymph mechanisms.

3.2.2.3   Otolith afferents

We shall now consider some of the recent advances in functional aspects of the peripheral otolith organs. The maculae of the vertebrate labyrinth appear to be functionally and structurally similar to the statocysts which are found throughout the animal kingdom. From the functional point of view all otolith receptors are best described as differential-density accelerometers which differ from the canals by the range of their frequency response. It has clearly been demonstrated that the old pressure or traction hypothesis still found in some textbooks[50] may be rejected. Instead it has been shown that the adequate stimulus for the macular hair cells is the tangential shearing force. On displacement of the head in one or the other direction the ciliary tufts become bent as a result of their attachment to the otolith membrane (Section 3.2.1). The shearing can be described by the equation $f = g \times \sin a$, where g is the gravitational force and a the tilting angle[51]. It appears that the otolith receptors serve a variety of functions. In addition to monitoring gravitational pull under static conditions, they are capable of measuring the velocity of changes in the direction of gravitational and linear translational acceleration in different spatial planes. Finally, in some vertebrates lacking the organ of Corti, they may respond to vibration[52]. The comparative physiology of the otolith system is still poorly understood, at least when it is compared with the relatively well-known canal system. Single unit recordings from the utriculus, sacculus and lagena—the otolith organs of fish—have demonstrated that some regions respond exclusively to vibrational stimuli (anterior part of sacculus, macula neglecta, lacinia utriculi) and others (otolith covered part of the macula utriculi, posterior sacculus, lagena) only to gravitational stimuli and to linear translation[52,53]. A special situation seems to have developed in the frog[36] in which the sacculus seems to be very sensitive to vibration, whereas the utricle responds to gravitational stimuli. Among the otolith responses in fish[52,53] those evoked from the utriculus and sacculus seem to be roughly synergistic, whereas the lagena responds antagonistically to both. Utricular units respond to static tilts about all horizontal axes (longitudinal, transverse and diagonal). This behaviour is to be expected on the basis of the spatial arrangement of the hair-cell groups in this organ (see earlier). The discharge frequency of the utricular fibres is minimal in the normal position of the head and reaches a maximum near 90 degrees head-up or down and side-up or down positions. With gravity sensitive saccular units different response maxima may be expected owing to their different spatial orientation. Besides the responses to static tilt, some otolith units of fish respond only during the tilt and are unable to maintain their increased discharge rate during static tilt. They have been described as out-of-position receptors and may have their receptors close to the marginal zone on the macula. Except for the out-of-position receptors similar responses have been recorded from utricular fibres of mammals[54]. Thus rolling movement about the longitudinal body axis causes a decrease in firing of most utricular units (66%) when the recording side moves upwards and an increase of the rate is noted on side-down movement. The rest of the units showed the opposite trend. Similar proportions have been described for neurones in the lateral vestibular nucleus (see Section 3.4.2.2). In the isolated labyrinth of fish the steady-state discharge characteristic for different head positions is related linearly to the angle of maintained tilt[52,53]. A somewhat more complicated situation exists in mammals*. Here many fibres show multivaluedness, i.e. the interval mean (and other statistics) from different stations at any given position covered a range greater than at each station[54]. Multivaluedness varies from fibre to fibre and was also found in secondary gravity sensitive neurones (see Section 3.4.2.2). It is suggested that multivaluedness may be due to forces which, like stiction, prevent complete relaxation of the otolith membrane under static but not under dynamic stimulus conditions. When sinusoids of low frequencies (up to 0.1 Hz) were applied, the spike trains showed a continuous mapping of the tilt angle into instantaneous frequency with little multivaluedness. However, in addition to the tonic response, phasic components were observed with a distinct unidirectional rate sensitivity that gave a phase lead of the response with respect to the input sine wave. Though the origin of this dynamic response is not known the finding suggests that utricular hair cells may have a dynamic function at least as important as their static function, which measures head position with respect to gravity. Theoretical models of the otolith system have been developed which include the phasic sensitivity of the otolith receptors[55]. In passing, it may be mentioned that the canals known to represent angular accelerometers also appear to be slightly sensitive to the position of the head in space, i.e. to gravitational accelerations[25,36]. Thus the resting discharge of canal units varies with different positions of the head in space. However, the fundamental role of the canals as accelerometers need not be affected by this finding except for a difference in base line[25]. Finally, a rather unusual experiment may be mentioned. Frogs have been launched into space with chronic electrodes implanted into the vestibular nerve[56]. Among other findings it was shown that weightlessness did not abolish the resting activity of utricular afferents.

3.3 EFFERENT INNERVATION OF VESTIBULAR RECEPTORS

It is well known that the control of sensory information can take place at different levels of a given sensory pathway. For example, higher centres may act on second-order sensory neurones directly or presynaptically on the afferent fibres in order to modulate the incoming information in accordance

* See 'Note added in Proof'.

with different functional requirements (see Refs 57–60). The present section, however, deals with another interesting aspect of centrifugal control of sensory activity, i.e. the action of fibres of central origin on receptors themselves. Since Rasmussen[61] first clearly demonstrated anatomically the efferent neurone to the auditory labyrinth, great interest has arisen in the physiology and function of such dual innervation of not only the labyrinth but other sense organs as well.

3.3.1 Morphology of efferent system

The peripheral efferent neurone to the vestibular portion of the labyrinth has been precisely described[62,63]. Efferent fibres enter the vestibular root in the brain stem. As the bundles course toward Scarpa's ganglion, the efferent vestibular fibres split off and run in the branches to each vestibular end organ. Efferent axons have a small diameter of *ca.* 2–3 μm a finding which may indicate that their cells of origin are also relatively small. The following may be stated concerning the central location of efferent neurones. The possible existence of a crossed origin for the efferent vestibular neurone[64] has now been ruled out by direct neuroanatomical evidence[63] indicating that the site of origin is entirely homolateral. In the cat a wide array of electrolytic lesions of various brain stem regions has narrowed the probable location of efferent neurones to the area occupying the caudal region of the ventral Deiters' nucleus and rostral end of the descending nucleus; the medial–lateral limits of the area would extend from the lateral aspect of the medial vestibular nucleus to the vestibular root. Unfortunately, methods utilising the phenomenon of retrograde cell changes following labyrinthectomy have so far failed to localise the cells of origin. The histochemical method localising acetylcholinesterase activity has been very useful in demonstrating efferents and their endings because of the very high content of this enzyme in efferent fibres[65]. Brain stem material studied with the same technique revealed a small area in the Deiters' nucleus which shows high Ache activity[66]. However, experimental confirmation by small selective lesion of this area is necessary before a definitive statement on these cells as the origin of the efferent vestibular component can be made. In the frog it has been demonstrated recently by physiological and anatomical methods that the ipsilateral vestibular nucleus contains cell bodies of efferent neurones[67,68]. The anatomical demonstration was based on the method of axonal iontophoresis of Procion yellow[69], a fluorescent dye which accumulates in the somata of efferent neurones following their peripheral axotomy. Furthermore, in the frog evidence has been provided that Purkinje cells located in the auricular lobe of the cerebellum send axons to the vestibular receptors[14,70]. It is clear that a proper combination of anatomical and physiological methods will eventually clarify the central location of efferent neurones in various vertebrates. The two types of nerve endings described in ultrastructural studies of the vestibular sensory epithelium[15,16] represent the two types of innervation to this organ. The vesiculated endings represent the terminals of the efferent nerve fibres while the non-vesiculated terminals are those of the afferent neurones (Figure 3.2e). It is interesting to note that afferent terminals always make direct contact with the hair cells (type I and type II), while efferent terminals reach only the type II. In the region of type I hair cells efferent terminals contact the afferent terminal rather than the receptor.

3.3.2 Physiology and functional importance

The presence of efferent fibres in the vestibular nerve of the frog[70,71], guinea-pig[72] and fish[73] was demonstrated physiologically by detaching the distal end of the nerve from the labyrinthine receptors and recording changes in single unit activity from the proximal end of the nerve in response to adequate and electrical stimulation of the contralateral intact labyrinth. It could be shown that stimulation of any of the three semicircular canals and the otoliths on the intact side, succeeded in evoking efferent spike activity on the deafferented side[71,74,75]. The strongest effects appear to arise from the horizontal canals. Evidence for an efferent feed-back to an ampulla from itself is also present[37,71,76]. Thus, it has been found that in bilateral intact frogs many efferent neurones show an increase in frequency of discharge in response to horizontal rotation in either direction (type III response) indicating that both horizontal canals converge on the efferent neurones[37]. Intracellular studies of efferent neurones located in the vestibular nuclei of the frog confirm this bilateral labyrinthine convergence[67,68,77]. Furthermore, it has been shown that when the vestibular nerve was stimulated at its peripheral branches which were detached from the receptor organs, action potentials can be recorded proximally in the same nerve with latencies as short as 3 ms[70]. In an attempt to measure the thresholds of efferent fibres to angular acceleration it was found that, in general, efferents have higher thresholds as compared to afferent fibres, although on occasion low threshold efferents were detected[37,76]. It has been a constant observation that efferent impulses are elicited by active or passive movements of the limbs, head and eyes or by gently pushing the eye in the region of Gasserion ganglion[37,71,73]. A question of paramount interest is related to the mode of action of the efferent fibres, i.e. are they excitatory or inhibitory in nature. At present no direct experimental evidence, based on intracellular recordings from receptor cells, is available. However, several investigators have studied the effect of electrical stimulation of efferent fibres on the resting activity of afferent fibres. In the cat, decrease of afferent discharge was noted following tetanic stimulation of the contralateral Deiters' nucleus[78,79] and in frogs a similar decrease was noted on caloric stimulation of the contralateral labyrinth[80]. Since no crossing efferent neurones have been described (see Section 3.3.1) this effect must be mediated by fibres crossing the midline and converging upon efferent neurones on the other side. From this it may be assumed that the efferents are inhibitory in nature. This assumption was further supported by recent studies in the frog. It was demonstrated that cerebellar Purkinje cells located in the ipsilateral auricular lobe were activated antidromically by stimulation of the ipsilateral vestibular nerve[70]. Stimulation of the auricular lobe resulted in a distinct inhibition of resting discharge of identified afferent vestibular fibres. Since it is known that Purkinje cells are inhibitory in nature[81] and that some efferent synaptic boutons undergo degeneration following cerebellar lesion[14], it may be assumed that the inhibitory effect is mediated by a monosynaptic cerebello–labyrinthine path. Interestingly, stimulation of the proximal part of the vestibular nerve had a similar inhibitory effect on afferent discharge, which suggests strongly that all efferent vestibular neurones are inhibitory in nature. Occasionally, increase of discharge of afferent fibres has been observed in response to stimulation of central structures. These findings may be explained, however, by assuming that a tonically-active inhibitory efferent neurone is subjected to convergence of inhibitory and excitatory inputs, which may result in inhibition of the inhibitory efferent neurone. Thus, the resulting disinhibition of the receptors could give rise to a relative excitation of afferent fibres. These mechanisms have to be kept in mind in further studies on the efferent system. It is known that d.c. potential shifts can be recorded extracellularly in the crista ampullaris during cupula deflection (Section 3.2.2). Attempts have been made to record d.c. potential changes in response to stimulation of the efferent system. Stimulation of the vestibular nuclei causes a positive d.c. shift which parallels the decrease of afferent discharge described above[78,79]. Of particular interest are the results obtained with caloric stimulation[79]. Warm-water irrigation of the ear causes a negative potential shift on the stimulated side and a positive d.c. shift in the opposite labyrinth, while cold-water irrigation had the opposite effects. The positive d.c. shift recorded in the contralateral labyrinth could be related to the activation of the inhibitory efferent system and its hyperpolarising action on peripheral structures, while the negative d.c. shift may be related to a disinhibitory effect mentioned earlier. As for the functional meaning of the efferent system, a few points will be discussed here. It has been shown that a feed-back loop exists from a given receptor organ in the labyrinth through the cerebellum and/or the vestibular nuclei back on the receptors. Such a negative feed-back may provide an inhibitory control mechanism which is operative in the case of strong sensory stimulation thus acting as a kind of overflow-preventing mechanism. The higher threshold for frequency increase of efferent neurones would support this view. Furthermore, frequency adaptation of primary vestibular fibres may be caused partially by the efferent system[37,82]. Efferent vestibular neurones are also activated by stimulation of the contralateral receptors. Given that the action of the efferent system is inhibitory in nature the interaction between the bilateral receptors may function to sharpen a given vestibular input by suppressing the activity on the other side. This mechanism may be of particular importance for the frog whose vestibular nuclei are lacking the commissural inhibition[77] which is found in the higher vertebrates[83].

A puzzling observation in regard to the efferent system is the fact that various extralabyrinthine sources are able to influence its activity. It appears that, in general, effective stimuli are those which tend to make the animal move the body or the eyes. In all these cases efferent activity changes *precede* movements meaning that frequency modulation is not caused by proprioceptice feed-back but rather by motor centres. Therefore, it may be assumed that during active head or body movements vestibular activity arising from the labyrinth which would cause movements opposite to the active ones is counterbalanced by the action of the efferent system as far peripheral as at the receptor level. It should be kept in mind, however, that the effect of the efferent system on the afferents is rather weak and often very difficult to detect[70,73,84] and may, therefore, by itself not be sufficient for the proper compensation of the vestibular input during active movements. Similar compensatory changes may occur in higher vestibular neurones which then would add to the direct effect on the receptors. It is clear that more experimental work is necessary for a more complete understanding of the function of the efferent vestibular system.

3.4 VESTIBULAR NUCLEI: FUNCTIONAL ORGANISATION OF LABYRINTHINE INPUT

The labyrinthine input to the vestibular nuclei (VN) is certainly of prime interest for the understanding of the functional organisation of this voluminous cellular complex in the brain stem. Sensory organs located in the labyrinth serve as receptors for linear and angular accelerations about different axes, thus providing the VN with a three-dimensionally-organised pattern of information about the position of the head and body in space. Other sensory systems such as somatosensory afferents and visual apparatus combine with the vestibular input in assuring the high fidelity of orientation in space. Part of this sensory integration is achieved by means of interaction in the VN which receive directly or indirectly information from these various sensory systems. Via their efferents the VN communicate with many other central structures and effector systems. Some of the integrative properties will be dealt with in the following sections. In the past, most investigators dealing with physiological aspects of the VN have studied the behavioural effects resulting from electrical stimulation and/or experimental lesions. More recently, however, the application of microphysiological techniques and refined morphological studies have greatly advanced our understanding of the VN. In the account given in this section, emphasis will be placed on recent studies and an attempt will be made to correlate the present physiological knowledge with the anatomical data.

3.4.1 Field and unitary potentials evoked by stimulation of the VIIIth nerve

Numerous anatomical studies have contributed to the present knowledge of the histological organisation of the VN. The VN have been subdivided into four nuclei: the lateral (Deiters), medial, superior and descending nuclei. Further subdivisions have been made on the basis of more sophisticated studies (see Ref. 85). For the physiologist, knowledge of the detailed projection of the VIIIth nerve into the VN is of great importance, since it will allow him to find the region of interest within reasonable time limits. Recent studies in the monkey[86] and cat[87] strongly support the idea of a distinctive as well as partially common distribution of primary fibres arising from different receptors. It appears that fibres innervating the cristae of the semicircular canals terminate mainly in the interstitial nucleus of the VIIIth nerve, the superior VN, oral parts of the medial and descending VN, whereas fibres coming from the otolithic organs end, for the most part, in the descending, medial, and ventral parts of the lateral nucleus and group 'Y'. As will be seen below, this pattern of distribution correlates very well with physiological data. Before entering into the description of the behaviour of vestibular neurones during natural stimulation it seems worth while to report findings that have been obtained with electrical stimulation of the VIIIth nerve. This type of stimulation has proven to be a powerful method for studying the synaptic organisation between afferents and central neurones. On the basis of such knowledge results obtained by natural stimulation can be more readily interpreted.

The field potentials recorded in the VN of the cat following VIIIth nerve stimulation will be described first. When a microelectrode is inserted into the VN, a characteristic field potential is evoked by single shock stimulation of the ipsilateral VIIIth nerve[41, 88-92]. Figure 3.4 shows the field potentials correlated with the location of the microelectrode tip. The potential consists of an initial positive–negative deflection (P) followed by a large negative wave (N_1) and a small negative potential (N_2). When the electrode tip moved through the border of the VN, the potentials decreased with fairly sharp gradients, especially at the ventral border (Figure 3.4). N_1 and N_2 potentials were evoked at similar threshold intensity. For obtaining fields restricted to the VN, the intensity of stimulation must be no more than twice the threshold intensity for the N_1 response, because with stronger stimulation, responses of complex shape were evoked in the adjacent reticular formation. When stimulating the whole VIIIth nerve the field potentials are of similar configuration in all VN, although differences in amplitudes of the various components can be seen in different recording positions. Thus, the amplitude of the P-wave is larger the more lateral the electrode is placed, due to the proximity of the primary vestibular fibres[92], and both P and N_1 potentials dominate in the ventral Deiters' nucleus[93] as one would expect from the distribution of primary fibres in this nucleus[87,94]. Attempts have been made to map the field potentials in the VN that have been evoked by stimulating individual branches of the VIIIth nerve. For example, after lateral ampullary nerve stimulation, the N_2 wave is large in the ventromedial part of the medial nucleus, whereas the N_1 potential has a larger amplitude in the ventrolateral part of this nucleus[91]. The latter part is known to receive primary afferents[94], whereas in the former primary afferent projection is scarce. As for the nature of the individual components of the field potential, the following can be said: the P-potential (latency 0.66 ± 0.14 ms) is generated by the compound action currents evoked conjointly in primary vestibular fibres and in the efferent fibres[92]. The N_1 potential (latency 1.06 ± 0.22 ms) consists of the synaptic and action currents generated, for the most part monosynaptically, by the exitatory action of vestibular fibres in secondary vestibular neurones[92]. As a peculiar feature of vestibular fibres, repetitive action potentials are triggered by single-shock stimulation. The action currents of these repetitively firing axons would also contribute to the N_1 and N_2 potentials[93]. Finally, the N_2 potential (latency 2.46 ± 0.26 ms) is composed of synaptic and action currents generated by polysynaptic activation of vestibular neurones[92]. Possible anatomical substrates for polysynaptic excitation of vestibular neurones may be either internuncial neurones in the VN or collaterals of the axons leaving the nuclei. Recording of these field potentials allows

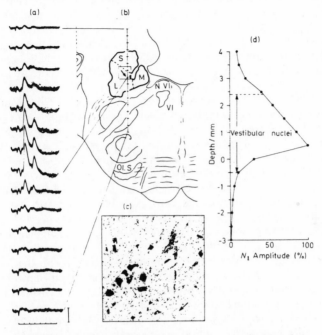

Figure 3.4 Field potentials generated by stimulation of the vestibular nerve and recorded by a microelectrode in the ipsilateral vestibular nuclei of unanaesthetised decerebrate cat: (a) potential fields evoked by single shocks of the vestibular nerve (the first downward deflection indicates stimulation artefact). Upward deflection indicates negativity of the microelectrode. Each record is composed of *ca.* 20 superimposed traces and was obtained from the site indicated by the scale in (b). Time: 1 ms; voltage calibration: 0.5 mV, (b) line drawing of histological section of the brain stem. The vertical line shows the insertion of the recording electrode. Scales on this line indicate 500 μm. Arrow indicates the site where coagulation was made with the microelectrode. S, superior nucleus; L, lateral nucleus; M, medial nucleus; D, descending nucleus; Ol.S., superior olive; N.VII, seventh cranial nerve; VI, sixth cranial motor nucleus, (c) microphotograph of the part surrounded by a square in (b). Arrow indicates the position of the tip of the electrode. (d) Diagram showing relative amplitude of N_1 potential in A, correlated with the location of the electrode. 0 mm in the depth scale corresponds to the level of the surface in the midline of the fourth ventricle. Upper and lower borders of the vestibular nuclei are indicated by the two vertical arrows. Note the sharp decrease in amplitude of N_1 as the electrode approaches the ventral border of the vestibular nuclei. (From Shimazu and Precht[41], by courtesy of *J. Neurophysiol.*, and American Physiol. Society.)

physiological identification of the VN. Furthermore, single-action potentials recorded in the VN can be properly identified as primary fibres or secondary neurones by their temporal relationship to the various components. Using threshold stimulation, one can decide whether a given second-order neurone has primarily a monosynaptic or polysynaptic connection with the periphery[92]. When the stimulus intensity is increased, most vestibular neurones show a double firing, the doublets being related in time to N_1 and N_2 potentials. Intracellular studies of vestibular neurones indicate that this double firing is caused by mono- and poly-synaptic EPSPs generated in these neurones[93,95]. It was found that unitary components of the EPSPs recorded in different vestibular neurones vary. Thus, non-Deiters' neurones have significantly larger unitary EPSPs as compared to Deiters' neurones. This would suggest that primary vestibular impulses activate some vestibular neurones more effectively than others, which means a smaller number of nerve fibres would be required in these neurones for the same synaptic efficacy[93,95]. While the peripheral vestibular system of lower vertebrates is well studied, only few experiments have dealt with the vestibular nuclei of lower forms. It has been shown in recent studies on the vestibular neurones of the frog that the dendrites of most of these neurones are excitable electrically, i.e. dendritic spikes were recorded after stimulation of the VIIIth nerve[68]. Dendritic spikes have not been observed in vestibular neurones of higher vertebrates. These spikes which are superimposed on the EPSPs may enhance the efficacy of synaptic excitation occurring at more distal parts of frog vestibular neurones which otherwise would be too small to generate full action potentials in the soma. Another distinct feature of frog vestibular neurones is the fact that electrotonic coupling between neurones or between afferents and neurones may be recorded easily[68,96]. Evidence for electrotonic coupling in the VN of higher vertebrates is scarce. Thus, so far only Deiters' neurones of the rat have been shown to have gap junction contacts[97]. Recent electrophysiological studies of this neurone strongly suggest that the giant cells of the Deiters' nucleus are coupled electrotonically[98]. Some of the early responses to VIIIth nerve stimulation recorded in the vestibular neurones of the pigeon are probably another example of electrically-mediated synaptic transmission[99]. It has been claimed that the functional meaning of electrotonic coupling mediates a synchronisation of firing of neurones[100,101] in various nuclei. It may be assumed that coupling of vestibular neurones provides a similar mechanism which may be useful for rapidly synchronising groups of neurones that are involved in various vestibular reflexes.

3.4.2 Responses to natural stimulation

It is generally accepted that angular and linear accelerations are the adequate stimuli for the semicircular canal and otolith receptors, respectively (see Section 3.2.2). Using various experimental apparatuses these stimuli can be applied in a well-controlled way and their magnitudes can be varied over a wide range so as to allow a complete input–output study. Any neuronal element along the vestibular pathway is amenable to this type of analysis. The data to be reported in this section will be based on this type of stimulation. Since various other forms of pseudo-natural stimulation are still used in physiological and clinical studies of the vestibular system, their value will be discussed briefly. *Caloric* stimulation of the labyrinth, by means of irrigation of the ear with hot or cold water causes convection in the endolymph of the semicircular canals which leads to deflection of the cupula in one or the other direction, depending on the relative temperature of the water used with respect to body temperature. As a result, the afferent discharge increases (hot irrigation) or decreases (cold irrigation), and the well-known caloric ocular nystagmus can be observed[102-107]. Proper placement of the head allows isolated stimulation of various semicircular canals. It is obvious that with this method precise input–output studies are limited and difficult to control but it may serve as a simple and convenient method for provoking vestibular unit activity and ocular movements in studies that are more interested in qualitative aspects or in diagnosis of vestibular dysfunction. Furthermore, this technique has the advantage over rotational stimulation in that it allows unilateral stimulation of a particular canal. *Galvanic* stimulation has been frequently used in physiological studies[26,106]. When cathodal or anodal d.c. currents are applied to the ear, the afferent discharge increases or decreases, respectively, and will remain more or less constant as long as the stimuli continue. No movements of the cupula will occur with this stimulation and the changes in frequency of firing are probably caused by the current acting somewhere on the junction between receptors and afferent nerve fibres. For precise studies of central vestibular neurones, this method is of little use since all receptors are stimulated simultaneously owing to current spread, thus allowing no correlation between unitary response and a particular receptor organ. It may be of some use for studies of experimental nystagmus and in experiments in which only the overall vestibular input is of interest. Finally, mechanical stimulation of the semicircular canals by means of compression and decompression deserves mention since in the past this procedure has given much information concerning the direction specific mechanisms of the cupula–endolymph system and the effects provoked thereby in related systems[7,47,108-111].

3.4.2.1 *Response to stimulation of semicircular canals*

(a) *Resting discharge*—As in the case of primary vestibular neurones (Section 3.2.2), many second-order neurones of higher vertebrates show a resting discharge in the absence of stimulation. In decerebrate, as well as in encephale insolé preparations, the activity is fairly regular and ranges from 2 to 30 Hz and only occasionally, the frequency amounts to 80–90 Hz[41,112,113]. It is important to note that under pentobarbital anaesthesia, the number of spontaneously-firing units is significantly decreased and the threshold to natural stimulation is dramatically increased[92,105]. It is only under light ether anaesthesia that the resting discharge appears to be in the range found in decerebrate animals[113]. Thus, central neurones behave in a distinctly different manner from peripheral neurones whose characteristics are not significantly changed by anaesthetics[38,39]. Extracellular recordings from single neurones in the VN performed in freely-moving animals confirm the presence of resting discharge[114]. Units recorded in the various nuclei

differ slightly in regard to their regularity of resting discharge which averages
ca. 40 impulses s^{-1}. It was also shown that the discharge frequencies of
many neurones tend to increase during arousing stimuli such as acoustic
click stimulation. While the units in the medial and descending nuclei show
high frequency bursts which are strictly associated with rapid eye movements occurring during desynchronised sleep, no change in resting discharge
is observed during spontaneous eye movements performed while awake.

While the origin of the 'spontaneous' discharge found in primary neurones
still remains a matter of conjecture as far as the physiological mechanism
is concerned, the resting discharge of central vestibular neurones is for the
most part not autochthonous in nature. It was shown that acute neurotomy
of the VIIIth nerve nearly abolishes resting discharge, suggesting that the
labyrinth is the main source for the tonic firing[83,115]. These findings confirm
the old notion of a 'vestibular tone' which was based on the observation of
loss of muscle tone following bilateral labyrinthectomy and on the presence
of tonic asymmetries resulting from unilateral removal of the labyrinths[108].
It is interesting to note that some weeks after neurotomy (Section 3.4.4.4),
units regain to some extent their resting activity, the origin of which is not
known[116].

(b) *Qualitative aspects*—As described in Section 3.2.2, the frequency of
unit discharge recorded from primary afferents of the horizontal canals
increases when the cupula is deflected in an utriculopetal direction and
spontaneous firing ceases when inertia movement of the endolymph causes
the cupula to move in an utriculofugal direction. The opposite is the case with
vertical canal units. The second- or higher-order neurones show a similar
response pattern. Thus, with the horizontal canal in the plane of rotation,
utriculopetal endolymph flow occurs on accelerated rotation towards the
side of recording and utriculofugal flow is generated when rotation is applied
to the opposite side. Correspondingly in tonically-active units firing increases
on ipsilateral and decreases on contralateral rotation. This response pattern
will be called type I[41,105,112,113].

In addition to type I neurones a less frequent type of neurone (type II)
has been found by several investigators[41,83,113,117]. It shows an increase in
firing on contralateral rotation and cessation of firing on ipsilateral angular
acceleration. Type II neurones are not found in the isolated peripheral
vestibular system[34,35] and, therefore, represent a new type of neuronal
pattern characteristic of the VN of vertebrates (frog, cat, rabbit). Their
thresholds for frequency increases during contralateral accelerations range
from 1.5 to 10 deg s^{-2} and are significantly higher than the thresholds of
type I neurones (see later). Other characteristics such as input–output
relationship, mode of increase and resting discharge are similar to type I[83].
For the most part, type II neurones receive their labyrinthine input from the
contralateral canal, a finding which explains their response pattern[83]. Their
functional role will be discussed in detail in Section 3.4.4. However, some
type II neurones can still be recorded after removal of the contralateral
labyrinth[83]. At present, it is not clear whether this response is the result of an
inhibitory interaction between central neurones of different canals[83] or
whether it is caused by concomitant stimulation of a vertical canal during
horizontal rotation. Two other types of neuronal responses have been found

in the VN. A certain group of neurones (type III) increases its firing on rotation in either direction, and other neurones decrease their discharge irrespective of the direction of rotation (type IV)[41,105,113,117,118]. The functional meaning of types III and IV is not known although some data seem to indicate that type III has a close relation to arousing stimuli[113]. As for the location of these various types of neurones, it has been shown that the majority of type I and type II neurones are found in the medial and superior VN, and type III and IV appear to be concentrated in the medial VN[41,112,113,118-120]. These findings are in good agreement with the anatomy described above[87].

Unlike the horizontal canal effects, the influences of vertical canal stimulation on vestibular neurones have not been studied in great detail[112,121--124] mainly because it is more difficult to place these canals in the plane of rotation while recording unit activity. Since the anterior canal on one side is approximately co-planar with the posterior canal on the other side, any attempt to bring one of them in the plane of a horizontally-rotating table will result in placing both of them in this plane. By recording from the side where the anterior canal is in the plane of rotation, it was found that most units increased and decreased their discharge during utriculofugal and utriculopetal endolymph flow, respectively[124]. These neurones probably represent the type I neurone of the anterior canal. Their location within the VN is similar to the horizontal canal units. They seem to have higher thresholds for frequency increase during angular acceleration, as compared to horizontal canal units, a finding which may explain the higher threshold of vertical nystagmus[125]. Also the number of neurones responding to vertical canal stimulation appears to be smaller than for the horizontal system[124]. This finding may explain the observation that eye-muscle tension developed by stimulation of the anterior canal nerve is smaller as compared to the one caused by stimulation of the horizontal canal nerve[126]. Adequate stimulation of the anterior canal reveals a group of neurones responding in an inverse manner (type II). It is very likely that these neurones receive their excitatory input from the contralateral posterior canal being also in the plane of rotation[124]. This neuronal group is similar to the type II neurones of the horizontal canals which receive input from the opposite side. Thus, the anterior canal on one side and the posterior canal on the opposite side can be considered as a pair of canals acting on central neurones in a way similar to the bilateral horizontal canals. Further evidence for this notion will be given in Section 3.4.4. Finally, neurones showing bilateral activation (type III) have also been found in the vertical canal system[124].

(c) *Quantitative aspects*—As described in Section 3.2.2, the response characteristics of primary vestibular neurones have been known for some years. Several attempts have been made to correlate sensation of rotation or ocular nystagmus directly with the activity of primary neurones[48,127]. These studies have treated the neuronal circuits intercalated between receptors and effectors as a 'black box'. We are now in the position to describe some of the characteristics of the neuronal links such as the vestibular and ocular motoneurones. Since type I vestibular neurones of the horizontal canals are the only neurones which are well studied at the present time, their responses to rotational stimulation will be described in detail.

In Figure 3.5 are plotted the serial changes of impulse frequencies of a tonic (a)/(b) and kinetic type I neurone caused by ipsilateral rotations at different magnitudes of acceleration[41]. As shown in each diagram of this figure, when the table was rotated in the ipsilateral direction with constant acceleration, the discharge frequency of both types of neurones initially

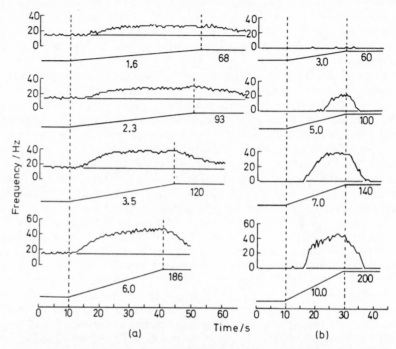

Figure 3.5 Frequency diagrams of discharges of a tonic (a) and a kinetic (b) type I vestibular neurone of decerebrate cat in response to ipsilateral horizontal constant angular accelerations. In each diagram, the ordinate represents spike per second of single unit discharges measured in each half-second. The horizontal line in each diagram represents the average frequency over 10 s before rotation. Onset of rotation is indicated by the left vertical broken line and the end of acceleration (or beginning of constant velocity rotation) by the right vertical broken line. Curve below each frequency diagram indicates velocity of rotation. The left-hand number in each diagram indicates magnitude of acceleration (deg s^{-2}) and the right-hand number indicates velocity (deg s^{-1}) of constant rotation. (From Shimazu and Precht[41], by courtesy of *J. Neurophysiol.* and American Physiol. Society.)

increased along an approximately exponential time course and then maintained a fairly constant value during the remainder of the acceleration. After the achievement of constant velocity, the frequency decreased gradually to the level of the resting discharge. This exponentional increase was confirmed in two-thirds of the responses tested. The following equation may, therefore, be applicable for the frequency response of vestibular neurones to angular acceleration[41]:

$$f = f_{max} (1 - \exp(-t/p))$$

where f = frequency increase per second; f_{max} = frequency at its maximum level; $p=$ time constant of response. Measurements of p values for a large number of tonic and kinetic neurones showed that kinetic neurones had smaller p values or steeper slopes (3.7 ± 0.8 s) than tonic neurones (8.1 ± 1.6 s). It is interesting to note that the coefficients of the equation for cupula deviation that have been calculated on the basis of data obtained from

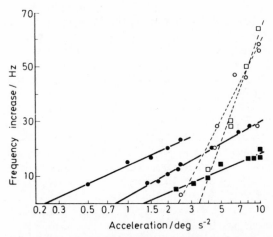

Figure 3.6 Relationship between angular acceleration and maximum frequency increase of type I vestibular neurones of the cat. Solid and broken lines indicate tonic and kinetic vestibular neurones, respectively. Each line gives the regression line of points obtained from single neurones with different magnitudes of acceleration. Note semilogarithmic plot. (From Shimazu and Precht[41], by courtesy of *J. Neurophysiol.* and American Physiol. Society.)

human sensation of rotation or nystagmus gave values very similar to the p-values obtained for tonic types I neurones[48]. The values obtained with primary vestibular neurones show a somewhat similar range (Section 3.2.2) although no separation in tonic and kinetic responses could be found indicating that this difference first occurs in the VN.

It can be seen from Figure 3.5 that the maximum frequency during acceleration is related to the magnitude of the stimulus. In Figure 3.6 the frequency increases for several neurones are plotted against the logarithm of acceleration. Each series of points appears to be distributed along a straight line[41]. In comparing these data with the theoretically-deduced equation for cupula deviation produced by constant angular acceleration[48], it may be stated that the maximal frequency increase of vestibular neurones during long-lasting constant acceleration is proportional to the logarithm of the maximal angular deviation of the cupula[41]. The linear stimulus–response relationship described in primary vestibular neurones[39] on the basis of acceleration step stimuli is not necessarily contradictory to the above non-linear relationship of central vestibular neurones. In the former case only brief stimuli have been applied and it was noted that with prolonged acceleration steps the response became progressively non-linear. Since prolonged accelerations rarely occur in normal life, the stimulus–response characteristics of peripheral and central neurones may be considered approximately linear for all practical purposes.

It can be seen in Figure 3.6 that the gradients of the regression lines are significantly steeper for kinetic as compared to the tonic type I neurones. Furthermore, this diagram shows that the thresholds of tonic neurones $(0.65\pm0.25$ deg s$^{-2})$ are lower than the ones for kinetic units $(4.65\pm1.84$ deg s$^{-2})$ (for further considerations on the problem of vestibular threshold see Section 3.2.2).

One may now ask: what is the functional meaning of tonic and kinetic neurones? The latter are characterised by lack of resting discharge, high threshold for frequency increase, rapid time course of frequency change and a steep gradient of the acceleration–frequency relationship, the former showing the opposite of these characteristics. It may be that the precise response of the vestibular system to head movement in space is secured with the help of a double safety mechanism. The threshold of tonic neurones assures the sensitivity of the response, and their resting activity provides the vestibular tone of related motor systems. The high-threshold kinetic neurones respond with high-frequency discharges and rapid changes in impulse frequency at higher stimulus intensities and may be a second factor essential for the high fidelity of the vestibular system. These characteristics may complement those of tonic neurones such as slow responsiveness and frequency saturation at higher accelerations. Interestingly, it has been found that the threshold of sensation of continued rotation after sudden stopping of the turntable is lower than that of afternystagmus, and with high stopping velocities duration of afternystagmus is larger than that of aftersensation[128]. The afternystagmus cupulogram, therefore, has a steeper slope than the aftersensation cupulogram and they are crossed with each other similarly to the crossing of acceleration–frequency curves of tonic and kinetic neurones (Figure 3.6). This may imply that the oculomotor system receives a strong influence from kinetic neurones in addition to the input from tonic units. Supportive evidence for this notion has been obtained by recording from ocular motoneurones under similar experimental conditions[129].

Recently, attempts have been made to study the characteristics of central vestibular neurones in response to sinusoidal stimulation. In central neurones the firing frequency was approximately in phase with the angular velocity of rotational stimulation[5,130]. This finding held for both tonic and silent neurones as well as for type I and type II units. As properly pointed out by the authors, the frequency range (0.25–1.7 Hz) used in these studies is rather narrow and no attempts have been made so far to study the full frequency response of the system. For this limited frequency range, however, it appears that the phase of the neuronal message established in the peripheral vestibular system has been transmitted to the second-order neurones with reasonable fidelity. It was also found that the mean gain of unit responses was 0.76 ± 0.08 action potentials s^{-1} per deg s^{-1} and that the gain varied as the (-0.28) power of stimulus angular velocity[130]. Surprisingly, this method did not reveal any differences in mean gain or phase between tonic and kinetic type I neurones suggesting that the cells studied belong to a homogeneous cell group. This discrepancy cannot be resolved at the present time since tonic and kinetic neurones identified with the procedures mentioned above have not been systematically analysed by sinusoidal stimulation. There is no question about the fact that these two distinct types exist and that their functional role has to be considered in any attempt to characterise the central vestibular system.

Frequency decrease of sensory impulses, following a transient maximal response during application of a long-lasting constant stimulation, may be called adaptation. Using a prolonged-period constant angular acceleration, most of the type I and type II vestibular neurones show no significant frequency adaptation as may be seen from Figure 3.5. In lower vertebrates, such as the frog, frequency adaptation is more frequently encountered in central[117] as well as in peripheral vestibular neurones[37]. It should be mentioned, however, that in cat vestibular neurones slight decreases in frequency are observed occasionally[41]. Only in these neurones was a clear undershoot of discharge frequency (secondary response) noted following a velocity step and in some of the neurones the firing returned from this undershoot and still increased beyond the basic rate. Similar results have been reported for primary neurones (Section 3.2.2). In vestibular adaptation models the secondary responses found with nystagmus and subjective sensation are considered evidence for adaptation[45]. Even if there is a slight tendency for adaptation in some vestibular neurones, it may not be sufficiently significant to explain the considerable 'adaptation' observed in human subjects under the condition of sustained cupula deflection[131]. The above data would suggest that this phenomenon is for the most part not produced by inherent mechanisms in the end organs and VN but rather may involve more complicated nervous activities such as habituation[132].

Finally, a few comments will be made on the functional connection of type I neurones. Using single near-threshold electrical pulse stimulation, it has been shown that most of the kinetic type I neurones were excited by VIIIth nerve stimulation with latencies in the monosynaptic range, i.e. the spikes were superimposed on the N_1 peak of the field potential[92]. On the other hand, most of the tonic type I neurones responded to the same stimulation with long and fluctuating latencies suggesting a polysynaptic linkage. With stronger stimulation both kinetic and about half of the tonic neurones showed mono- and poly-synaptic activation. As for the pathway involved in polysynaptic activation interneurones in the VN or axon collaterals of axons leaving the VN may be responsible. Given that several regions of the VN receive no vestibular fibres[86, 87, 133], it is not surprising that some vestibular neurones lack monosynaptic activation.

3.4.2.2 *Stimulation of otolith organs*

Whereas the peripheral neurones of the otolith system have been investigated in the past (see Section 3.2.2), it was only recently that similar investigations have been performed on second-order neurones. The most frequent type of unit response found in the VN shows an increase in firing on tilting of the head towards the side of the recording position and a decrease on tilt in the opposite direction provided that there is resting discharge. Linear acceleration in the horizontal plane away from the recording side also excited these neurones. In some cases, the same neurones were influenced by both lateral and fore and aft tilt[112,121,134]. The majority of neurones, however, are sensitive to displacement about only one of the axes, thus showing 'orthogonality' which seems to enable the nervous system to analyse head positions into different perpendicular components[135]. Investigations in fish[136] and higher vertebrates[121,134,135,137,138] demonstrated the existence of a less common type of neurone that behaved opposite to the one described above and others which increased or decreased firing on tilting in either direction. The latter responses were mainly found in neurones which showed polysynaptic activation following stimulation of the VIIIth nerve.

In dealing with the time course of the responses of central neurones to tilt, it is essential to realise that the type of preparation used is of critical importance. Thus, it has been shown that in non-anaesthetised cats with intact cerebellum, vestibular stimulation resulted in a perfect dynamic response in the majority of Deiters' neurones[139] while in the decerebellated cat a static response with a small dynamic component could be observed[138,140]. In anaesthetised cats many vestibular neurones show a phasic–tonic pattern characterised by an initial increase, followed by a tonic or steady level of discharge which is different from that found in the horizontal plane and is stationary or non-adapting as long as the animal is held at a particular position[112,135]. Some neurones, however, also show a predominantly phasic character. It appears, therefore, that anaesthesia has an effect similar to cerebellectomy on central vestibular neurones that respond to tilt. The fact that in the intact animal Deiters' neurones show mainly dynamic characteristics should not lead to the conclusion that all gravity-sensitive neurones in the VN behave the same way. One has to postulate a good number of neurones with static response characteristics to account for tonic vestibular reflexes. It could well be that these neurones are independent of cerebellar control. The interspike interval histograms of gravity sensitive. Deiters' neurones at zero level allow a classification of the neurones into asymmetric, symmetric and multimodal types[135]. When the head of the cat is tilted laterally into different positions, the histograms are usually shifted along the interval axis, leaving their general shape unchanged. Figure 3.7 displays examples of vestibular neurones whose stationary mean interval has been measured at different angles, showing that one particular position occurred more than once during the test. Connecting the points in the order in which they were reached during the experiments resulted in three different forms (Figure 3.7). It is concluded that 'multivaluedness', i.e. several values of mean intervals correspond to each position, is a characteristic feature of gravity-sensitive second-order neurones. Multivaluedness implies that on the basis of just one statistic of a particular cell only a probabilistic statement about angular displacement of the head can be made. It is probably the combination of several statistics in a large number of cells which eventually will provide the means to determine more exactly the position in space. The shearing force acting on the hair cells of the maculae has been shown to represent a sinusoidal function of the angular displacement of the head[51]. A similar relation has been found psychophysically by comparing the actual angular displacement of the head with the perception of position in space[141].

Many primary and secondary neurones of fish[53,136] show a similar sinusoidal function when subjected to different lateral displacements.

The distribution of neurones responding to otolithic stimulation fits approximately with the distribution of fibres from the otolith organs in the VN, i.e. they are mainly found in the Deiters' nucleus, the descending nucleus and the more caudal parts of the medial nucleus[135, 137, 138]. As for the Deiters'

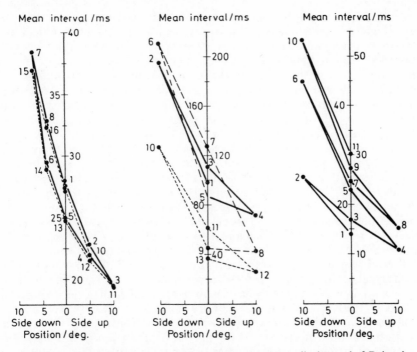

Figure 3.7 Forms of the relationship between mean interspike interval of Deiters' neurones and position of the head. Each point in the three diagrams derived from three different cells corresponds to a different station of angular displacement of the head whose order in the cycle is indicated by a number. For a given station the abscissa of the point is the position of the head with respect to gravity measured in degrees (recording side down or recording side up) by the angle between the basal stereotaxic reference plane and the horizontal. The ordinates are the mean interval in ms calculated over the stationary part of the spike train. The three curves represent recordings from three single cells responding in three different ways to the same kind of stimulation procedure. Their mode of response has been designated as (from the left to the right): 'stable loop', 'loop and creep' and 'creep'. For further details, see text. (From Fujita et al.[135], by courtesy of *J. Physiol.* (*London*) and Cambridge University Press.)

nucleus in anaesthetised animals, the most sensitive neurones are located in the ventral part and a high percentage of them are activated monosynaptically[93,138]. This is in good agreement with the anatomical finding that only the ventral part of Deiters' nucleus receives primary afferents[87, 94]. In unanaesthetised cats, however, many neurones in dorsal and middle Deiters' nucleus were found to be highly sensitive to lateral tilting of the head[142]. Apparently, monosynaptic linkage of vestibular neurones with primary afferents is not essential for sensitivity of the response to natural stimulation. A similar conclusion has been reached for tonic type I vestibular neurones (see Section 3.4.2.1).

3.4.3   Receptor convergence on vestibular neurones

In recording from single neurones in the VN during natural stimulation, it was found that they may be influenced by activity arising in more than one labyrinthine receptor. Thus, some horizontal type I units of rabbit[121], cat[143] and frog[117] can be influenced by stimulation of otoliths and vertical canals. In the rabbit, most of the responses evoked by stimulation of the otoliths and vertical canals had the same sign, i.e. they showed homonymous coupling. Such type of convergence of otoliths and canals may be very useful for the conpensatory adjustment of the eyes when the head is moved in space. Most of the type I neurones of rabbits also receive an excitatory input from the ipsilateral otolith system and some of them from the ipsilateral posterior canal too. Type II and III neurones receive influences from the otoliths and vertical canals[121]. On natural stimulation of otolith receptors and the vertical canals in the cat, *ca*. 40% of type I and II horizontal canal neurones showed no convergence at all; 35% only from otolith receptors; 10% from one or two vertical canals; and 10% from otolith plus one or two canals. Tonic neurones received convergence about twice as often as kinetic neurones[143]. It is interesting to note that in the cat some horizontal type II neurones can still be recorded after contralateral labyrinthectomy[83]. These neurones are monosynaptically activated by VIIIth nerve stimulation which implies that they must be second-order neurones of a canal other than the horizontal. The data, therefore, suggest an inhibitory interaction within the VN between different labyrinthine receptors of the same side. Convergence in this case could function to sharpen incoming impulses from one organ. It may well be that disynaptic and polysynaptic IPSPs evoked in vestibular neurones following ipsilateral VIIIth nerve stimulation are responsible for this kind of interaction[93, 95]. In the frog only *ca*. 20% of the horizontal type I neurones showed no convergence at all[117]. These neurones were characterised by an approximately linear input–output relationship, whereas most of the neurones showing convergence had a non-linear input–output characteristic. Among the various combinations of convergence on type I neurones that of the posterior canal of the same side occurred most frequently.

   Natural stimulation has thus shown considerable receptor convergence on central neurones. It should be emphasised, however, that in some animals a considerable percentage shows no convergence at all, i.e. in these cases a high specificity of receptor projection is present. The question arises now, what pathways are responsible for convergence? Electrical stimulation of individual receptor organs should solve this problem. Such studies have been performed in the cat[144,145] and pigeon[146]. The interesting point of these investigations is the fact that short latency convergence of different labyrinthine receptors on a given vestibular neurone occurs only rarely. Thus, only 6% of the neurones of the pigeon showed convergence from more than one ampulla. The rest of the neurones showed the expected mono- and/or poly-synaptic activation from only one receptor organ. This figure seems to be similar in the cat[144]. Obviously, we are faced with an enormous discrepancy between the results obtained with natural and electrical stimulation. The conclusion from this finding would be that the high degree of convergence taking place when natural stimuli are used involve pathways through other centres such as the reticular formation and the cerebellum, which in turn would feed-back onto vestibular neurones.

At present we are far from knowing the exact organisation and functional implications of convergence. Earlier observations have shown that each canal may be able to provoke nystagmus in all of the eye muscles, and that position of the head can also affect nystagmic eye movements[147,148]. In man the recognition of the subjective vertical is influenced by activity arising from the canals[149] and the intensity and duration of caloric nystagmus increases in direct proportion to higher values of gravitational forces[150,151]. While an influence of stimulation of otolith organs on canal-evoked nystagmus can be demonstrated clearly, this influence is not essential for its generation since nystagmus occurs also during weightlessness[152]. Receptor convergence on central neurones may thus play an important role in the precise control of ocular movements supporting the rather stereotyped three-neuronal vestibulo-ocular reflex which connects one ampulla with pairs of eye muscles (see Section 3.5). Similarly, precise regulation of body posture may require this convergence.

3.4.4 Interaction between the two labyrinths

There is anatomical evidence that the VN are interconnected by commissural fibres crossing the midline beneath the fourth ventricle[153-156]. Indirect vestibulo–reticulo–vestibular paths may serve as additional morphological substrates for the mutual interaction between the VN[156]. Earlier physiological studies have shown that some Deiters' neurones can be influenced by galvanic stimulation of the contralateral labyrinth[107,157,158]. Recent more sophisticated physiological studies have added much detailed information on the organisation of the crossed influences[83,116,124,145,159,160].

3.4.4.1 Field potentials

After weak stimulation of the contralateral VIIIth nerve a field potential can be recorded in the VN consisting of an initial positive-negative deflection (latency of positive peak 2.4 ms) and a later slow negative wave (latency 3.2 ms)[83]. This field potential is mainly found in the ventral part of the medial and ventromedial part of the superior and lateral nuclei, which is in good agreement with the anatomy of the commissural projection[156]. From the analysis of the field potential it appears that the summit of the initial positive wave corresponds in time to the arrival of the earliest impulses arriving in the contralateral VN along the commissural system and that the slow negative wave represents the synaptic and action currents generated in vestibular neurones by the action of commissural fibres. It has further been shown that the commissural fibres are axons of secondary neurones and that no primary fibres cross the midline. After sagittal incision of the dorsal brain stem (about 2 mm deep) the field potential disappeared, suggesting that it is produced exclusively by the commissural path and not by vestibulo-reticular connections. However, when the intensity of nerve stimulation is raised to more than twice that of N_1 threshold, complex potentials are observed throughout the VN and reticular formation, which are not altered by midline incisions[83].

3.4.4.2 Contralateral excitation of single neurones

As already mentioned in Section 3.4.2.1, some neurones are connected exclusively to the contralateral labyrinth. In the horizontal canal system these neurones have been called type II and they are activated by weak single-shock stimulation of the contralateral VIIIth nerve with latencies as short as 3.2 ms provided that the commissural path is intact[83]. It was shown that some type II neurones were monosynaptically activated by the commis-

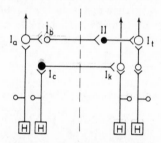

Figure 3.8 Diagram showing neuronal circuitry of commissural vestibular pathways. *Abbreviations:* I, type I neurone; II, type II neurone; H, horizontal canal; filled circles, inhibitory neurones; open circles, excitatory neurones. For explanation see text

sural fibres (Figure 3.8). Type II neurones excited by contralateral stimulation are found in the region where the field potential can be recorded. These regions are for the most part free of primary vestibular afferents[94]; however, degenerating terminals of commissural fibres were described to terminate in these areas[156].

It should be added that many of the Deiters' neurones, in particular the ones responding to tilt and not to angular rotation, are activated by contralateral stimulation[142,157,161]. This crossed activation is mediated by extracommissural polysynaptic pathways through the reticular formation[142]. It is clear from the above discussion that, unless the stimulus intensities are carefully controlled, crossed effects cannot be attributed to one or the other pathway. Furthermore, the functional interpretation of crossed effects will be greatly enhanced by proper identification of the neurones studied.

3.4.4.3 *Contralateral inhibition of single neurones*

Whereas type II neurones are excited via the commissural pathway type I neurones are strongly inhibited by weak stimulation of the contralateral VIIIth nerve[83]. This crossed inhibitory influence on type I neurones is abolished after interruption of the commissural fibres and replaced by excitatory responses mediated through the reticular formation provided stronger stimuli are applied[83]. In tonic type I neurones, the inhibition of the resting discharge occurs with a latency of *ca.* 4.0 ms[83,124,159] and lasts for *ca.* 20–40 ms after single-shock stimulation, which is in agreement with the time course of the IPSPs generated in tonic vestibular neurones[162] by contralateral stimulation. When the value of the latency of type I inhibition is compared with the latency of type II excitation it may be concluded that some of the type II neurones are inhibitory to type I. In Figure 3.8 is summarised the simplest neuronal circuit that may lead to inhibition of tonic type I neurones (I_t). As can be seen, primary afferents activate a type I neurone (I_a) which activates a second type I neurone (I_b), the actual commissural neurone. This neurone activates type II on the other side which inhibits the tonic type I (I_t) neurone[83]. Recent intracellular studies led to the conclusion that kinetic type I neurones are inhibited with shorter latencies than tonic neurones[159,160,162]. Intracellular recordings from these neurones revealed IPSPs occurring with latencies of *ca.* 2.0 ms after contralateral stimulation. Stimulation of the contralateral medial VN produced in the same neurones IPSPs with latencies ranging from 1.0 to 1.3 ms. Including the measurements for conduction time, the wiring diagram, shown in Figure 3.8, for inhibition of kinetic type I neurones has been obtained. An inhibitory type I commissural neurone (I_c) is activated by nerve stimulation and it directly inhibits kinetic type I units (I_k) on the other side. Hence, the commissural system is composed of both inhibitory and excitatory fibres.

Further studies of the commissural system have demonstrated that reciprocal inhibition is not restricted to the horizontal canal system but appears to be a general property of the canal system. Thus, separate stimulation[145] of the three canal nerves in each labyrinth has shown that second-order neurones of the anterior and posterior canals were inhibited by stimulation of the contralateral posterior and anterior canal nerves, respectively. This means that, in general, antagonistic pairs of canals are linked across the midline by the commissural pathway. The neuronal circuits interconnecting the vertical canal system appear to be the same as in the case of the horizontal canals[124,145].

3.4.4.4 *Functional aspects of crossed inhibition*

Given the geometrical arrangement of the six semicircular canals, the specific mode of inhibition among pairs of canals should be helpful in enhancing the sensitivity of secondary vestibular neurones to angular accelerations of the head. Indeed, after removal of the contralateral labyrinth, the average threshold for frequency increase of type I neurones on the intact side to horizontal angular acceleration is significantly higher as compared to animals with bilaterally intact labyrinths[83]. This effect occurs in spite of the fact that the average discharge of these neurones appears to be slightly higher due to removal of tonic inhibition. It may be concluded from these results that during ipsilateral angular acceleration, discharge frequencies of type I neurones are enhanced not only by the increased activity of the ipsilateral horizontal canal but also by decrease of tonic inhibition resulting from decreased activity of the contralateral canal. In other words, withdrawal of inhibitory influence from the other side elevates the excitability of type I. On the other hand, during contralateral acceleration, both crossed inhibition and disfacilitation assure the depression of type I neurones. As a result, the lateralisation of the response may be enhanced. Given that many of the excitatory type I neurones project to the contralateral abducens nucleus, commissural inhibition may support the decrease of firing of the antagonistic or ipsilateral motoneurones, thereby enhancing the smooth performance of canal induced conjugate eye movements[129] (for details see Section 3.5). The same functional considerations are, of course, applicable to crossed inhibition in the vertical canal system.

Interestingly, comparative physiological studies have shown that amphibia lack the commissural inhibition and only crossed excitation has been noted in canal units[77]. In reptiles, however, commissural inhibition is present (unpublished observation). It may tentatively be assumed that the presence of commissural inhibition is related to the functional state of development of the vestibular-induced eye movements which are known to be rather primitive in amphibia[77] and highly developed in higher vertebrates such as reptiles and mammals. Teleologically speaking, the commissural system would be an ideal instrument to allow only one labyrinth to control neurones on both sides. It has been shown[116] that in the process of compensation of vestibular-induced eye movements following hemilabyrinthectomy type I neurones on the deafferented side regain their tonic discharge. This discharge can be modulated by rotation in a way similar to the intact cat, i.e. type I neurones can be recorded on the deafferented side. In this chronic experimental situation, the increase in frequency of type I neurones during ipsilateral rotation is achieved by withdrawal of inhibition which occurs as a result of decrease of the input on the intact side. The decrease of type I neurones, of course, is caused by the inhibitory action of the commissural system. It is clear that the maximum increase in firing is determined by the resting discharge of the neurone whose true value will be revealed by removal of tonic inhibition. Since no excitation arrives from the destroyed side the maximum value of frequency increase will be less than in intact preparations[116]. Also, the threshold for frequency increase will be slightly higher on the deafferented side since type II neurones mediating crossed effects have a slightly higher threshold as compared to type I. It is interesting to note that in the stage of compensation the threshold for commissural inhibition is significantly lower as compared to acute preparations[116]. This finding may explain the surprising functional recovery of type I neurones. The finding that in decerebrate cats the rigidity decreases in the ipsilateral forelimb after labyrinthectomy and that a fairly symmetrical muscle tone is obtained after destruction of the remaining labyrinth would indicate crossed inhibitory mechanisms[163,164]. Since gravity sensitive vestibular neurones are not inhibited but rather excited by contralateral stimulation this may further indicate that tonic canal units are at least in part responsible for extensor tone in peripheral muscle.

3.5 VESTIBULO–OCULAR RELATIONS

It has long been recognised that labyrinthine receptor organs are capable of influencing the extraocular muscles in a precise way. The eye movements caused by labyrinthine stimulation are for the most part compensatory in nature, i.e. they oppose head movements and act to stabilise the visual axis in space. In as much as proprioceptive and vestibular integration is important for the regulation of body posture, vestibular and visual co-operation appears to be essential for the maintenance of the optimal angle of the retina in space. In this brief review only the recent development of vestibulo–ocular relations can be discussed. Most of the older work has been extensively reviewed elsewhere[165,166]. Furthermore, this chapter will be restricted to the vestibular control of eye movements. The reader interested in the general aspects of the oculomotor system, in particular the saccadic system, is referred to recent reviews of these subjects[166–168].

3.5.1 Synaptology of vestibulo–ocular reflex

Many studies have shown that electrical or natural stimulation of a given semicircular canal evokes, after a short delay, strong contractions of at least one muscle in each eye leading to the well-known conjugate eye movements[108,109,169–173]. It was demonstrated that short pathways exist between the horizontal canal and the ipsilateral medial and contralateral lateral rectus muscle, the superior canal and the ipsilateral superior rectus and contralateral inferior oblique, the posterior canal and the ipsilateral superior oblique and contralateral inferior rectus muscle. In the past indirect evidence has led to the conclusion that the shortest reflex connection between the receptors and the ocular muscles consists of three neurones, i.e.

   (a) the primary vestibular neurone;
   (b) the secondary vestibular neurone projecting to the ocular motor nuclei via the MLF;
   (c) the motoneurones innervating the various ocular muscles.
As will be shown below, this postulate has been confirmed fully by anatomical and physiological studies. In addition to this powerful basic circuit connecting labyrinth and eye muscles, any semicircular canal can establish functional contact with any one of the extraocular muscles by means of complex polysynaptic connections through the reticular formation. Because of the complexity of these extra MLF pathways their synaptology is far from being known at present[172,173].

Many attempts have been made in the past to study the anatomical basis of the well-known vestibulo–ocular reflex, by investigating the distribution of degenerations of secondary vestibular fibres in the ocular motor nuclei following lesions of the various subdivisions of the VN. Since the somato-topical distribution of motoneurones of different ocular nerves has also been studied[174-177], a meaningful interpretation of the degeneration patterns will be possible. This type of study has been performed in great detail in monkeys[178] and cats[179]. Since physiological studies of the synaptology of the vestibulo–ocular connection so far have been restricted mainly to cats, details will be described only for this animal. In the cat, vestibular projections to the ocular motor nuclei arise only in the superior VN and in rostral portions of the medial VN, both of which receive projections from primary vestibular afferents. The majority of fibres from the superior VN join the ipsilateral MLF from which they enter the ipsilateral IV and III nuclei. Fibres passing to the contralateral motor nuclei cross the midline within the III nuclei. From the rostral medial VN, ascending fibres project to the ipsi- and contra-lateral VI and through the contralateral MLF to the IV and III nuclei bilaterally[179]. Thus, only relatively small regions in the VN participate in the ascending projections to the motoneurones.

Recent physiological investigations of the vestibulo–ocular connections of the cat have elucidated the precise neuronal circuitry of the short latency pathways from the labyrinth to the motoneurones (Figure 3.9). Stimulation of the contralateral VIIIth nerve (V_c) causes disynaptic EPSPs in abducens, trochlear and those oculomotor neurones which are connected to V_c[180-184]. Similar results have been obtained in rabbits[185-187]. A comparison between the latencies of the V_c evoked EPSPs and those that have been evoked in motoneurones by direct stimulation of the medial VN indicates that the latter are evoked monosynaptically. This disynaptic nature of the vestibulo–ocular reflex has further been corroborated by the comparison of the latencies of action potentials of vestibular axons terminating in the motor nuclei with those of the postsynaptic potentials. This comparison demonstrates that in the motor nuclei no interneurones are intercalated between vestibular axons and motoneurones[182]. Single-shock stimulation of the VIIIth nerve generally produces double activation of secondary vestibular neurones terminating in the motor nuclei[182]. This double firing corresponds well with the double activation of vestibular neurones described earlier (Section 3.4.2) and indicates that both N_1 and N_2 components of the vestibular field potential are also represented in the output to the oculomotor system. The rapid succession of this double firing will add to the efficacy of synaptic transmission through temporal summation of PSPs in the motoneurones. In brief, it may be stated that the above results are in complete agreement with the anatomical data and fully support the interpretations given on the basis of previous experiments monitoring eye movements and/or muscle contraction. Interestingly, comparative physiological studies have shown that in teleost fish the vestibulo–ocular reflex may be monosynaptic[188] a finding which is clearly different from higher vertebrates.

A second even more interesting finding has emerged from recent intra-cellular studies of mammalian ocular motoneurones. Whereas the intra-cellular studies of the excitatory vestibulo–ocular reflex basically-confirmed and directly proved previous conclusions obtained with less sophisticated methods, these studies revealed for the first time the existence of a disynaptic inhibitory vestibulo–ocular reflex (Figure 3.9). From recordings of mechano-grams and electromyograms from extraocular muscles, it has long been recognised that a given conjugate eye movement is accompanied not only by the contraction of a pair of eye muscles but also by the relaxation of the antagonistic pair[169, 171, 172]. As will be shown in this section, at least three mechanisms assure the effective depression of the muscle tone in the antagonists. One of them is the inhibitory vestibulo–ocular reflex which, in contrast to the previous notion[172], appears to be organised in the same way as its excitatory counterpart[180-182, 184, 185]. Following stimulation of the ipsilateral vestibular nerve (V_i), disynaptic IPSPs have been recorded in abducens,

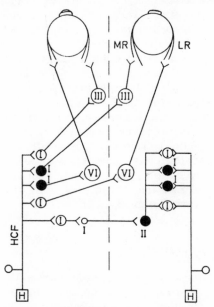

Figure 3.9 Diagram of neuronal circuitry of vestibulo–ocular reflex for horizontal eye movements. *Abbreviations:* I,II, type I and II neurones; VI, abducens nucleus; III, oculomotornucleus (region of medial rectus); LR, lateral rectus; MR, medial rectus; HCF, horizontal canal fibre. Open and filled circles indicate excitatory and inhibitory neurones, respectively. Note that reticular connections are not shown. The vestibulo–ocular projection of the right VN is omitted; instead the commissural connections are shown

trochlear and certain oculo–motoneurones. As in the case of the EPSPs, the latencies become monosynaptic following stimulation of the ipsilateral VN. It appears that for the IPSPs recorded in the abducens motoneurones the medial VN is the relay nucleus, whereas trochlear and oculomotor neurones are monosynaptically inhibited following stimulation of the superior VN. The presence of inhibitory vestibular neurones projecting all the way up to the oculomotor nuclei also explains some of the anatomical findings which so far have been difficult to reconcile with the results obtained from stimulation experiments. Now it is clear that the degenerations found in the ipsilateral abducens and trochlear nuclei (see earlier) represent the degenerated inhibitory axons. In brief, reciprocal organisation between semicircular canals and pairs of eye muscles via the MLF path appears to be a general principle in the oculo–motor system. It is interesting to note that the importance of both contracting and extending eye muscles for the direction of a given eye excursion has also been theoretically deduced on the basis of measurements of the effective origins and insertions of the six extraocular muscles[189].

As with the semicircular canals, the otolith organs can influence the position of the eyes, a phenomenon which is known as compensatory counter-rolling[50,166,190–193]. Compensatory counter-rolling acts to maintain the visual axis in space when the head and/or body is subjected to static tilt. At present the synaptology of the otolith reflex on the eyes is not well understood. Mechanical[194] and electrical stimulation of the utricle itself produced distinct eye movements whose characteristics would suggest a more complex pathway as compared to the canal evoked eye movements. However, the patterns of eye movements and latencies of muscle contraction evoked by electrical stimulation of the utricular nerve[195,196] are not so different from canal-induced contractions. This may suggest that similar short latency connections exist between otolith and ocular motoneurones. Microphysiological studies are needed to clarify this point*. On the basis of anatomical studies it may be assumed that the relay stations in the VN are different from the canal pathways (Section 3.4.2.2).

3.5.2 Natural stimulation

The responses of abducens motoneurones of cat[129] and rabbit[197] to horizontal rotation have been investigated. Spontaneously active motoneurones increase their firing to contralateral angular acceleration and decrease firing to ipsilateral rotation. When the quick phase of the nystagmus is not suppressed by anaesthesia or acute decerebration, the smooth frequency increase is rhythmically interrupted by sudden decreases in firing; the opposite effect, rhythmic burst-like increases of discharge frequency, are seen during the decrease of firing occurring on ipsilateral rotation. This response pattern of abducens motoneurones is, of course, in agreement with the direction of conjugate eye movements observed during horizontal rotation. On the basis of the synaptology described above it is clear that the frequency increase on contralateral rotation is brought about by the increased activity in the contralateral horizontal canal nerve and the resulting activation of type I neurones in the VN which project to the abducens nucleus on the other side (Figure 3.9). The decrease in firing on ipsilateral rotation may be explained by several mechanisms:

(a) disfacilitation of motoneurones as a result of frequency decrease in the contralateral VIIIth nerve;

(b) disfacilitation of motoneurones caused by the commissural inhibition acting on contralateral type I neurones which are facilitory on motoneurones (see Section 3.4.4); and

(c) direct inhibition of abducens motoneurones by inhibitory type I neurones located in the ipsilateral VN.

  * See 'Note added in Proof'.

All three mechanisms are always operant during horizontal rotation. Experiments in which the brain stem was split along a midsaggital plane to eliminate all influences on abducens neurones from the contralateral side show that the inhibitory vestibulo–ocular reflex alone can modify the discharge of motoneurones[181,184]. In this experimental situation motoneurones respond qualitatively the same way as in the intact preparation, a finding which clearly shows the functional importance of direct inhibition. It also means that frequency decrease and increase on ipsilateral and contralateral rotation is caused by inhibition and disinhibition, respectively. In recording from the abducens nucleus, units were observed frequently which increased their firing on ipsilateral rotation and ceased to fire on contralateral rotation[129]. It has been shown that for the most part these action potentials were generated by axons of inhibitory vestibular neurones terminating in the motor nucleus. A comparison of the results obtained by natural and electrical stimulation has shown that the excitatory and inhibitory vestibulo–ocular reflex path running in the MLF can explain the canal induced slow compensatory eye movements. As mentioned above, pathways through the reticular formation are probably involved although not essential for the slow conjugate eye deviations.

A few quantitative studies of the vestibulo–ocular relation deserve mention. The thresholds of abducens motoneurones for frequency increase during horizontal rotation[129] are practically identical with those reported for secondary vestibular neurones (see Section 3.4.2.1). Furthermore, the time course of the frequency increase, the non-adaptive properties in response to prolonged acceleration steps and the input–output relationship are surprisingly similar to the values obtained in the VN[129]. These findings may also indicate that secondary vestibular neurones impose their influences directly onto motoneurones. This notion is further supported by experiments employing sinusoidal rotatory stimulation of the labyrinth. As in the case of vestibular neurones, the results have shown clearly that within a certain frequency range tested the discharge of ocular motoneurones is related to the velocity of the sinusoidal stimulus (maximum discharge lags velocity by ca. 30 degrees)[130,198]. Since the end organs are stimulated by the accelerations of the head, two successive integrations should occur along the vestibulo–ocular pathway to obtain the correct change in position of the eyes[167,199]. The fact that the discharge of primary[40] and secondary vestibular neurones[41,130] as well as of ocular motoneurones[5,198] are related approximately to velocity of the input (within a certain frequency range) may suggest that the second integration possible does not occur along the central pathway as suggested by Robinson[199] but rather in the eye. It was shown that motoneurone discharge is slightly lagging velocity; if an additional phase lag is introduced by the eye muscles and the viscoelastic properties of the tissue surrounding the eye[199], the final eye movement may be related to the displacement of the head. After acute hemilabyrinthectomy a large increase of tonic background firing was observed in those ocular motoneurones which were connected to the intact side. This effect may be due to both removal of direct vestibulo–ocular inhibition and commissural inhibition. The observations that the phasic character of the motor activity during sinusoidal stimulation was diminished and that ocular motoneurone firing leads velocity in hemilabyrinthectomised animals indicate that the inhibitory mechanisms contribute to the dynamic properties of the vestibular induced ocular compensatory movements[198].

3.5.3 Cerebellar influence on vestibulo–ocular reflex

The precise knowledge of both the vestibulo–ocular reflex and the vestibulo–cerebellar relationship (Section 3.6) presents an ideal situation to study cerebellar influences on central oculomotor pathways. As summarised in

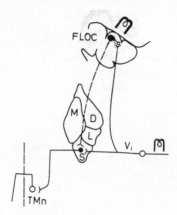

Figure 3.10 Diagram of vestibulo–cerebellar inter-relationship in cat. *Abbreviations:* FLOC flocculus; L, lateral VN; M, medial VN; S, superior VN; TMn, trochlear motoneurone; V_i, ipsilateral VIIIth nerve. Filled and open circles denote inhibitory and excitatory neurones respectively; broken line indicates axons of Purkinje cell

Figure 3.10, primary vestibular fibres terminate monosynaptically on both secondary vestibular neurones[182,185] which project to the ocular motoneurones (see earlier) and on cerebellar granule cells which excite the inhibitory Purkinje cells[200,201]. The latter project monosynaptically onto vestibulo–ocular neurones[202]. In lower vertebrates having a monosynaptic vestibulo–ocular reflex connection, Purkinje cells project directly on ocular motoneurones[188]. Thus, in both vertebrates the pathway through the cerebellum converges at the site at which primary vestibular neurones exert their influences. The connections shown in Figure 3.10 strongly suggest that the vestibulo–ocular reflex may be under direct control of the vestibulo–cerebellar cortex. This suggestion has been proved experimentally[203, 204]. Floccular stimulation produced a strong monosynaptic suppression of both the excitatory and inhibitory vestibulo–ocular transmission as evidenced by the depression of field and intracellular potentials evoked in ocular motor nuclei by V_i and V_c

stimulation. In chronic experiments in which the vestibular nerve had been transected to eliminate axon reflex activation, ipsilateral floccular stimulation generated disinhibition in motoneurones through its suppression of the tonic inhibitory vestibular neurones projecting onto the motoneurones. Contralateral stimulation produced a distinct disfacilitation of motoneurones by the inhibition of tonic excitatory vestibular neurones. Furthermore, it could be shown that the reverberatory-like tendency of synaptic potentials occurring in motoneurones following V_i and V_c stimulation (e.g. disynaptic IPSP followed by disinhibition and later IPSPs) was absent in cerebellectomised animals. It appears, from the above studies in mammals, that one of the functions of the vestibulo–cerebellum is to influence the transmission of canal activity to ocular motoneurones at the level of the VN. Ablation experiments suggest that otolith influences on eye position are likewise affected by the cerebellum[205]. Information being processed in the vestibulo–cerebellum may, therefore, be important for the optimal regulation of vestibular induced eye movements. In terms of control theory, the vestibulo–cerebello–vestibular system appears to be similar to a feed-forward control system, since no evidence is present for a negative feed-back loop from the eye to the vestibular organ. At present we do not know the characteristics of the cerebellar output to the VN under biological conditions. Probably the flocculus not only uses vestibular but also visual information for its regulation of the vestibulo–ocular transmission in the VN (see Section 3.6). Some of the effects of stimulation and ablation of the vestibulo–cerebellum will be mentioned in Section 3.6.

3.5.4 Vestibular nystagmus

At rest the output from the VN to the ocular motor nuclei via the MLF is symmetrical and the eyes are held in a certain position characteristic for each animal. Stimulation or destruction of the semicircular canals or the VN (for references see Ref. 206) on one side will produce an asymmetric outflow which, in the awake animal, generates rhythmic eye movements. This vestibular nystagmus consists of two phases, i.e. the slow compensatory ocular movement in one direction and the quick return movement to the other side. There is reason to assume that the slow phase is generated by the classical vestibulo–ocular reflex path, thus reflecting the activities of the primary and secondary vestibular neurones which are mediated to the motoneurones mainly via MLF[172,173,207]. The quick phase, however, appears to be entirely central in origin. In brief, regarding the mechanism and precise origin of the quick phase two main concepts have emerged in the past which may be called vestibular and reticular theory. The latter theory claims that the quick component originates in the reticular formation (RF) since destruction of parts of the bulbopontine RF abolished the quick phase[173]. On the contrary, other investigators provided experimental evidence which led them to conclude that the VN are the site of rhythm formation[207]. In the 30 years following the formulation of these controversial theories many investigators have tried to prove or disprove one or the other theory and it appeared that until recently the general tendency was in favour of the reticular theory (for a summary see Ref. 166). It should be emphasised, however, that convincing direct experimental evidence is still missing in both cases. In the following, the main data obtained with single-neurone recording during nystagmus will be summarised briefly and their respective contribution to the vestibular and reticular theory will be evaluated. It is to be expected that this approach combined with well-controlled lesions will eventually settle the problem. The detailed knowledge of the synaptology of the vestibulo–ocular reflex (see earlier and Figure 3.9) represents a solid basis for studies of the neurophysiological mechanisms underlying the generation of nystagmus. Since in the ocular motor nuclei recording can be obtained not only from motoneurones but also from identified axons of secondary vestibular neurones terminating on motoneurones, a comparison between the timing of impulses in presynaptic axons and the synaptic events generated in motoneurones during nystagmus will be possible. Such studies have been performed during spontaneous nystagmus in the trochlear and oculomotor nuclei[208] and during evoked vestibular nystagmus in the abducens nuclei[209]. The results obtained by these studies are summarised in Figure 3.11 for the left (LIO) and right (RIO) inferior oblique motor nuclei. The data, however, are representative for the nystagmic events occurring in any pair of antagonistic motor nuclei. It can be seen that the membrane potential rhythms in the antagonistic pair of motoneurones show a symmetric configuration, i.e. the quick depolarisation in RIOMn is highly synchronous with the quick hyperpolarisation in LIOMn. RIO and LIO are recordings of the mass discharge of corresponding motor nerves and show the time course of quick and slow nystagmus. After the quick phase, the membrane potential in RIOMn moves in the hyperpolarising direction leading to the cessation of discharge in RIO during the slow phase. In LIOMn, however, a slowly-increasing depolarisation is noted which leads to a slow increase of firing of the cell (not shown) and as a result of that the slow phase of the nystagmus is generated in the LIO. When the discharge frequency of identified secondary vestibular axons are recorded in the right nucleus during nystagmus, it can be easily seen that they show a similar rhythmic modulation. The two excitatory V_c axons (line 1 and 3 from the top) increase their discharge whereas the inhibitory V_i axon ceases to fire during the quick depolarisation. During the slow phase V_i and V_c axons also show a reciprocal behaviour. Thus it may be concluded that the quick depolarisation is the combined result of excitation (V_c) and disinhibition (V_i) and that the relative hyperpolarisation that follows is caused by inhibition (V_i) and disfacilitation (V_c). On the other hand, presynaptic V_i and V_c axons in the left nucleus increase and decrease their firing during the quick hyperpolarisation, respectively. The opposite is the case during the slow depolarisation potential. Thus, the quick hyperpolarising potential is due to active inhibition (V_i) and disfacilitation (V_c), and the slow depolarising event is caused by excitation (V_c) and disinhibition (V_i). These results demonstrate beyond any doubt that secondary vestibular neurones participate in the generation of synaptic events occurring in motoneurones not only during the slow phase but also during the quick phase of nystagmus. Interestingly, earlier studies of vestibular neurones recorded in the VN have already shown some correlation between the nystagmic rhythm[113–118] although in these studies the functional connections of the units were not known.

Do these results indicate that the VN are the site of rhythm formation? A definite answer can certainly not be given at the present time. It has been pointed out, however, that the excitatory and inhibitory vestibulo–ocular reflex in conjunction with the commissural inhibition interconnecting the vestibulo–ocular neurones may be able to form rhythmic activity[210]. In this

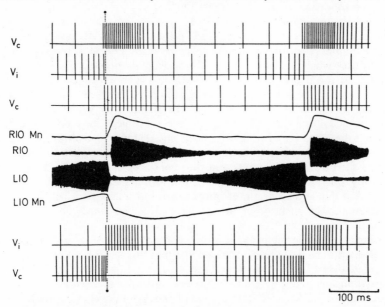

Figure 3.11 Diagram of neuronal activity recorded from secondary vestibular and ocular motoneurones of the unanaesthetised cat during nystagmus. This diagram is based on many recordings from vestibular axons and ocular motoneurones during spontaneous nystagmus produced by labyrinthine lesion. Action potentials are not shown in the intracellular tracings (RIOMn; LIOMn). *Abbreviations:* V_i, V_c, ipsilateral (inhibitory) and contralateral (excitatory) secondary vestibular axons; RIO and LIO, gross activity of right and left inferior oblique nerves during nystagmus; RIOMn, LIOMn, synaptic events in right and left inferior oblique motoneurones during slow and quick phases of nystagmus. Vertical dotted line is drawn through the beginning of the quick phase EPSP (agonist) and quick phase IPSP (antagonist). Note simultaneous onset of the two events. (By courtesy of Drs Baker and Berthoz.)

hypothesis the role of the RF would be to provide the general excitatory background for the rhythm generated in the VN. Reticular lesions or anaesthesia removing this background activation may then lead to the disappearance of the quick phase, i.e. the rhythm. The reticular hypothesis, of course, assumes that the rhythm is generated in the RF and that vestibular neurones receive that rhythm from this site. In fact, it has been shown that reticular neurones fire in close correlation with vestibular-induced nystagmus[211] but unfortunately their functional connection is not known. It may thus well be that they receive the rhythm from the VN. Even if they were the structures responsible for the rhythm it would have to be shown whether they act through the VN or directly on to motoneurones, or both. Evidently, much work remains to be done in this field. It may be mentioned that occasionally recordings from axons are obtained in motoneurone pools which are activated from V_c with long latencies indicating polysynaptic activation. Such a unit is shown in Figure 3.11 (trace 1). It shows that polysynaptic pathways are involved but it does not reveal the site of origin of this neurone, i.e. it could be a vestibular or reticular neurone since both can be polysynaptically activated following vestibular stimulation[92].

An interesting observation has been made in ocular motoneurones of teleost fish during vestibular induced nystagmus[101,212]. It has been shown that the impulses occurring in motoneurones during the slow phase originate in dendrites whereas action potentials associated with the quick phase are initiated in the soma. In addition, in these ocular motoneurones the cell bodies but not the dendrites are electrotonically coupled. The absence of coupling in the dendrites allows the cells to fire independently following dendritic activation, and the resulting eye movement may be of the slow graded type observed during the slow phase. On the contrary, coupling between cell bodies provides a significant synchronisation when the neurones are activated by somatic inputs and thus enhances the rapid eye movements occurring during the quick phase. These differential inputs may suggest that in fish the sites of origin of fibres causing the slow and fast phase may be different. No such observations have been obtained in mammalian motoneurones.

Firing of vestibular neurones not only correlates with vestibular nystagmus but also with the occurrence of rapid eye movements (REM) during desynchronised sleep[213]. It seems that in this case vestibular neurones are excited by rhythmically-active reticular neurones and are an essential link in the production of REM since destruction of the VN abolishes all REM burst in extra-ocular muscles. At least, in this situation, reticular neurones do not project directly onto motoneurones but yet seem to be the site of rhythm generation. Whether a similar mechanism is also applicable to the generation of vestibular nystagmus remains to be shown.

3.6 VESTIBULO–CEREBELLAR INTERACTION

Phylogenetic and ontogenetic studies of the cerebellum have shown that its development is characterised by a close relationship to the vestibular system[214–216]. In all vertebrates, this close relationship is represented by the presence of primary and secondary vestibular fibres projecting to the cerebellar cortex and to some of the cerebellar nuclei[217,218]. The vestibular fibres are in fact the only sensory fibres having direct access to the cerebellar cortex. On the other hand, the cerebellar cortex sends a significant number of Purkinje-cell axons to the VN thus establishing the basis for a mutual interaction (Figure 3.10).

3.6.1 Vestibulo–cerebellar input

Recent physiological studies have shown that in the frog, primary vestibular fibres end monosynaptically as climbing fibres on Purkinje cells and as mossy fibres on granule cells in the flocculus of the cerebellar cortex.

Secondary vestibulo–cerebellar fibres terminate exclusively as mossy fibres on granule cells[200]. In the cat and pigeon, however, both primary and secondary vestibulo–cerebellar fibres end exclusively as mossy fibres in the vestibulo–cerebellum[200,219], which is in agreement with anatomical studies[218,220,221]. The pure mossy fibre nature of the vestibulo–cerebellar input in higher vertebrates is of great functional importance. It seems to suggest that the two afferent systems to the cerebellum, the mossy and climbing fibres, act as parallel channels carrying entirely different information to the vestibulo–cerebellum. There is experimental evidence suggesting that the climbing fibre input to the vestibulo–cerebellum carries visual information arriving via the accessory optic system[222]. This interesting dual sensory projection to the vestibulo–cerebellum using mossy and climbing systems independently deserves particular attention in future studies on the functional role of vestibulo–cerebellar interaction in the regulation of eye movements.

One may now ask: what kind of vestibular receptors project to the cerebellum? Using electrical stimulation of individual canal nerves in the pigeon, it has been shown that canal fibres were able to activate single Purkinje cells via the mossy fibre–granule cell pathway[219]. As in the case of the VN this projection appears to be rather specific, i.e. little convergence of different canals occurs at a given Purkinje cell. Similarly, in the frog it has been shown that Purkinje cells of the vestibulo–cerebellum responded very well to rotational stimulation of the horizontal canals[223]. Interestingly, the four types of unit responses (type I–IV) found in the VN of various vertebrates on horizontal rotation (Section 3.4.2.1) have also been recorded from cerebellar Purkinje cells of the frog. Whereas, the type I responses are restricted to the flocculus, particularly type III neurones are found along the posterior rim of the entire cerebellum[200,223]. The latter type shows polysynaptic activation following stimulation of both vestibular nerves and may, therefore, be mainly influenced by the secondary vestibular input. At present it is not known whether otolith receptors also have access to the cerebellum. Given the fact that secondary vestibulo–cerebellar fibres in part originate in the descending nucleus[224] which is known to receive afferents from the utricle (see Section 3.4.2.2), one may assume that gravity sensitive neurones project to the cerebellum.

Besides the direct vestibular projection to the vestibulo–cerebellum, other parts of the cerebellum appear to receive indirect vestibular information via vestibulo–reticulo–cerebellar pathways. The potentials recorded in the lobulus simplex and culmen have longer latencies than those in the vestibulo–cerebellum and are probably mediated by these indirect pathways[225]. Finally, it should be added that the fastigial nucleus and parts of the dendate nucleus also receive primary and secondary vestibular fibres[85,216]; this has been confirmed physiologically[226,227].

3.6.2 Cerebello–vestibular projection

The cerebellum not only receives information from the vestibular system, but it also controls the VN by means of direct corticofugal fibres (Purkinje cell axons) and by fibres arising in the nuclei fastigii. The latter nuclei are in turn under the control of the cerebellar cortex (for anatomical details see Refs. 217, 228). Recent physiological work has shown that the Purkinje cells—the only output of the cerebellar cortex—are inhibitory in nature[81], and that the neurones of the cerebellar nuclei are excitatory on their target neurones. In fact, the inhibitory action of Purkinje cells was demonstrated first by recording monosynaptic IPSPs from neurones in the dorsal Deiters' nucleus which is known to receive direct corticofugal fibres from the anterior lobe of the cerebellum[81, 229, 230]. Only EPSPs were recorded in ventral Deiters' neurones after cerebellar stimulation. They were shown to be caused by axon reflexes through collaterals of cerebellar afferents[231]. Thus, ventral and dorsal Deiters' nucleus are clearly different in their synaptology: whereas the former receives primary vestibular afferents[94], fastigial afferents[85] and Purkinje axons from the flocculus[232], the dendrites and somata of the latter are supplied by Purkinje axons from the anterior lobe and lack vestibular afferents[85, 233]. Inhibition of gravity-sensitive Deiters' neurones following anterior-lobe stimulation has been demonstrated experimentally[142]. This effect may, in part, explain the disappearance of the dynamic response characteristic of Deiters' neurones following cerebellectomy (see Section 3.4.2.2). Furthermore, the direct inhibitory action of Purkinje cells on postural centres in the brain stem and their indirect disfacilitatory action on these centres through the inhibition of the cerebellar nuclei may explain the well-known suppressory action of cerebellar stimulation on postural tone[85, 234, 235], which is so clearly seen by the disappearance of decerebrate rigidity after anterior-lobe stimulation[236]. Occasionally, excitatory effects have been observed in brain stem neurones following cerebellar stimulation[157, 237]. These effects may be explained either by the activation of axon reflexes (see earlier) through cerebellar afferents and/or by disinhibition occurring in cerebellar target neurones as a result of depression of tonic Purkinje cell discharge by the activation of the interneurones in the cerebellar cortex[238].

Whereas gravity sensitive Deiters' neurones may be inhibited by stimulation of the anterior lobe, second-order neurones of the semicircular canals are not influenced by this stimulation[142]. Stimulation of the flocculus, however, distinctly inhibits the second-order neurones of horizontal (type I) and vertical canals[142,203], whereas utricular units are not influenced. Thus, canal units receive inhibition via the commissural vestibular system (Section 3.4.4) and from the vestibulo–cerebellum. On the other hand, otolith units lack the commissural inhibition, which is replaced by polysynaptic excitation across the midline and receive cerebellar inhibition mainly from the anterior lobe. It has been shown that inhibitory and excitatory vestibular neurones projecting to the ocular motor nuclei are among the ones that are inhibited by floccular stimulation[203]. Physiological and anatomical studies show that floccular Purkinje cells exert their inhibition monosynaptically on vestibular neurones which receive primary vestibular afferents from the canals[87,202,203,232]. These findings clearly indicate that the vestibulo–ocular reflex is under inhibitory cerebellar control (Figure 3.10). Inhibition of vestibular nystagmus on stimulation of the flocculus[239] may now be explained on the basis of the neuronal circuit described above (see also Section 3.5.3). Similarly, enhancement of nystagmus, appearance of spontaneous nystagmus, and lack of habituation of nystagmus observed following lesions of the vestibulo–

cerebellum may in part be due to the removal of the inhibitory action of Purkinje cells from their target neurones[240-243]. In comparing the two mutually exclusive modes of direct cerebellar control of the VN, it is apparent that the vestibulo–cerebellum not only projects directly to the VN but it also receives primary and secondary vestibular fibres, whereas the anterior lobe projecting to the Deiters' nucleus does not receive any direct or short latency vestibular input but rather information from the spinocerebellar paths. These two systems, therefore, serve different functions. In the case of the former the function may be more related to control of vestibular induced eye movements; the control of the VN by the anterior lobe appears to serve the organisation of postural activities in which the vestibulo–spinal system originating in part in Deiters' nucleus is of some importance (for details see Ref. 85).

A few recent studies dealing with the effects of stimulation of the fastigial nucleus deserve mention (for a summary of the older literature see Ref. 85). Following stimulation of the contralateral fastigial nucleus type I vestibular neurones of the horizontal canal were inhibited with disynaptic latencies. The same neurones were monosynaptically excited by stimulation of the ipsilateral fastigial nucleus[142]. It is very likely that the disynaptic inhibition of type I neurones is mediated by type II inhibitory neurones which are also responsible for commissural inhibition of tonic type I neurones (Section 3.4.4). In general, the excitatory nature of the cerebellar nuclei on their target neurones is well established experimentally (see Ref. 229). Since these nuclei are under the inhibitory control of Purkinje cells, the latter may indirectly influence vestibular neurones by this pathway. At any given time the influence of cerebellar nuclei on vestibular neurones depends on the activity level of Purkinje cells, i.e. an increase in their activity will depress vestibular neurones by disfacilitation, and a decrease in Purkinje-cell firing will result in disinhibition of cerebellar-nuclei neurones and consequently in an increase in firing of vestibular neurones. Thus, the pathway from the cerebellar cortex through the cerebellar nuclei complements the direct corticofugal path to the brain stem and gives various other regions of the cerebellar cortex access to the vestibular neurones.

3.7 VESTIBULO–SPINAL INTERACTION

It is well known from classical investigations that the vestibular system plays an important role in the regulation of body posture[50,236]. Much of this earlier work can be found in textbooks and previous monographs[85]. In this section only the recent neurophysiological and anatomical work will be reviewed and an attempt will be made to elucidate the role of the VN in vestibulo–spinal interactions. Vestibular and proprioceptive activity may converge at various levels of the nervous system:

(a) in the spinal cord and

(b) in the brain stem, in particular in the VN and associated structures. During locomotion and postural regulation both sites are linked intimately together by pathways descending from the brain stem to the spinal cord and by various ascending connections informing the higher centres about the activity in the periphery.

3.7.1   Spino–vestibular input

A relatively small number of spinal afferents ascending mainly with the dorsal spinocerebellar tract have been described to end in the caudalmost region of the descending and medial VN, the dorsal part of Deiters' nucleus (hind limb region) and in the cell group x and z[244,245]. These parts of the VN do not receive primary vestibular afferents. In addition to this direct spino–vestibular pathway, spino–reticulo–vestibular paths and collaterals of the spino–olivo–cerebellar tract provide multiple opportunities for spinal activity to reach the VN[246,247]. It is important to note that some of the vestibular regions receiving direct afferents also project to the cerebellum, as do, of course, the indirect pathways through the reticular formation and inferior olive. Thus, VN and cerebellum appear to be closely linked in spino–vestibular interactions.

According to the anatomical connection briefly outlined above, it is not surprising that many neurones in the VN can be influenced by stimulation of the spinal cord and afferent nerves. In general, it may be stated that the earliest spinal input to most neurones of the VN is mainly excitatory[96, 161, 248-250]. In Deiters' nucleus both hind-limb and fore-limb areas receive excitatory influences, which also suggests that indirect spino–vestibular paths are involved in the transmission of spinal signals. On direct stimulation of the cord at C_3, about half of the antidromically activated vestibulo–spinal neurones received monosynaptic excitation and to a lesser degree poly- and mono-synaptic IPSPs[248]. These spinal evoked IPSPs may partly explain the inhibitory effects caused by conditioning stimulation of the sciatic nerve on utricular-evoked test responses in decerebellate animals[251]. Recently, the synaptic events occurring in Deiters' neurones after peripheral nerve stimulation have been analysed by intracellular recordings[247,252,253]. To exemplify the complex nature of spino–vestibular inputs arriving via direct and indirect pathways at the level of vestibular neurones these data will be briefly described. Deiters' neurones were classified as fore-limb or hind-limb cells according to the site of the most effective nerve. Antidromic identification of these neurones showed that for the most part hind-limb cells projected to lumbosacral levels of the cord and fore-limb cells to cervico thoraric regions. In Deiters' neurones, stimulation of peripheral nerves of the dominant limb causes a combination of earlier EPSP (d_2) and later IPSP (h_3), whereas stimulation of the non-dominant limb was ineffective or produced small EPSPs. It was shown that all of these responses were mediated by the spino–olivo–cerebellar tract which has excitatory collaterals to the Deiters' neurones (d_2 EPSP) and which causes IPSPs (h_3) through spino–olivo–cerebello–vestibular paths. This indicates that there are two types of excitatory convergence on Deiters' neurones from the inferior olive; one is activated from the nerves of the dominant limb and is always associated with the convergence of inhibition from Purkinje cells, and the other is activated from the non-dominant limb and free from the inhibitory effects. The same experiments were performed in unanaesthetised decerebrate cats in which olivo–cerebellar fibres were severed in order to study the effects of mossy fibres and their collaterals on Deiters' neurones. In this preparation, early EPSPs (d_1) and early (h_1) and later (h_2) IPSPs were found. The d_1

potentials are caused by mossy fibre collaterals to the Deiters' neurones and h_2 by the inhibitory action of Purkinje cells activated through the mossy fibre pathway. The latency of h_1 IPSP was too short to be mediated through the cerebellum and, therefore, was probably produced by reticulo–vestibular connections. In summary, following stimulation of the peripheral nerves of the dominant limb in decerebrate cats with intact olivo–cerebellar tract the sequence of synaptic events in Deiters' neurones is as follows: d_1, h_1, h_2, d_2, h_3. Whereas d_1 EPSP and h_1, h_2 IPSPs are produced by the fast mossy fibre pathway, d_2 and h_3 are mediated by the slowly-conducting climbing fibres. The stimulus intensity necessary to evoke the above responses indicates that group I and II muscle afferents and low- and high-threshold cutaneous afferents may be involved. Experiments with natural stimulation of different types of somatosensory receptors, however, indicate that skin and deep receptors, particularly the joint receptors, may excite vestibular neurones, whereas muscle spindle afferents are apparently ineffective[254,255]. Only the nucleus z appears to represent an exception, since it is a medullary relay in the low threshold group I muscular path from the hind-limb to the cerebral cortex[256]. This finding seems to emphasise the importance of joint receptors in supplying postural information to the VN. Summative convergence of somatic (joint movements) and vestibular stimulation on single vestibular neurones was indeed demonstrated[158]. Furthermore, proprioceptive influences arising in the joints of the neck can produce eye movements[50,196] and seem to alter vestibular induced eye movements[257]. Much of this interaction between neck and vestibular receptors seems to occur in the VN. This interaction is, of course, of prime importance in animals whose head moves with respect to the body. Thus, when the head is tilted to one side with the rest of the body remaining in an upright position, otolith receptors signal a change in head position. This message would be the same if the whole body together with the head would have been tilted. Therefore, in the former case meaningful reflex correction can only be initiated by vestibulo–spinal mechanisms if information from the neck simultaneously cancels vestibular information by means of summative convergence on vestibular neurones.

Finally, it should be mentioned that the general facilitation of vestibular neurones located in various subdivisions of the VN by impulses arising in the periphery of the body may contribute to the tonic resting discharge of vestibular units, which in turn may be modified by changes occurring in the periphery. The detailed description of the behaviour of Deiters' neurones during peripheral stimulation has exemplified to some extent how a given group of vestibular neurones which projects to the spinal cord may be informed by ascending pathways about activities in the periphery.

3.7.2 Vestibulo–spinal projection

The VN can influence the spinal cord by means of two direct pathways: the lateral and medial vestibulo–spinal tracts[85, 258]. Deiters' nucleus gives origin to the uncrossed lateral tract so that its rostroventral part projects to cervico–thoracic levels and the dorsocaudal part to lumbosacral segments, thus indicating a clear somatotopical arrangement[85]. Neurones of the medial, and to some extent, the descending nucleus constitute the medial tract, which is found in the MLF in the lower brain stem[258].

As for the lateral tract physiological experiments have confirmed the somatotopical arrangement in the Deiters' nucleus mentioned above, though most authors noted overlapping between the two regions of origin[161,248–250]. The percentage of cells being driven monosynaptically by vestibular nerve stimulation is much higher in the rostroventral area of Deiters' nucleus[249, 250], a finding which is also in good agreement with the anatomy[94]. This means that Deiters' nucleus can transmit labyrinthine activity more directly to rostral segments of the cord. On the other hand, the dorsocaudal Deiters is under direct inhibitory control of the anterior lobe of the cerebellum (see Section 3.6). It may also be recalled that only a modest number of canal units are found in Deiters' nucleus, whereas many cells respond to otolith stimuli. These findings may suggest that the lateral vestibulo–spinal tract is for the most part involved in the mediation of otolith evoked labyrinthine reflexes on the head, body and eyes. As for the mode of action of the lateral tract, its excitatory nature on extensor muscles has been noted for some time (for references see Ref. 85). Recently, microphysiological studies have confirmed and extended this early notion[259–263]. It has been shown that all monosynaptic connections of vestibulo–spinal fibres on motoneurones are excitatory. Provided that given motoneurones show short latency effects by stimulation of the lateral tract, extensor motoneurones show mono-synaptic excitation and flexor motoneurones disynaptic inhibition. In general, excitatory monosynaptic pathways are dominant in axial extensor motoneurones (neck, back) while polysynaptic pathways more frequently link Deiters' nucleus and limb extensors. Interestingly, axial motoneurones are also more readily excited by labyrinthine stimulation as compared to limb extensors[262]. The latter, in particular those projecting to the fore-limbs are more easily influenced by the cerebellar vermis, which projects to the dorsal Deiters' nucleus (see Section 3.6). In addition to the direct influence on motoneurones the vestibulo–spinal tract can alter segmental activity via its action on interneurones[264–266]. Direct evidence for convergence of cortical, proprioceptive and vestibular impulses on spinal interneurones has been obtained[265]. These findings further support the importance of the interaction of proprioceptive and vestibular impulses at different levels of the CNS for the maintenance of postural reflexes. Also the gamma moto-neurones of the extensor muscles receive an excitatory influence from Deiters' nucleus[267–269]. This influence represents another indirect pathway for excitation of a-motoneurones.

Whereas the facilitatory action of the lateral vestibulo–spinal tract has been known and proven for some time, it is only recently that the mode of action of the medial vestibulo–spinal tract has been studied. It originates for the most part in the medial VN and extends as far as to midthoracic levels[258]. Since the medial VN has a strong monosynaptic vestibular input, this pathway may be well suited to relay labyrinthine influences to the spinal cord. It has been reported that interruption of this path did not affect the vestibular transmission to the limb motoneurones[270]. These negative results have been supported by recent more refined studies showing that its action is mainly inhibitory and that limb motoneurones are poorly affected[263]. It may be safely stated that the components of the medial vestibulo–spinal tract which originate in the medial VN are inhibitory on axial motoneurones. Many of these extensor neurones showed mono- and di-synaptic IPSPs after stimulation of the medial VN and vestibular nerve, respectively. EPSPs that were also recorded on stimulation of the caudal MLF are presumably caused by reticulo–spinal fibres joining the MLF[263]. Inhibitory and excitatory effects mediated by the two vestibulo–spinal tracts represent the neural basis for reciprocal innervation occurring during vestibular-induced postural reflex. It is obvious that other pathways such as vestibulo-reticulo–spinal paths combine with the more direct vestibulo–spinal efferents in the transmission of vestibular information to the cord. Besides the post-synaptic effects that these tracts exert on spinal neurones, presynaptic influences on dorsal-root afferents certainly also play a role[254].

In contrast to the wealth of new data concerning the neuronal organisation of the vestibulo–spinal tract relatively little new work has been done regarding the overall function of this system. A few pilot studies will be mentioned. Activity of Deiters' neurones has been recorded during locomotion produced in mesencephalic and thalamic cats[271]. Many of the Deiters' neurones were modulated in phase with the locomotor cycle during walk or trot. The activity changes coincide with the activity of extensor muscles and disappear completely after cerebellectomy. Since destruction of Deiters' nucleus, does not abolish locomotion, it can be concluded that the vestibulo–spinal tract is not responsible for this rhythm. It may be that the function of this pathway is to co-ordinate and adjust extensor activity, presumably through afferent information involving the cerebellum. Another interesting finding has emerged from these studies. It has been shown that the response of Deiters' neurones to vestibular stimulation is reduced during locomotion irrespective of the presence or absence of the cerebellum[140]. This effect may in part be mediated by the efferent vestibular system to the labyrinth receptors (see Section 3.3.2), and/or by inhibition arriving via spinal afferents[251]. It is assumed that this depressory action on the vestibular response during locomotion protects the rhythmic firing frequency of Deiters' neurones occurring during stepping from irregular disturbances that would result from head movements.

As for the interaction of neck and labyrinthine afferents an interesting observation has been made in recording from α-motoneurones of the hind-limb[272]. Passive head movements caused a brief increase in discharge of extensor α-motoneurones regardless of the direction of the movement. After the neck afferents were eliminated the facilitation of these neurones observed previously during the movement was now abolished and marked facilitation for the period of maintained head position appeared. In flexor motoneurones decrease of firing was the rule. The neck afferents, therefore, appear to have an inhibitory influence on labyrinthine reflexes arising in the otolith organs (see earlier). The effect of periodic oscillations about the longitudinal axis on fore-limb and neck extensor muscles of the cat have been tested in preparations in which the neck receptors have been elimi-nated[273,274]. It was shown that the final dynamic vestibular motor control of these muscles is related to velocity of sinusoidal rotation and is for the most part linearly related to its magnitude. Interestingly, studies comparing vestibular effects on neck and fore-limb extensor muscles have also demonstrated that the responses in ipsilateral fore-limbs are in phase with those in the contralateral neck extensors, a finding which clearly shows the precise functional organisation of the vestibulo–spinal reflex path.

3.8 VESTIBULAR INTERACTION WITH OTHER SYSTEMS

In the preceding sections the major input and output stations of the vestibular system have been described. There are, however, several other systems whose mutual connection with the vestibular system deserves our interest, although relatively little detailed work has been devoted to them in the past. Nevertheless, it is our hope that this account will stimulate future work in these fields.

3.8.1 Vestibulo–reticular interaction

Anatomical studies have shown that only very few primary vestibular fibres end in the reticular formation (RF). Secondary vestibular fibres to the RF originate from all major VN (for details see Ref. 275). The majority of vestibular efferents terminate in the nucleus reticularis gigantocellularis and in the nucleus reticularis pontis caudalis both of which give rise to ascending fibres (beyond the mesencephalon) and to reticulo–spinal fibres. Those reticular nuclei which project to the cerebellum (lateral reticular nucleus, nucleus reticularis tegmenti pontis) receive afferents from the superior and lateral VN. Certain regions of the paramedian pontine RF have been related to vestibulo–reticular interactions occurring during nystagmus[173]. It should be emphasised that the connections between VN and RF are mutual although detailed anatomical information concerning the RF projections to the VN is still missing.

Neurones in the RF have long been known for being influenced by a great variety of sense modalities, which are integrated in this system before they reach their target systems[59]. The importance of the labyrinthine input to the RF appears to be related to the co-ordination of both postural and ocular movements and probably to the mediation of vestibular activity to the cerebral cortex. Single neurones in the bulbopontine RF on both sides are influenced by natural stimulation of the semicircular canals[115]. In addition, many of them can be activated by acoustic, somatosensory and visual stimuli[276]. Such types of multisensory convergence are generally not found in the VN except for the so-called type III neurones (Section 3.4.2.1). Electrical stimulation of the vestibular nerve shows that above a certain threshold (Section 3.4.2) complex field potentials are generated in the RF surrounding the VN on both sides[92]. Reticular neurones are likely to mediate the excitatory effects on certain vestibular neurones across the midline after VIIIth nerve stimulation[83] and may serve as an additional source for the tonic activity of vestibular neurones. The fact that small doses of barbiturates reduce the resting discharge of secondary but not of primary vestibular neurones may thus be partly explained by the reduction of the reticular input to the VN under the influence of the drug. At this stage little more can be said about the functional meaning of the vestibular efferents to the RF of the lower brain stem since detailed studies are missing. In Sections 3.4–3.6, some of the possible functional aspects have already been mentioned, in particular the role of the RF for vestibular induced eye movements, and its mediating role for vestibular induced spinal and cerebellar activity.

Somewhat more refined studies have been performed on the function of the reticular nuclei in the midbrain such as the interstitial nucleus of Cajal and adjacent structures. Pathways ascending from the VN to these structures have been described by various authors (for summary see Ref. 277), and it has been noted that the interstitio–spinal tract sends off collaterals to the ipsilateral VN[85]. Single neurones in the interstitial nucleus were influenced by natural stimulation[278]. This effect may be caused by the action of certain secondary vestibular neurones projecting to the interstitial nucleus[279].

Stimulation of the interstitial nucleus produced a distinct inhibition of the main secondary vestibular neurones of the horizontal and vertical canals[124,279]. This inhibitory effect on type I neurones was restricted to the ipsilateral VN and probably mediated through the activation of type II inhibitory neurones. Previous authors have shown that the interstitial nucleus appears to be involved in the co-ordination of vertical and rotatory eye and head movements[109,280]. Since this nucleus has direct fibre connections to various ocular motor nuclei[109], stimulation-evoked ocular movements would not necessitate activation of pathways through the VN. However, the VN are often involved in the production of ocular movements induced from higher centres. This notion is further supported by the finding that cortical induced eye movements change their direction following destruction of the VN[281]. It has been shown that single vestibular neurones were activated with polysynaptic latencies following stimulation of both ipsilateral and contralateral areas, 2 pri and $6a\delta$[282]. This response may be conducted to the VN via the interstitial nucleus or adjacent structures in the midbrain. Anatomical studies suggest that descending and reticular afferent fibres to the VN take their origin only from the interstitial nucleus and the pontine and medullary reticular formation. Lesions of the RF rostral to the pons gives no degeneration in the VN[277]. Changes in firing of vestibular neurones during optokinetic nystagmus are likely to be mediated by similar reticular influences on the VN. In addition, interaction between vestibular and visual activity appears to occur in the visual centres such as the visual cortex[283] and lateral geniculate nucleus. It has been shown that during the large bursts of REM the latter receives a strong input from the medial VN[213]. Vestibular and visual interactions may contribute to the visual stabilisation of the environment during eye movements.

3.8.2 Vestibulo–cortical projection

Conscious orientation in space would require vestibular signals to reach the cerebral cortex, i.e. a primary vestibular projection area should be present. Furthermore, it may be expected that motor co-ordination occurring in the cerebral cortex needs the vestibular information for its optimal performance in addition to the somatosensory inputs from the rest of the body. With these logical postulates in mind it is not surprising that many investigators have succeeded in recording vestibular evoked· activity in various regions of the cerebral cortex. It is only a slight exaggeration to say that a review of the pertinent literature has revealed that the number of cortical vestibular areas is about as large as the number of investigators dealing with the problem. Part of the discrepancies in the localisation are certainly due to the types of preparations that were used (anaesthesia; encephale insolée). For the most part, however, differences in the stimulation procedures may have contributed to the confusion. The proximity of the auditory and vestibular receptors in the labyrinth, and the neighbourhood of the brain stem requires a very careful control of the vestibular stimulation parameters. Most of the work performed before 1962 has been summarised critically elsewhere[85] and need not be repeated here. Instead, several of the recent careful studies performed in cat and monkey will be summarised.

It appears that in the cat certain regions surrounding the contralateral rostral part of the anterior suprasylvian sulcus and parts of the ectosylvian gyrus receive short latency (4–8 ms) vestibular activation[225,284–286]. Whereas most studies agree on this location, a second area has recently been claimed to receive short latency vestibular projection[286,287]. This field is located in the sensorimotor cortex in the upper part of the posterior sigmoid gyrus, at the level of the postcruciate dimple and may correspond to area 3a. Strong input from muscle spindles of the fore-limb[288] has been recorded in the same area. Many single units in the motor cortex, in fact, respond to vestibular stimulation with latencies as short as 5 ms. In contrast to the neurones in the primary vestibular field, these responses are direction specific[289]. It is of some functional interest that the areas surrounding the vestibular field also receive afferent paths from receptors in muscle, joints and skin, which provide information concerning movement and position of limbs[285]. They may co-operate with the vestibular field by mutual connections. In fact, convergence of vestibular and somatosensory afferents in vestibular cortex has been found in cat and monkey[88,290]. In contrast to the short latency responses found in the vestibular and parts of the sensory motor cortex vestibular evoked activities in the visual cortex[283] generally have long and variable latencies and are not considered specific vestibular projection areas.

In the Rhesus monkey, the primary cortical projection area of the vestibular nerve is found in the postcentral gyrus at the lower end of the intraparietal sulcus, at the level of the first somatosensory projection of the mouth[290]. Thus, the location of this area in the monkey between the first and second somatic field is approximately the same as in the cat. As in the cat, the projection is bilateral, although the ipsilateral responses are more susceptible to barbiturates. Whether or not this area corresponds to Brodmann's area 2 is still a matter of conjecture[290, 291]. It is of great functional importance, however, that single neurones in the primary vestibular projection field are influenced by two sensory modalities, namely, vestibular and proprioceptive, somatosensory stimuli (joint afferents; deep muscle pressure). This finding is in contrast to findings in other primary sensory projection fields[291]. Similar findings have been obtained in the cat (see earlier). Since perception of body in space requires the collaboration of vestibular input (head position) and somatosensory afferents (joint receptors) from the rest of the body it may be assumed that, functionally speaking, the dual projection to the vestibular cortex may be considered as specific.

A few comments will be made regarding the pathways carrying vestibular information from the labyrinth to the cerebral cortex. It is clear that all information reaching higher centres has to pass through the VN. Short latency potentials have been recorded around the anterior descending limb of the suprasylvian sulcus following stimulation of the medial and descending VN[292]. No data are given on the other nuclei which likewise give origin to ascending projections. Several authors agree that section of the MLF does not abolish vestibular evoked cortical activity (see Ref. 85). This finding may suggest that various extra MLF paths are mainly responsible for the activation of certain thalamic nuclei which in turn project to the cerebral cortex. It has been suggested that the fasciculus tegmenti dorsolateralis receives impulses from the VN (ipsilateral lateral and superior VN, contralateral descending VN) and is continued in Forel's tegmental fasciculi. These fasciculi are found lateral to the MLF and have terminations in the thalamus[293]. In the cat, thalamic degenerations have in fact been demonstrated with the Nauta method after electrolytic lesions of the VN[294]. It appears that the main relay nucleus is the internal part of the intermediate ventral nucleus (V. im. i.) which projects to the area 6aδ of the motor cortex. A small integrative nucleus (Z. im. i.) receives some collateral degeneration of vestibular fibres. The multisensory magnocellular part of the medial geniculate nucleus receives vestibular projections in addition to somatosensory visual and acoustic afferents and projects to the anterior ectosylvian gyrus in which vestibular evoked potentials have been recorded (see earlier). Recent physiological studies in the cat have demonstrated short latency responses in the dorsomedian part of the VPL and in the middle section of the VL of the thalamus after well controlled stimulation of the vestibular nerve[286]. In the monkey, ascending vestibular fibres terminate in the ventralis posterior inferior and ventralis medial nuclei[295]. Vestibular evoked responses recorded in the monkey thalamus were located in a region between the inferior medial part of the VPL and VPM[296]. This nucleus (VPI) receives a short latency vestibular evoked response (2.5 ms) whereas longer latency responses (5 ms) were recorded in the magnocellular part of the medial geniculate body, the VPL, the VPM and the medial and posterior nuclei. It is very likely that the VPI represents the relay station for the vestibular field in the cortex since stimulation of the latter antidromically-evoked cells in the VPI.

3.8.3 Vestibular effects on autonomic functions

Contrary to the rather detailed knowledge of the functional organisation of vestibular influences on the somatic system, relatively little is known on the pathways by which the labyrinth affects the autonomic nervous system. Most studies in the past have been restricted to the recording of physiological manifestations of vestibular stimulation. Thus it has been shown that vestibular stimuli may evoke responses from the vasomotor system, sweat and salivary glands, pupils, digestive tracts, etc. but more detailed studies concerning the pathways have only been recently carried out. Most of the previous literature related to autonomic effects has been extensively summarised by two major reviews on motion sickness[297,298] and the reader interested in this field is referred to them. In this paragraph only a few very recent studies will be discussed.

It has been known for some time that various types of labyrinthine stimulation in rabbits caused a distinct vaso-depressor reaction resulting in a fall of blood pressure[299,300]. Recent neurophysiological studies have shown that weak stimulation of the vestibular nerve ($1.5–1.9 \times N_1$ threshold) inhibited the spontaneous discharge recorded from the sympathetic ganglionic renal nerve. Simultaneously a fall in systemic arterial blood pressure was noted[301,302]. Strong vestibular stimulation exciting high threshold vestibular afferents and possibly adjacent structures caused excitation followed by inhibition as evidenced by recording from sympathetic nerves. Furthermore, it was noted that stimulus intensities causing a fall in blood pressure had little effect on respiration, whereas clear-cut respiratory responses were always accompanied by an increase in blood pressure[303]. The inhibition of sympathetic activity and fall of blood pressure were almost completely abolished after lesion of the ipsilateral medial VN[300,301]. This finding may indicate that neurones in the medial VN project to the bulbar reticular depressor area which eventually produces the depression of sympathetic firing. Evidence for ample vestibulo–reticular projection has been given in Section 3.8.1.

As mentioned above, vestibular stimulation increased both rate and depth of respiration as demonstrated by recordings from motor fibres of the phrenic and recurrent laryngeal nerves[303]. Although specific neuronal connections are not known at present, it is likely that these influences may be mediated by pathways involving the VN and their projections to the bulbar reticular formation. The latter may be the mediating link between VN and respiratory centre.

It appears from the recordings at different levels (neck and chest) of the vagus nerve that the strong vestibular activation in the neck vagus nerve is conducted exclusively in the recurrent laryngeal nerve and not in the vagus nerve proper. This means that the effects of vestibular stimulation upon the autonomic system are mediated only by its sympathetic portion, as demonstrated by recordings from splanchnic nerve[302], abdominal sympathetic chain, cardiac sympathetic nerves[304], renal nerve[301] and neck sympathetic fibres[303]. The discharge in the latter follows strong vestibular stimulation of varying frequencies. Thus, the resulting increase in blood pressure may be properly explained by a widespread excitatory effect of strong vestibular stimulation on the sympathetic outflow.

Notes added in proof

1. Recent studies describing the responses of primary otolith neurones in monkey[305] and cat[306] to static tilts about different axes deserve mention. In monkey[305], the functional polarisation vectors for most superior nerve units (utriculus) lie near the horizontal plane; those for most inferior nerve

units, near the sagittal plane (sacculus). On the contrary, in the cat the majority of otolith afferents are maximally sensitive to position changes when the head is at or near its normal position[306]. The reason for this remarkable difference is not clear at present and future studies are needed to solve this discrepancy.

Further discrepancies between the otolith system of cat and monkey appear to arise when the stimulus-response relationship of statoreceptor afferents are compared: Whereas a more or less linear relationship has been found in the monkey[305] the discharge rate in statoreceptor afferents of the cat varied as a power function of the sine of angular head position[306]. It has been suggested[306] that in part these differences may be explained by the fact that measurements at too few head positions have been performed in monkey. As pointed out earlier, however, the linear relationship holds also for the otolith system of lower vertebrates[52, 53].

2. Recent studies in cat abducens motoneurones have, in fact, shown that disynaptic EPSPs may be evoked in motoneurones upon selective stimulation of the utricular nerve[307].

References

1. Lowenstein, O. (1966). The functional significance of the ultrastructure of the vestibular end organs. *The Role of the Vestibular Organs in Space Exploration*. NASA SP **115**, 73
2. Blanks, R. H. I., Curthoys, I. S. and Markham, C. H. (1972). Planar relationships of semicircular canals in the cat. *Amer. J. Physiol.*, **223**, 55
3. Fernández, C. and Valentinuzzi, M. (1968). A study on the biophysical characteristics of cat labyrinth. *Acta Oto-laryng.* (*Stockholm*), **65**, 293
4. Valentinuzzi, M. (1967). An analysis of the mechanical forces in each semicircular canal of the cat under single and combined rotations. *Bull. Mathem. Biophysics*, **29**, 267
5. Melvill Jones, G. (1972). Transfer function of labyrinthine volleys through the vestibular nuclei. *Progress in Brain Research*. Vol. 37, *Basic Aspects of Central Vestibular Mechanisms* (A. Brodal and O. Pompeiano, editors) (Amsterdam: Elsevier)
6. Oman, C. M. and Young, L. R. (1972). Physiological range of pressure difference and cupula diflections in the human semicircular canal: theoretical consideration. *Progress in Brain Research*, Vol. 37, *Basic Aspects of Central Vestibular Mechanisms* (A. Brodal and O. Pompeiano, editors) (Amsterdam: Elsevier)
7. Steinhausen, W. (1931). Über den Nachweis der Bewegung der Cupula in der intakten Bogengangsampulle des Labyrinthes bei der natürlichen rotatorischen und calorischen Reizung. *Pflügers Arch. Ges. Physiol.*, **228**, 322
8. Hillman, D. E. (1972). Observation on morphological features and mechanical properties of the peripheral vestibular receptor system in the frog. *Progress in Brain Research*. Vol. 37, *Basic Aspects of Central Vestibular Mechanisms* (A. Brodal and O. Pompeiano, editors) (Amsterdam: Elsevier)
9. Melvill Jones, G. and Spells, K. E. (1963). A theoretical and comparative study of the functional dependence of the semicircular canal upon its physical dimensions. *Proc. Roy. Soc.* (*London*), **B157**, 403
10. Lindeman, H. H. (1969). Studies on the morphology of the sensory regions of the vestibular apparatus. *Ergebn. Anat. Entwickl. Gesch.*, **42**, 1
11. Wersäll, J. (1972). Morphology of the vestibular receptors in mammals. *Progress in Brain Research*, Vol. 37, *Basic Aspects of Central Vestibular Mechanisms* (A. Brodal and O. Pompeiano, editors) (Amsterdam: Elsevier)
12. Lowenstein, O. and Wersäll, J. (1959). A functional interpretation of the electron microscopic structure of the sensory hairs in the cristae of the elasmobranch Raja Clavata in terms of directional sensitivity. *Nature* (*London*), **184**, 1807

13. Hillman, D. E. and Lewis, E. R. (1971). Morphological basis for a mechanical linkage in otolithic receptor transduction in the frog. *Science*, **174**, 416

14. Hillman, D. E. (1969). Light and electron microscopical study of the relationship between the cerebellum and the vestibular organ of the frog. *Exp. Brain Res.*, **9**, 1

15. Engström, H. (1958). On the double innervation of the inner ear. *Acta Oto-laryng. (Stockholm)*, **40**, 5

16. Wersäll, J. (1956). Studies on the structure and innervation of the sensory epithelium of the cristae ampullares in the guinea pig. A light and electron microscopic investigation. *Acta Oto-laryng. (Stockholm)*, **126**, 1

17. Lowenstein, O., Osborne, M. P. and Wersäll, J. (1964). Structure and innervation of the sensory epithelia of the labyrinth in the thornback ray (Raja clavata). *Proc. Roy. Soc. (London)*, **B160**, 1

18. Hama, K. (1969). A study on the fine structure of the saccular macula of the gold fish. *Z. Zellforsch.*, **94**, 155

19. Goldberg, J. M. and Fernandez, C. (1971). Physiology of peripheral neurons innervating semicircular canals of the squirrel monkey. III. Variations among units in their discharge properties. *J. Neurophysiol.*, **34**, 676

20. Spoendlin, H. H. (1965). Ultrastructural studies of the labyrinth in squirrel monkeys. *The Role of the Vestibular Organs in the Exploration of Space*. NASA SP 77, 7

21. Dohlman, G. (1971). The attachment of the cupula, otolith and tectorial membranes to the sensory cell areas. *Acta Oto-laryng. (Stockholm)*, **71**, 89

22. Ballantyne, J. and Engström, H. (1969). Morphology of the vestibular ganglion cells. *J. Laryng.*, **83**, 19

23. Gazek, R. R. and Rasmussen, G. L. (1961). Fiber analysis of the stato-acoustic nerve of guinea pig, cat and monkey. *Anat. Rec.*, **139**, 455

24. Burlet, H. M. de (1929). Zur vergleichenden Anatomie der Labyrinthinnervation. *J. Comp. Neurol.*, **47**, 155

25. Lowenstein, O. (1972). Physiology of the vestibular receptors. *Progress in Brain Research*. Vol. 37, *Basic Aspects of Central Vestibular Mechanisms* (A. Brodal and O. Pompeiano, editors) (Amsterdam: Elsevier)

26. Trincker, D. (1965). Physiologie des Gleichgewichtsorgans. *Hals-Nasen-Ohren-Heilkunde*, Band III, Teil 1 (J. Berendes, R. Link and F. Zöllner, editors) (Stuttgart: Thieme)

27. Dohlman, G. (1960). Some aspects of the mechanism of vestibular hair cell stimulation. *Confin. Neurol. (Basel)*, **20**, 169

28. Dohlman, G. and Ormerod, F. C. (1960). The secretion and absorption of endolymph. *Acta Oto-laryng. (Stockholm)*, **51**, 435

29. Christiansen, J. A. (1964). On hyaluronate molecules in the labyrinth as mechanoelectrical transducers and as molecular motors acting as resonators. *Acta Oto-laryng. (Stockholm)*, **57**, 33

30. Smith, C. A., Lowry, O. H. and Wu, M. L. (1954). The electrolytes of the labyrinthine fluids. *Laryngoscope (St. Louis)*, **64**, 141

31. Loewenstein, W. R. (1961). Excitation and inactivation in receptor membrane. *Ann. N. Y. Acad. Sci.*, **94**, 510

32. Lowenstein, O. (1936). The equilibrium function of the vertebrate labyrinth. *Biol. Rev.*, **11**, 113

33. Lowenstein, O. (1950). Labyrinth and equilibrium. *Symp. Soc. Exp. Biol.*, **4**, 60

34. Lowenstein, O. and Sand, A. (1940). The individual and integrated activity of the semicircular canals of the elasmobranch labyrinth. *J. Physiol. (London)*, **99**, 89

35. Lowenstein, O. and Sand, A. (1940). The mechanism of the semicircular canal. A study of the responses of single-fibre preparation to angular accelerations and rotation at constant speed. *Proc. Roy. Soc. (London)*, **129**, 256

36. Ledoux, A. (1949). Activité électrique des nerfs des canaux semicirculaires du saccule et de l'utricle chez la grenouille. *Acta Oto-rhino-laryng. belg.*, **3**, 335

37. Precht, W., Llinás, R. and Clarke, M. (1971). Physiological responses of frog vestibular fibres to horizontal angular rotation. *Exp. Brain Res.*, **13**, 378

38. Rupert, A., Moushegian, G. and Galambos, R. (1962). Microelectrode studies of primary vestibular neurons in cat. *Exp. Neurol.*, **5**, 100
39. Goldberg, J. M. and Fernandez, C. (1971). Physiology of peripheral neurons innervating semicircular canals of the squirrel monkey. Resting discharge and response to constant angular accelerations. *J. Neurophysiol.*, **34**, 635
40. Fernandez, C. and Goldberg, J. M. (1971). Physiology of peripheral neurons innervating semicircular canals of the squirrel monkey. II. Response to sinusoidal stimulation and dynamics of peripheral vestibular system. *J. Neurophysiol.*, **34**, 661
41. Shimazu, H. and Precht, W. (1965). Tonic and kinetic responses of cat's vestibular neurons to horizontal angular acceleration. *J. Neurophysiol.*, **28**, 991
42. Lowenstein, O. (1956). Peripheral mechanisms of equilibrium. *Brit. Med. Bull.*, **12**, 114
43. Clark, B. (1967). Thresholds for the perception of angular acceleration in man. *Aerospace Med.*, **38**, 443
44. Ek, J., Jongkees, L. B. W. and Klijn, A. J. (1959). The threshold of the vestibular organ. *Acta Oto-laryng. (Stockholm)*, **50**, 292
45. Young, L. R. and Oman, C. M. (1969). Model of vestibular adaptation to horizontal rotations. *Aerospace Med.*, **40**, 1076
46. Groen, J. J., Lowenstein, O. and Vendrik, A. J. H. (1952). The mechanical analysis of the responses from the end organs of the horizontal semicircular canal in the isolated elasmobranch labyrinth. *J. Physiol. (London)*, **117**, 329
47. Steinhausen, W. (1933). Über die Beobachtung der Cupula in den Bogengangsampullen des lebenden Hechts. *Pflügers Arch. Ges. Physiol.*, **232**, 500
48. Van Egmond, A. A. J., Groen, J. J. and Jongkees, L. B. W. (1949). The mechanism of the semicircular canal. *J. Physiol. (London)*, **110**, 1
49. Young, L. R. (1969). Biocybernetics of the vestibular system. *Biocybernetics of the Central Vestibular System* (L. D. Proctor, editor) (Boston: Little, Brown and Co.)
50. Magnus, R. (1924). *Körperstellung* (Berlin: Springer)
51. Holst, E. von (1950). Die Tätigkeit des Statolithenapparates im Wirbeltierlabyrinth. *Naturwissenschaften*, **37**, 265
52. Lowenstein, O. and Roberts, T. D. M. (1951). The localization and analysis of the responses to vibration from the isolated elasmobranch labyrinth. A contribution to the problem of the evolution of hearing in vertebrates. *J. Physiol. (London)*, **114**, 471
53. Lowenstein, O. and Roberts, T. D. M. (1949). The equilibrium function of the otolith organs of the thornback ray. *J. Physiol. (London)*, **110**, 392
54. Vidal, J., Jeannerod, M., Lifschitz, W., Levitan, H., Rosenberg, J. and Segundo, J. P. (1971). Static and dynamic properties of gravity-sensitive receptors in the cat vestibular system. *Kybernetik*, **9**, 205
55. Mayne, R. (1966). The mechanics of the otolith organs. *Reports, Manned Spacecraft Center, NASA, Houston, GERA*, **112**, 1
56. Gualtierotti, T. and Bracchi, F. (1971). Spontaneous and evoked activity of bullfrogs vestibular statoreceptors in weightlessness. Four units sampled continuously during a six-day orbital flight. *Proc. 11th Int. Congr. Physiol. Sci. (Munich)*, IX, 635
57. Hernández-Peón, R. (1955). Central mechanisms controlling conduction along central sensory pathways. *Acta neurol. Lat.-amer.*, **1**, 256
58. Granit, R. (1955). *Receptors and Sensory Perception*. (New Haven, Conn.: Yale University Press)
59. Rossi, G. F. and Zanchetti, A. (1957). The brain stem reticular formation. Anatomy and Physiology. *Arch. Ital. Biol.*, **95**, 199
60. Hagbarth, K. E. (1960). Centrifugal mechanisms of sensory control. *Ergebn. Biol.*, **22**, 47
61. Rasmussen, G. L. (1946). The olivary peduncle and other fibre projections of the superior olivary complex. *J. Comp. Neurol.*, **84**, 141
62. Rasmussen, G. L. and Gazek, R. R. (1958). Concerning the question of the efferent fibre component of the vestibular nerve of the cat. *Anat. Rec.*, **130**, 361

63. Gacek, R. R. (1960). Efferent component of the vestibular nerve. *Neural Mechanism of the Auditory and Vestibular Systems*. (Springfield, Ill.: Thomas)
64. Petroff, A. E. (1955). An experimental investigation of the origin of efferent fibre projections to the vestibular neuroepithelium. *Anat. Rec.*, **121**, 352
65. Gazek, R. R., Nomura, Y. and Balogh, K. (1965). Acetylcholinesterase activity in the efferent fibres of the stato-acoustic nerve. *Acta Oto-laryng.* (*Stockholm*), **59**, 541
66. Rossi, G. and Cortesina, G. (1962). The efferent innervation of the inner ear. *Panminerva Med.*, **4**, 478
67. Precht, W., Richter, A. and Ozawa, S. (1972). Antidrome and synaptische Aktivierung von Vestibularisneuronen des Frosches durch Reizung des Nervus vestibularis. *Pflügers Arch. Ges. Physiol.*, **R101**, 332
68. Precht, W., Richter, A., Ozawa, S. and Shimazu, H. (1973). Intracellular study of frog's vestibular neurons in relation to the labyrinth and spinal cord. *Exp. Brain Res.*, in the press.
69. Iles, J. F. and Mulloney, B. (1971). Procion yellow staining of cockroach motor neurones without the use of microelectrodes. *Brain Res.*, **30**, 397
70. Llinás, R. and Precht, W. (1969). The inhibitory vestibular efferent system and its relation to the cerebellum in the frog. *Exp. Brain Res.*, **9**, 16
71. Schmidt, R. F. (1963). Frog labyrinthine efferent impulses. *Acta Oto-laryng.* (*Stockholm*), **56**, 51
72. Trincker, D. (1968). Analyse des afferenten Informationsflusses von Labyrinth-Receptoren, seiner Stabilisierung durch Rückkoppelung und der Kriterien für Konstanz der Raum- und Zeitkoordinaten zentraler Datenverarbeitung. *Biokybernetik*, Vol. 2 (H. Drischel and N. Tiedt, editors) (Leipzig: Karl Marx Universität)
73. Dichgans, J., Schmidt, C. L. and Wist, E. R. (1972). Frequency modulation of afferent and efferent unit activity in the vestibular nerve by oculomotor impulses. *Progress in Brain Research*, Vol. 37, Basic aspects of central vestibular mechanisms. (A. Brodal and O. Pompeiano, editors) (Amsterdam: Elsevier)
74. Bertrand, R. A. and Veenhof, V. B. (1964). Efferent vestibular potentials by canalicular and otolithic stimulations in the rabbit. *Acta Oto-laryng.* (*Stockholm*), **58**, 515
75. Klinke, R. and Schmidt, C. L. (1968). Efferente Impulse im Nervus vestibularis bei Reizung des kontralateralen Otolithenorgans. *Pflügers Arch. Ges. Physiol.*, **304**, 183
76. Gleissner, L. and Hendriksson, N. G. (1963). Efferent and afferent activity pattern in the vestibular nerve of the frog. *Acta Oto-laryng.* (*Stockholm*), **58**, 90
77. Ozawa, S., Shimazu, H. and Precht, W. (1973). Absence of crossed inhibition of central vestibular neurons in the horizontal canal system of the frog. *Exp. Brain Res.*, in the press
78. Sala, O. (1962). Modificazioni dell'attivita del nervo vestibolare a seguito della stimulazione del sistema vestibolare efferente. *Boll. Soc. Ital. Biol. Sper.*, **38**, 1048
79. Sala, O. (1965). The efferent vestibular system. *Acta Oto-laryng.* (*Stockholm*), **197**, 1
80. Ledoux, A. (1958). Les canaux semi-circulaires. Etude électrophysiologique. Contribution à l'effort d'uniformination des épreuvés. Essai d'interprétation de la semiologie vestibulaire. *Acta Oto-rhino-laryng. Belg.*, **12**, 109
81. Ito, M. and Yoshida, M. (1964). The cerebellar-evoked monosynaptic inhibition of Deiters neurones. *Experientia* (*Basel*), **20**, 515
82. Goetmakers, R. (1968). Adaptation of the vestibular organ. (Thesis). (Utrecht: Grafisch Bedrijf Schotanus+Jens Utrecht N.V.)
83. Shimazu, H. and Precht. W. (1966). Inhibition of central vestibular neurons from the contralateral labyrinth and its mediating pathway. *J. Neurophysiol.*, **29**, 467
84. Klinke, R. (1970). Efferent influence on the vestibular organ during active movements of the body. *Pflügers Arch. Ges. Physiol.*, **318**, 325
85. Brodal, A., Pompeiano, O. and Walberg, F. (1962). *The Vestibular Nuclei and Their Connections: Anatomy and Functional Correlations*. (London: Oliver and Boyd)
86. Stein, B. M. and Carpenter, M. B. (1967). Central projection of portions of the vestibular ganglia innervating specific parts of the labyrinth in the rhesus monkey. *Amer. J. Anat.*, **120**, 281

87. Gacek, R. R. (1969). The course and central termination of first order neurons supplying vestibular endorgans in the cat. *Acta Oto-laryng.* (*Stockholm*), **254**, 1

88. Mickle, W. A. and Ades, H. W. (1954). Rostral projection pathway of the vestibular system. *Amer. J. Physiol.*, **176**, 243

89. Gernandt, B. E. (1960). Generation of labyrinthine impulses, descending vestibular pathway, and modulation of vestibular activity by proprioceptive, cerebellar, and reticular influences. *Neural Mechanisms of the Auditory and Vestibular Systems.* (Springfield, Ill.: Thomas)

90. Kumoi, T., Hosomi, H. and Matsumura, H. (1963). An analysis of the vestibular evoked potentials in response to stimulation of the ampullar nerve. *Kobe J. Med. Sci.*, **9**, 79

91. Kumoi, T., Hosomi, H., Matsumura, H., Amatsu, M. and Asai, R. (1965). An analysis of the vestibular evoked potentials in response to stimulation of the vestibular nerve branches. *International Symposium on Vestibular and Oculomotor Problems* (Tokyo: Auspices of University of Tokyo)

92. Precht, W. and Shimazu, H. (1965). Functional connections of tonic and kinetic vestibular neurons with primary vestibular afferents. *J. Neurophysiol.*, **28**, 1014

93. Ito, M., Hongo, T. and Okada, Y. (1969). Vestibular-evoked postsynaptic potentials in Deiters' neurones. *Exp. Brain Res.*, **7**, 214

94. Walberg, F., Bowsher, D. and Brodal, A. (1958). The termination of primary vestibular fibres in the vestibular nuclei in the cat. An experimental study with silver methods. *J. Comp. Neurol.*, **110**, 391

95. Kawai, N., Ito, M. and Nozue, M. (1969). Postsynaptic influences on the vestibular non-Deiters nuclei from primary vestibular nerve. *Exp. Brain Res.*, **8**, 190

96. Richter, A., Ozawa, S. and Precht, W. (1972). Elektrotonische Kopplung zwischen vestibulans neuronen des Frosches. *Pflügers Arch. Ges. Physiol.*, **332** (Suppl.) R102

97. Sotelo, C. and Palay, S. L. (1970). The fine structure of the lateral vestibular nucleus in the rat. II. Synaptic organization. *Brain Res.*, **18**, 93

98. Korn, H., Sotelo, C. and Crepel, F. (1973). Electrotonic coupling between neurones in the rat lateral vestibular nucleus. *Exp. Brain Res.*, **16**, 255

99. Wilson, V. J. and Wylie, R. M. (1970). A short-latency labyrinthine input to the vestibular nuclei in the pigeon. *Science*, **168**, 124

100. Bennett, M. V. L., Pappas, G. D., Gimenez, M. and Nakajima, Y. (1967). Physiology and ultrastructure of electrotonic junctions. IV. Medullary electromotor nuclei in gymnotid fish. *J. Neurophysiol.*, **30**, 236

101. Korn, H. and Bennett, M. V. L. (1972). Electrotonic coupling between teleost oculomotor neurons; restriction to somatic regions and relation to function of somatic and dendritic sites of impulse initiation. *Brain Res.*, **38**, 433

102. Breuer, J. (1889). Neue Versuche an den Ohrbogengängen. *Pflügers Arch. Ges. Physiol.*, **44**, 135

103. Barany, R. (1907). *Physiologie und Pathologie des Bogengangsapparates beim Menschen.* (Wien: Franz Deuticke)

104. Dohlmann, G. (1925). Physikalische und physiologische Studien zur Theorie des Kalorischen Nystagmus. *Acta Oto-laryng.* (*Stockholm*), Suppl. 5
Dohlman, G. (1929). Experimentelle Untersuchungen über die galvanische Vestibularisreaktion. *Acta Oto-laryng.* (*Stockholm*), Suppl. 8, 1

105. Gernandt, B. E. (1949). Response of mammalian vestibular neurons to horizontal rotation and caloric stimulation. *J. Neurophysiol.*, **12**, 173

106. Lowenstein, O. (1955). The effect of galvanic polarization on the impulse discharge from sense endings in the isolated labyrinth of the Thornback ray (Raja clavata). *J. Physiol.* (*London*), **127**, 104

107. Weber, G. and Steiner, F. A. (1965). Labyrinthär erregbare Neurone im Hirnstamm und Kleinhirn der Katze. *Helv. Physiol. Pharmacol. Acta*, **23**, 61

108. Ewald, J. R. (1892). *Physiologische Untersuchungen über das Endorgan des N. Oktavus* (Wiesbaden: Bergmann)

109. Szentágothai, J. (1943). Die zentrale Innervation der Augenbewegungen. *Arch. Psychiat. Nervenkr.*, **116**, 721

110. Szentágothai, J. (1952). *Die Rolle der einzelnen Labyrinthrezeptoren bei der Orientation von Augen und Kopf im Raume* (Budapest: Akadémiai Kiado)

111. Trincker, D. (1957). Bestandspotentiale im Bogengangssystem des Meerschwein-chens und ihre Änderung bei experimentellen Cupula Ablenkungen. *Pflügers Arch. Ges. Physiol.*, **264**, 351

112. Adrian, E. D. (1943). Discharges from vestibular receptors in the cat. *J. Physiol. (London)*, **101**, 389

113. Duensing, F. and Schaefer, K. P. (1958). Die Aktivität einzelner Neurone im Bereich der Vestibulariskerne bei Horizontalbeschleunigungen unter besonderer Berücksichtigung des vestibulären Nystagmus. *Arch. Psychiat. Nervenkr.*, **198**, 225

114. Bizzi, E., Pompeiano, O., Somogyi, J. (1964). Spontaneous activity of single vestibular neurons of unrestrained cats during sleep and wakefulness. *Arch. Ital. Biol.*, **102**, 308

115. Gernandt, B. E. and Thulin, C. A. (1952). Vestibular connections of the brain stem. *Amer. J. Physiol.*, **171**, 121

116. Precht, W., Shimazu, H. and Markham, C. H. (1966). A mechanism of central compensation of vestibular function following hemilabyrinthectomy. *J. Neurophysiol.*, **29**, 996

117. Richter, A. and Precht, W. (1972). Responses of frog vestibular neurons to physiological stimulation of the labyrinth. *Pflügers Arch. Ges. Physiol.*, **339** (Suppl.) 335 R79

118. Eckel, W. (1954). Elektrophysiologische und histologische Untersuchungen im Vestibulariskerngebiet bei Drehreizen. *Arch. Ohr.-, Nas.-, u. Kehlk.-Heilk.*, **164**, 487

119. Ryu, J. H. and McCabe, B. F. (1971). Types of neuronal activity in the lateral vestibular nucleus. *Acta Oto-laryng. (Stockholm)*, **72**, 288

120. Ryu, J. H., McCabe, B. F. and Funasaka, S. (1969). Types of neuronal activity in the medial vestibular nucleus. *Acta Oto-laryng. (Stockholm)*, **68**, 137

121. Duensing, F. and Schaefer, K. P. (1959). Über die Konvergenz verschiedener labyrinthärer Afferenzen auf einzelne Neurone des Vestibulariskerngebietes. *Arch. Psychiat. Nervenkr.*, **199**, 345

122. Duensing, F. (1968). Die Aktivität der von den vertikalen Bogengängen abhängigen Neurone im Hirnstamm des Kaninchens. I. Mitteilung. Drehbeschleunigungen in Seitenlage. *Arch. Ohr.-, Nas.-, u. Kehlk.-Heilk.*, **192**, 32

123. Duensing, F. (1968). Die Aktivität der von den vertikalen Bogengägen anhängigen Neurone im Hirnstamm des Kaninchens. II. Mitteilung. Drehbeschleunigungen in verschiedenen Positionen. *Arch. Ohr.-, Nas.-, u. Kehlk.-Heilk.*, **192**, 51

124. Markham, C. H. (1968). Midbrain and contralateral labyrinth influences on brainstem vestibular neurons in the cat. *Brain Res.*, **9**, 312

125. Decher, D. (1963). Neues zur Labyrinthphysiologie. Die Drehreiz-Schwellen der verticalen Bogengänge. *Arch. Ohr.-, Nas.-, u. Kehlk.-Heilk.*, **181**, 395

126. Suzuki, J. I. and Cohen, B. (1966). Integration of semicircular canal activity. *J. Neurophysiol.*, **29**, 981

127. Hallpike, C. S. and Hood, J. D. (1953). The speed of the slow component of ocular nystagmus induced by angular acceleration of the head: its experimental determination and application to the physical theory of the cupular mechanism. *Proc. Roy. Soc. (London)*, **B141**, 216

128. Hulk, J. and Jongkees, L. B. W. (1948). The turning test with small regulable stimuli. II. The normal cupulogram. *J. Laryng.*, **62**, 70

129. Precht, W., Richter, A. and Grippo, J. (1969). Responses of neurones in cat's abducens nuclei to horizontal angular acceleration. *Pflügers Arch. Ges. Physiol.*, **309**, 285

130. Melvill Jones, G. and Milsum, J. H. (1970). Characteristics of neural transmission from the semicircular canal to the vestibular nuclei of cats. *J. Physiol. (London)*, **209**, 295

131. Hallpike, C. S. and Hood, J. D. (1953). Fatigue and adaptation of the cupular mechanism of the human horizontal semicircular canal: an experimental investigation. *Proc. Roy. Soc. (London)*, **B141**, 542

132. Albert, H. H. von (1965). Untersuchungen zur Habituation des postrotatorischen Nystagmus. *Dtsch. Z. Nervenheilk.*, **187**, 503

133. Lorente de Nó, R. (1933). Anatomy of the eighth nerve. The central projection of the nerve endings of the internal ear. *Laryngoscope*, **43**, 1

134. Hiebert, T. G. and Fernandez, C. (1965). Deitersian response to tilt. *Acta Oto-laryng.* (*Stockholm*), **60**, 180.
135. Fujita, Y., Rosenberg, J. and Segundo, J. P. (1968). Activity of cells in the lateral vestibular nucleus as a function of head position. *J. Physiol.* (*London*), **196**, 1
136. Schoen, L. (1957). Mikroableitungen einzelner zentraler Vestibularisneurone von Knochenfischen bei Statolithenreizen. *Z. Vergl. Physiol.*, **39**, 399
137. Peterson, B. W. (1967). Effect of tilting on the activity of neurons in the vestibular nuclei of the cat. *Brain Res.*, **6**, 606
138. Petersen, B. W. (1970). Distribution of neural responses to tilting within the vestibular nuclei of the cat. *J. Neurophysiol.*, **33**, 750
139. Orlovsky, G. N. and Pavlova, G. A. (1972). Response of Deiters' neurons to tilt during locomotion. *Brain Res.*, **42**, 212
140. Orlovsky, G. N. and Pavlova, G. A. (1973). Vestibular reactions of different descending pathways in cats with intact cerebellum and in decerebrated cats. *J. Neurophysiol.*, in the press
141. Schöne, H. (1962). Über den Einfluß der Schwerkraft auf die Augenrollung und die Wahrnehmung der Lage im Raum. *Z. Vergl. Physiol.*, **46**, 57
142. Shimazu, H. and Smith, C. M. (1971). Cerebellar and labyrinthine influences on single vestibular neurons identified by natural stimuli. *J. Neurophysiol.*, **34**, 493
143. Curthoys, I. S. and Markham, C. H. (1971). Convergence of labyrinthine influences on units in the vestibular nuclei of the cat. I. Natural stimulation. *Brain Res.*, **35**, 469
144. Markham, C. H. and Curthoys, I. S. (1972). Labyrinthine convergence on vestibular nuclear neurons using natural and electrical stimulation. *Progress in Brain Research*. Vol. 37, *Basic Aspects of Central Vestibular Mechanisms*. (Amsterdam: Elsevier)
145. Kasahara, M. and Uchino, Y. (1971). Selective mode of commissural inhibition induced by semicircular canal afferents on secondary vestibular neurons in the cat. *Brain Res.*, **34**, 366
146. Wilson, V. J. and Felpel, L. P. (1972). Specificity of semicircular canal input to neurons in the pigeon vestibular nuclei. *J. Neurophysiol.*, **35**, 253
147. Lorente de Nó, R. (1931). Ausgewählte Kapitel aus der vergleichenden Physiologie des Labyrinths. Die Augenmuskelreflexe beim Kaninchen und ihre Grundlagen. *Ergebn. Physiol.*, **32**, 71
148. Koella, W. (1950). Gleichgewichtsorgan und Augenmuskelsystem im Lichte der Koordinationslehre. *Vjschr. Naturforsch. Ges. Zurich. Beiheft*, **95**,
149. Holst, E. von, and Grisebach, E. (1951). Einfluß des Bogengangsystems auf die "subjektive Lotrechte" beim Menschen. *Naturwissenschaften*, **38**, 67
150. Bergstedt, M. (1961). The effect of gravitational force on the vestibular caloric test. *Acta Oto-laryng.* (*Stockholm*), **53**, 551
151. Bergstedt. M. (1961). Studies of postiional nystagmus in the human centrifuge. *Acta Oto-laryng.* (*Stockholm*), Suppl. 165, 1
152. Jackson, M. M. and Sears, C. W. (1966). Effect of weightlessness upon the normal nystagmic reaction. *Aerospace Med.*, **37**, 719
153. Gray, L. P. (1926). Some experimental evidence on the connections of the vestibular mechanism in the cat. *J. Comp. Neurol.*, **41**, 319
154. Rasmussen, A. T. (1932). Secondary vestibular tracts in the cat. *J. Comp. Neurol.*, **54**, 143
155. Ferraro, A., Pacella, B. L. and Barrera, S. E. (1940). Effects of the lesions of the medial vestibular nucleus. An anatomical and physiological study in macacus Rhesus monkeys. *J. Comp. Neurol.*, **73**, 7
156. Ladpli, R. and Brodal, A. (1968). Experimental studies of commissural and reticular formation projections from the vestibular nuclei in the cat. *Brain Res.*, **8**, 65
157. Vito, R. V. de, Brusa, A. and Arduini, A. (1956). Cerebellar and vestibular influences on Deitersian units. *J. Neurophysiol.*, **19**, 241
158. Fredrickson, J. M., Schwarz, D. and Kornhuber, H. H. (1966). Convergence and interaction of vestibular and deep somatic afferents upon neurons in the vestibular nuclei of the cat. *Acta Oto-laryng.* (*Stockholm*), **61**, 168
159. Kasahara, M., Mano, M., Oshima, T., Ozawa, S. and Shimazu, H. (1968).

Contralateral short latency inhibition of central vestibular neurones in the horizontal canal system. *Brain Res.*, **8**, 376

160. Mano, M., Oshima, T. and Shimazu, H. (1968). Inhibitory commissural fibres interconnecting the bilateral vestibular nuclei. *Brain Res.*, **8**, 378

161. Precht, W., Grippo, J. and Wagner, A. (1967). Contribution of different types of central vestibular neurons to the vestibulo-spinal system. *Brain Res.*, **4**, 119

162. Shimazu, H. (1967). Mutual interactions between bilateral vestibular nuclei and their significance in motor regulation. *Neurophysiological Basis of Normal and Abnormal Motor Activities* (New York: Raven Press)

163. Moruzzi, G. and Pompeiano, O. (1957). Inhibitory mechanisms underlying the collapse of decerebrate rigidity after unilateral fastigial lesions. *J. Comp. Neurol.*, **107**, 1

164. Batini, C., Moruzzi, G. and Pompeiano, O. (1957). Cerebellar release phenomena. *Arch. Ital. Biol.*, **95**, 71

165. Kornhuber, H. H. (1966). *Physiologie und Klinik des zentralvestibulären Systems (Blick- und Stützmotorik)*. Hals-Nasen-Ohrenheilkunde. Band III/Teil 3 (J. Berendes, R. Link and F. Zöllner, editors) (Stuttgart: Thieme)

166. Cohen, B. (1971). Vestibulo-ocular relations. *The Control of Eye Movements* (P. Bach-y-Rita, editor) (New York: Academic Press)

167. Fuchs, A. F. (1971). The saccadic system. *The Control of Eye Movements* (P. Bach-y-Rita, editor) (New York: Academic Press)

168. Robinson, D. A. (1968). Eye movement control in primates. *Science*, **161**, 1219

169. Cohen, B. and Suzuki, J. I. (1963). Eye movements induced by ampullary nerve stimulation. *Amer. J. Physiol.*, **204**, 347

170. Cohen, B., Suzuki, J. I., Shanzer, S. and Bender, M. B. (1964). Semicircular canal control of eye movements. *The Oculomotor System.* (New York: Hoeber)

171. Fluur, E. (1959). Influences of semicircular ducts on extraocular muscles. *Acta Oto-laryng. (Stockholm)*, Suppl. 149, 1

172. Szentágothai, J. (1950). The elementary vestibulo–ocular reflex arc. *J. Neurophysiol.*, **13**, 395

173. Lorente de Nó, R. (1933). Vestibulo-ocular reflex arc. *Arch. Neurol. Psychiat.*, **30**, 245

174. Szentágothai, J. (1942). Die innere Gliederung des Oculomotorius-Kernes. *Arch. Psychiat. Nervenkr.*, **115**, 127

175. Bender, M. B. and Weinstein, E. A. (1943). Functional representation in the oculomotor and trochlear nuclei. *Arch. Neurol. Psychiat.*, **48**, 98

176. Warwick, R. (1953). Representation of the extraocular muscles in the oculomotor nuclei of the monkey. *J. Comp. Neurol.*, **98**, 449

177. Tarlov, E. (1972). Anatomy of the two vestibulo-oculomotor projection systems. *Progress in Brain Research*, Vol. 37, *Basic Aspects of Central Vestibular Mechanisms* (A. Brodal and O. Pompeiano, editors) (Amsterdam: Elsevier)

178. McMasters, R. E., Weiss, A. H. and Carpenter, M. B. (1966). Vestibular projections to the nuclei of the extra-ocular muscles. Degeneration resulting from discrete partial lesions of the vestibular nuclei in the monkey. *Amer. J. Anat.*, **118**, 163

179. Tarlov, E. (1970). Organization of vestibulo–oculomotor projections in the cat. *Brain Res.*, **20**, 159

180. Baker, R. G., Mano, N. and Shimazu, H. (1969). Postsynaptic potentials in abducens motoneurons induced by vestibular stimulation. *Brain Res.*, **15**, 577

181. Richter, A. and Precht, W. (1968). Inhibition of abducens motoneurones by vestibular nerve stimulation. *Brain Res.*, **11**, 701

182. Precht, W. and Baker, R. (1972). Synaptic organization of the vestibulotrochlear pathway. *Exp. Brain Res.*, **14**, 158

183. Berthoz, A. and Baker, R. (1972). Localisation électrophysiologique des motoneurones du noyau oculomoteur innervant le petit oblique, et nature des influences d'origine labyrinthique sur ces motoneurones. *C.R. Acad. Sci. (Paris)*, **275**, 425

184. Precht, W. (1972). Vestibular and cerebellar control of oculomotor functions. *Bibl. Ophthal. (Basel)*, **82**, 71

185. Highstein, S. M., Ito, M. and Tsuchiya, T. (1971). Synaptic linkage in the vestibulo-ocular reflex pathway of rabbit. *Exp. Brain Res.*, **13**, 306

186. Highstein, S. M. and Ito, M. (1971). Differential localization within the vestibular nuclear complex of the inhibitory and excitatory cells innervating IIIrd nucleus oculomotor neurons in rabbit. *Brain Res.*, **29**, 358
187. Highstein, S. M. (1971). Organization of the inhibitory and excitatory vestibulo–ocular reflex pathways to the third and fourth nuclei in rabbit. *Brain Res.*, **32**, 218
188. Kidokoro, Y. (1969). Cerebellar and vestibular control of fish oculomotor neurones. *Neurobiology of Cerebellar Evolution and Development*. (R. Llinás, editor) (Chicago: Amer. Med. Assoc. Educ. and Res. Fed.)
189. Boeder, P. (1962). Co-operative action of extraocular muscles. *Brit. J. Ophthal.*, **46**, 397
190. Kleyn, A. de and Magnus, R. (1920). Tonische Labyrinthreflexe auf die Augenmuskeln. *Pflügers Arch. Ges. Physiol.*, **178**, 179
191. Lorente de Nó, R. (1928). *Die Labyrinthreflexe auf die Augenmuskeln nach einseitiger Labyrinthextirpation nebst einer kurzen Angabe über den Nerven-mechanismus der vestibulären Augenbewegungen* (Berlin and Wien: Urban und Schwarzenberg)
192. Miller, E. F. (1962). Counter-rolling of the human eyes produced by head tilt with respect to gravity. *Acta Oto-laryng.* (*Stockholm*), **54**, 479   %
193. Cohen, B., Krejcova, A. and Highstein, S. (1970). Ocular counter-rolling induced by static head tilt in the monkeys. *Fed. Proc.* (*Fed. Amer. Soc. Exp. Biol.*), **29**, 454
194. Szentágothai, J. (1964). Pathways and synaptic articulation patterns connecting vestibular receptors and oculomotor nuclei. *The Oculumotor System* (New York: Hoeber)
195. Suzuki, J. I., Tokumasu, K. and Goto, K. (1969). Eye movements from single utricular nerve stimulation in the cat. *Acta Oto-laryng.* (*Stockholm*), **68**, 350
196. Suzuki, J. I. (1972). Vestibulo–oculomotor relations: static responses. *Progress in Brain Research*, Vol. 37, *Basic Aspects of Central Vestibular Mechanisms* (A. Brodal and O. Pompeiano, editors) (Amsterdam: Elsevier)
197. Schaefer, K. P. (1965). Die Erregungsmuster einzelner Neurone des Abducens-Kernes beim Kaninchen. *Pflügers Arch. Ges. Physiol.*, **284**, 31
198. Berthoz, A., Baker, R. and Precht, W. (1973). Labyrinthine control of inferior oblique motoneurons. *Exp. Brain Res.*, in the press
199. Robinson, D. A. (1971). Models of oculomotor neural organization. *The Control of Eye Movements* (P. Bach-y-Rita *et al.*, editors) (New York: Academic Press)
200. Precht, W. and Llinás, R. (1969). Functional organization of the vestibular afferents to the cerebellar cortex of the frog. *Exp. Brain Res.*, **9**, 30
201. Precht, W. and Llinás, R. (1969). Comparative aspects of the vestibular input to the cerebellum. *Neurobiology of Cerebellar Evolution and Development* (R. Llinás, editor) (Chicago: Amer. Med. Assoc. Educ. Res. Fed.)
202. Ito, M., Highstein, S. M. and Fukuda, J. (1970). Cerebellar inhibition of the vestibulo-ocular reflex in rabbit and cat and its blockage by picrotoxin. *Brain Res.*, **17**, 524
203. Baker, R., Precht, W. and Llinás, R. (1972). Cerebellar modulatory action on the vestibulo–trochlear pathway in the cat. *Exp. Brain Res.*, **15**, 364
204. Fukuda, J., Highstein, S. M. and Ito, M. (1972). Cerebellar inhibitory control of the vestibulo–ocular reflex investigated in rabbit IIIrd nucleus. *Exp. Brain Res.*, **14**, 511.
205. Manni, E. (1950). Localisazzioni cerebellari corticali nella cavia. II. Effeti di lesioni delle parti vestibolari del cervelletto. *Arch. Fisiol.*, **50**, 110
206. Uemera, T. and Cohen, B. (1972). Vestibulo–ocular reflexes: effects of vestibular nuclear lesions. *Progress in Brain Research*, Vol. 37, *Basic Aspects of Central Vestibular Mechanisms* (A. Brodal and O. Pompeiano, editors) (Amsterdam: Elsevier)
207. Spiegel, E. A. and Price, J. B. (1939). Origin of the quick component of laby-rinthine nystagmus. *Arch. Otolaryng.*, **30**, 576
208. Baker, R. and Berthoz, A. (1971). Spontaneous nystagmus recorded in trochlear motoneurons following labyrinthine lesion. *Brain Res.*, **32**, 239
209. Maeda, M., Shimazu, H. and Shinoda, Y. (1972). Nature of synaptic events in cat abducens motoneurons at slow and quick phase of vestibular nystagmus. *J. Neurophysiol.*, **35**, 279

210. Shimazu, H. (1972). Vestibulo-oculomotor relations: dynamic responses. *Progress in Brain Research*, Vol. 37, *Basic Aspects of Central Vestibular Mechanisms* (A. Brodal and O. Pompeiano, editors) (Amsterdam: Elsevier)

211. Duensing, F. and Schaefer, K. P. (1957). Die Neuronenaktivität in der Formatio reticularis des Rhombencephalons beim vestibulären Nystagmus. *Arch. Psychiat. Nervenkr.*, **196**, 265

212. Korn, H. and Bennett, M. V. L. (1971). Dendritic and somatic impulse initiation in fish oculomotor neurons during vestibular nystagmus. *Brain Res.*, **27**, 169

213. Pompeiano, O. (1972). Reticular control of the vestibular nuclei: physiology and pharmacology. *Progress in Brain Research*, Vol. 37, *Basic Aspects of Central Vestibular Mechanisms* (A. Bordal and O. Pompeiano, editors) (Amsterdam: Elsevier)

214. Larsell, O. (1923). The cerebellum of the frog. *J. Comp. Neurol.*, **36**, 89

215. Larsell, O. (1929). The comparative morphology of the membraneous labyrinth and the lateral-line organs in their relation to the development of the cerebellum. *The Cerebellum* (Baltimore: William and Wilkins)

216. Herrick, C. J. (1924). Origin and evolution of the cerebellum. *Arch. Neurol. Psychiat. (Chicago)*, **11**, 621

217. Jansen, J. and Brodal, A. (1954). *Aspects of Cerebellar Anatomy* (Oslo: Johan Grundt Tanum)

218. Brodal, A. and Hoivik, B. (1964). Site and mode of termination of primary vestibulo-cerebellar fibres in the cat· An experimental study with silver impregnation methods. *Arch. Ital. Biol.*, **102**, 1

219. Wilson, V. J., Anderson, J. A. and Felix, D. (1972). Semicircular canal input pigeon vestibulocerebellum. *Brain Res.*, **45**, 230

220. Snider, R. S. (1936). Alterations which occur in mossy terminals of the cerebellum following transection of the brachium pontis. *J. Comp. Neurol.*, **65**, 417

221. Szentágothai, J. and Rajkovits, K. (1959). Über den Ursprung der Kletterfasern des Kleinhirns. *Z. Anat. Entwickl.-Gesch.*, **121**, 130

222. Maekawa, K. and Simpson, J. I. (1972). Climbing fibre activation of Purkinje cell in the flocculus by impulses transferred through the visual pathway. *Brain Res.*, **39**, 245

223. Llinás, R., Precht, W. and Clarke, M. (1971). Cerebellar Purkinje cell responses to physiological stimulation of the vestibular system in the frog. *Exp. Brain Res.*, **13**, 408

224. Brodal, A. and Torvik, A. (1957). Über den Ursprung der sekundären vestibulo-cerebellaren Fasern bei der Katze. Eine experimentellanatomische Studie. *Arch. Psychiat. Nervenkr.*, **195**, 550

225. Anderson, S. and Gernandt, B. E. (1954). Cortical projection of vestibular nerve in cat. *Acta Oto-laryng. (Stockholm)*, Suppl. 116, 10

226. Arduini, A. and Pompeiano, O. (1957). Microelectrode analysis of units of the rostral portion of the nucleus fastigius. *Arch. Ital. Biol.*, **95**, 56

227. Precht, W. and Llinás, R. (1968). Direct vestibular afferents to cat cerebellar nuclei. *Proc. XXIVth Internat. Congr. Physiological Sci.*

228. Jansen, J. and Brodal, A. (1958). *Das Kleinhirn. v. Möllendorffs Handbuch der mikroskopischen Anatomie des Menschen* IV/8 (Berlin, Gottingen, Heidelberg: Springer Verlag)

229. Eccles, J. C., Ito, M. and Szentágothai, J. (1967). *The Cerebellum as a Neuronal Machine* (Berlin, Heidelberg and New York: Springer-Verlag)

230. Walberg, F. and Jansen, J. (1961). Cerebellar cortico–vestibular fibres in the cat. *Exp. Neurol.*, **3**, 32

231. Ito, M., Kawai, N., Udo, M. and Mano, N. (1969). Axon reflex activation of Deiters neurones from the cerebellar cortex through collaterals of the cerebellar afferents. *Exp. Brain Res.*, **8**, 249

232. Angaut, P. and Brodal, A. (1967). The projection of the 'vestibulocerebellum' onto the vestibular nuclei in the cat. *Arch. Ital. Biol.*, **105**, 441

233. Mugnaini, E. and Walberg, F. (1967). An experimental electron microscopical study on the mode of termination of cerebellar cortico–vestibular fibres in the cat lateral vestibular nucleus (Deiters' nucleus). *Exp. Brain Res.*, **4**, 212

234. Moruzzi, G. (1950). *Problems in Cerebellar Physiology*. (Springfield, Ill.: C. C. Thomas)

235. Brookhardt, J. M. (1960). *The Cerebellum. Handbook of Physiology*, Sect. I, *Neurophysiology*, II (Washington, D.C.: American Physiological Society)

236. Sherrington, C. S. (1898). Decerebrate rigidity and reflex co-ordination of movements. *J. Physiol.* (*London*), **22**, 319

237. Pompeiano, O. and Cotti, G. (1959). Analisi microelettrodica delle proiezioni cerebello-deitersiane. *Arch. Sci. Biol.* (*Bologna*), **43**, 57

238. Ito, M., Kawai, M., Udo, M. and Sato, N. (1968). Cerebellar evoked disinhibition in dorsal Deiters neurones. *Exp. Brain Res.*, **6**, 247

239. Fernandez, C. and Fredrickson, J. M. (1963). Experimental cerebellar lesions and their effect on vestibular function. *Acta Oto-laryng.* (*Stockholm*), Suppl. 192, 52

240. Halstead, W. (1935). The effects of cerebellar lesions upon the habituation of postrotational nystagmus. *Comp. Psychol. Monogr.*, **12**, 1

241. Spiegel, E. A. and Scala, N. P. (1942). Positional nystagmus in cerebellar lesions. *J. Neurophysiol.*, **5**, 247

242. Grant, G., Aschan, G. and Ekvall, L. (1964). Nystagmus produced by localized cerebellar lesions. *Acta Oto-laryng.* (*Stockholm*), **58**, Suppl. 192, 78

243. Aschan, G., Ekvall, L. and Grant, G. (1964). Nystagmus following stimulation in the central vestibular pathways using permanently implanted electrodes. *Acta Oto-laryng.* (*Stockholm*), **192**, 63

244. Pompeiano, O. and Brodal, A. (1957). Spino-vestibular fibres in the cat. An experimental study. *J. Comp. Neurol.*, **108**, 353

245. Brodal, A. and Angaut, P. (1967). The termination of spinovestibular fibres in the cat. *Brain Res.*, **5**, 494

246. Lorente de Nó, R. (1924). Etudes sur le cerveau postérieur. III. Sur les connexions extracérébelleuses des fascicules afférents au cerveau, et sur la fonction de cet organe. *Trav. Lab. Rech. Biol.*, **22**, 51

247. Allen, G. I., Sabah, N. H. and Toyama, K. (1972). Synaptic actions of peripheral nerve impulses upon Deiters neurones via the mossy fibre afferents. *J. Physiol.* (*London*), **226**, 335

248. Ito, M., Hongo, T., Yoshida, M., Okada, Y. and Obata, K. (1964). Antidromic and trans-synaptic activation of Deiters' neurones induced from the spinal cord. *Jap. J. Physiol.*, **14**, 638

249. Wilson, V. J., Kato, M., Thomas, R. C. and Peterson, B. W. (1966). Excitation of lateral vestibular neurones by peripheral afferent fibres. *J. Neurophysiol.*, **29**, 508

250. Wilson, V. J., Kato, M., Petersen, B. W. and Wylie, R. M. (1967). A single-unit analysis of the organization of Deiters' nucleus. *J. Neurophysiol.*, **30**, 603

251. Gernandt, B. E. (1970). Discharges from utricular receptors in the cat. *Exp. Neurol.*, **26**, 203

252. Allen, G. I., Sabah, N. H. and Toyama, K. (1972). Synaptic actions of peripheral nerve impulses upon Deiters neurones via the climbing fibre afferents. *J. Physiol.* (*London*), **226**, 311

253. Bruggencate, G. Ten, Sonnhof, U., Teichmann, R. and Weller, E. (1971). A study of the synaptic input to Deiters' neurones evoked by stimulation of peripheral nerves and spinal cord. *Brain Res.*, **25**, 207

254. Pompeiano, O. (1972). Spinovestibular relations, anatomical and physiological aspects. *Progress in Brain Research*. Vol. 37, *Basic Aspects of Central Vestibular Mechanisms*. (A. Brodal and O. Pompeiano, editors) (Amsterdam: Elsevier)

255. Pompeiano, O. and Barnes, C. D. (1971). Effect of sinusoidal muscle stretch on neurones in medial and descending vestibular nuclei. *J. Neurophysiol.*, **34**, 725

256. Landgren, S. and Silfvenius, H. (1971). Nucleus Z, the medullary relay in the projection path of the cerebral cortex of group I muscle afferents from cat's hind limb. *J. Physiol.* (*London*), **218**, 551

257. Koella, W. P., Nakao, H., Evans, R. L. and Wada, J. (1956). Interaction of vestibular and proprioceptive reflexes in the decerebrate cat. *Amer. J. Physiol.*, **185**, 607

258. Nyberg-Hansen, R. (1964). Origin and termination of fibres from the vestibular nuclei descending in the medial longitudinal fasciculus. An experimental study with silver impregnation methods in the cat. *J. Comp. Neurol.*, **122**, 355

259. Lund, S. and Pompeiano, O. (1965). Descending pathways with monosynaptic action on motoneurones. *Experientia (Basel)*, **21**, 602

260. Grillner, S., Hongo, T. and Lund, S. (1966). Descending pathways with monosynaptic action on motoneurones. *Acta Physiol. Scand.*, **68**, Suppl. 277, 60

261. Grillner, S., Hongo, T. and Lund, S. (1970). The vestibulospinal tract. Effects on α-motoneurons in the lumbosacral spinal cord in the cat. *Exp. Brain Res.*, **10**, 94

262. Wilson, V. J. and Yoshida, M. (1969). Comparison of effects of stimulation of Deiters' nucleus and medial longitudinal fasciculus on neck, forelimb, and hindlimb motoneurons. *J. Neurophysiol.*, **32**, 743

263. Wilson, V. J. and Yoshida, M. (1969). Monosynaptic inhibition of neck motoneurons by the medial vestibular nucleus. *Exp. Brain Res.*, **9**, 365

264. Bruggencate, G. Ten, Burke, R., Lundberg, A. and Udo, M. (1969). Interaction between vestibulospinal tract and Ia afferents. *Brain Res.*, **14**, 529

265. Erulkar, S. D., Sprague, D. M., Whitsel, B. L., Dogan, S. and Jannetta, P. J. (1966). Organization of the vestibular projection to the spinal cord of the cat. *J. Neurophysiol.*, **29**, 626

266. Grillner, S. and Hongo, T. (1972). Vestibulospinal effects on motoneurones and interneurones in the lumbosacral cord. *Progress in Brain Research*, Vol. 37, *Basic Aspects of Central Vestibular Mechanisms*. (A. Brodal and O. Pompeiano, editors) (Amsterdam: Elsevier)

267. Carli, G., Diete-Spiff, K. and Pompeiano, O. (1967). Responses of the muscle spindles and of the extrafusal fibres in an extensor muscle to stimulation of the lateral vestibular nucleus in the cat. *Arch. Ital. Biol.*, **105**, 209

268. Diete-Spiff, K., Carli, G. and Pompeiano, O. (1967). Comparison of the effects of stimulation of the VIIIth cranial nerve, the vestibular nuclei or the reticular formation on the gastrocnemius muscle and its spindles. *Arch. Ital. Biol.*, **105**, 243

269. Grillner, S., Hongo, T. and Lund, S. (1969). Descending monosynaptic and reflex control of γ-motoneurones. *Acta Physiol. Scand.*, **75**, 592

270. Gernandt, B. E. (1968). Functional properties of the descending medial longitudinal fasciculus. *Exp. Neurol.*, **22**, 326

271. Orlovsky, G. N. (1972). The effect of different descending systems on flexor and extensor activity during locomotion. *Brain Res.*, **40**, 359

272. Ehrhardt, K. J. and Wagner, A. (1970). Labyrinthine and neck reflexes recorded from spinal single motoneurons in the cat. *Brain Res.*, **19**, 87

273. Berthoz, A. and Anderson, J. H. (1971). Frequency analyses of vestibular influence on extensor motoneurons. I. Response to tilt in forelimb extensors. *Brain Res.*, **34**, 370

274. Berthoz, A. and Anderson, J. H. (1971). Frequency analysis of vestibular influence on extensor motoneurons. II. Relationship between neck and forelimb extensors. *Brain Res.*, **34**, 376

275. Brodal, A. (1972). Anatomy of the vestibuloreticular connections and possible 'vestibular' ascending pathways from the reticular formation. *Progress in Brain Research*, Vol. 37, *Basic Aspects of Central Vestibular Mechanisms*. (A. Brodal and O. Pompeiano, editors) (Amsterdam: Elsevier)

276. Potthoff, P. C., Richter, H. P. and Burandt, H. R. (1967). Multisensorische Konvergenzen an Hirnstammneuronen der Katze. *Arch. Psychiat. Nervenkr.*, **210**, 36

277. Walberg, F. (1972). Descending and reticular relations to the vestibular nuclei: anatomy. *Progress in Brain Research*, Vol. 37, *Basic Aspects of Central Vestibular Mechanisms*. (A. Brodal and O. Pompeiano, editors) (Amsterdam: Elsevier)

278. Duensing, F., Schaefer, K. P. and Trevisan, C. (1963). Die Raddrehung vermittelnde Neurone in der zentralen Funktionsstruktur der Labyrinthstellreflexe auf Kopf und Augen. *Arch. Psychiat. Nervenkr.*, **204**, 113

279. Markham, C. H., Precht, W. and Shimazu, H. (1966). Effect of stimulation of interstitial nucleus of Cajal on vestibular unit activity in the cat. *J. Neurophysiol.*, **29**, 493

280. Hassler, R. and Hess, W. R. (1954). Experimentelle und anatomische Befunde über die Drehbewegungen und ihre nervösen Apparate. *Arch. Psychiat. Nervenkr.*, **192**, 488

281. Spiegel, E. A. (1933). Role of vestibular nuclei in cortical innervation of the eye muscles. *Arch. Neurol. Psychiat.*, **29**, 1084

282. Gildenberg, P. L. and Hassler, R. (1971). Influence of stimulation of the cerebral cortex on vestibular nuclei units in the cat. *Exp. Brain Res.*, **14**, 77

283. Grüsser, O. J. and Grüsser-Cornehls, U. (1972). Interaction of vestibular and visual inputs in the visual system. *Progress in Brain Research*, Vol. 37, *Basic Aspects of Central Vestibular Mechanisms* (Amsterdam: Elsevier)

284. Walzl, E. W. and Mountcastle, V. (1949). Projection of vestibular nerve to cerebral cortex of the cat. *Amer. J. Physiol.*, **159**, 595

285. Landgren, S., Silfvenius, H. and Wolsk, D. (1967). Somato-sensory paths to the second cortical projection area of the group I muscle afferents. *J. Physiol. (London)*, **191**, 543

286. Sans, A., Raymond, J. and Marty, R. (1970). Résponses thalamiques et corticales à la stimulation électrique du nerf vestibulaire de chat. *Exp. Brain Res.*, **10**, 265

287. Boisacq-Schepens, N. and Hanus, M. (1972). Motor cortex vestibular responses in the chloralosed cat. *Exp. Brain Res.*, **14**, 539

288. Oscarsson, O. and Rosén, I. (1966). Short-latency projections to the cat's cerebral cortex from skin and muscle afferents in the contralateral forelimb. *J. Physiol. (London)*, **182**, 164

289. Kornhuber, H. H. and Aschoff, J. C. (1964). Somatisch-vestibuläre Integration an Neuronen des motorischen Cortex. *Naturwissenschaften*, **51**, 62

290. Frederickson, J. M., Figge, U., Scheid, P. and Kornhubber, H. H. (1966). Vestibular nerve projection to the cerebral cortex of the Rhesus monkey. *Exp. Brain Res.*, **2**, 318

291. Schwarz, D. W. F. and Fredrickson, J. M. (1971). Rhesus monkey vestibular cortex: a bimodal primary projection field. *Science*, **172**, 280

292. Massopust, L. C. Jr. and Daigle, H. J. (1960). Cortical projection of the medial and spinal vestibular nuclei in the cat. *Exp. Neurol.*, **2**, 179

293. Hassler, R. (1948). Forels Haubenfascicel als vestibuläre Empfindungsbahn mit Bemerkungen über einige andere sekundäre Bahnen des Vestibularis und Trigeminus. *Arch. Psychiat. Nervenkr.*, **180**, 23

294. Hassler, R. (1972). Hexapartition of inputs as a primary role of the thalamus. *Corticothalamic projections and sensorymotor activities:* (T. Frigyesi, E. Rinvik and M. D. Yahr, editors) (New York: Raven Press)

295. Carpenter, M. B. and Strominger, N. L. (1964). Cerebello-oculomotor fibres in the rhesus monkey. *J. Comp. Neurol.*, **123**, 211

296. Deecke, L., Schwarz, D. W. F. and Fredrickson, J. M. (1972). VPI, the vestibular thalamic nucleus in the Rhesus monkey. *Pflügers Arch. Ges. Physiol.*, **R80**, 159

297. Tyler, J. B. and Bard, B. (1949). Motion sickness. *Physiol. Rev.*, **29**, 311

298. Money, K. E. (1970). Motion sickness. *Physiol. Rev.*, **50**

299. Spiegel, E. A. and Demetriades, T. D. (1922). Beitrag zum Studium des vegetativen Nervensystems. 3. Mitteilung: Der Einfluβ des Vestibularapparates auf das Gefäβsystem. *Pflügers Arch. Ges. Physiol.*, **196**, 185

300. Spiegel, E. A. and Demetriades, T. D. (1924). Beiträge zum Studium des vegetativen Nervensystems. 7. Teil: Der zentrale Mechanismus der vestibulären Blutdrucksenkung und ihre Bedeutung für die Entstehung desLabyrinths chwindels. *Pflügers Arch. Ges. Physiol.*, **205**, 329

301. Uchino, Y., Kudo, N., Tsuda, K. and Iwamura, Y. (1970). Vestibular inhibition of sympathetic nerve activities. *Brain Res.*, **22**, 195

302. Megirian, D. and Manning, J. W. (1967). Input-output relations of the vestibular system. *Arch. Ital. Biol.*, **105**, 15

303. Tang, P. C. and Gernandt, B. E. (1969). Autonomic responses to vestibular stimulation. *Exp. Neurol.*, **24**, 558

304. Cobbold, A. F., Megirian, D. and Sherrey, J. H. (1968). Vestibular evoked activity in autonomic motor outflows. *Arch. Ital. Biol.*, **106**, 113

305. Fernandez, C., Goldberg, J. M. and Abend, W. K. (1972). Response to static tilts of peripheral neurons innervating otolith organs of the squirrel monkey. *J. Neurophysiol.*, **35**, 978

306. Loe, P. R., Tomko, D. L. and Werner, G. (1973). The neural signal of angular head position in primary afferent vestibular nerve axons. *J. Physiol.*, **230**, 29

307. Schwindt, P. C., Richter, A. and Precht, W. (1973). Short latency utricular and canal input to ipsilateral abducens motoneurons. *Brain Res.*, **59**.

4
The Neurophysiology of Movement Performance

R. PORTER
Monash University, Clayton, Victoria

4.1	INTRODUCTION	151
4.2	MOTONEURONES	152
	4.2.1 *Reflex activation of motoneurones*	154
	4.2.2 *Effects of supraspinal activity on spinal motoneurones*	157
	4.2.3 *The effects of cortical stimulation on spinal motoneurones*	158
	4.2.4 *Corticospinal actions on individual motoneurones*	160
	4.2.5 *The effects of destruction of pathways which influence motoneurones*	162
4.3	RECORDING FROM NEURONAL ELEMENTS DURING MOVEMENT	164
4.4	AFFERENT SYSTEMS IN MOVEMENT PERFORMANCE	170

4.1 INTRODUCTION

In his book, *Integrative Action of the Nervous System*, Sherrington[1] discussed 'Movement as an outcome of the working of the brain' (p. 307) and he developed the concept of motoneurones as the 'final common path' for movement. He pointed out that movement occurred by the activation of muscles and that this activation, in turn, resulted from the discharge of nerve impulses along axons of motoneurones which were the foci of convergence of all reflex-arcs capable of influencing muscle. This is still a convenient starting point for considerations of the nervous system's involvement in management of muscles and movement. From it, the properties of motoneurones and the muscle fibres they innervate may be examined. The anatomical connections between afferent fibres or central brain structures and these motoneurones may be studied to reveal details of the influences produced on motoneurones. Moreover, attempts may be made to describe and evaluate the probable function of these influences and their interactions during movement performance.

Although a great deal of experimental work has been devoted to these areas of study, the available information is limited in a number of ways. Most of the work has concerned the motoneurones supplying the musculature of the cat's hind limb[2]. There is very little detailed information about other motoneurones in other animals. But there are enough experimental observations to show that, even in the cat's spinal cord, not all motoneurones have identical properties[3], that the actions exerted by different afferent systems may vary with the different properties of the motoneurones and that some of this specialisation may be related to the functional development of muscles and movement performance in particular situations.

4.2 MOTONEURONES

The concept of different populations of motoneurones with different physical properties and connections with different functional groups of motor units has been reviewed recently by Granit in his book *The Basis of Motor Control*[4]. Individual motoneurones in the spinal cord of the cat, when activated by muscle stretch, show either a tonic (i.e. maintained discharge) or phasic (i.e. discharge only at the onset of stretch) response. Evidence that these responses reflect, at least in part, the nature and properties of the individual motoneurones has been collected and has led to the view that there are specific 'tonic' and 'phasic' motoneurones. Both with weak reflex activation and when driven to produce a maximum response, these different classes of motoneurones remain true to type. The maintained discharge of the tonic motoneurones responding to muscle stretch has been shown to be independent of reinforcement from concomitant fusimotor fibre activation because it persists after section of ventral roots. Moreover, when activated over a number of different reflex pathways, the response of an individual motoneurone maintains its tonic or its phasic character[5].

For the most part, tonic motoneurones tend to have slowly conducting axons of small diameter and phasic motoneurones have rapidly conducting axons. The cells of the tonic motoneurones have higher input resistance and need weaker currents passed across their membranes from an intracellular electrode in order to achieve threshold depolarisation for repetitive discharge. But, when these cells are made to discharge in response to applied currents, the relationship between current strength and firing rate differs from that of phasic motoneurones in that larger increments in current strength are required in order to produce a given increase in discharge frequency in the tonic motoneurones[6]. When caused to discharge, the duration of the after-hyperpolarisation tends to be longer in tonic than in phasic motoneurones[7]. Whether or not this hyperpolarisation plays a major role in limiting the firing frequency of motoneurones under natural conditions is not established. Moreover, the function of Renshaw cells, which could also tend to prevent high-frequency discharge of motoneurones, requires to be evaluated in relation to natural movement.

There is a good correlation between the electrical measurements of such parameters as motoneurone input resistance and membrane time constant and histological estimates of cell size and the numbers and the diameters of dendritic branches[6]. Direct correlates for individual motoneurones have recently been obtained by labelling cells in which electrical measurements have been made and then estimating cellular dimensions[8]. It may be demonstrated by electrical stimulation of individual motoneurones with pulses of current passed through an intracellular microelectrode that tonic motoneurones supplying the cat's hind-limb tend to supply slow-twitch muscle fibres while phasic motoneurones tend to supply fast-twitch muscle fibres.

In a number of recent studies some of the electrotonic characteristics of alpha motoneurones supplying the cat's hind-limb have been examined[9-11]. An indication of some of the differences in different populations of motoneurones supplying the cat *triceps surae* muscles is contained in the following summary from Burke and ten Bruggencate[10]. It reveals that while the membrane time constants and input resistance measurements varied with cell size and the innervation of fast-twitch and slow-twitch muscle fibers, the characteristic electrotonic length of the equivalent dendritic cable[12] was similar for the two populations.

Table 4.1 Cat triceps surae a-motoneurones supplying fast- and slow-twitch muscle units

	Fast-twitch muscle units ($N = 13$)	Slow-twitch muscle units ($N = 12$)
Time constant (T_m)	5.58 ± 1.93 ms	6.70 ± 2.05 ms
Electrotonic length (L)	1.57 ± 0.35 λ	1.49 ± 0.21 λ
Input resistance (R_N)	0.78 ± 0.17 MΩ	1.87 ± 0.74 MΩ

It is likely that there is a gradation in properties of motoneurones between the largest alpha motoneurones and the smallest. These properties will determine in part the responsiveness of the individual motoneurone to a particular afferent influence[3]. But other factors such as the density and distribution of afferent terminals and the magnitude of the synaptic action exerted by these may also influence responsiveness[13, 14].

In studying the functional connections of motoneurones, it has been important to understand the arrangement of these cells in the anterior horn of the spinal cord. Thorough mapping of the territories occupied by particular pools of motoneurones in the lumbosacral spinal cord of the cat was carried out by Romanes[15] who localised the motoneurones for individual muscles by identifying chromatolysis in their cell bodies after section of muscle nerves. A similar study of the monkey spinal cord has also been carried out. As a result of such investigations and many similar ones[16], it has been possible to give a general account of the organisation of a-motoneurones which has been useful in interpreting the connections of central nervous pathways which are afferent to the motor pools[17]. In general, the motoneurones destined to inner-vate distal limb musculature are situated in the lateral parts of the anterior horn. Intermediate cell groups in the anterior horn supply proximal limb musculature, while the most medial cell groups send their axons into axial and girdle musculature[18].

4.2.1   Reflex activation of motoneurones

As Sherrington and his colleagues discovered[19], the same pool of motoneu-rones is capable of being influenced over a large number of reflex pathways for which the afferent systems may arise either locally and be delivered within a segment of the spinal cord, or they may arise in other segments or even supraspinally. My colleague, Professor A. K. McIntyre, has prepared a summary of some of the segmental reflex actions in tabular form and this is reproduced in Table 4.2. This table provides a simplified view of the general features of some of the reflexes described by Creed et al.[19]. A detailed con-sideration of the functional role of such receptors as Golgi tendon organs during active muscle contraction[20] may require that the simple view be con-siderably modified, however.

Both excitatory and inhibitory influences may be exerted on the moto-neurones and reciprocal effects may be demonstrated on the motoneurones of antagonist muscles. The mechanisms by which these are produced have been studied extensively (see a review by Eccles[2]) and the role of interneuronal activity in allowing the demonstration of certain effects has come to be realised[21]. But, largely for technical reasons, no other reflex pathway has commanded the same attention as that given to the monosynaptic phasic stretch reflex which is produced by the activation of primary endings of muscle spindles in the stretched muscle. An extensive review of this important area has recently been presented by Matthews[22] and the reader is referred to Chapter 7 of that book for a full discussion of the reflex actions produced by different groups of muscle afferents.

It has been important to attempt to understand differences in the magnitude of the monosynaptic reflex responses of, for example, a slow twitch and a fast-twitch muscle[23]. Under a given set of conditions and with a particular 'bias' produced by interneuronal activity, different responses could be due, at the simplest level, to different numbers of active synapses or to different distributions of these synapses over the soma-dendritic surface of the moto-neurone with resulting differences in attenuation of the action exerted at the impulse-generating region of the cell. These matters have been investi-gated[14, 24-26] and it has been deduced that, for the group Ia influences, differ-ent numbers of active contacts are responsible for the differences seen when synchronous electrical stimulation of muscles afferents is used to set up synaptic potentials in individual motoneurones. For different single afferent fibres, the statistical chance of monosynaptic contact depends on the nature of the motoneurone under study, i.e. whether it is innervating the muscle in which the afferent fibre originates or one of its synergists. But the distribution of synapses tends to be to similar electrotonic distances on the motoneurone cable in either case. This conclusion is consistent with Conradi's observation[27]

Table 4.2 Characteristics of some major segmental spinal reflexes

Reflex	*Stretch (myotatic) reflex*	*Lengthening reaction*	*Flexor reflex*	*Crossed extensor reflex*	*Extensor thrust reflex*
Receptor(s)	Spindle primary (Ia) (length monitors: in parallel with extrafusal fibres)	Golgi tendon organs (tension monitors: in series with extrafusal fibres)	Various superficial and deep receptors in skin, muscles, joints, etc.	Similar to flexor reflex	Unknown—? tactile of foot-pad, plus toe and foot proprioceptors together with stretch of extensors of limb
Adequate stimulus	(a) Stretch of muscle (b) Contraction of intrafusal fibres by fusimotor impulses	Strong extension of muscle. But threshold is lowered during active contraction	Many stimuli to most tissues; notably strong and potentially damaging ones	Similar to flexor, but in opposite limb	Pressure between toes and footpad with spreading of toes and tendency to flex limb
Pathway: **(a) Afferent**	Fast group Ia	Fast group Ib	Fairly fast, medium and slow myelinated fibres (skin and joint Aα to δ); muscle groups II and III; dorsal root C fibres	Similar to flexor reflex but largely slow (Aδ or group III) fibres	Unknown
(b) Central 'circuitry'	Monosynaptic	Disynaptic	Polysynaptic—3 (or more) neurones. (Inter-neurones and 'reverberating' chains)	As for flexor, but longer 'shortest' path.	Unknown
(c) Efferent	Fast α-motor fibres	α-Motor fibres (reduction of discharge, i.e. inhibition of muscle stretched)	α-Motor (and fusi-motor)	α-Motor (and fusi-motor)	α-Motor

Table 4.2 (*continued*)

Reflex	Stretch (myotatic) reflex	Lengthening reaction	Flexor reflex	Crossed extensor reflex	Extensor thrust reflex
Receptive field	Restricted	Restricted	*Wide:* whole limb	*Wide:* whole limb	Limited: special stimulation of foot needed
Effector field	Restricted (myotatic unit)	Spreads outside myotatic unit	*Wide:* whole flexor musculature	*Wide:* whole extensor musculature	*Wide:* extensor muscles
Synergic pattern	Muscle stretched contracts, synergists facilitated, antagonists inhibited	Muscle stretched inhibited. Synergists inhibited (other actions complex)	*Extensors* inhibited Contralateral extensors? excited	*Extensors* excited. Flexors inhibited	*Extensors* excited. Flexors inhibited
Temporal characteristics	Short latency. Prompt onset. Well sustained. Rapid decline. No after discharge	Fairly short latency. Prompt onset, rapid decline with little after effect	Longer latency. Slow climb to max. Less well sustained. More gradual decline when stimulation ceases. After discharge	Still longer latency, slower build-up and more gradual decline than flexor. After discharge prominent	Shortish latency. Fairly prompt onset. Brief in action, and not well sustained
Functions	Posture—'length-servo'. Movement—'follow-up', servo	? protective	Limb withdrawal as in stepping, or removal from noxious stimulus	Limb extension—to support body when opposite limb is flexed	? to boost extensor phase of step when running

that only 0.5 % of the boutons on the surface of a lateral motoneurone in the cat's spinal cord were monosynaptic contacts from dorsal-root fibres and that these were aggregated particularly on the proximal parts of the motoneurone dendrites.

A great deal of experimental effort has been devoted to the separation of the reflex effects of primary (group Ia) and secondary (group II) muscle spindle afferent endings. In addition it has been important to distinguish the individual influences of Golgi tendon organs (group Ib afferents) from those of primary muscle spindle endings with similar afferent-fibre conduction velocities. A detailed resume of these considerations has been given by Matthews[22].

Recently, the individual influences of primary and secondary endings of muscle spindles have been investigated using intracellular recording from the motoneurones of the muscle when the spindle afferents were being influenced by a combination of small amplitude vibration (to 'drive' the primary endings) and stretch (to activate additionally secondary endings). Westbury[28] showed that, under optimal conditions for driving the primary endings, there was no occlusion between the effects of vibration and of stretch for the maintained component of the response to stretch (see also Matthews[22]). The phasic response to the dynamic component of the stretch was, however, occluded by vibration and could therefore have been produced by the same afferents and the same mechanism. In general, the depolarisations produced by maintained stretch and by vibration were greater in motoneurones which innervated slow-twitch motor units than in those which innervated fast-twitch motor units and the former motoneurones were more sensitive to changes in the amplitude of stretch or the frequency of vibration.

Such results lead to the suggestion that different afferent inputs and/or different mechanisms are involved in the responses of individual motoneurones to stretch of a muscle and to vibration. It may be that the secondary endings of the muscle spindles are involved in the excitation of motoneurones in the tonic stretch reflex. This is a different view of the role of secondary endings to that which resulted from the early experiments of Lloyd[29] which suggested that the reflex effect of stimulation of group II muscle afferents was a general flexor response, and it differs from the suggestions made by some other workers that group II muscle afferents cause inhibition of extensor motoneurones (see Cangiano and Lutzemberger[30]). The regulating role of spinal interneurones in these processes must, however, be appreciated and the capacity of descending pathways to switch interneuronal 'bias' may be of great importance in assessing the results of natural or unnatural (electrical) activation of afferent pathways.

4.2.2 Effects of supraspinal activity on spinal motoneurones

In spite of the serious disadvantages of electrical stimulation as a tool for studying the function of the nervous system, synchronous electrical activation of descending fibre pathways has been used in combination with intracellular recording in motoneurones to study the actions exerted on these cells and their mechanisms. Reticulospinal[31], vestibulospinal[32-34], tectospinal[35] and rubrospinal[36, 37] pathways have all been examined to define the influences exerted on spinal motoneurones of the cat following electrical stimulation. It is very difficult to be certain that these pathways were stimulated in isolation. The possibility exists that the current could spread to nearby structures in a region densely packed with fibre bundles. It is also conceivable that collaterals of such through-pathways as the pyramidal tract were being activated in some of these experiments, although, in a number of cases, lesions were made in other pathways to limit such effects. Moreover, the meaningfulness of synchronous volleys of nerve impulses may be questioned when it is realised that the natural influences brought to bear on the motoneurones are spatially and temporally dispersed and may normally achieve their effects by virtue of this patterned activity.

The conclusion has been reached that, in the cat, both excitatory and inhibitory influences converge on to spinal motoneurones from reticular nuclei[38], that the vestibulospinal tract exerts excitatory influences on hindlimb extensor motoneurones over both monosynaptic and polysynaptic pathways and that the rubrospinal tract exerts mainly polysynaptic excitatory effects on flexor motoneurones. However, it is clear that in other species these broad generalisations need not apply, for Shapovalov et al.[39] have shown monosynaptic EPSPs in spinal motoneurones of the monkey on stimulation of the red nucleus. Moreover, it is necessary, in order to understand the meaning of the connections made by these pathways, to examine activities in these regions during movement (Orlovsky, see later).

Although study of the influences exerted on individual motoneurones allows the fine detail of subcorticospinal actions to be examined by the neurophysiologist, it is necessary to appreciate that indirect actions are also possible during natural function. It has been demonstrated that some of the same brain stem structures which influence a-motoneurones are also capable of modifying the function of fusimotor neurones[40-44]. Hence an effect on spinal a-motoneurones during movement in the intact animal could be produced by a change in fusimotor drive to muscle spindles and the consequent alteration in muscle afferent convergence on to motoneurones. Further than this, a number of the brain stem structures which have been demonstrated to exert effects on spinal motoneurones are also capable of producing primary afferent depolarisation in the spinal cord and could modify motoneurone function by an influence on cutaneous, joint or muscle afferents[45].

4.2.3   The effects of cortical stimulation on spinal motoneurones

Since the pioneer experiments of Fritsch and Hitzig[46] and of Ferrier[47], it has been clear that electrical stimulation of a region of cerebral cortex (the motor area) results in movements of the muscles of the contralateral side of the body. The cortex is organised topographically so that stimulation applied to a particular region of the motor area produces movements in one body part while stimulation of an adjacent cortical zone gives rise to movement in an adjacent body part. In animals, this topographical organisation may be revealed by careful local stimulation of many points within a large cortical zone and recording of the movements produced[48]. In many cases, the results of such experiments have been presented as figurine maps such as those which show that movements of the hind-limb, fore-limb and face are represented in successively more lateral regions of the monkey's precentral gyrus. Much larger areas of cortical surface contain the representations of the distal musculature of the limbs (e.g. wrist and finger movements) than are concerned with proximal musculature (shoulder movements)[49,50]. A large variety of movement responses may be produced by appropriate repetitive stimulation of the cortical surface and the map of these responses is relatively fixed, i.e. the same stimulus applied to the same point on a number of separate occasions always produces the same movement. Similar maps of the topographical organisation of the motor areas of the cerebral cortex have been prepared for man. But, in this case, the maps are composite and the observations have been collected from the study of many patients[51].

Again, while recognising the limitations of electrical stimulation as a method for revealing aspects of natural function, localised stimuli have been applied within particular parts of the topographically organised motor cortex and the effects of this stimulation have been investigated on spinal cord function to examine the mechanisms by which motoneurones are caused to discharge and movement results. Lloyd[52] pioneered these investigations with studies of corticospinal influences on motor pools in the cat spinal cord. Lloyd established that volleys of nerve impulses conducted from the cortex to the spinal cord along fibres of the pyramidal tract, when all other connections between the forebrain and the spinal cord had been severed, were capable of facilitating electrically-elicited monosynaptic spinal reflexes. He further demonstrated that the pathways for this facilitatory influence in the cat involved activation of interneurones in an intermediate region of the spinal cord.

Preston and his colleagues[53-56] have elaborated this experimental approach and have shown that different effects are demonstrable in motoneurone pools which have connections with different functional groups of muscles. They used localised electrical stimulation of motor areas of the cerebral cortex after they had divided all brain stem structures other than the pyramidal tracts in their experimental animals. These 'pyramidal' preparations required no subsequent anaesthesia because the brainstem damage produced coma. The influence of the cortical activation was assessed by measuring the amplitudes of monosynaptic reflex discharges set up in circumscribed motoneurone populations by stimulation of group I afferent fibres in a variety of muscle nerves at a number of time delays after the cortical stimulus.

Repetitive volleys in the pyramidal tract of the cat produced facilitation of flexor motoneurones and inhibition of extensor motoneurones in both the fore-limb and the hind-limb. These effects resulted from pyramidal tract actions on local spinal interneurones[57]. In the pyramidal baboon, however, the effects were more complex and depended on the functional connections of the motoneurone populations. Hence many motoneurone pools, whether of flexor or extensor muscles, received an early facilitation from pyramidal tract volleys. This short latency effect could have been produced by monosynaptic connections of cortical efferent fibres[17,58-60]. The early facilitation was most effective for flexor motoneurones and for extensor motoneurone populations supplying fast-twitch muscle fibres. Less facilitatory action was exerted on extensor motoneurones innervating slow-twitch muscles.

The early facilitation from cortical stimulation in the pyramidal baboon was succeeded by a later brief inhibitory effect which then gave rise to a prolonged phase of facilitation of flexor motoneurone populations and some extensor motoneurones supplying fast-twitch muscles. Other extensor motoneurones were markedly inhibited during this late phase of the cortical effect and in those the inhibitory influence of cortical stimulation was dominant.

These rather complex patterns of cortical effects on populations of motoneurones led Preston and his colleagues to suggest that the influence of the motor cortex on a given pool of motoneurones depends on the function of those motoneurones in movement performance. The dominant facilitation of flexor motoneurones would allow the cerebral cortex to activate flexor motor units in skilled motor performance, while the preponderant inhibition of extensor motoneurones would provide a mechanism through which the cortex could curtail antigravity extensor contractions at the onset of a movement pattern. When a survey was made of the cortical influences exerted on the motoneurones for particular muscles serving an antigravity function in both the cat and the baboon, this view seemed to receive considerable support because, in both species, these motoneurone populations were inhibited by cortical stimulation in the pyramidal animal. Further evidence in support of this generalisation has been obtained by studying cortical influences conveyed through the pyramidal tract to motoneurone groups in the lumbar spinal cord of an arboreal marsupial (*Trichosurus vulpecula*). In this animal also, the motoneurones of a muscle which serves a postural function in clamping the animal to branches of the tree (*flexor digitorum longus*) are inhibited by cortically-initiated nerve volleys in the pyramidal tract[61].

Although these technically-difficult experiments have not been conducted in many animal species and although the information available relates only to a small number of motoneurone populations, it is possible to conclude that the average effect exerted on a spinal motoneurone by the cerebral cortex, even when the cortex is operating only through a single anatomical pathway (the pyramidal tract) depends to considerable degree on the functional connections made by that motoneurone. If the muscle unit supplied by the motoneurone is normally tonically active in the habitual static posture of the animal, it may be inhibited by the cerebral cortex at the onset of movement. But if the muscle unit is one involved in the phasic movement task, its motoneurone will be excited by the cortical activity. However, cortical units capable of producing excitation of a motor unit and cortical units capable of producing inhibition of the same motor unit exist. The mechanism by which these are differentially activated by the motor programmes for different movements remains to be investigated.

4.2.4 Corticospinal actions on individual motoneurones

Electrophysiological experiments have confirmed that the direct influence produced on individual spinal motoneurones in primates by pyramidal tract volleys is an excitatory one[59, 60]. No such short-latency, monosynaptic effect has been observed in the cat[62]. The results of Landgren, Phillips and Porter[60] indicated convergence, on to individual spinal motoneurones in the baboon, of excitatory effects from a group of corticomotoneuronal pyramidal cells and the name 'colony' was used to distinguish this group of functionally-related cells[63]. The magnitude of the excitatory effect produced by maximal simultaneous activation of the colony varied for different motoneurones.

Much more corticomotoneuronal excitation was revealed in motoneurones supplying distal musculature of the fore-limb of the baboon than in motoneurones supplying proximal musculature. Indeed some motoneurones innervating proximal fore-limb muscles received no direct excitation from the motor cortex[64]. The maximal size of the corticomotoneuronal EPSP which could be produced in a given motoneurone by electrical activation of the motor cortex varied with the functional characteristics of the muscle innervated. Hence the motoneurones of certain finger muscles (*extensor digitorum communis* and the intrinsic muscles of the hand) received much more depolarisation from the cerebral cortex than the motoneurones of other forearm muscles and frequently the size of the corticomotoneuronal EPSPs in these cells exceeded the size of the monosynaptic EPSPs set up by maximal stimulation of group I afferent fibres in the homonymous muscle nerve[65].

From a study of minimal synaptic potentials set up in lumbar spinal motoneurones of the monkey by weak cortical stimulation and by stimulation of one or a few group I afferent fibres in motor-nerve filaments supplying the muscle or one of its synergists, Porter and Hore[66] concluded that, in general, the corticomotoneuronal synapses were likely to be situated on more peripheral parts of the motoneurone dendritic processes than the synapses from group I afferent fibres (see also Valverde[67]). It had been established that corticomotoneuronal EPSPs were usually of small amplitude and subthreshold for initiating cell firing[60, 64]. The question of their efficacy in causing motoneurone discharge and hence muscle contraction therefore required evaluation.

It had been found that, when corticomotoneuronal synapses were activated repetitively, increasing depolarising effects were recorded in motoneurones following the later volleys in the train[60, 64, 68, 69]. This potentiation of synaptic effectiveness by a preceding volley in a train was reminiscent of the facilitation of transmission which is revealed under certain conditions of diminished transmitter release at neuromuscular junctions[70-72]. A similar facilitation phenomenon is also evident at the synapses made on motoneurones by some spinal interneurones[73]. It was reasoned that this facilitation of synaptic action could provide a mechanism for the build-up of excitation during natural repetitive corticomotoneuronal activity and that this could make the corticomotoneuronal synapses effective[64].

The time course of corticomotoneuronal facilitation has been examined using paired corticospinal volleys in the monkey. The onset of an EPSP is associated with the development of facilitation which may be revealed by an increase in amplitude of a subsequent EPSP generated by activity at those synapses. This corticomotoneuronal facilitation decays approximately exponentially with a time constant of *ca.* 10 ms[69]. Recently, it has been possible to investigate the influence, on the amplitude of an EPSP, of a pair of preceding volleys with different intervals between them and delivered at

varying times before the test volley. These studies have revealed that a corticomotoneuronal EPSP is facilitated by both of the preceding nerve volleys in
the presynaptic pathway and that the facilitation seems to add in a simple
manner in relation to the time delays between each of the preceding volleys
and the test volley[74]. The facilitation (f) of a third EPSP (3) with respect to
the size of a control, first EPSP (1) in a train of 3 in which the times of
occurrence of the EPSPs are t_1, t_2 and t_3 may then be approximated by the
expression:

$$f_{3-1} = 0.85 \exp \left[\frac{-(t_3 - t_1)}{10} \right] + 0.85 \exp \left[\frac{-(t_3 - t_2)}{10} \right]$$

If the time interval between the corticomotoneuronal volleys was 50 ms or
greater, no significant facilitation effect was revealed.

The significance of these properties of corticomotoneuronal synapses
may be investigated by studying the effects of temporal patterns of activity
in corticospinal fibres. It has been found that the timing of onset of electromyographic activity in a muscle, when this is produced by cortical stimulation,
is very dependent on the temporal pattern of nerve impulses in a corticospinal
volley, even when the overall mean frequency is held constant. It has also
been demonstrated that the synaptic depolarisation produced in sample
motoneurones of the monkey's spinal cord depends markedly, in the timing
of its peak and in the amplitude of depolarisation produced, on the temporal
sequence of nerve volleys in corticomotoneuronal fibres[75]. These experimental
observations may be mimicked in a model of corticomotoneuronal activity
which includes a definition of the time course of individual EPSPs on motoneuronal dendrites and the description of facilitation occurring at these
synapses with successive presynaptic volleys.

An understanding of the processes operating at the motoneurone in the
automatic decoding of the pulsed signals arriving along corticomotoneuronal
fibres is important in studying the significance of particular patterns of
naturally-occurring activity in these fibre pathways. From an examination of
the real transduction of presynaptic impulse activity to graded synaptic
depolarisation, an interpretation may be made of the significance of the
various temporal patterns of signals which are found to occur naturally.
The prediction may be made, for example, that a major determinant of the
timing of onset of muscle contraction initiated from the cerebral cortex under
natural conditions will be the time of occurrence of the short impulse intervals within the bursts of corticomotoneuronal discharge associated with the
movement. This prediction has been tested for some natural discharges of
pyramidal tract neurones associated with self-initiated movements in a
conscious monkey and a high correlation has been demonstrated[76, 77].

4.2.5 The effects of destruction of pathways which influence motoneurones

Although a very large number of studies have been undertaken to demonstrate
the deficits of movement performance produced by damage to particular
central nervous structures, interpretation of the results of these experiments

is fraught with difficulties[78-84]. Deficits in movement performance tend to be greater following damage to central nervous structures in adult animals than they do when the same structures are damaged in immature or juvenile animals[85, 86]. Recovery of function after nervous-system damage is common and the degree of this recovery depends to a large extent on the training schedules used during recovery[87]. Tests of motor performance must be carefully planned to reveal particular deficits and, if the tests are insufficiently refined, important disorders of movement control may not be appreciated[88, 89].

A recent reinvestigation of the involvement of the pyramidal tract and of non-pyramidal influences in movement control in the monkey has been conducted by Lawrence and Kuypers[90, 91]. Their investigation employed rigid control of the limits of the anatomical extent of the surgical lesions. It utilised sophisticated tests of the animal's manual dexterity before and after the lesions and it followed the performance of the animals for long periods of time (up to a year) after the lesions had been made, using cinematographic recording of motor performance. Lawrence and Kuypers found that, after bilateral complete pyramidal-tract section, monkeys were still able to carry out many movements such as walking and climbing in a manner indistinguishable from normal. However, section of the pyramidal tracts had produced deficits in movement performance. The animals lacked agility, their movements were slowed and it appeared that they tired more readily. The dramatic disability experienced by these animals was a loss of skill in manipulative tasks. These monkeys permanently lost the ability to use their digits independently in such movement tasks as retrieving a morsel of food from a small hole in a board. They could use the hand for grasping when all the fingers were used together and the whole hand was flexed around an object. But the precision grip using opposition only of forefinger and thumb could not be performed. Moreover, once the hand had grasped an object such as a piece of food, some difficulty in relaxation was experienced and the animal sometimes had a problem releasing the food again. Monkeys were seen to muzzle into their closed fist in order to eat the food which had been grasped.

Woolsey et al.[92] have repeated the tests of manipulative skill in monkeys with unilateral pyramidal-tract section. It was possible then to compare motor performance in the affected with that in the normal hand and it was found that pyramidotomy made it impossible for the monkey to use the digits of the affected hand independently for skilled manipulative tasks. These observations were paralleled by a striking alteration in the motor map defined by electrical stimulation of the cerebral cortex in these animals with pyramidal-tract section. The cortex was stimulated on both sides after corticospinal (pyramidal tract) fibres had completely degenerated unilaterally. Thresholds for eliciting movement with electrical stimuli were elevated on the apyramidal side. But also the movements elicited were different. No movements of distal parts of the limbs could be produced after pyramidal-tract degeneration and there was a considerable reduction in the variety of movements elicited. The responses which remained were confined to proximal musculature.

These ablation and stimulation experiments highlight the probable role of the corticomotoneuronal system in primate movement performance requiring skill and agility[93]. This system is directed more effectively to the motoneurones supplying distal musculature[17, 64]. Moreover, Lawrence and

Hopkins[94] have shown that interruption of the pyramidal tract in infant monkeys, before corticomotoneuronal connections have been formed, produces a permanent disability in fine control of distal musculature in which the animals, even though reared with other normally-developing monkeys, never achieve the ability to manipulate their digits independently. Other less direct pathways by which the cerebral cortex could influence spinal motoneurones are not competent to initiate independent control of digital movements, even when they alone are able to develop unhindered and establish exclusive contacts with motoneurones.

But section of the pyramidal tracts leaves intact the subcorticospinal pathways (rubrospinal, etc.) through which the motor areas of the cerebral cortex may exercise executive management of other movement functions. Lawrence and Kuypers investigated the role of these other systems in movement performance by sectioning them in animals which had previously been subjected to bilateral pyramidal-tract interruption (see also Kuypers[95]). They came to the conclusion that a laterally-situated system of descending fibre tracts in the spinal cord (corticospinal plus rubrospinal and possibly other fibres) engaged both directly (in the monkey) and indirectly (via interneurones) the laterally situated motoneurone pools destined to innervate distal limb musculature[18, 96]. These lateral fibre tracts could be involved in the control of movements of distal musculature and, when damage to a lateral tract such as the rubrospinal was superimposed on pyramidotomy, the deficit in movement ability at the distal joints of the limb became more severe. Independent movements of the peripheral part of the extremity and the hand were severely impaired and the animal's capacity to flex its extended limb was reduced. However, movements of the whole limb about the proximal joint and combined movements of the body and limbs were relatively unaffected.

In contrast, when the descending fibres of the ventromedial system (vestibulospinal and reticulospinal fibres) which engage interneurones associated mainly with the motor supply of proximal and axial musculature were interrupted, severe disturbances of control of the trunk and proximal limb muscles resulted and a flexed posture of the trunk and limbs was usual. Lawrence and Kuypers concluded that the basic control of movement concerned with the maintenance of posture, the integrated movements of body and limbs and the directing of progression were all served by the ventromedial system of subcorticospinal fibres[91]. On this basic control, the lateral brain stem pathways superimposed the capacity to produce independent movement of the limbs and control of the distal extremities of the limbs. The refinement added by the direct corticospinal part of the lateral fibre system was to confer the capacity to fractionate these distal movements and to control individual and independent movements of the digits with precision.

4.3 RECORDING FROM NEURONAL ELEMENTS DURING MOVEMENT

Because of the problems associated with the assessment of results obtained in experiments utilising electrical stimulation or ablation of the central nervous system to study central nervous management of movement performance, attention has been directed to the need to study the neuronal activities which accompany spontaneous movement[97]. It has long been possible to register the output from individual units in the 'final common path' by recording muscle unit electromyographical (EMG) activity during muscle contraction. The concept of grading of force of muscle contraction by changes in frequency of firing of individual motor units and by recruitment of additional motor units to the task is well established. But it is only recently that quantitative information has been obtained concerning the functional role of the stretch reflex and the involvement of fusimotor activation and muscle-spindle afferent 'feed-back' in voluntary movement in man. Concomitant with this, increasing attention has been given to the recording of natural activity in single neurones of strategic brain structures of animals during spontaneous self-initiated movements.

These investigations have shed new light on the meaning of the anatomical and physiological connections which have been described. But limits are imposed on the interpretation of these findings also. Natural movements are extremely complex. They involve muscular contraction for a postural set of the whole body, they involve fixation of some joints with co-contraction of agonists and antagonists and they involve quite different reciprocal actions in muscles acting about joints where change in position occurs[98]. The demonstration of a relationship between discharge of a cell in the brain and one or more of these muscle actions does not preclude another statistical correlation with other quite different muscle actions. Very few attempts have been made to devise tests for causality in a demonstrated correlation between neuronal firing and muscle contraction. Even the movement tasks involving simple repetitive flexion and extension about a single joint are in fact so complex that it is difficult to evaluate correlations which are observed. The stage has been reached where attention to the mechanics of the movement itself is of great importance, and further understanding of the functional role of nervous structures in producing this movement is likely to be obtained in proportion to refinements and sophistication introduced into the motor task itself.

In spite of the limitations of the method, in the last few years a dramatic increase in understanding of the functional significance of the brain's involvement in muscle management has been obtained. Melvill Jones and Watt[99, 100] investigated the involvement of the stretch reflex in the muscular contractions of the human calf during stepping and during landing on the soles of the feet from a short unexpected vertical fall. They found that electromyographic activity began in the calf muscles *before* the feet made contact with the ground and before these muscles could have been stretched. Hence the muscle contractions were not produced by a stretch reflex and were not responses to contact and ankle extension. Rather they were produced by central nervous activation of α-motoneurones preparatory to the load-bearing contact of the foot with the ground.

But muscle stretch receptors (muscle spindles) may be activated during movement. Vallbo[101-103] recorded from single muscle-spindle afferent fibres in the median nerve of conscious human subjects while these individuals carried out small voluntary isometric contractions using finger muscles containing the spindles from which recordings were being made. The spindle afferents demonstrated *increased* firing during muscle contraction and were not unloaded and silenced during the voluntary development of isometric force. Spindle discharge increased as the force developed increased. Such results suggested that the central nervous signals for execution of the voluntary motor task were directed both to the a-motoneurones and to the fusimotor neurones of the muscle concerned. The central signals produced co-activation of these two groups of ventral horn cells. Co-activation could cause the muscle spindle 'feed-back' onto a-motoneurones to reinforce the a-activity in servo-assistance of the movement (Matthews[104]). In these particular experiments the change in firing of the muscle spindles lagged behind the onset of electromyographic activity of the muscle. Hence, for these movement tasks at least, the muscle contraction was not being *initiated* by way of the 'γ-loop'[105] but the muscle spindle 'servo' was being activated during the contraction and could be contributing to its maintenance.

In a number of experiments on chronically-prepared thalamic or mesencephalic decorticate cats which were capable of demonstrating apparently normal sequences of muscle contractions involved in stepping and walking, Orlovsky[106, 107] recorded from neuronal units in vestibulospinal, reticulospinal and rubrospinal pathways. The cats were made to walk by mid-brain stimulation or by movement backwards of a treadmill on which their foot-pads rested. Neurones in Deiters' (lateral vestibular) nucleus, which have been shown to have an excitatory influence on the motoneurones of extensor muscles, showed bursts of firing or modulated discharge frequencies in which increased activity was associated in time with the contractions of extensor muscles during locomotion. The maximum discharge in these vestibulospinal neurones accompanied the end of the swing phase or the early stance phase of limb movements in locomotion. But the activity in vestibulospinal neurones was dependent on afferent feed-back from the moving limb because, if the limb was stopped by force from moving, the modulation disappeared. Moreover, the feed-back could well have occurred via the cerebellum, because, if the cerebellum was ablated the modulation with locomotor activity disappeared.

Rubrospinal neurones also demonstrated periodic alterations in activity with stepping in these cats if the cerebellum was intact. The peak discharge of the rubrospinal neurones occurred during the swing phase of the movements of the contralateral hindlimb when the flexor muscles were active. This periodicity is consistent with a role for rubrospinal excitation of flexor muscles in normal limb movements during progression. Once again, interference with the movement, by forceful prevention of it, removed the phasic modulation of rubrospinal activity.

Arshavsky *et al.*[108, 109] recorded the discharges of neurones in the dorsal spinocerebellar tracts (D.S.C.T.) which could have been involved in the afferent feed-back from the moving limb during this form of locomotion in mesencephalic or thalamic cats. They found that D.S.C.T. neurones became active during the phase of the step involving the muscles which fed afferent impulses to the D.S.C.T. cell under investigation. Moreover, the more muscle activity generated in the step, the more discharge was registered in the D.S.C.T. cell.

The most quantitative studies of neuronal correlates of movement performance have been those which examined the behaviour of pyramidal tract neurones in the motor cortex of conscious monkeys while these animals carried out self-initiated learned movement tasks. It was found that pyramidal tract neurones altered their activity during movement[110, 111]. Those pyramidal tract neurones which had short antidromic response latencies tended to be phasically active in association with movements of a contralateral limb. When the animal was not moving this limb, the unit was silent. Pyramidal-tract neurones which had longer antidromic response latencies and, one would deduce, smaller cell bodies and thinner axons, tended to be tonically active. But this activity was modulated with movement of a contralateral limb. The change in frequency of cellular discharge associated with the movement was greater for the pyramidal-tract cells with short antidromic latencies than for those with longer antidromic latencies[110].

In a conditioned response test in which monkeys were taught to perform a brisk extension movement of the wrist in response to a visual stimulus, some pyramidal-tract neurones were found which always discharged in relation to the response (and were not discharging in association with the stimulus) and these neurones began to fire *before* electromyographic activity occurred in the extensor muscles of the wrist[112]. In many of the neurones whose activity was most closely related to the response, the unit's discharge began *ca.* 80 ms before the beginning of electromyographic change[113]. Most of the pyramidal tract neurones in the arm area of the motor cortex showed responses only in relation to movements of the contralateral wrist and not to ipsilateral movements.

For these units which began to fire before muscle contraction, it was important to attempt to assess whether they were signalling the position to be taken up by the limb (irrespective of loads or forces opposing this) or the force to be generated by the prime movers in order to achieve the desired position. Evarts tested this matter in an experiment in which, during the learned repetitive flexion–extension movement of the wrist, a given single wrist position could be associated with a number of different loads requiring different force development in the muscles producing this position[114]. Flexion of the wrist, for example, could be carried out in a 'no load' test in which the monkey simply moved a vertical lever to a flexor stop. Alternatively, by means of pulleys and weights, movement of the lever to the flexor stop could be assisted by, or opposed by, a variety of additional loads requiring less or more force to be generated in the forearm flexor muscles for accomplishment of the task.

While recordings were being made from single pyramidal-tract neurones in the arm area of the motor cortex, the animals were required to produce the learned repetitive wrist flexion–extension task against a number of different load conditions. It was demonstrated that the mean frequency of discharge of some pyramidal-tract neurones was related to the *force* required to be generated by the prime-movers and not to the position achieved. Many units also appeared to code changes in force development with time. In a later study, Evarts[115] showed that pyramidal-tract units could also demonstrate activity during postural fixation of the wrist against changing forces. The discharges of the pyramidal-tract neurones were related to the patterns of muscular contraction acting about a joint rather than to the resultant displacement of the joint. Because of this relationship to activity in a muscle, a given pyramidal-tract cell could be seen to discharge during many different movements with which the muscle was associated[116].

Humphrey, Schmidt and Thompson[117] studied the behaviour of sets of 3–8 simultaneously-recorded discharge patterns in pyramidal-tract neurones of conscious monkeys performing wrist movements. They showed that by weighting and summing the discharge frequencies of each cell in the co-operating set, it was possible to predict the time course of some of the movement response characteristics with considerable accuracy. Although the predictions were most accurate for force characteristics, over a number of different load conditions, the summed activity of groups of neurones gave only slightly less accurate estimates of the time course of the force trace, of displacement and of velocity of movement. Therefore, cortical activity, as represented by these groups of co-operating neurones, could be coding much more than force development. Indeed Humphrey[118] noted that the theoretical transfer functions necessary to convert a pattern of cellular discharge into a time course of torque development with which the cellular discharge was associated varied for different cells. He suggested that a mathematical statement for cortical activity in movement might express the cortical control signal $(F_{(t)})$ in relation to net muscular tension or torque $(T_{(t)})$ in the following way:

$$F_{(t)} = a\,\frac{\mathrm{d}^2 T}{\mathrm{d}t^2} + \beta\,\frac{\mathrm{d}T}{\mathrm{d}t} + \mu T$$

where a, β and μ are constants. He further suggested that different cortical units might be concerned in signalling with different emphasis the 'derivative' or 'proportional' components of torque development and that the phasic 'derivative' signals of cortical units might allow compensation for the slow dynamic properties of muscle and the mechanical loads of the limb system in movement.

Arguing from the properties of corticomotoneuronal synapses in transforming impulse activity in corticospinal fibres to synaptic depolarisation of motoneurones, it was suggested by Porter et al.[75, 76, 77, 119] that the time of onset of muscular contraction might be determined by the temporal sequence of impulses in the bursts of cortical activity associated with movement. They produced evidence for a high correlation between the time of occurrence of short impulse intervals in a burst of pyramidal-cell activity and the time of onset of contraction after the beginning of the burst. This possibility, that the precise timing of muscle contractions as well as the force to be generated is signalled by pyramidal-tract neurones, would be consistent with the function of these cells in conferring speed, skill and agility on movement performance[90], because much of movement skill involves precise timing of sequences of muscle contraction. It was further shown that the same pyramidal-tract neurone was capable of demonstrating discharge characteristics which were correlated with force development *and* with time of onset of movement (Lewis and Porter, 1973, unpublished observations).

Recordings have been made from many other brain regions and in relation to many other aspects of movement performance[120, 121]. Bizzi[122, 123] and Bizzi and Schiller[124] recorded from single units in the frontal eye fields of the cerebral cortex. Cells in this region discharged *after* the voluntary or involuntary eye movements which occurred naturally. Kubota and Niki[125] examined the behaviour of prefrontal neurones in relation to delayed response tasks and found that neurones could become active 200 ms before the delayed motor response and maintain their activity throughout the movement performance. Luschei, Garthwaite and Armstrong[126] found that precentral neurones in the 'face area' of the motor cortex began to discharge *ca* 50 ms before jaw movements but did not demonstrate a clear relationship between firing pattern and force or displacement of the jaw movement.

Evarts[127] examined the activities of cells in nucleus ventralis lateralis of the thalamus in relation to movements performed by conscious monkeys. He found that these cells increased or decreased their discharge as much as 100 ms before the onset of movement, a time not dissimilar to that found for precentral neurones[113, 117, 119, 128]. Strategically situated as this nucleus is on the pathway to the motor cortex from both the cerebellum and the basal ganglia, it is possible that some of the programming of the motor cortex for the execution of movement is relayed through this zone[129]. A search for the structures and the mechanisms upstream of the motor cortex which must be involved in the selection and direction of appropriate pyramidal tract action in skilled movement performance has only just begun.

Cerebellar neuronal discharges have also been found to be associated with movement performance[130-132]. Conscious monkeys were required to maintain a given posture (e.g. wrist flexion) until a signal was presented upon which they made a sudden ballistic movement to the next posture (wrist extension) and held this new position. Many cells in the deep nuclei of the cerebellum and in the cerebellar cortex changed their discharge in relation to these movements. Many of the changes occurred 50–100 ms before the onset of the movement. They were related to the movement, not the signal to move, but the maintained discharge of the cells was not significantly different in the two extremes of posture of the wrist. This could be consistent with a function of cerebellar neurones in starting and stopping ballistic movements rather than in positional control[133] and such a view has arisen from clinical observations in disorders of cerebellar function[134-136].

De Long[137] recorded from cells in the internal and external segments of globus pallidus of conscious monkeys during repetitive motor tasks performed with either hand or with the contralateral foot. Cells in the lateral parts of both segments of the globus pallidus changed their firing in relation to contralateral limb movements. Many of the cells discharged differently in relation to different phasic movements but very little relationship between cellular activity and posture was noted. It is not clear whether these cells in the globus pallidus which were in regions receiving topographically-organised projections from sensorimotor cortex by way of the caudate nucleus and putamen[129, 138, 139] were responding to activity in the motor cortex or were concerned in the input to the motor cortex and hence its modulation (by way of connections through nucleus ventralis lateralis of the thalamus)[140, 141]. De Long and Evarts[142] reported that pallidal neurones discharged before the beginning of movement performance. But the precise temporal relationships between the discharges of these cells and those in other regions concerned in movement function is not clear.

Such studies as the ones referred to above are capable of demonstrating a relationship between neuronal activity and movement performance. This relationship may be interpreted in the light of other evidence such as the demonstration of a consistent deficit of motor performance when the structure from which recordings have been made is damaged. But the only serious attempt to demonstrate the stability of the relationship between cellular function and motor response has been that of Fetz and Finnochio[143, 144]. They trained monkeys to contract only one of a group of muscles from which electromyographic recordings were made while suppressing, more or less completely, concomitant electromyographic activity in the others. They rewarded the monkey for relatively-isolated isometric contraction of a muscle with which cortical unit activity was normally strongly associated. Then, when they changed the reinforcement criteria, they were able to demonstrate that the animal could be retrained to produce bursts of cortical cell activity without contractions in that isolated muscle. Conversely, the animal could be taught to produce the particular muscle contractions with less associated discharge in the sample cortical cell. But full suppression of cortical unit discharge was not achieved in relation to contractions of a muscle with which that unit's activity was normally strongly associated.

These observations were interpreted in terms of a 'flexibility' of the coupling between cortical unit activity and movement performance and it was concluded that the temporal correlations revealed between activity of precentral cells and components of the motor response may depend as much on the response pattern that is reinforced as on the underlying physiological connections. In order to demonstrate a 'cause and effect' relationship it would, on this hypothesis, be necessary to test the stability of any correlations established by attempting dissociation of the relationship using operant-conditioning techniques. But, of course, a fixed anatomical and physiological relationship may be made more or less effective, and may be prevented from functioning at all, by the operation of other systems converging on to the final common path with additional excitatory or inhibitory influences. So 'flexibility' does not imply lack of functional or even of causal capability and the results of the experiments just referred to do not deny an important executive function for precentral neurones in movement performance.

Such experiments do, however, demonstrate the need to bear in mind the motor 'programme' which the animal has been taught to perform. It is well known that, for skilled movements of the distal part of the limb, adequate *performance* requires the intactness of the precentral motor cortex. But the programme survives damage to this area and may readily be used to direct another non-paralysed limb in the same task after the motor cortex of one side is ablated[87, 145]. If, during training, a programme for isometric development of force is built up, it is likely that correlation between cortical unit discharge and isometric force development will be revealed when cellular activity is examined in relation to this learned task. But it is conceivable that a different correlation, for example with speed of movement, might be revealed in the same cells if the learned programme had been one involving movements at different speeds.

4.4 AFFERENT SYSTEMS IN MOVEMENT PERFORMANCE

Afferent systems which are presumably capable of detecting aspects of movement performance converge on motor regions of the central nervous system at all levels—at a segmental level in the spinal cord, on to reticular, cerebellar, striatal and cortical neurones, to give a few of the most important examples[146-161]. There has been a great deal of speculation about the importance for the control of movement of this afferent feed-back to motor regions. Dexterity in the performance of skilled manipulative tasks is impaired when human subjects are blindfolded or when the moving limb is made anaesthetic. Moreover, the experiments of Mott and Sherrington[162] showed that the forelimb of a monkey, deafferented by dorsal root section, was not used in normal motor tasks but became a useless paralysed appendage even though its motor nerve supply was intact. Such a deafferented limb could be made to move by stimulation of the motor cortex and it could be used in stressful situations when the animal struggled to escape from the experimenter (see also Ref. 163). But the precise actions exerted by afferent systems and the levels at which they operate to influence motor function and to allow animals normal use of their limbs in motor performance require detailed evaluation.

In view of the fact that so much quantitative information has been collected about the activities of pyramidal-tract neurones in association with movement performance, it has been of interest to assess the effects of feed-back on to pyramidal-tract neurones from receptors capable of being influenced by the movement[152, 159-164]. Parallel investigations have examined afferent influences on cerebellar Purkinje cells and other relevant structures[149, 150, 151]. It remains possible that afferent modulation of the discharges of precentral neurones occurs by way of influences relayed through the cerebellum and indeed Brooks et al.[165, 166] found that cooling of the dentate nucleus of the cerebellum altered the relationship between the phasic discharges of cortical units and the movement being executed. The cortical discharges fell below those which would have been expected to accompany movement of the designated load at the higher velocities which were produced after dentate cooling. But a number of parallel pathways exist, all of which could be involved in the central organisation of management of movement.

In view of the fact that pyramidal-tract cell activity precedes the onset of movement and is related to the force *to be developed*, it is difficult to imagine how feed-back from a load detector in the limb could be responsible for the correlations observed by Evarts[114]. Cutaneous, visual and auditory afferents are able to cause pyramidal-tract neurones in chloralose anaesthetised cats to discharge[167]. Some pyramidal-tract cells in the cat have very localised cutaneous 'receptive fields' from which they may be activated, but the role of these influences in 'positive feed-back' during movement is not at all clear (see a review by Brooks and Stoney[159]).

Considerable debate has surrounded the question of the influences exerted on pyramidal-tract neurones by joint afferents. There may be considerable species differences in the effects observed. However, it is clear that a large proportion of pyramidal-tract neurones in the monkey are influenced by joint movement[168]. Moreover, it has been demonstrated recently, for a limited sample of precentral neurones in conscious man, that passive joint movement caused the cells to discharge[169]. This discharge was produced by movement in the same direction as that with which the cell's activity was associated during active voluntary movements. Of 30 cells which were tested, 16 responded to active or passive movement of the contralateral hand, but none responded to tactile or auditory stimulation, suggesting a dominance of afferent influence from the moving part. This contrasts with experimental observations in the cat, for example[167]. Four of the 16 precentral neurones responded to passive movement of both the ipsilateral and the contralateral hand[169].

It is still not clear whether muscle afferents are importantly concerned in response feed-back to the motor cortex and a closely-coupled direct influence of muscle spindle afferents on pyramidal-tract neurones in the primate has not been demonstrated. Afferent fibres from primary endings of muscle spindles have been shown to produce a short-latency influence on area 3a of the cerebral cortex (between 'somatosensory' receiving zones and the motor cortex)[170-172]. It is also possible that muscle afferents may project to other zones of somatosensory cortex such as area 2 and area 5 in the primate[173]. But it has not been shown that motor zones within area 4 receive a short-latency influence from group Ia fibres and microstimulation within area 3a did not directly influence these motor zones in area 4[172].

Although peripheral response feed-back may be important in the guiding of movement performance and, although it is essential to attempt to understand the pathways and mechanisms involved in this feed-back, it is clear from recent repetitions of the Mott and Sherrington experiment that movement performance may be accomplished without significant peripheral feed-back and utilising only the central programme for management of muscles. Knapp, Taub and Berman[174] and Taub, Ellman and Berman[175] demonstrated that monkeys could use a totally deafferented limb in a conditioned avoidance task. The animals could maintain a forceful grasp with this affected limb, developing full power and they could release the grasp normally. Moreover, they could learn and perform these movement tasks in the absence of vision.

In the free situation, monkeys did not use a deafferented limb. But, if the other normal limb was strapped and immobilised, a hungry monkey could learn to reach out with a deafferented limb to collect food from outside the cage. If both limbs were deafferented, spontaneous movements of these limbs returned after a few weeks and, over a period of months, the capacity to use the limbs in walking, climbing, grasping and holding was regained. It has been reported that such movements could be performed quite well even when the animals were blindfolded[176]. With visual control, dextrous manipulations like collecting a small piece of food from a hole in a board could be accomplished and the movements were said to be smooth and well co-ordinated[177]. The time course of recovery of movement ability after dorsal rhizotomy has been studied by Bossom[178]. He found that, during the days immediately following the surgery, the animals were very dependent on visual control to produce any movements. Between 2 weeks and 3 months after deafferentation, they regained dexterity in movement performance and were able to perform tasks without visual aid.

Such observations naturally lead to the view that the central programme of movement direction is all important. But it is incorrect to conclude, from experiments in which nervous structures such as peripheral afferents are damaged, that these structures had no function in movement performance when they were present and able to act. The fact that motor performance is preserved in the absence of a large part of natural afferent inflow to the central nervous system demonstrates the remarkable power of compensatory mechanisms in the brain, but it does not reveal the subtle influences which the sensory fibres might have produced in normal circumstances.

In quantitative tests, it was possible to demonstrate that temporary interruption of pedal afferents in dogs produced disturbances in their postural control and in their postural recovery mechanisms following a sudden displacement[179]. When temporary impairment of afferent feed-back from the moving hand was produced in a monkey trained to carry out a brisk flexor movement with this hand, the discharges of precentral neurones whose activity was correlated with the flexor phase of the task was increased in association with the movement performance. The cells began to fire even earlier before the movement and more discharge was associated with the movement task than before partial local anaesthesia of the hand had been produced[180, 181]. So an effect of afferent feed-back from the moving limb could be demonstrated. But this afferent feed-back was not essential for the signalling by pyramidal tract cells of the force to be generated in the flexor muscles or of the time of onset of contraction in these muscles, because pyramidal tract neurones still demonstrated changes in discharge with changes in load to be moved and the same correlation between temporal pattern of impulse activity and time of initiation of movement existed before and after partial local anaesthesia of the hand (Lewis and Porter, 1973, unpublished observations).

In both monkeys and man it has been possible, using computer averaging techniques, to detect a potential change in scalp electroencephalograph (EEG) recordings which is associated with movement performance, occurs in a localised zone overlying the appropriate part of the contralateral precentral motor cortex and precedes the beginning of the movement by a time interval of the order of 80 ms[182-184]. Vaughan, Gross and Bossom[185] studied the effect of total limb deafferentation on the relationship between this EEG motor potential and the onset of a self-initiated movement (wrist extension) in trained monkeys. They found that the motor potential itself was not altered by limb deafferentation. But the loss of afferent signals produced a longer delay between the cortical potential change and the onset of movement as detected electromyographically. Since the dorsal-root section would have affected the excitability of spinal centres, the longer delay could be accounted for by diminished spinal excitability and the need for more temporal summation before motor units could be activated.

The increased firing of pyramidal tract neurones seen in the experiments of Lewis, Porter and Horne[180, 181] when a small temporary reduction in afferent inflow to the spinal cord was produced, could also represent an automatic compensatory change in descending excitatory actions associated with a reduction in spinal cord excitability. It has been shown by Asanuma and Rosén[186] in the conscious monkey that cortical efferent cylinders of functionally-related cells received excitatory inputs from peripheral receptors in skin and joints. The fields containing these receptors were related to the movement which intracortical microstimulation within the cortical cylinder evoked. The excitatory influences were directed on to superficial cells within the cylinder which then projected excitatory influences on to deeper units within the same cylinder and produced depolarisation of cells in lamina V. In neighbouring cylinders, the effect of the same afferent stimulation was to produce inhibition of the deeply-situated cells. Whether or not this surround inhibition of neighbouring cortical units was produced over recurrent collaterals of pyramidal neurones is not clear. But, whatever the mechanism, it is certain that afferent discharges arising in receptor zones related to a movement which is cortically directed are capable of producing both excitatory and inhibitory influences on cells in cortical efferent zones.

The relevence of such findings for control of voluntary movement requires to be further evaluated. In studies on voluntary movement of the terminal joint of the thumb in man, Marsden, Merton and Morton[187-189] examined the influences of suddenly loading and suddenly unloading the movement on the electromyographic activity of the contracting muscles. Approximately 50 ms after a sudden perturbation of the movement, a change in electromyographic activity occurred. The same proportional changes occurred whether the muscles were contracting against a large load or a small and they also occurred when the muscle fibres were fatigued. These findings were consistent with the view that a muscle spindle servo system was operating in the regulation of the muscle contraction. But the gain of this servo system could be automatically increased to compensate for extra load or to offset muscle fatigue[188,189]. The interesting finding in these studies was that sensation in the moving thumb itself was 'necessary for that part of servo activation which turns up gain and focuses spindle excitation' on the muscle needed for movement. These authors indicate that this action of thumb sensibility (presumably exerted by skin and joint afferents) could be exerted at a spinal or a cerebral level (or presumably at both). It may be that the cutaneous and joint afferent influences on pyramidal-tract neurones, demonstrated in experiments on monkeys performing movement tasks, are operating to allow the cerebral cortex to focus its output on the a- and γ-motoneurones of contracting muscles[190,191]. It may even be that a long transcortical loop is involved in the responses of muscle to stretch during voluntary movement[192].

But the pathways by which these afferent influences exert their effects are not known. Disturbance of dorsal column function in humans may lead, among other things, to disorders of motor co-ordination, and dorsal-column section in experimental animals has been reported to produce disturbances of motor function[193-196]. But the precise involvement of this or of other afferent systems in co-ordinated movement performance still requires quantitative evaluation. Reynolds, Talbott and Brookhart[197] concluded that dogs subjected to bilateral surgical interruption of the dorsal columns showed a systematic decrease in their capability to produce precise symmetrical weight distribution in quiet stance. But the postural adjustments of these animals to a sudden step displacements of the platform on which they stood were not consistently altered. Spinocerebellar or other afferent pathways could have conveyed the signals which allowed the brain to produce these postural adjustments.

Not only do the pathways for input to the central nervous system require further study to reveal the significance of this input for movement control and the subtleties of the effects exerted on evolving motor performance[198], but a major effort will be required if a search is to be made for the structural and functional correlates of the movement 'programmes' which are elaborated for the many aspects of motor behaviour of which an animal is capable. Information has now been collected about the interrelations of some of the efferent systems through which the programme operates[199]. But the mechanisms involved in elaborating the programme, the methods by which the programme gains access to the efferent machinery and the manner in which it may operate through a number of separate and distinct effector channels (e.g. to the hand or to the whole arm in writing the letter 'a' with a pencil or describing it in the air with whole arm action) all require imaginative thought and incisive experiments.

References

1. Sherrington, C. S. (1906). *The Integrative Action of the Nervous System* (New York: Scribners)
2. Eccles, J. C. (1964) *The Physiology of Synapses* (Berlin, Gottingen, Heidelberg: Springer-Verlag)
3. Henneman, E., Somjen, G. and Carpenter, D. O. (1965). Functional significance of cell size in spinal motoneurons. *J. Neurophysiol.*, **28**, 560
4. Granit, R. (1970). *The Basis of Motor Control* (London: Academic Press)
5. Granit, R., Phillips, C. G., Skoglund, S. and Steg, G. (1957). Differentiation of tonic from phasic alpha ventral horn cells by stretch, pinna and crossed extensor reflexes. *J. Neurophysiol.*, **20**, 470
6. Kernell, D. (1966). Input resistance, electrical excitability and size of ventral horn cells in cat spinal cord. *Science* **152**, 1637
7. Eccles, J. C., Eccles, R. M. and Lundberg, A. (1957). Durations of after-hyperpolarization of motoneurones supplying fast and slow muscles. *Nature (London)*, **179**, 866
8. Lux, H. D., Schubert, P. and Kreutzberg, G. W. (1971). Direct matching of morphological and electrophysiological data in cat spinal motoneurons. *Excitatory Synaptic Mechanisms*, 189 (P. Anderson and J. K. S. Jansen, editors) (Oslo: Universitetsforlaget)
9. Burke, R. E. (1967). Motor unit types of cat triceps surae muscle. *J. Physiol. (London)*, **193**, 141
10. Burke, R. E. and ten Bruggencate, G. (1971). Electrotonic characteristics of alpha motoneurones of varying sizes. *J. Physiol. (London)*, **212**, 1
11. Jack, J. J. B., Miller, S., Porter, R. and Redman, S. J. (1971). The time course of minimal excitatory post-synaptic potentials evoked in spinal motoneurones by group Ia afferent fibres. *J. Physiol. (London)*, **215**, 353
12. Rall, W. (1967). Distinguishing theoretical synaptic potentials computed for different somadendritic distributions of synaptic input. *J. Neurophysiol.*, **30**, 1138
13. Burke, R. E. (1968). Group Ia synaptic input to fast and slow twitch motor units of cat triceps surae. *J. Physiol. (London)*, **196**, 605
14. Jack, J. J. B., Miller, S., Porter, R. and Redman, S. J. (1970). The distribution of group Ia synapses on lumbosacral spinal motoneurones in the cat. In *Excitatory Synaptic Mechanisms*, 199 (P. Anderson and J. K. S. Jansen, editors) (Oslo: Universitetsforlaget)
15. Romanes, G. J. (1951). The motor cell columns of the lumbo-sacral spinal cord of the cat. *J. Comp. Neurol.*, **94**, 3i3
16. Sprague, J. M. (1951). Motor and propriospinal cells in the thoracic and lumbar ventral horn of the rhesus monkey. *J. Comp. Neurol.*, **95**, 105
17. Kuypers, H. G. J. M. (1964). The descending pathways to the spinal cord, their anatomy and function. *Progress in Brain Research: Organization of the Spinal Cord*, 178 (J. C. Eccles and J. P. Schade, editors) (Amsterdam: Elsevier)
18. Nyberg-Hansen, R. and Brodal, A. (1963). Sites of termination of corticospinal fibers in the cat. An experimental study with silver impregnation methods. *J. Comp. Neurol.*, **120**, 369
19. Creed, R. S., Denny-Brown, D., Eccles, J. C., Liddell, E. G. T. and Sherrington, C. S. (1932). *Reflex Activity of the Spinal Cord* (Oxford: Clarendon Press)
20. Houk, J. and Henneman, E. (1967). Responses of Golgi tendon organs to active contractions of the soleus muscle of the cat. *J. Neurophysiol.*, **30**, 466

21. Holmqvist, B. and Lundberg, A. (1961) Differential supraspinal control of synaptic actions evoked by volleys in the flexion reflex afferents in alpha motoneurones. *Acta Physiol. Scand.*, **54**, Suppl. 186

22. Matthews, P. B. C. (1972). *Mammalian Muscle Receptors and their Central Actions* (Baltimore: Williams and Wilkins)

23. Eccles, J. C., Eccles, R. M. and Lundberg, A. (1957). The convergence of monosynaptic excitatory afferents on to many different species of alpha motoneurones. *J. Physiol. (London)*, **137**, 22

24. Mendell, L. M. and Henneman, E. (1968). Terminals of single Ia fibres: distribution within a pool of 300 homonymous motor neurons. *Science*, **160**, 96

25. Kuno, M. and Miyahara, J. T. (1969). Analysis of synaptic efficacy in spinal motoneurons from 'quantum' aspects. *J. Physiol. (London)*, **201**, 479

26. Rall, W., Burke, R. E., Smith, T. G., Nelson, P. G. and Frank, K. (1967). Dendritic location of synapses and possible mechanisms for the monosynaptic EPSP in motoneurones. *J. Neurophysiol.*, **30**, 1169

27. Conradi, S. (1969). On motoneuron synaptology in adult cats. *Acta Physiol. Scand.*, Suppl. 332

28. Westbury, D. R. (1972). A study of stretch and vibration reflexes of the cat by intracellular recording from motoneurones. *J. Physiol. (London)*, **226**, 37

29. Lloyd, D. P. C. (1943). Reflex action in relation to pattern and peripheral source of afferent stimulation. *J. Neurophysiol.*, **6**, 111

30. Cangiano, A. and Lutzemberger, L. (1972). The action of selectively activated group II muscle afferent fibers on extensor motoneurons. *Brain Res.*, **41**, 475

31. Llinas, R. and Terzuolo, C. A. (1965). Mechanisms of supraspinal actions upon spinal cord activities. Reticular inhibitory mechanisms upon flexor motoneurons. *J. Neurophysiol.*, **28**, 412

32. Grillner, S. and Lund, S. (1968). The origin of a descending pathway with monosynaptic action on flexor motoneurones. *Acta Physiol. Scand.*, **74**, 274

33. Grillner, S., Hongo, T. and Lund, S. (1970). The vestibulospinal tract. Effects on alpha-motoneurones in the lumbosacral spinal cord in the cat. *Expl. Brain Res.*, **10**, 94

34. Wilson, V. J. and Yoshida, M. (1969). Comparison of effects of stimulation of Deiters' nucleus and medial longitudinal fasciculus on neck, forelimb and hindlimb motoneurons. *J. Neurophysiol.*, **32**, 743

35. Anderson, M. E., Yoshida, M. and Wilson, V. J. (1972). Tectal and tegmental influences on cat forelimb and hindlimb motoneurons. *J. Neurophysiol.*, **35**, 462

36. Hongo, T., Jankowska, E. and Lundberg, A. (1969). The rubrospinal tract. I. Effects on alpha-motoneurones innervating hindlimb muscles in cats. *Expl. Brain Res.*, **7**, 344

37. Hongo, T., Jankowska, E. and Lundberg, A. (1969). The rubrospinal tract. II. Facilitation of interneuronal transmission in reflex paths to motoneurones. *Expl. Brain Res.*, **7**, 365

38. Terzuolo, C. and Llinas, R. (1966). Distribution of synaptic inputs in the spinal motoneurone and its functional significance. In *Muscular Afferents and Motor Control*, 373 (R. Granit, editor) (Stockholm: Almquist and Wiksell)

39. Shapovalov, A. I., Karamjan, O. A., Kurchavyi, G. G. and Repina, Z. A. (1971). Synaptic actions evoked from the red nucleus on the spinal alpha-motoneurons in the rhesus monkey. *Brain Res.*, **32**, 325

40. Granit, R. and Kaada, B. R. (1952). Influence of stimulation of central nervous structures on muscle spindles in cat. *Acta Physiol. Scand.*, **27**, 130

41. Granit, R., Holmgren, B. and Merton, P. A. (1955). The two routes for excitation of muscle and their subservience to the cerebellum. *J. Physiol. (London)*, **130**, 213

42. Fidone, S. J. and Preston, J. B. (1969). Patterns of motor cortex control of flexor and extensor fusimotor neurons. *J. Neurophysiol.*, **32**, 103

43. Yokota, T. and Voorhoeve, P. E. (1969). Pyramidal control of fusimotor neurons supplying extensor muscles in the cat's forelimb. *Expl. Brain. Res.*, **9**, 96

44. Grigg, P. and Preston, J. B. (1971). Baboon flexor and extensor fusimotor neurons and their modulation by motor cortex. *J. Neurophysiol.*, **34**, 428

45. Chan, S. H. H. and Barnes, C. D. (1972). A presynaptic mechanism evoked from brainstem reticular formation in the lumbar cord and its temporal significance. *Brain Res.*, **45**, 101

46. Fritsch, G. and Hitzig, E. (1870). Ueber die elektrische Erregbarkeit des Grosshirns. *Archs. Anat. Physiol. Wiss. Med.* **37**, 300 Translation by G. von Bonin in *The Cerebral Cortex*, 73 (Springfield: C. C. Thomas)

47. Ferrier, D. (1873). Experimental researches in cerebral physiology and pathology. *West Riding Lunatic Asylum med. Rep.* 3, 1

48. Grünbaum, A. S. F. and Sherrington, C. S. (1903). Observations on the physiology of the cerebral cortex of the anthropoid apes. *Proc. Roy. Soc. (London)*, **B72**, 152

49. Woolsey, C. N., Settlage, P. H., Meyer, D. R., Sencer, W., Hamuy, T. P. and Travis, A. M. (1952). Patterns of localization in precentral and 'supplementary' motor areas and their relation to the concept of a premotor area. *Res. Publs Ass. Res. Nerv. Ment. Dis.*, **30**, 238

50. Woolsey, C. N. (1965). Organisation of somatic sensory and motor areas of the cerebral cortex. *Biological and Biochemical Bases of Behaviour*, 63 (H. F. Harlow and C. N. Woolsey, editors) (Madison: Univ. of Wisconsin Press)

51. Penfield, W. and Boldrey, E. (1937). Somatic motor and sensory representation in the cerebral cortex of man as studied by electrical stimulation. *Brain*, **60**, 389

52. Lloyd, D. P. C. (1941). The spinal mechanism of the pyramidal system in cats. *J. Neurophysiol.*, **4**, 525

53. Agnew, R. F., Preston, J. B. and Whitlock, D. G. (1963). Patterns of motor cortex effects on ankle flexor and extensor motoneurons in the 'pyramidal' cat preparation. *Expl. Neurol.*, **8**, 248

54. Agnew, R. F. and Preston, J. B. (1965). Motor cortex-pyramidal effects on single ankle flexor and extensor motoneurons of the cat. *Expl. Neurol.*, **12**, 384

55. Uemura, K. and Preston, J. B. (1965).Comparison of motor cortex influences upon various hindlimb motoneurons in pyramidal cats and primates. *J. Neurophysiol.*, **28**, 393

56. Preston, J. B., Shende, M. C. and Uemura, K. (1967). The motor cortex–pyramidal system: patterns of facilitation and inhibition on motoneurons innervating limb musculature of cat and baboon and their possible adaptive significance. *Neurophysiological Basis of Normal and Abnormal Motor Activities* 61 (M. D. Yahr and D. P. Purpura, editors) (New York: Raven Press)

57. Lundberg, A., Norrsell, V. and Voorhoeve, P. (1962). Pyramidal effects on lumbosacral interneurones activated by somatic afferents. *Acta. Physiol. Scand.*, **56**, 220

58. Bernhard, C. G., Bohm, E. and Petersen, I. (1953). Investigations on the organization of the corticospinal system in monkeys (*Macaca mulatta*). *Acta Physiol. Scand.*, **29**, Suppl. 106, 79

59. Preston, J. B. and Whitlock, D. G. (1961). Intracellular potentials recorded from motoneurons following precentral gyrus stimulation in primate. *J. Neurophysiol.*, **24**, 91

60. Landgren, S., Phillips, C. G. and Porter, R. (1962). Minimal synaptic actions of pyramidal impulses on some alpha motoneurones of the baboon's hand and forearm. *J. Physiol. (London)*, **161**, 91

61. Hore, J. and Porter, R. (1972). Pyramidal and extrapyramidal influences on some hindlimb motoneuron populations of the arboreal brushtailed possum *Trichosurus vulpecula*. *J. Neurophysiol.*, **35**, 112

62. Hern, J. E. C., Phillips, C. G. and Porter, R. (1962). Electrical thresholds of unimpaled corticospinal cells in the cat. *Quart. J. Exp. Physiol.*, **47**, 134

63. Landgren, S., Phillips, C. G. and Porter, R. (1962). Cortical fields of origin of the monosynaptic pyramidal pathways to some alpha motoneurones of the baboon's hand and forearm. *J. Physiol. (London)*, **161**, 112

64. Phillips, C. G. and Porter, R. (1964). The pyramidal projection to motoneurones of some muscle groups of the baboon's forelimb. In *Progress in Brain Research: Physiology of Spinal Neurons*, 222 (J. C. Eccles and J. P. Schade, editors) (Amsterdam: Elsevier)

65. Clough, J. F. M., Kernell, D. and Phillips, C. G. (1968). The distribution of monosynaptic excitation from the pyramidal tract and from primary spindle afferents to motoneurones of the baboon's hand and forearm. *J. Physiol. (London)*; **198**, 145

66. Porter, R. and Hore, J. (1969). The time course of minimal corticomotoneuronal excitatory postsynaptic potentials in lumbar motoneurons of the monkey. *J. Neurophysiol.*, **32**, 443

67. Valverde, F. (1966). The pyramidal tract in rodents. A study of its relations with the posterior column nuclei, dorsolateral reticular formation of the medulla oblongata, and cervical spinal cord. (Golgi and electron microscopic observation.) *Z. Zellforsch. Mikrosk. Anat.*, **71,** 297

68. Kernell, D. and Wu, Chien-ping (1967). Post synaptic effects of cortical stimulation on forelimb motoneurones in the baboon. *J. Physiol. (London)*, **191,** 673

69. Porter, R. (1970). Early facilitation at corticomotoneuronal synapses. *J. Physiol. (London)*, **207,** 733

70. Castillo, J. Del and Katz, B. (1954). Statistical factors involved in neuromuscular facilitation and depression. *J. Physiol. (London)*, **124,** 574

71. Mallart, A. and Martin, A. R. (1967). An analysis of facilitation of transmitter release at the neuromuscular junction of the frog. *J. Physiol. (London)*, **193,** 679

72. Katz, B. and Miledi, R. (1968). The role of calcium in neuromuscular facilitation. *J. Physiol. (London)*, **195,** 481

73. Kuno, M. and Weakly, J. N. (1972). Facilitation of monosynaptic excitatory synaptic potentials in spinal motoneurones evoked by internuncial impulses. *J. Physiol. (London)*, **224,** 271

74. Muir, R. B. and Porter, R. (1973). The effect of a preceding stimulus on temporal facilitation at corticomotoneuronal synapses. *J. Physiol. (London)*, **228,** 749

75. Porter, R. and Muir, R. B. (1971). The meaning for motoneurones of the temporal pattern of natural activity in pyramidal tract neurones of conscious monkeys. *Brain Res.*, **34,** 127

76. Porter, R. (1972). Relationship of the discharges of cortical neurones to movement in free-to-move monkeys. *Brain Res.*, **40,** 39

77. Porter, R., Lewis, M.McD., and Muir, R. B. (1972). The relationship between pattern of neuronal discharge in the precentral gyrus and the time of onset of movement in conscious monkeys. *Proc. Aust. Physiol. Pharmacol. Soc.* 3, No. 2, p. 190

78. Tower, S. S. (1940). Pyramidal lesion in the monkey. *Brain*, **63,** 36

79. Liddell, E. G. T. and Phillips, C. G. (1944). Pyramidal section in the cat. *Brain*, **67,** 1

80. Denny-Brown, D. (1950). Disintegration of motor function resulting from cerebral lesions. *J. Nerve. Ment. Dis.*, **112,** 1

81. Bucy, P. C., Ladpli, R. and Ehrlich, A. (1966). Destruction of the pyramidal tract in the monkey. The effects of bilateral sections of the cerebral peduncles. *J. Neurosurg.*, **25,** 1

82. Chambers, W. W. and Liu, C. N. (1957). Corticospinal tract of the cat. An attempt to correlate the pattern of degeneration with deficits in reflex activity following neocortical lesions. *J. Comp. Neurol.*, **108,** 23

83. Gilman, S. and Marco, L. A. (1971). Effects of medullary pyramidotomy in the monkey. I. Clinical and electromyographic abnormalities. *Brain*, **94,** 495

84. Castro, A. J. (1972). The effects of cortical ablations on digital usage in the rat. *Brain Res.*, **37,** 173

85. Kennard, M. A. (1938). Reorganisation of motor function in the cerebral cortex of monkeys deprived of motor and premotor areas in infancy. *J. Neurophysiol.*, **1,** 477

86. Kennard, M. A. (1942). Cortical reorganization of motor function. Studies on series of monkeys of various ages from infancy to maturity. *Archs. Neurol. Psychiat. (Chicago)*, **48,** 227

87. Glees, P. and Cole, J. (1950). Recovery of skilled motor functions after small repeated lesions of motor cortex in macaque. *J. Neurophysiol.*, **13,** 137

88. Beck, C. H. and Chambers, W. W. (1970). Speed, accuracy, and strength of forelimb movement after unilateral pyramidotomy in rhesus monkeys. *J. Comp. Physiol. Psychol.*, **70,** Monograph No. 2, Pt. 2, 1

89. Hepp-Reymond, M. C. and Wiesendanger, M. (1972). Unilateral pyramidotomy in monkeys: effect on force and speed of a conditioned precision grip. *Brain Res.*, **36,** 117

90. Lawrence, D. G. and Kuypers, H. G. J. M. (1968). The functional organization of the motor system in the monkey. I. The effects of bilateral pyramidal lesions. *Brain*, **91,** 1

91. Lawrence, D. G. and Kuypers, H. G. J. M. (1968). The functional organization of the motor system in the monkey. II. The effects of lesions of the descending brain-stem pathways. *Brain*, **91,** 15

92. Woolsey, C. N., Gorska, T., Wetzel, A., Erickson, T. C., Earls, F. J. and Allman, J. M. (1972). Complete unilateral section of the pyramidal tract at the medullary level in *Macaca mulatta. Brain Res.*, **40,** 119

93. Phillips C. G. (1971). Evolution of the corticospinal tract in primates with special reference to the hand. *Proc. 3rd. Int. Congr. Primat., Zurich,* **2,** 2

94. Lawrence, D. G. and Hopkins, D. A. (1970). Bilateral pyramidal lesions in infant rhesus monkeys. *Brain Res.* **24,** 543

95. Kuypers, H. G. J. M. (1963). The organization of the 'motor system'. *Int. J. Neurol.,* **4,** 78

96. Liu, C. N. and Chambers, W. W. (1964). An experimental study of the corticospinal system in the monkey (*Macaca mulatta*). The spinal pathway and preterminal distribution of degenerating fibres following discrete lesions of the pre- and post-central gyri and bulbar pyramid. *J. Comp. Neurol.,* **123,** 257

97. Engberg, I. and Lundberg, A. (1969). An electromyographic analysis of muscular activity in the hindlimb of the cat during unrestrained locomotion. *Acta. Physiol. Scand.,* **75,** 614

98. Beevor, C. E. (1904). *The Croonian Lectures on Muscular Movements and their Representation in the Central Nervous System,* 84, 86 (London: Adlard)

99. Melvill Jones, G. and Watt, D. G. D. (1971). Observations on the control of stepping and hopping movements in man. *J. Physiol. (London),* **219,** 709

100. Melvill Jones, G. and Watt, D. G. D. (1971). Muscular control of landing from unexpected falls in man. *J. Physiol. (London),* **219,** 729

101. Vallbo, Å. B. (1970). Slowly adapting muscle receptors in man. *Acta Physiol. Scand.* **78,** 315

102. Vallbo, Å. B. (1970). Discharge patterns in human muscle spindle afferents during isometric voluntary contractions. *Acta Physiol. Scand.* **80,** 552–566

103. Vallbo, Å. B. (1971). Muscle spindle response at the onset of isometric voluntary contractions in man. Time difference between fusimotor and skeletomotor effects. *J. Physiol. (London),* **218,** 405

104. Matthews, P. B. C. (1964). Muscle spindles and their motor control. *Physiol. Rev.,* **44,** 219

105. Merton, P. A. (1953). Speculations on the servo-control of movement. In *Ciba Foundation Symp. on the Spinal Cord,* 247 (London: Churchill)

106. Orlovsky, G. N. (1972). Activity of vestibulospinal neurons during locomotion. *Brain Res.,* **46,** 85

107. Orlovsky, G. N. (1972). Activity of rubrospinal neurons during locomotion. *Brain Res.,* **46,** 99

108. Arshavsky, Y. I., Berkinblit, M. B., Fukson, O. I., Gelfand, I. M. and Orlovsky, G. N. (1972). Recordings of neurones of the dorsal spinocerebellar tract during evoked locomotion. *Brain Res.,* **43,** 272

109. Arshavsky, Y. I., Berkinblit, M. B., Fukson, O. I., Gelfand, I. M. and Orlovsky, G. N. (1972). Origin of modulation in neurones of the ventral spinocerebellar tract during locomotion. *Brain Res.,* **43,** 276

110. Evarts, E. V. (1965). Relation of discharge frequency to conduction velocity in pyramidal tract neurons. *J. Neurophysiol.,* **28,** 216

111. Hardin, W. B. (1965). Spontaneous activity in the pyramidal tract of chronic cats and monkeys. *Archs. Neurol. Psychiat. (Chicago),* **13,** 501

112. Evarts, E. V. (1966). Pyramidal tract activity associated with a conditioned hand movement in the monkey. *J. Neurophysiol.,* **29,** 1011

113. Evarts, E. V. (1972). Contrasts between activity of precentral and postcentral neurons of cerebral cortex during movement in the monkey. *Brain Res.,* **40,** 25

114. Evarts, E. V. (1968). Relation of pyramidal tract activity to force exerted during voluntary movement. *J. Neurophysiol.,* **31,** 14

115. Evarts, E. V. (1969). Activity of pyramidal tract neurons during postural fixation. *J. Neurophysiol.,* **32,** 375

116. Evarts, E. V. (1971). Central control of movement. *Neurosciences Res., Prog. Bull.,* **9,** 1

117. Humphrey, D. R., Schmidt, E. M. and Thompson, W. D. (1970). Predicting measures of motor performance from multiple cortical spike trains. *Science,* **170,** 758

118. Humphrey, D. R. (1972). Relating motor cortex spike trains to measures of motor performance. *Brain Res.,* **40,** 7

119. Porter, R., Lewis, M.McD. and Horne, M. (1971). Analysis of patterns of natural activity of neurones in the precentral gyrus of conscious monkeys. *Brain Res.*, **34**, 99

120. Luschei, E. S. and Fuchs, A. F. (1972). Activity of brain stem neurons during eye movements in alert monkeys. *J. Neurophysiol.*, **35**, 445

121. Wurtz, R. H. and Goldberg, M. E. (1972). Activity of superior colliculus in behaving monkey. III. Cells discharging before eye movements. *J. Neurophysiol.*, **35**, 575

122. Bizzi, E. (1967). Discharge of frontal eye field neurons during eye movements in unanesthetized monkeys. *Science*, **157**, 1588

123. Bizzi, E. (1968). Discharge of frontal eye field neurons during saccadic and following eye movements in unanesthetized monkeys. *Expl. Brain Res.*, **6**, 69

124. Bizzi, E. and Schiller, P. H. (1970). Single unit activity in the frontal eye fields of unanesthetized monkeys during eye and head movement. *Expl. Brain Res.*, **10**, 151

125. Kubota, K. and Niki, H. (1971). Prefrontal cortical unit activity and delayed alternation performance in monkeys. *J. Neurophysiol.*, **34**, 337

126. Luschei, E. S., Garthwaite, C. R. and Armstrong, M. E. (1971). Relationship of firing patterns of units in face area of monkey precentral cortex to conditioned jaw movements. *J. Neurophysiol.*, **34**, 552

127. Evarts, E. V. (1970). Activity of ventralis lateralis neurons prior to movement in the monkey. *Physiologist (Washington)*, **13**, 191

128. Luschei, E. S., Johnson, R. A. and Glickstein, M. (1968). Response of neurones in the motor cortex during performance of a simple repetitive arm movement. *Nature (London)*, **217**, 190

129. Kemp, J. M. and Powell, T. P. S. (1971). The connexions of the striatum and globus pallidus: synthesis and speculation. *Phil. Trans. Roy. Soc. (London)*, **B262**, 441

130. Evarts, E. V. and Thach, W. T. (1969). Motor mechanisms of the CNS: cerebro-cerebellar interrelations. *Annu. Rev. Physiol.*, **31**, 451

131. Thach, W. T. (1970). Discharge of cerebellar neurons related to two maintained postures and two prompt movements. II. Purkinje cell output and input. *J. Neurophysiol.*, **33**, 537

132. Thach, W. T. (1970). Discharge of cerebellar neurons related to two maintained postures and two prompt movements. I. Nuclear cell output. *J. Neurophysiol.*, **33**, 527

133. Kornhuber, H. H. (1971). Motor functions of cerebellum and basal ganglia: The cerebellocortical saccadic (ballistic) clock, the cerebellonuclear hold regulator, and the basal ganglia ramp (voluntary speed smooth movement) generator. *Kybernetik*, **8**, 157

134. Walshe, F. M. R. (1929). Oliver–Sharpey lectures on physiological analysis of some clinically observed disorders of movement. *Lancet*, **1**, 963

135. Walshe, F. M. R. (1929). Oliver–Sharpey lectures on physiological analysis of some clinically observed disorders of movement; tremor–rigidity symptom-complex. *Lancet* **1**, 1024

136. Holmes, G. (1939). The cerebellum of man. *Brain*, **62**, 1

137. DeLong, M. R. (1971). Activity of pallidal neurons during movement. *J. Neurophysiol.*, **34**, 414

138. Webster, K. E. (1961). Cortico-striate interrelations in the albino rat. *J. Anat.*, **95**, 532

139. Webster, K. E. (1965). The cortico-striatal projection in the cat. *J. Anat.*, **99**, 329

140. Wilson, S.A.K. (1928). *Modern Problems in Neurology* (London: Arnold)

141. Denny-Brown, D. (1962) *The Basal Ganglia and Their Relation to Disorders of Movement*. (London: Oxford Univ. Press)

142. DeLong, M. R. and Evarts, E. V. (1971). Activity of basal ganglia neurons prior to movement. *Fed. Proc. (Fed. Amer. Soc. Exp. Biol.)*, **30**, 433

143. Fetz, E. E. and Finocchio, D. V. (1971). Operant conditioning of specific patterns of neural and muscular activity. *Science*, **174**, 431

144. Fetz, E. E. and Finocchio, D. V. (1972). Operant conditioning of isolated activity in specific muscles and precentral cells. *Brain Res.*, **40**, 19

145. Denny-Brown, D. (1966). *The Cerebral Control of Movement* (Liverpool: Liverpool Univ. Press)

146. Snider, R. S. and Stowell, A. (1944). Receiving areas of the tactile, auditory and visual systems in the cerebellum. *J. Neurophysiol.*, **7**, 331

147. Bell, C. C. and Dow, R. S. (1967). Cerebellar circuitry. *Neurosciences Res. Prog. Bull.*, **5**, 121

148. Eccles, J. C., Ito, M. and Szentagothai, J. (1967). *The Cerebellum as a Neuronal Machine* (New York: Springer-Verlag)

149. Eccles, J. C., Faber, D. S., Murphy, J. T., Sabah, N. H. and Táboříková, H. (1970). The integrative performance of the cerebellar Purkinje cell. *Excitatory Synaptic Mechanisms*, 223 (P. Andersen and J. K. S. Jansen, editors) (Oslo: Universitetsforlaget)

150. Eccles, J. C., Sabah, N. H., Schmidt, R. F. and Táboříková, H. (1971). Cerebellar Purkinje cell responses to cutaneous mechanoreceptors. *Brain Res.*, **30**, 419

151. Purpura, D. P., Frigyesi, T. L., McMurtry, J. G. and Scarff, T. (1966). Synaptic mechanisms in thalamic regulation of cerebello-cortical projection activity. *The Thalamus*, 153 (D. P. Purpura and M. D. Yahr, editors) (New York: Columbia Univ. Press)

152. Li, C. -L. (1959). Some properties of pyramidal neurones in motor cortex with particular reference to sensory stimulation. *J. Neurophysiol.*, **22**, 385

153. Brooks, V. B., Rudomin, P. and Slayman, C. L. (1961). Peripheral receptive fields of neurons in the cat's cerebral cortex. *J. Neurophysiol.*, **24**, 302–325.

154. Albe-Fessard, D. and Liebeskind, J. (1966). Origine des messages somato-sensitifs activant les cellules du cortex moteur chez le singe. *Expl. Brain Res.*, **1**, 127

155. Welt, C., Aschoff, J. C., Kameda, K. and Brooks, V. B. (1967). Intracortical organization of cat's motosensory neurons. *Neurophysiological Basis of Normal and Abnormal Motor Activities*, 255 (M. D. Yahr and D. P. Purpura, editors) (New York: Raven Press)

156. Asanuma, H., Stoney, S. D., Jr. and Abzug, C. (1968). Relationship between afferent input and motor outflow in cat motosensory cortex. *J. Neurophysiol.*, **31**, 670

157. Sakata, H. and Miyamoto, J. (1968). Topographic relationship between the receptive fields of neurons in the motor cortex and the movements elicited by focal stimulation in freely moving cats. *Jap. J. Physiol.*, **18**, 489

158. Wettstein, A. and Handwerker, H. O. (1970). Afferente Verbindungen zu schnell- and langsam-leitenden Pyramidenbahnneuronen der Katze. *Pflugers Arch. Ges Physiol.*, **320**, 247

159. Brooks, V. B. and Stoney, S. D., Jr. (1971). Motor mechanisms: The role of the pyramidal system in motor control. *Annu. Rev. Physiol.*, **33**, 337

160. Asanuma, H. and Rosén, I. (1972). Functional role of afferent inputs to the monkey motor cortex. *Brain Res.*, **40**, 3

161. Rosén, I. and Asanuma, H. (1972). Peripheral afferent inputs to the forelimb area of the monkey motor cortex: input-output relations. *Expl. Brain Res.*, **14**, 257

162. Mott, F. W. and Sherrington, C. S. (1895). Experiments upon the influence of sensory nerves upon movement and nutrition of the limbs. Preliminary communication. *Proc. Roy. Soc. (London)*, **B57**, 481

163. Lewis, M.McD. and Porter, R. (1971). Lack of involvement of fusimotor activation in movement of the foot produced by electrical stimulation of monkey cerebral cortex. *J. Physiol. (London)*, **212**, 707

164. Wiesendanger, M. (1969). The pyramidal tract. Recent investigations on its morphology and function. *Ergebn. Physiol.*, **61**, 72

165. Brooks, V. B., Kozlovskaya, I., Atkin, A., Horvath, F. E. and Uno, M. (1971). Experimental analysis of cerebellar dysfunction. *Proc. 14th Int. Congr. Physiol. Sciences*, 84

166. Brooks, V. B., Adrien, J. and Dykes, R. W. (1972). Task-related discharge of neurons in motor cortex and effects of dentate cooling. *Brain Res.*, **40**, 85

167. Buser, P. and Imbert, M. (1961). Sensory projections to the motor cortex in cats: a microelectrode study. *Sensory Communication*, 607 (W. A. Rosenblith, editor) (Cambridge, Mass: M. I. T. Press)

168. Fetz, E. E. and Baker, M. A. (1969). Response properties of precentral neurons in awake monkeys. *Physiologist (Washington)* **12**, 223P

169. Goldring, S. and Ratcheson, R. (1971). Human motor cortex: Sensory input data from single neuron recordings. *Science*, **175**, 1493

170. Oscarrson, O. and Rosén, I. (1966). Short-latency projections to the cat's cerebral cortex from skin and muscle afferents in the contralateral forelimb. *J. Physiol. (London)* **182**, 164

171. Landgren, S. and Silfvenius, H. (1969). Projection to cerebral cortex of Group 1 muscle afferents from the cat's hindlimb. *J. Physiol. (London)*, **200**, 353

172. Phillips, C. G., Powell, T. P. S. and Wiesendanger, M. (1971). Projection from low threshold muscle afferents of hand and forearm to area 3a of baboon's cortex. *J. Physiol.* (*London*), **217**, 419
173. Burchfiel, J. L. and Duffy, F. H. (1972). Muscle afferent input to single cells in primate somatosensory cortex. *Brain Res.*, **45**, 241
174. Knapp, H. D., Taub, E. and Berman, A. J. (1963). Movements in monkeys with deafferented forelimbs. *Expl. Neurol.*, **7**, 305
175. Taub, E., Ellman S. J. and Berman, A. J. (1966). Deafferentation in monkeys: Effect on conditioned grasp response. *Science.* **151**, 593
176. Taub, E. and Berman, A. J. (1963). Avoidance conditioning in the absence of relevant proprioceptive and exteroceptive feedback. *J. Comp. Physiol. Psychol.*, **56**, 1012
177. Taub, E. and Berman, A. J. (1968). Movement and learning in the absence of sensory feedback. *The Neuropsychology of Spatially Oriented Behaviour*, 173 (J. Freedman, editor) (Illinois: Dorsey Press)
178. Bossom, J. (1972). Time of recovery of voluntary movement following dorsal rhizotomy. *Brain Res.*, **45**, 247
179. Mori, S., Reynolds, P. J. and Brookhart, J. M. (1970). Contribution of pedal afferents to postural control in the dog. *Amer. J. Physiol.*, **218**, 726
180. Lewis, M.McD., Porter, R. and Horne, M. (1971). The effects of impairment of afferent feedback from the moving limb on the natural activities of neurones in the precentral gyrus of conscious monkeys: a preliminary investigation. *Brain Res.*, **32**, 467
181. Lewis, M.McD. and Porter, R. (1972). The effects of local anaesthesia of the moving hand on the discharges of precentral neurones associated with hand movements. *Proc. Aust. Physiol. Pharmacol. Soc.*, **3**, No. 1, 56
182. Gilden, L., Vaughan, H. G. Jr. and Costa, L. D. (1966). Summated human EEG potentials with voluntary movement. *Electroenceph. Clin. Neurophysiol.* **20**, 433
183. Deecke, L., Scheid, P. and Kornhuber, H. H. (1969). Distribution of readiness potential, pre-motion positivity and motor potential of the human cerebral cortex preceding voluntary finger movements. *Expl. Brain Res.*, **7**, 158
184. Kato, M. and Tanji, J. (1972). Cortical motor potentials acompanying volitionally controlled single motor unit discharges in human finger muscles. *Brain Res.*, **47**, 103
185. Vaughan, H. G., Jr., Gross, E. G. and Bossom, J. (1970). Cortical motor potential in monkeys before and after upper limb deafferentation. *Expl. Neurol.*, **26**, 253
186. Asanuma, H. and Rosén, I. (1972). Topographical organization of cortical efferent zones projecting to distal forelimb muscles in the monkey. *Expl. Brain Res.*, **14**, 243
187. Marsden, C. D., Merton, P. A. and Morton, H. B. (1971). Servo action and stretch reflex in human muscle and its apparent dependence on peripheral sensation. *J. Physiol.* (*London*), **216**, 21P
188. Marsden, C. D., Merton, P. A. and Morton, H. B. (1972). Changes in loop gain with force in human muscle servo. *J. Physiol.* (*London*), **222**, 32P
189. Marsden, C. D., Merton, P. A. and Morton, H. B. (1972). Servo action in human voluntary movement. *Nature,* (*London*), **238**, 140
190. Vedel, J. P. and Mouillac-Baudevin, J. (1970). Pyramidal control of the dynamic and static fusimotor fibres activity in the cat. *Expl. Brain Res.*, **10**, 39
191. Clough, J. F. M., Phillips, C. G. and Sheridan, J. D. (1971). The short-latency projection from the baboon's motor cortex to fusimotor neurones of the forearm and hand. *J. Physiol.* (*London*), **216**, 257
192. Phillips, C. G. (1969). The Ferrier Lecture, 1968. Motor apparatus of the baboon's hand. *Proc. Roy. Soc.* (*London*), **B173**, 141
193. Ferraro, A. and Barrera, S. E. (1935). Summary of clinical and anatomical findings following lesions in the dorsal column system of *Macacus rhesus* monkeys. *Proc. Ass. Res. Nerv. Ment. Dis.*, **15**, 371
194. Denny-Brown, D. and Gilman S. (1963). Behavioural effects of dorsal column lesions. *Trans. Amer. Neurol. Assoc.*, **88**, 95
195. Cook, A. W. and Browder, E. J. (1965). Functions of posterior columns in man. *Archs. Neurol.* (*Chicago*), **12**, 72
196. Gilman, S. and Denny-Brown, D. (1966). Disorders of movement and behaviour following dorsal column lesions. *Brain*, **89**, 397

197. Reynolds, P. J., Talbott, R. E. and Brookhart, J. M. (1972). Control of postural reactions in the dog: the role of the dorsal column feedback pathway. *Brain Res.*, **40**, 159

198. Eccles, J. C. (1969). The dynamic loop hypothesis of movement control. In *Information Processing in the Nervous System*, 245–269 (K. N. Leiboric, editor) (New York: Springer-Verlag)

199. Burke, R. E. (1971). Control systems operating on spinal reflex mechanisms. *Neurosciences Res. Prog. Bull.*, **9**, 60

5
Superior Colliculus: Structure, Physiology and possible Functions

BARBARA GORDON
University of Oregon

5.1   INTRODUCTION   187

5.2   ANATOMY   188
      5.2.1   *Optic nerve projection*   188
      5.2.2   *Projection from visual cortical areas*   190
      5.2.3   *Topographic organisation*   190
      5.2.4   *Synaptic organisation*   192
      5.2.5   *Non-visual inputs*   193
      5.2.6   *Ascending efferents*   194
      5.2.7   *Descending efferents*   194
      5.2.8   *Summary of collicular anatomy*   195

5.3   RECEPTIVE FIELDS IN SUPERFICIAL LAYERS OF CAT AND MONKEY
      COLLICULUS   195
      5.3.1   *Cat colliculus*   195
            5.3.1.1   *Requirements for moving stimuli*   196
            5.3.1.2   *Size and shape of optimal stimuli*   196
            5.3.1.3   *Directional selectivity*   197
            5.3.1.4   *Mechanisms of directional selectivity*   199
            5.3.1.5   *Receptive field size*   199
            5.3.1.6   *Binocular interaction*   200
            5.3.1.7   *Laminar structure*   200
            5.3.1.8   *Summary and interpretation*   200
      5.3.2   *Primate colliculus*   201
            5.3.2.1   *Rhesus monkey*   201
                   (a) *Attention cells*   201
            5.3.2.2   *Cebus monkey*   203
                   (a) *Cells requiring precisely orientated stimuli*   203
                   (b) *Cells requiring real objects*   203
            5.3.2.3   *Squirrel monkey*   203

5.4   RECEPTIVE FIELDS OF CELLS IN DEEP LAYERS OF CAT AND MONKEY
      SUPERIOR COLLICULUS   203
      5.4.1   *Cat colliculus*   203
              5.4.1.1   *Visual receptive fields*   204
              5.4.1.2   *Auditory receptive fields*   204
              5.4.1.3   *Somatic receptive fields*   206
      5.4.2   *Primate colliculus*   206
              5.4.2.1   *Rhesus colliculus*   206
              5.4.2.2   *Cebus colliculus*   207

5.5   COLLICULAR RECEPTIVE FIELDS IN LOWER MAMMALS   207
      5.5.1   *Rabbit colliculus*   208
      5.5.2   *Ground squirrel colliculus*   208
      5.5.3   *Summary of interspecies comparisons*   209

5.6   ELABORATION OF COLLICULAR RECEPTIVE FIELDS   209
      5.6.1   *Properties of the cortico-collicular pathway in cats*   209
              5.6.1.1   *Antidromic recording of cortical cells*   209
              5.6.1.2   *Orthodormic driving of collicular cells by stimulation
                        of the visual cortex*   210
              5.6.1.3   *Elimination of visual cortex input*   210
                        (a) *Superficial units*   210
                        (b) *Deep units*   211
              5.6.1.4   *Modification of visual cortex input by visual
                        deprivation*   211
      5.6.2   *Function of various inputs to cat colliculus*   212
      5.6.3   *The cortico-collicular pathway in other species*   213
              5.6.3.1   *Primates*   213
              5.6.3.2   *Rabbit*   213
              5.6.3.3   *Ground squirrel*   213

5.7   COLLICULAR CELL ACTIVITY RELATED TO EYE MOVEMENT   213
      5.7.1   *Primates*   213
      5.7.2   *Cats*   215
      5.7.3   *Interpretation*   215

5.8   ELECTRICAL STIMULATION OF THE SUPERIOR COLLICULUS   215
      5.8.1   *Cats*   216
      5.8.2   *Rabbits*   217
      5.8.3   *Primates*   217

5.9   EFFECTS OF COLLICULAR LESIONS   219
      5.9.1   *Effects of collicular lesions on orientation to visual, auditory
              and somatic stimuli*   219
      5.9.2   *Effects of collicular lesions on pattern discrimination*   221
      5.9.3   *Effects of collicular lesions on eye movement*   222

5.10 SUMMARY AND CONCLUSIONS   223

      NOTE ADDED IN PROOF   225

5.1 INTRODUCTION

Ever since Kuffler's[1] pioneering work on receptive fields in the mammalian retina, a tremendous amount of effort has gone into understanding the processing of visual information in the geniculo-cortical system. The single unit analysis of receptive fields in the retina, lateral geniculate nucleus and areas 17, 18 and 19 of the cortex has provided a great deal of information about how the illumination of single receptors in the retina is transformed into information about the size, shape, orientation and location of real objects in the visual field[2-4]. Until recently, the role of the optic tectum or superior colliculus has received little attention. This structure on the dorsal surface of the midbrain is the primary site of optic tract termination in lower vertebrates. In spite of the development of the geniculo-cortical system in higher mammals, the superior colliculus continues to receive substantial optic tract input. It also receives massive input from the visual cortex as well as ascending and descending inputs from many other areas of the brain and spinal cord.

Ever since the end of the nineteenth century there have been sporadic attempts to study the anatomy and physiology of the superior colliculus. The general notion emerging from these early studies (reviewed by Whitteridge[5]) is that the superior colliculus may be involved in the control of visual orientation and eye movements. Many of these early studies, however, produced conflicting results. Moreover, they did not produce compelling arguments for any particular function of the superior colliculus. For example, although they demonstrated that eye movements can be evoked by collicular stimulation, eye movements can also be evoked by stimulation of many other portions of the brain.

In the last 6 or 7 years several laboratories have concentrated their efforts on understanding the anatomy, physiology, and function of the superior colliculus. In my review of this work. I will concentrate on cat and primate colliculus because we do not have detailed anatomical, physiological, and behavioural data about other species. Work on other mammalian species will be described where the experiments make points that have not been made by work on cat and monkey, or when interspecies comparisons suggest important interspecies differences in the organisation and function of the colliculus. (Except where the context might cause ambiguity, the superior colliculus will, in this paper, be referred to as the 'colliculus'.)

The experiments will be described under the following headings:

Anatomy. Degeneration studies have identified a large number of afferent and efferent collicular pathways. The synaptic structure of the superficial collicular layers has been investigated with the electron microscope and the anatomical relationships among the retinal and cortical inputs have been studied in some detail.

Receptive field structure. Single unit studies of collicular receptive fields have shown that the properties of collicular cells are quite different from the properties of cells in the visual cortex. These differences are quite suggestive of functional differences.

Elaboration of receptive field structure. Collicular anatomy can account for some of the properties of collicular receptive fields. The role of the cortical input to the colliculus can be examined by eliminating it.

Cells that fire before eye movements. Some of these cells also have visual receptive fields, suggesting that sensory information may be translated into motor commands in the colliculus. A comparison of collicular and occulo-motor neurones allows us to describe the transformations that must occur between the commands issued by the superior colliculus and the movements executed by the occulomotor neurones. A comparison of collicular and cortical cells firing in relation to eye movements also suggests functional differences between these two structures.

Electrical stimulation of the colliculus. These experiments corroborate the conclusions derived from experiments on collicular cells responding before eye movements. They also demonstrate that the activity of the colliculus and its efferent pathways is sufficient to initiate eye movements.

Collicular ablation. Behavioural deficits following collicular ablation suggest some functions that the colliculus might perform in normal animals. The effects of collicular lesions are quite different from the effects of lesions of the visual cortex.

Although this preview has emphasised the contrasts between the colliculus and the visual cortex, the two structures are probably mutually dependent. The colliculus receives much of its visual input from the visual cortex and the colliculus feeds back to cortical areas adjacent to the visual cortex via thalamic nuclei.

5.2 ANATOMY

The mammalian superior colliculus consists of alternating cell and fibre layers. From dorsal to ventral these are: zonal layer, superficial grey, optic layer, intermediate grey, intermediate white, deep grey and deep white[6]. The three dorsal layers will be referred to as the superficial layers and the four ventral layers will be referred to as the deep layers.

5.2.1 Optic nerve projection

Both crossed and uncrossed optic tract fibres enter the superior collicnuls via its brachium. The crossed projection is much larger than the uncrossed projection[6]. In fact, P. Sterling (personal communication), has examined over 1200 optic nerve terminals in the colliculus and has found only five originating in the ipsilateral eye.

After entering the colliculus through the optic layer, the optic tract fibres turn upwards to terminate primarily in the superficial grey. The distribution of the optic nerve terminals varies among species. In rat, these fibres terminate primarily in the upper part of the superficial grey, but are scattered through-out the entire superficial grey[7, 8]. In cat, optic nerve terminals are confined to the upper 100 μm of the superficial grey[9, 10] (P. Sterling, personal communi-cation).

In monkey, optic nerve terminals are confined exclusively to the caudal two-thirds of the colliculus[11-13] (see Section 5.2.3). Lund[8, 12] finds optic nerve terminals only in the upper half of the superficial grey, while Hendrickson et al.[11] finds such terminals throughout the entire thickness of the superficial grey, especially in the caudal portions of the colliculus.

A number of investigators have attempted to determine whether the optic tract fibres to the colliculus are branches of optic tract fibres to the geniculate or whether there is a separate population of retinal ganglion cell axons destined for the colliculus. Studies in both rat[14] and cat[15] have demonstrated that at least some optic nerve fibres send branches to both geniculate and colliculus. The experiments involved recording antidromic responses from the optic nerve during the electrical stimulation of optic nerve terminals in colliculus and geniculate. The optic nerve potential in response to a geniculate stimulus is reduced by a conditioning stimulus to the colliculus a few milliseconds earlier. This experiments suggests that some of the optic nerve fibres do not respond to the geniculate stimulus because they are refractory as a result of previous collicular stimulation. Sefton[14] has convincing arguments that these results are not an artifact of current spread.

Hoffman[16] has attacked this problem by recording from cat retinal ganglion cells while attempting to stimulate their axons antidromically from the colliculus. He finds that retinal X cells do not project to the colliculus. Retinal Y cells project to both colliculus and geniculate, but whether a single Y cell projects to both structures cannot be determined from Hoffmann's experiments*. Hoffmann has found a third category of retinal units (W units) that probably projects only to the colliculus. They have a conduction velocity of about 6 m s^{-1}, slower than the optic nerve units that project to geniculate. They respond to both the 'on' and 'off' of a small spot of light presented anywhere in their receptive field. Optic nerve units with these receptive field properties have not been found to project to geniculate, although the possibility that they project sparsely to very small geniculate cells cannot be eliminated.

In the ground squirrel separate populations of optic nerve cells project to geniculate and colliculus[17]. This species has three different types of optic nerve fibre receptive fields: contrast sensitive, colour coded and directionally selective. Only the first two project to geniculate while only the directionally selective optic nerve fibre project to colliculus.

In monkey there is no physiological evidence available on the distribution of optic tract fibres to geniculate and colliculus, but electron microscope studies have shown that following optic tract section one sees only dense degeneration in the colliculus and only primary filamentous degeneration in the geniculate[12]. Lund[12] suggests that a single optic nerve fibre does not produce one type of degeneration at one terminal and one type at another terminal. Therefore separate populations of optic tract fibres probably project to the geniculate and the colliculus. This argument is made more convincing by studies of the rat where physiological evidence[14] suggests that some fibres project to both structures and where both dense and filamentous degeneration are seen in both structures[7, 18].

Although the observations made on cat, rat, monkey and ground squirrel are not really comparable, available data suggest that in cat and rat at least some of the optic nerve fibres go to both geniculate and colliculus. In cat, a

* See 'Note added in proof'.

slowly conducting population of fibres probably goes only to colliculus. In ground squirrel and monkey, on the other hand, completely separate populations of optic nerve fibres probably project to colliculus and to geniculate. (The evidence on the monkey is, however, weak.) Unfortunately, there is no obvious physiological and behavioural significance to the interspecies variation in optic nerve input to the colliculus.

5.2.2 Projection from visual cortical areas

The visual areas of the cortex all project to the superficial layers of the ipsilateral colliculus via its brachium. The exact pattern of termination is species dependent. In Rhesus monkey[8, 12, 13, 19] and cat[10, 20, 21] (and P. Sterling, personal communication) lesions of areas 17 and 18 result in dense degeneration in the ipsilateral superior colliculus throughout the zonal layer and the superficial grey. Thus, in these species the retinal and cortical projections completely overlap. In the monkey, the cortical terminals are rather evenly distributed throughout the superficial grey[8], while in the cat they are most concentrated in the lower portion of the superficial grey[10]. If a lesion in cat cortex is extended to include area 19 and the lateral suprasylvian gyrus (Clare–Bishop area), degeneration is seen in the optic layer and the top portion of the intermediate grey as well as in the bottom of the superficial grey[20, 21]. In rat[7, 8], the visual cortex projection to the colliculus is less dense and terminates primarily in the bottom half of the superficial grey. Ascending the phylogenetic scale from rat to cat to monkey, the density of the corticocollicular projection increases relative to the density of the retino-collicular projection.

In cat, a single collicular cell may receive input from both cortex and retina[83*]. The distributions of cortical and retinal projections overlap extensively and Sterling[10] shows at least one micrograph in which both cortical and retinal presynaptic profiles terminate on the same dendrite.

In monkey, there is no direct evidence that a single collicular cell receives input from both retina and the cortex. However, cells in the rostral portion of the monkey colliculus receive only cortical input[11-13].

5.2.3 Topographic organisation

The topographic organisation of the superior colliculus has been studied both anatomically and physiologically. The details of the map vary substantially among species but, in general, each colliculus contains a map of the contralateral visual field. Thus retinal and cortical fibres with receptive fields in the same portion of the visual field project to the same part of the colliculus. The vertical meridian of the visual field is mapped onto the rostral portion of the colliculus while the peripheral visual field projects to the caudal colliculus. The superior visual field projects medially and the inferior visual field laterally.

In cat[22, 23] and monkey[24], although not in rat[25], the map of the contralateral visual field onto the colliculus is non-linear; the representation

* See 'Note added in proof'.

of the area of central vision is greatly expanded at the expense of the peripheral visual field. In rhesus monkey, this large representation of the fovea and perifoveal area receives input only from the cortex. Eye removal produces degenerating terminals only in the caudal two-thirds of the colliculus[12, 13]. Lesions of the central 5 degrees of the retina do not result in any degeneration in the colliculus[13]. In contrast, lesions of the portions of the striate cortex representing the fovea do result in substantial degeneration in the rostral portion of the colliculus[13].

Although the colliculus receives its visual input primarily from the contralateral visual field, the portion of the visual field mapped onto the superior colliculus is not always identical to the portion of the visual field mapped onto the corresponding visual cortex. In primates, animals with frontal vision and substantial binocular overlap, each colliculus, like each visual cortex, receives input only from the contralateral nasal retina and the ipsilateral temporal retina; that is, from the contralateral visual field[24, 26, 27, 61].

Although the receptive fields of cells in the cat visual cortex rarely extend into the ipsilateral visual field, the anterior edge of the cat colliculus contains a representation of the central 8–12 degrees of the ipsilateral visual field[23, 28]. Kruger and his colleagues[23] report that units with ipsilateral receptive fields are driven only by the contralateral eye. These collicular cells may be innervated by fibres from the temporal retina that have crossed in the optic chiasm. Stone[29] has provided anatomical evidence for the existence of such fibres. Alternatively, collicular cells with ipsilateral receptive fields might receive input from the contralateral colliculus via the intercollicular commissure.

In animals with lateral vision and little binocular overlap, e.g. rat[25] and ground squirrel[30], each colliculus contains a map of the entire visual field of the contralateral eye. Lane, Allman and Kaas[31] have examined the map of the visual field onto both cortex and colliculus of grey squirrel and tree shrew. They find that the geniculo-cortical system receives input from the contralateral nasal retina and the ipsilateral temporal retina. In contrast, each colliculus contains a map of the entire field of the contralateral eye.

The above descriptions of the map of the visual field onto the colliculus are based on electrophysiological mapping experiments. Degeneration experiments may show a projection from the ipsilateral retina to the colliculus even when mapping experiments do not. In the hooded rat no portion of the field of the ipsilateral eye is mapped onto the colliculus, yet enucleation causes degeneration in the ipsilateral colliculus[32]. Perhaps projections from the retina to the ipsilateral colliculus also exist in other animals with lateral vision. The fact that the ipsilateral retino-collicular pathway in the rat cannot drive collicular cells raises the possibility that this pathway is also incapable of driving collicular cells in cat and monkey; perhaps the ipsilateral eye can drive collicular cells only via the cortico-collicular pathway. This possibility is supported by the effects of decortication on cat collicular cells[33]. Following this procedure, superficial units receive inputs only via the retino-collicular pathway and they are driven only by the contralateral eye (see Section 5.6.1.3 for a more detailed description of the effects of decortication).

5.2.4 Synaptic organisation

The zonal layer and superficial grey of the cat[10,123], rat[8] and monkey[12] colliculus have been studied with the electron microscope. Although the pattern of termination of the cortical and retinal afferents varies among species (Section 5.2.2), the synaptic organisation of the colliculus is basically similar in all three species. Most afferent axons terminate on dendrites and dendritic spines although a few axosomatic synapses are also observed. Axonal terminals contain either pale or dark mitochondria and spherical synaptic vesicles. Degeneration studies have shown that the terminals with pale mitochondria are retinal afferents while those with dark mitochondria are cortical afferents.

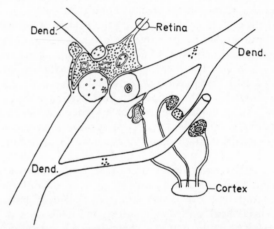

Figure 5.1 Diagram of synaptic connections in superficial grey. Note that retinal and cortical fibres terminate on dendrites of the same collicular cell and that dendrites may be presynaptic as well as post-synaptic, thus forming the intermediate elements in serial synapses. (From Sterling[10], Figure 13 by courtesy of *Vision Res.* and Pergamon Press.)

Serial synapses are frequently observed in the colliculus (Figure 5.1). In these synapses the first synaptic element is usually an axonal terminal. It may be of either retinal or cortical origin. The intermediate profile, which is postsynaptic to the axonal terminal and presynaptic to a third terminal, usually contains flattened vesicles. Although it is usually difficult to identify the intermediate profile with certainty, it is often clearly dendritic. The final profiles in serial synapses are also dendritic. Lund[8,12] finds that all identified presynaptic dendrites in rat and monkey colliculus contain flattened vesicles. By analogy with other preparations, Lund suggests that these vesicles contain inhibitory transmitters. Although Sterling[10], studying the cat colliculus, has not observed reliable variations in vesicle morphology, he comes to the same conclusion by arguing that only inhibitory denidro-dendrite synapses could account for the receptive field properties of cat superior colliculus (Section 5.6.2).

5.2.5 Non-visual inputs

Like the visual system, the auditory and somatic systems send both ascending and descending input to the superior colliculus. Lesions of the inferior colliculus result in degeneration in the deep layers of the ipsilateral superior colliculus[34-36]. The degeneration is primarily in the caudolateral portion of the colliculus. but some degeneration extends over its entire length. A few degenerating fibres enter the contralateral superior colliculus via the commissure of the superior colliculus. Input from the inferior to the superior colliculus has also been demonstrated physiologically[37]; between a third and half of the cells in the intermediate grey layers of the superior colliculus respond both to acoustical stimulation and to electrical stimulation of the inferior colliculus. The short latency (less than 5 ms) of the response of some neurones is consistent with the notion that there are monosynaptic connections from the inferior to the superior colliculus. Some superior colliculus neurones, however, respond with much longer latencies, suggesting that there are alternative longer pathways by which activity in the inferior colliculus is relayed to the superior colliculus.

The degenerating fibres that result from lesions of the auditory cortex enter the colliculus via the ipsilateral cerebral peduncle. In the monkey these fibres terminate in the lateral two-thirds of the colliculus over the entire rostro-caudal extent[19]. Degenerating terminals are found primarily in the optic layer and the intermediate grey.

In the cat, investigators disagree somewhat on both the origin and termination of auditory cortex-colliculus fibres. Paula-Barbosa and Sousa-Pinto[121] report that area AII and the suprasylvian fringe provide most of the auditory cortex input to the superior colliculus. In contrast, Garey et al.[20] and Diamond et al.[122] do not differentiate among different auditory cortical areas in describing the pathway from auditory cortex to superior colliculus. According to Paula-Barbosa and Sousa-Pinto[121], virtually the entire colliculus receives input from one or more auditory cortical areas. Other investigators[20, 21], however, find that lesions of auditory cortex produce degeneration primarily in the posterior portion of the intermediate and deep grey. Since the descriptions of the lesioned areas are not always directly comparable, the disagreements may result from differences in the exact areas damaged by the lesions.

Ascending somatic input from the face can be demonstrated by lesions of the spinal trigeminal nucleus[38]. Such lesions result in bilateral degeneration deep in the rostrolateral portion of the colliculus. Superficial cells in this region have visual receptive fields near the area centralis, occasionally extending into the ipsilateral visual field. Ascending somatic input from the forelimbs and trunk can be demonstrated by spinal cord hemisection[39] or by lesions in dorsal column nuclei[19]. Such lesions cause degeneration deep in the caudolateral portion of the colliculus. Visually responsive cells in this region of the colliculus have receptive fields in the periphery of the visual field.

The somatic cortex also projects to the deep layers in the lateral portion of the ipsilateral colliculus[19, 20]. In the monkey, this projection is primarily from the ventral part of the postcentral gyrus, the part representing the face. While a detailed map of the somatic cortex projection to the colliculus has not been made, the location of preterminal degeneration in the colliculus varies with the location of the cortical lesion.

Proprioceptive input from the eye muscles also terminates in the superior colliculus[40, 41]. Stretching extraocular muscles of cat and goat evokes multi-unit responses in the deep layers of the superior colliculus.

Two motor areas, motor cortex and frontal eye fields, also provide input to the deep layers of the monkey superior colliculus[19]. The ventral portion of the precentral gyrus, representing the face and neck, provides input to the lateral portion of the colliculus. The dorsal portion of the precentral gyrus, representing trunk and hind limbs, does not project to the superior colliculus. Lesions of the frontal eye fields[42] in monkeys also result in degeneration in the colliculus, primarily in the intermediate grey layer.

5.2.6 Ascending efferents

Ascending fibres headed for the thalamus leave the colliculus via its brachium. These ascending fibres probably originate in the superficial collicular layers[43]. Following lesions of cat colliculus, degeneration is found in several sensory nuclei; the ventral lateral geniculate, lamina C_2 of the dorsal lateral geniculate and the magnocellular portion of the medial geniculate[45, 46]. Degeneration in non-specific thalamic nuclei is confined primarily to the lateral posterior nucleus, although earlier reports[43] also described degeneration in the pulvinar.

The cat lateral posterior nucleus, in turn, sends fibres to several cortical areas, including area 19 and the Clare–Bishop area. It does not, however, project to the striate cortex or to other primary sensory areas[49]. Thus some of the connections between the colliculus and cortex are reciprocal, although the cortico-collicular connections from primary sensory areas are not. The significance of these reciprocal connections is not clear.

The projection of the primate colliculus has not been studied in as much detail[46, 47]. Rhesus colliculus projects to dorsal and ventral lateral geniculate nuclei. Both Rhesus and squirrel monkey colliculus project to non-specific thalamic nuclei. In squirrel monkey this projection is restricted to the posterior nucleus and the inferior pulvinar.

5.2.7 Descending efferents

One hopes that a study of the descending fibres will reveal an anatomical basis for the notion that the colliculus is involved in the control of head and eye movements. Unfortunately, the superior colliculus does not connect directly to any of the oculomotor nuclei (to the nuclei of cranial nerves III, IV or VI)[48]. Indirect pathways between the colliculus and the oculomotor nuclei are poorly understood. Descending collicular output originates mainly from the deep layers[43]. Following lesions of the deep collicular layers, pre-terminal degeneration is seen bilaterally in the Interstitial Nucleus of Cajal and Nucleus of Darkschewitsch[43,48]. Both of these nuclei have been impli-cated in the control of eye movements (see review by Carpenter[48]). These nuclei send fibres to the third and fourth cranial nerve nuclei, but there is no evidence that they innervate the sixth cranial nucleus[48]. This is unfortunate, since the sixth cranial nerve nuclei controls the lateral rectus muscles, and stimulation studies indicate that the eye movements generated in the colliculus are predominantly horizontal (Section 5.8). Some descending collicular fibres terminate, primarily homolaterally, in the pontine nuclei and the mesencephalic reticular formation. The colliculus also provides crossed fibres to the medial regions of the pontine and medullary reticular forma-tions[43,47-49]. Neurones in this region may project to portions of the oculomotor nuclei, but the evidence for this projection is not compelling (Carpenter[48]). The colliculus also gives rise to a crossed tectospinal tract. Fibres of the tecto-spinal tract terminate in laminae 6 through 8 of Rexed (the dorsal part of the ventral horn)[43,49,50]. Although tectospinal fibres do not end directly on motoneurones, this projection may be involved in the control of neck move-ments[51] (Section 5.8.1).

5.2.8 Summary of collicular anatomy

The superior colliculus receives topographically organised visual projections from both retina and visual cortex. The deep collicular layers also receive both ascending and descending input from the auditory and somatic systems. These cells are ideally suited to integrate visual, auditory and somatic infor-mation. The cells of the superficial layers project to cortical association areas via the lateral posterior nucleus of the thalamus. Descending collicular out-puts do not go directly to the oculomotor nuclei but may project there indirect-ly via other brain stem nuclei. The collicular projection to the cervical spinal cord may be involved in the control of neck movements.

5.3 RECEPTIVE FIELDS OF NEURONES IN SUPERFICIAL LAYERS OF THE CAT AND MONKEY SUPERIOR COLLICULUS

5.3.1 Cat colliculus

Both the geniculo-striate system and the superior colliculus have been studied more extensively in the cat than in any other species. Most studies have used paralysed animals in conjunction with barbiturate anaesthesia, local anaes-thesia or midpontine section. Receptive fields are usually investigated by moving a variety of light and dark bars, edges and spots within the visual field. A comparison of cortical and collicular receptive fields suggests that the colliculus is probably not involved in pattern perception but in detecting stimulus position and direction of movement.

5.3.1.1 Requirement for moving stimuli[52-55]

Most collicular cells produce a more sustained and vigorous response to stimuli moved across the receptive field than to stimuli flashed on and off within the receptive field. Responses to stationary stimuli frequently cannot be evoked from all points within the receptive field boundaries that are mapped with moving stimuli. The optimum speed of movement varies considerably from cell to cell. Several laboratories report that it is usually between 0.5 and 20 degrees per second[53-55] although at least one laboratory has reported that the optimal speed frequently exceeds 50 degrees per second[52]. The reason for this discrepancy is not clear.

5.3.1.2 Size and shape of optimal stimuli[28,52,55]

The receptive field of most collicular units consists of an activating region flanked by one or more suppressive regions. The activating region is the portion of the visual field from which responses can be evoked. If the stimulus is enlarged to invade a suppressive region, the response is decreased. Thus the presence of suppressive regions imposes the major limitation on the size

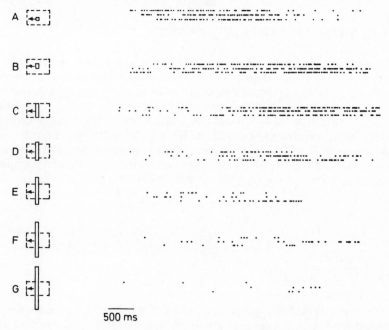

Figure 5.2 Responses of a collicular unit responding well over a wide range of stimulus sizes. The response is, however, suppressed when the stimulus extends into the suppressive regions above and below the activating region. Activating region 2.5° × 1.5°. Stimulus sizes: A. 1/16° square, B. 1/4° × 1/2°, C. 1/4° × 1½°, D. 1/4° × 2°, E. 1/4° × 3°, F. 1/4° × 4°, G. 1/4° × 5°. (From Sterling and Wickelgren[55], Figure 9, by courtesy of *J. Neurophysiol.* and American Physiol. Society.)

of effective stimuli. Although the strength and distribution of suppressive regions varies from unit to unit, at least two-thirds of the units have suppressive regions outside one or more borders of the activating region.

Although both collicular and hypercomplex cortical receptive fields have suppressive regions bordering the activating region, the stimulus requirements for collicular and cortical cells are otherwise quite different. Most units in the visual cortex respond only to light or only to dark stimuli within a very narrow range of size, shape and orientation. (Some, however, are less specific in their stimulus requirements.) Most collicular units, in contrast, respond to both light and dark stimuli and are rather insensitive to stimulus size, shape and orientation, as long as the stimulus does not invade the suppressive regions of the receptive field. About two-thirds of the collicular units respond equally well to stimuli less than half the size of the activating region and to stimuli filling the activating region (Figure 5.2). About one-sixth of the units responds maximally only to stimuli filling the activating region, while another one-sixth responds maximally only to stimuli smaller than the activating region. If a stimulus is within the appropriate size range, collicular units are insensitive to the exact shape of the stimulus and to the orientation of its leading edge; changing a small square to a circle or a straight edge to a serrated edge makes no detectable difference in the response.

5.3.1.3   Directional selectivity[28,52,53,55-57]

About three-quarters of the collicular units are directionally selective in that they respond better to stimuli moving in one direction than to stimuli moving in the diametrically opposite direction. (If a unit responds maximally to both of two opposite directions of movement but fails to respond to movement perpendicular to these directions, it is not classified here as directionally selective, e.g. a unit responding to left-right movement and to right-left movement, but not to up-down or down-up movement is not directionally selective.) The exact proportion of directionally selective units reported by different laboratories varies somewhat, perhaps because the proportion of directionally selective units varies with depth in the colliculus. Differences in the criteria used to determine directional selectivity probably cannot account for the discrepancies. Sterling and Wickelgren[55] did not distinguish between directional selectivity confined to the activating region and directional selectivity due to asymmetries in the surround. Berman and Cynader[28] designated a unit as directionally selective only if it was selective to stimuli moved entirely within the activating region. Yet these two laboratories report almost identical percentages of directionally selective units.

The properties of directionally selective collicular units are somewhat different from the properties of directionally selective cortical units[55]. First, collicular units respond over a much wider range of directions than do cortical units. In fact, for collicular units, the null direction of movement is often much easier to determine than the preferred direction. Second, collicular units respond least to movement opposite to the preferred direction; they often respond moderately well to movement perpendicular to the preferred direction. In contrast, cortical units respond least to movement

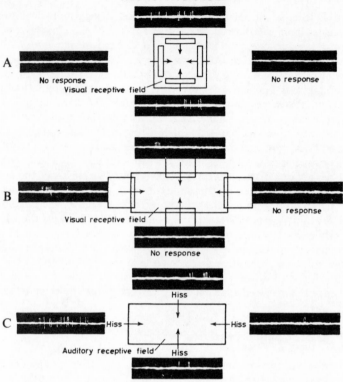

Figure 5.3 Directional selectivity in a A. visual cortex unit, B. and C. deep collicular unit with activating region 10° × 3°. A. Responses of cortical unit to dark bar. The unit responds well to both upward and downward movement, but not to right-left or left-right movement. B. Response of collicular unit to dark tongue. Collicular unit responds best to left-right movement but also responds to downward movement. It does not respond to right-left or upward movement. (Both deep and superficial collicular units often respond to two directions of movement 90 degrees apart). C. Response of collicular unit to a hiss (made by a partially constricted air hose moved across the activating region). Note that the preferred direction is the same for both visual and auditory stimuli. (From Gordon[58], by courtesy of *Sci. Amer.*)

perpendicular to the preferred direction. Movement opposite to the preferred direction often produces an intermediate response (Figure 5.3a and b). Third, most collicular units prefer movement away from the area centralis and toward the periphery of the visual field[28, 55, 57]. Thus most units in the right colliculus have receptive fields in the left visual field and prefer movement from right to left, and vice versa. In contrast, there is no indication that the distribution of directional selectivities of cortical units in non-uniform. Experiments on the Siamese cat[28] suggest that the preferred direction of a collicular unit is determined by its location in the brain rather than by the position of its receptive fields. The colliculus of this breed contains many units with receptive fields confined entirely to the ipsilateral field. For these units the preferred direction is toward the vertical meridian; that is, these units have the same preferred direction as other collicular units on the same side of the brain.

The distribution of vertical components of the preferred direction is in more dispute. Sterling and Wickelgren[55] report that most units preferred movements that are horizontal or almost so. Two other laboratories report a much larger number of units with strong vertical components to their preferred directions. Straschill and Hoffman[57] report that units with receptive fields in the upper portion of the visual field (units in the medial colliculus) prefer upward movement. Conversely, units with inferior receptive fields prefer downward movement. Berman and Cynader[28] find many more units preferring upward rather than downward movement, but do not attempt to correlate the vertical component of the preferred direction with receptive field location.

5.3.1.4 Mechanisms of directional selectivity

The directional selectivity of collicular units probably results from discrimination of the sequence in which different portions of the activating region are stimulated rather than from the arrangement of 'on' and 'off' regions within the receptive field. Most units are directionally selective in response to stimuli confined solely to the activating regions[28,53], and the activating regions do not have discrete 'on' and 'off' areas[55]. The preferred direction is independent of contrast between stimulus and ground[53,55].

Directional selectivity in the colliculus probably results both from inhibitory mechanisms decreasing the response to movement in the null direction and from excitatory mechanisms increasing the response to movement in the preferred direction. See Straschill and Tagavy[54] and McIlwain and Buser[52] for detailed presentations of the arguments.

5.3.1.5 Receptive field size

Receptive fields in the superficial layers of the cat colliculus are substantially bigger than those in the visual cortex. In animals under barbiturate anaesthesia, cortical fields within 30 degrees of the area centralis average about eight (degrees of arc)^2 [3], while the activating regions of collicular fields in the same region of the visual field average about 20 (degrees of arc)^2 [28,52,55,56]. In the unanaesthetised cat, activating regions of collicular receptive fields are larger still[55]. Receptive field size is loosely correlated with the distance of the receptive field from the area centralis. Within 10 degrees of the area centralis activating regions are frequently as small as four (degrees of arc)^2 and may be as large as 36 (degrees of arc)^2. More than 20 degrees from the area centralis, the activating regions are never smaller than 16 (degrees of arc)^2 and may be as large as several hundred (degrees of arc)^2. (The exact size of very large fields is quite difficult to determine.)

5.3.1.6   Binocular interaction[28-55]

Most collicular cells can be driven by either eye. The two eyes are not always
equally effective and the contralateral eye dominates more units than does
the ipsilateral eye. The dominance of the contralateral eye is more striking
in the colliculus than in the visual cortex, perhaps because the crossed retinal
projection to the colliculus contains many more fibres than does the uncrossed
projection. The approximate receptive field location and stimulus requirements are the same for the two eyes. A detailed search for units with binocular
disparity has not been made. Such cells would, however, be difficult to detect
because collicular units have much less precise stimulus requirements and
less reliable responses than cortical cells have.

5.3.1.7   Laminar structure

Straschill and Hoffman[57] have made the most detailed studies of changes in
receptive field properties as the electrode goes through the superficial layers
from the top of the superficial grey to the bottom of the optic layer. The
proportion of units responding to diffuse light, the proportion of directionally
selective units, and the proportion of binocularly driven units have been
reported to change with depth. Responses to diffuse light are more common
in the upper than in the lower portion of the superficial grey. Some investigators[55], however, find very few units anywhere in the colliculus that respond
well to diffuse light. Directionally selective units increase in frequency with
depth[56, 57]. There is, however, some disagreement regarding the percentage
of directionally selective units found at each level. Straschill and Hoffman[57]
report that binocularly driven units are found only below the upper third
of the superficial grey. In contrast, other laboratories[28, 55] report that almost
all units throughout the colliculus are binocularly driven.

These changes in receptive field properties are consistent with the anatomy.
The optic nerve terminals in the cat colliculus are found primarily in the
upper portion of the superficial grey while the cortical terminals are found
in the bottom half of this layer[10, 12]. In addition, Golgi studies show that
the shapes of cells in the upper part of the superficial grey are quite different
from the shapes of cells in the lower portion of this layer[10, 59].

5.3.1.8   Summary and interpretation

Cells in the superficial layers of the cat superior colliculus respond to a wide
variety of small stimuli moving from the area centralis toward the periphery
of the visual field. The loose requirements for stimulus size and shape and
the large receptive fields of collicular cells suggest that this structure is not
used in the identification of visual stimuli or in their exact localisation. The
properties of collicular cells are more consistent with the notion that activity
of cells in this structure can direct the direction of movement of an animal's
gaze so that the animal can keep a moving stimulus within his visual field.

5.3.2 Primate colliculus

5.3.2.1 Rhesus monkey

The receptive fields of cells in the superficial layers of the Rhesus superior colliculus are very similar to those found in the cat. For most of these cells the receptive field consists of an activating region flanked by suppressive regions[24, 60, 61]. The activating region shows little spatial summation. Many units respond to both light and dark stimuli with a wide variety of sizes and shapes[24, 62]. Others require stimuli much smaller than the activating region. Stimuli extending beyond the activating region usually suppress the response. Suppressive regions do show some spatial summation; the suppression increases as the stimuli extend father into the surround.

In the paralysed monkey, moving stimuli are much more effective than stationary ones[24, 62]. In the alert, unparalysed monkey, however, moving stimuli are not dramatically better than stationary ones[61]. Perhaps most collicular cells require some movement of the retinal image within the activating region, and this movement can be provided either by stimulus movement or by the small eye movements that occur during natural fixation.

The receptive fields in the superficial layers of the Rhesus colliculus do, however, differ from those found in the cat in two respects. First, the activating regions in the monkey superior colliculus are much smaller[24, 63]. They range from less than one (degree of arc)^2 to approximately 25 (degrees of arc)^2. Fields as large as 25 (degrees of arc)^2 are found only in the peripheral visual field, more than 30 degrees away from the fovea. Second, directionally selective cells comprise only about 10% of the cells in the monkey colliculus[61]. These units are similar to directionally selective units found in the cat colliculus in that the null direction is opposite to the preferred direction, not perpendicular to it. There is, however, no indication that cells preferring movement in one direction are any more common that cells preferring movement in any other direction.

(a) 'Attention' cells—About half the cells in the superficial layers of the alert Rhesus colliculus increase their response to a receptive field stimulus if this stimulus acquires a behavioural significance for the animal[64]. Goldberg and Wurtz demonstrated this phenomenon by the following training procedure: The animals are first trained to fixate a small spot of light. Then a second spot of light is introduced in the receptive field. If, simultaneously with the introduction of the receptive field stimulus, the initial fixation stimulus is turned off, the animal must make a saccade toward the receptive field stimulus (saccade condition). If both stimuli remain on, the animal is required to maintain fixation on the original stimulus (no saccade condition). In the saccade condition, either the initial response of the cell to the receptive field stimulus becomes more reliable or the train of spikes in response to the receptive field stimulus lengthens (Figure 5.4). Some cells show both these types of enhancement. The following control experiment demonstrates that the enhanced response is specific to stimuli presented within the cell's receptive field. The animal is presented with two possible spots as targets for saccades. One is within the receptive field and one is somewhere else in the visual field. The monkey randomly distributes his saccades between these two spots.

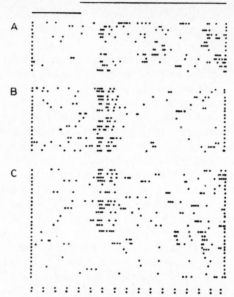

Figure 5.4 Enhancement of the response of a cell in the superficial layers of monkey colliculus. The line above the figure indicates when the receptive field stimulus came on. Each dot, except those at the beginning and end of a line, represents a spike. Each line shows the response to a single presentation of the stimulus. A. No-saccade condition. B. Saccade condition: the fixation stimulus went off when the receptive field stimulus went on, and the monkey made a saccade to the receptive field stimulus. C. Return to no-saccade condition. Note that the enhanced response does not disappear immediately upon return to the no-saccade condition. (From Goldberg and Wurtz[64], Figure 2, by courtesy of *J. Neurophysiol.* and American Physiol. Society.)

The response shows substantial enhancement only when the monkey saccades to the receptive field stimulus. The enhancement is not dependent solely on eye movement because: (1) the response is not enhanced when the eyes move toward the receptive field in darkness, (2) the timing of the units' firing is much more closely related to the stimulus onset than to the eye movement onset, (3) following a change from the saccade condition to the no saccade condition, the units give an enhanced response to the first few presentations of the receptive field stimulus even though the monkey did not use the stimulus as a target for a saccade. This experiment demonstrates that the physical features of a stimulus are only one of the determinants of the response of many collicular cells. The response is also determined by the behavioural significance of the stimulus; thus, such cells might be thought of as signalling both the fact that there is a visual stimulus in the receptive field and that the animal is paying attention to that stimulus.

5.3.2.2 Cebus monkey[65]

Like units in the Rhesus colliculus, most units in the Cebus colliculus respond to a wide variety of stimulus sizes and shapes and most of their receptive fields consist of an activating region bordered by one or more suppressive regions. Two types of postsynaptic units seen in Cebus colliculus have not been described in detail in other species. (This does not, of course, imply that these two types of cells are unique to the Cebus colliculus.)

(a) *Precisely orientated stimuli* are required by 17% of the cells. These units can be distinguished from cortical afferents because their receptive fields are considerably larger than receptive fields in the visual cortex of cats and primates (Cebus cortex has not been studied), and because they respond well to small unorientated stimuli moved in any direction. These cells have stringent orientation requirements only for large stimuli.

(b) *Real objects* are the only adequate stimuli for a few other cells. These cells respond to a wide variety of objects and do not respond well to any stimuli projected onto the tangent screen. The precise stimulus requirements of these cells have not been determined. Perhaps cells responding to object stimuli are similar to the 'attention' cells studied by Goldberg and Wurtz. Real objects may have more behavioural significance for the animal than do silhouettes projected onto a screen. Perhaps object requiring cells would respond to projected stimuli, if the projected stimuli acquired behavioural significance through training.

5.3.2.3 Squirrel monkey[66]

A single study on the superficial layers of the squirrel monkey colliculus has found three different populations of units at three different depths within the superficial collicular layers. In the top part of the superficial grey many units respond to diffuse light. In the middle of the superficial grey, diffuse light is no longer effective but most units can be mapped by flashing stationary stimuli on and off within the activating region. Most of these units have suppressive surrounds. In the bottom of the superficial grey and in the optic layer, the cells require moving stimuli and over half are directionally selective. These directionally selective units resemble those found in the cat colliculus in that the preferred direction is diametrically opposite to the null direction. More than half of these units prefer movements away from the fovea toward the periphery of the contralateral visual field.

5.4 RECEPTIVE FIELDS OF CELLS IN DEEP LAYERS OF CAT AND MONKEY SUPERIOR COLLICULUS

5.4.1 Cat colliculus

When the electrode leaves the stratum opticum and penetrates the intermediate grey layer, the visually evoked background activity decreases abruptly, the visual receptive fields become very large, and units responding to auditory and somatic stimuli appear[57, 67-71]. Units responding to auditory and somatic stimuli are most common in the lateral portion of the colliculus[68]. This finding is consistent with the anatomy; lesions of the auditory and somatic pathways projecting to the colliculus result in degeneration primarily in the lateral portion of the colliculus (see Section 5.2.4).

Some cells respond only to a single stimulus modality. Others are bimodally responsive, e.g. they respond to both visual and auditory stimuli. The percentage of bimodally responsive cells has been reported to be as low as 10%[69] and as high as 62%[68]. (The laboratory reporting the lowest figure probably included superficial cells in computing the percentage.)

5.4.1.1 Visual receptive fields[56, 68]

Deep layer cells, like those in the superficial layers, respond well to tongue- or edges moved across their receptive fields, but the optimal speed of movements is usually faster for deep than for superficial units. The activating regions of these units are often extremely large, sometimes comprising an entire quadrant or even the entire contralateral half of the visual field. For many of these large field units only the receptive field border nearest the area centralis can be mapped precisely. When the upper or lower field border can be mapped, there is usually a suppressive region outside of it. As long as the stimulus does not invade the suppressive region, most cells do not have stringent requirements for stimulus size and shape. Because these units have such large fields, they often respond over a much wider range of stimulus sizes than do superficial cells. A tongue 1 degree high and a tongue 30 degrees high frequently evoke approximately equal responses. As in the superficial layers, a few units respond maximally only to stimuli filling the activating region and a few respond maximally only to stimuli smaller than the activating region.

About three-quarters of the units are directionally selective and almost all of these prefer movement with the horizontal component toward the periphery of the visual field. The directional selectivity is more stringent for deep than for superficial cells in that most of the directionally selective cells in the deep layers fail completely to respond to movement in the null direction[57, 68]. In contrast most superficial cells respond weakly to movement in the null direction.

Cells in the deep collicular layers also differ from those in the superficial layers in that the majority do not respond consistently to repeated presentations of the same stimulus[56, 57, 68]. Such cells are seen occasionally in the superficial layers but are quite rare there. Although this unreliability of deep collicular cells has been called habituation by a number of authors, only a few collicular cells show a regular decrease in response with repeated stimulus presentation[53], and no one has shown that the decrement fulfills other traditional criteria[72] for habituation.

5.4.1.2 Auditory receptive fields[68, 69]

Some cells responding to auditory stimuli respond well to pure tones within a rather small range of frequencies. Other units appear to be driven by

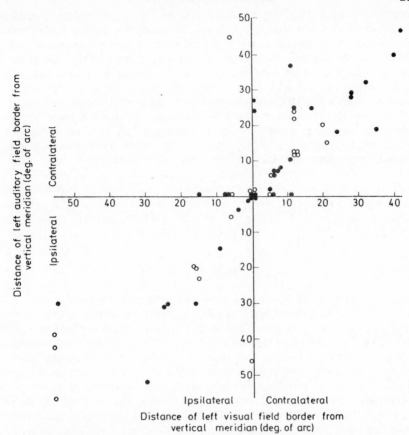

Figure 5.5 Horizontal distance from the vertical meridian of the visual field to the leading edges of visual and auditory receptive fields. The filled circles represent bimodally responsive units. The open circles represent units responding only to auditory stimuli. For these units the position of the visual receptive field was taken to be that of the nearest unit responding to visual stimuli. (From Gordon[68], Figure 14, by courtesy of *J. Neurophysiol.* and American Physiol. Society.)

complex noises such as the jangling of keys or the hiss of a partially constricted air hose. It is, however, possible that the appropriate frequency range was not explored for cells that appeared to require complex sounds.

If auditory stimuli are delivered by ear phones, most of the cells can be driven only from the contralateral ear[69]. If the stimuli are presented in real space, however, the cells have auditory receptive fields just as they have visual receptive fields[68]. Like the visual receptive fields in the deep collicular layers, the auditory receptive fields are often very large, and frequently only the medial border of the receptive field (the border nearest the vertical meridian of the visual field) can be accurately mapped. Nevertheless, there is a rough topographic map of the auditory field on the colliculus. For cells near the rostral edge of the colliculus the medial border of the auditory receptive field is near the area centralis. For cells located more caudally in the colliculus, the medial border of the auditory receptive field is in the periphery. Thus, for bimodally responsive cells, the position of the medial border of the auditory receptive field is closely correlated with the position of the medial border of the visual receptive field. Similarly, if a cell responds only to auditory stimuli, the position of the medial border of the auditory field is closely correlated with the position of the medial receptive field border of nearby visually responsive cells (Figure 5.5). The auditory receptive fields resemble the visual receptive fields of collicular cells in three other ways. First, most auditory cells respond much better to moving than to stationary stimuli. Stein and Agribede's[69] failure to use moving stimuli may explain why they found so few units responsive to auditory stimuli. Second, many cells responding to auditory stimuli are directionally selective and the horizontal component of the preferred direction is usually toward the periphery of the contralateral field (Figure 5.3b and c). Third, the auditory responses of deep collicular cells, like the visual responses, are often quite unreliable.

5.4.1.3   Somatic receptive fields[68,69,73]

Units responding to somatic stimuli have discrete receptive fields, most commonly on the contralateral face or forelimb. The somatic field is roughly mapped onto the collicular surface so that units in the most rostral part of the colliculus have somatic receptive fields primarily on the face and forelimbs, often bilaterally. When the electrode is placed more caudally, the somatic receptive fields become less frequent on the face and ipsilateral forelimbs and become more frequent on the contralateral forelimbs. With still more caudal electrode placement, somatic fields move to the trunk. Many somatic receptive fields are extremely difficult to map accurately and some are discontinuous. This physiological map is consistent with the anatomy. The ascending somatic projection from the face terminates rostrally in the colliculus, while the ascending somatic projection from the limbs and trunk terminates more caudally (see Section 5.2.4).

Gordon[68] found that most units responding to somatic stimuli have low thresholds, responding well to moving light touch or hair movement. Stein and Agribede[69], in contrast, used stationary stimuli and found that most of these units require pinch or electrical stimulation. Perhaps many somatic cells have a higher threshold to stationary than to moving stimuli.

5.4.2   Primate colliculus

5.4.2.1   Rhesus colliculus

Cells in the deep layers of the Rhesus colliculus respond to a wide variety of stimuli moved across the receptive field. They resemble cells in the deep layers of the cat colliculus in that they have much larger receptive fields than do superficial cells and they respond unreliably to repeated presentations of the same stimulus. They resemble cells in the superficial layers of the primate colliculus in that very few are directionally selective.

The intermediate grey layer of the Rhesus colliculus contains two types of units that have not been described elsewhere. The first responds only to short jerky movements within the receptive field and the second requires dark tongues (limited edges) entering the receptive field; light stimuli of similar size and shape are ineffective. Both types of receptive fields have suppressive flanks. The flanks of the units requiring tongues are unusual in that the response is suppressed not only when the dark tongue extends into the surround, but also when the illimunated area that the tongue enters is larger than the activating region.

Cells in the deep grey layers of the monkey colliculus are rather non-specific, responding well to a wide variety of large dark objects entering the receptive field. About 10% of these cells are polymodal, but their auditory and somatic receptive fields have not been studied in detail.

5.4.2.2 Cebus colliculus[65]

Receptive fields in the deep layers of Cebus colliculus are rather similar to those in Rhesus, but jerks detectors and units specific for tongues have not been described. The number of units requiring object stimuli increases to about 20% in the deep layers and a few of these units require objects moving toward the monkey, that is, perpendicular to the tangent screen. These units respond monocularly to stimuli approaching the animal and so are not responding to changing binocular disparity. The exact stimulus requirement for such units have not been determined.

In addition to units requiring object stimuli, the deep layers of Cebus colliculus contain another unusual type of unit. This type has non-uniform receptive fields. The portion of the activating region near the vertical meridian is much more sensitive than is the peripheral portion of the activating region. Although not directionally selective in the usual sense, such units may provide some information about the direction of stimulus movement. They respond with increasing discharge frequency to stimuli moved toward the vertical meridian and with decreasing discharge frequency to stimuli moved (along the same path) away from the vertical meridian.

5.5 COLLICULAR RECEPTIVE FIELDS IN LOWER MAMMALS

The visual systems of cat and monkey differ in many ways from the visual systems of rabbit and ground squirrel. Cat and monkey have frontal vision and a large area of binocular overlap, while rabbit and ground squirrel have primarily lateral vision with little or no binocular overlap. The genico-striate system is much more highly developed in the cat and monkey. The retinal ganglion cells of these species have centre-surround receptive fields, and the complex processing of visual information occurs in the visual cortex. In the rabbit and the ground squirrel, on the other hand, a great deal of complex processing of visual information occurs in the retina[17,74].

Comparisons among species are difficult because different investigators use entirely different schemes for categorising units. Nevertheless, many of the features characteristic of cat and monkey colliculus are also exhibited by rabbit and ground squirrel colliculus. The afferent connections generating these receptive field properties do, however, differ considerably among species.

5.5.1 Rabbit colliculus[75-78]

Some of the units seen in rabbit colliculus are similar or identical to the concentric, uniform and directionally selective units of rabbit optic nerve[76,77]. The criteria for distinguishing collicular units of these types from optic nerve afferents are not clear. Some collicular units clearly are not optic nerve fibres because they respond only to moving stimuli, or have an elongated receptive field with the long axis of the receptive field parallel to the visual streak. Many of these units have suppressive surrounds and some are directionally selective. For directionally selective units, the preferred direction is always opposite to the null direction. Because the rabbit visual pathway is almost entirely crossed, these units are all monocularly driven.

In the deep layers receptive fields are frequently difficult to map; many cells respond unreliably to repeated stimulus presentation and half the cells are responsive to sound and touch[75-77]. Occasional units responding to non-visual stimuli are also found in superficial layers[77].

Schaefer[78], using unparalysed and unanaesthetised animals, has found an interesting difference between the superficial and deep layer units. Units in the superficial layers respond both to movements of a visual stimulus and during head movements. Cells in the lower layer, however, respond only to movements of the visual stimulus and fail to respond during head movements. A few deep units are actually inhibited during head movements. Perhaps such units play a role in the stability of the visual world during movements of the head and eyes.

5.5.2 Ground squirrel colliculus[17]

The ground squirrel colliculus contains two categories of units. Superficial units are directionally selective. They can be mapped with small spots of stationary light, but respond much better to stimuli moved across the field in the preferred direction. For all of these units, the preferred direction is 180 degrees to the null direction but there is no indication that the preferred directions are not uniformly distributed. These units are orientated in the sense that they respond optimally to stimuli filling the long axis of the receptive field and moved in the preferred direction, perpendicular to the long axis of the receptive field. Most receptive fields have suppressive regions.

The deep layers of the ground squirrel colliculus are composed primarily of hypercomplex units. These units do not respond to stationary stimuli, and they respond poorly to small light or dark moving stimuli. They are maximally excited only by a specifically orientated edge, light bar, or dark bar that fills the activating region of the receptive field but does not extend into suppressive areas on either edge of the activating region.

Any given hypercomplex unit responds maximally only to light bars, only to dark bars or only to edges, and thus these units are much more specific in their stimulus requirements than are directionally selective units. The suppressive regions are also sensitive to stimulus orientation and their orientation is the same as that of the activating region. Changing the orientation of a stimulus in a suppressive region decreases its suppressive effect. Since many hypercomplex units are also directionally selective, hypercomplex units can be distinguished from directionally selective units primarily by the greater specificity of their requirements for stimulus size, shape and orientation.

5.5.3 Summary of interspecies comparisons

All mammals studied contain many units that require moving stimuli, many units that have large receptive fields, and many units that respond to both dark and light stimuli over a rather wide range of stimulus size, shape and orientation. In all species except the ground squirrel, the deep units have large receptive fields, less stringent stimulus requirements and less reliable responses than do superficial units. Many deep units also have polymodal responses.

The only striking difference among species is in directional selectivity. In the cat, approximately three-quarters of the units are directionally selective. The ground squirrel colliculus contains somewhat fewer directionally selective units; the rabbit colliculus contains fewer still, and the primate colliculus contains fewest of all. (It is impossible to make quantitative comparisons between species, because different investigators use different criteria for directional selectivity.) Only in cat is the distribution of preferred directions non-uniform.

5.6 ELABORATION OF COLLICULAR RECEPTIVE FIELDS

5.6.1 Properties of the cortico-collicular pathway in cats

5.6.1.1 Antidromic recording of cortical cells

By stimulating the cat superior colliculus electrically and recording antidromic action potentials in the visual cortex, Palmer et al.[79] has located cortical cells contributing to the cortico-tectal pathway. These cells are located in layer V of areas 17 and 18 (cf. Hayashi et al.[80]). The cortical cells projecting to the colliculus are mostly complex (perhaps including a few hypercomplex cells), but do not constitute a uniform cross-section of cortical cells. Cortico-tectal cells are much more likely to be binocularly driven and directionally selective than are complex cortical cells that do not project to the colliculus. When driven with long slits, most cortico-tectal cells appear normally orientated. Their preferred and null directions of movement are perpendicular, as is typical for cortical cells. Cortico-tectal cells, in contrast to other complex cells, frequently fire quite well to small spots. When tested with small spots, the preferred direction of these units remains constant, but the null direction is now opposite to the preferred direction rather than perpendicular to it.

5.6.1.2 Orthodromic driving of collicular cells by stimulation of the visual cortex[81,82,83]

Most units in the cat superior colliculus produce one or a few spikes in response to a shock to the visual cortex. This excitation is followed by a period of inhibition. This inhibition can be seen as a decreased response to a second shock delivered either to the visual cortex or to the optic nerve. Cells in a particular portion of the colliculus can only by driven by electrical stimulation of cortical areas representing the same portion of the visual field. The most effective stimulating points appear to be in areas 18, but the available evidence does not exclude the possibility that electrical stimulation of areas 17 and 19 can also activate collicular units.

5.6.1.3 Elimination of visual cortex input

(a) *Superficial units*—Three different laboratories[28,33,84] have reported that following ablation of areas 17, 18 and 19 collicular cells become more responsive to stationary stimuli, become monocularly driven and lose their directional selectivity. However, Rizzolatti *et al.*[85] report that cortical ablation causes only a slight decrease in the number of directionally selective and binocularly driven units, and Hoffmann and Straschill[81] report that the properties of collicular units are completely unaltered by cortical ablation.

The reason for these discrepancies is obscure. Variations in the size of the lesion probably cannot account for them because the above effects can be produced by lesions confined to area 17. (Large lesions of the visual cortex leaving area 17 intact, produce no changes in collicular receptive fields[84].) The lesions illustrated by Rizzolatti *et al.*[85] and by Straschill and Hoffmann[81] included most, if not all of area 17. Variations in the time between cortical ablation and recording from the colliculus also cannot account for the discrepancy; Rosenquist and Palmer[84] found the same effects of cortical lesions when they recorded 1 h after the lesion and when they recorded 16 months after the lesion. Differences in the definition of directional selectivity are also an unlikely explanation; rather different criteria for directional selectivity (see Section 5.3.1.3) have produced similar proportions of directionally selective cells both in normal animals and in animals with visual cortex ablations.

The spatial properties of collicular receptive fields are not altered as a result of cortical ablation[28,84]. Most receptive fields still have suppressive surrounds and many still respond optimally only to stimuli much smaller than the activating region. Wickelgren and Sterling[33] had suggested that cortical lesions decreased the percentage of units with spatial summation within the activating region, but this suggestion was based on rather little data and has not been confirmed by other laboratories.

The effects of cooling the visual cortex are somewhat less dramatic. Wickelgren and Sterling[33] found that many collicular units fail to respond to visual stimulation during cooling of the visual cortex. The receptive field properties of these units do not, however, change as long as the units continue to respond to visual stimulation. Other units remain active, directionally selective and binocularly driven in spite of cooling large areas of the visual cortex. Presumably, these units are driven by cortical units that are deep in a sulcus and are not adequately cooled. Hoffmann and Straschill[81], on the other hand, report that although cortical lesions clearly abolish the responses of collicular cells to electrical stimulation of the visual cortex, the lesions do not alter the responsiveness of these units to visual stimuli. Again, the reasons for the discrepancy between laboratories is obscure.

(b) *Deep units*—Rizzolatti *et al.*[85], in the only discussion of the effects of visual cortex ablation on the visual receptive fields of deep layer units, state that their lesions alter neither the ocular dominance nor the directional selectivity of these units. Since their description of the effects of cortical ablation on superficial units remains in some dispute, these results need confirmation.

Although some units in the visual cortex receive specific input from other sensory systems[86], the auditory and somatic responses of deep layer units are probably not mediated by the visual cortex. Trimodal units in the deep collicular layers respond to cooling of the visual cortex by ceasing to respond to visual stimuli while continuing to respond to auditory and somatic stimuli[69]. In contrast, the evoked potential produced by electrical stimulation of the skin is altered by the ablation of the visual cortex[87]. The use of chlorolose anaesthesia makes this study difficult to interpret.

The effects of ablation or cooling of auditory and somatic cortex has not been investigated.

5.6.1.4 Modification of visual cortex input by visual deprivation

The effects of modifying the properties of cat visual cortex cells support the notion that the ocular dominance and directional selectivity of collicular units requires cortical input. If an animal is raised for the first 3 months of life with one eye sewn shut, almost all units in both visual cortex and colliculus are driven only by the eye that has remained open. Subsequent removal of the visual cortex causes a dramatic reversal of eye dominance in the colliculus contralateral to the deprived eye. All the units in this colliculus are now driven by retinal input from the deprived eye. The retinal input from the deprived eye can drive collicular units only in the absence of cortical input dominated by the normal eye[88].

The cortical input to the colliculus can be weakened by raising animals for the first 3 months of life with both eyes sewn shut. As a result of this procedure many cortical cells fail to respond to visual stimuli or respond only very weakly. This procedure seems to decrease the effectiveness of the corticocollicular pathway. Collicular units in binocularly deprived animals resemble those in decorticate animals; most are driven only by the contralateral eye and very few are directionally selective[89].

Although a normally active cortex controls the ocular dominance histogram in the colliculus, the ocular dominance histograms of the two structures may differ considerably. If an animal is raised with artificial squint (one extraocular muscle is cut during the first or second month of life), most cortical cells are driven monocularly, some by one eye and some by the other. The colliculus, however, still contains a large number of binocularly driven units[90]. This result suggests that cortical units driven by the right eye and cortical units driven by the left eye converge on the same collicular cell. Alternatively, the few remaining binocularly driven cortical units may project to the colliculus. Each of these explanations could be tested by examining the ocular dominance of cortical cells antidromically activated from the colliculus of squint animals.

5.6.2 Function of various inputs to cat colliculus

The spatial properties of the receptive fields found in the superficial layers must be elaborated within the colliculus from the retinal and cortical inputs. These properties are unchanged by visual cortex ablations[28, 84] and are quite different from the spatial properties of optic nerve units[55]. Dendrodendritic synapses between collicular cells may produce both the lack of spatial summation and the suppressive flanks of collicular receptive fields[10].

The large receptive fields of deep layer cells probably result from a convergence of superficial cells onto a single deep layer cell. Although Ramon Cajal[59] draws some deep layer cells with dendrites sticking up into the optic layer and even into the lower regions of the superficial grey, Sterling (personal communication) finds that the dendrites of deep layer cells rarely reach into the superficial layers. Hence deep cells probably do not receive direct input from retina or from visual cortex.

In contrast, the weight of the evidence in dicates that directional selectivity and binocular interaction are dependent on input from area 17. These properties may be simply transmitted to the colliculus from binocularly driven directionally selective cortical cells. This view is supported by the fact that cortical cells projecting to the colliculus seem to be a special subpopulation with receptive fields somewhat like those of collicular cells[79].

Alternatively, binocular driving and directional selectivity may be elaborated in the colliculus as a result of synaptic connections between cortical and collicular cells. This view is consistent with the fact that following cortical lesions collicular units respond to stimuli moved in all directions[28, 33, 84]. Perhaps the major effect of cortical input is inhibition of the response in the null direction. The large number of binocularly driven collicular cells in animals with artificial squint[90] is also consistent with the notion that cortical cells with varying degrees of binocular input converge on a single collicular cell.

Little is known about the elaboration of auditory and somatic fields of deep layer cells. The anatomical inputs from these sensory systems have already been described. The only relevant physiological experiment[71] suggests that the inferior colliculus may be an important source of auditory input. Many superior colliculus units with auditory receptive fields can be activated by electrical stimulation of the inferior colliculus. In addition, many cells in the inferior colliculus are sensitive to sound location and direction of movement[91-94].

5.6.3 The cotrico-collicular pathway in other species

5.6.3.1 *Primates*

A single study on the squirrel monkey[66] examined the effects of electrical stimulation of the visual cortex. Some collicular units could be driven by visual stimuli and others responded to stimulation of area 17, but these two categories of units were mutually exclusive. This finding is extremely difficult to understand since studies in other laboratories have shown that almost all units in the superficial layers of the colliculus can be driven by visual stimuli.

5.6.3.2 *Rabbit*

Visual cortex ablation does not seem to cause any changes in the receptive field properties of collicular units[75, 77].

5.6.3.3 *Ground squirrel* [30]

Although the ground squirrel colliculus and the cat colliculus share many receptive field properties, the retinal and cortical inputs appear to have quite different functions in the two species. Simultaneous recordings from a directionally selective collicular cell and one of its afferents or from a hypercomplex cell and one of its afferents suggests that the cells classified as directionally selective are innervated solely by the retina while hypercomplex cells receive cortical inputs. The effects of visual cortex ablation are consistent with this notion. Following cortical removal, hypercomplex units are abolished while directionally selective units remain completely normal.

5.7 COLLICULAR CELL ACTIVITY RELATED TO EYE MOVEMENT

5.7.1 Primates[60,95,96]

The deep layers of Rhesus monkey colliculus contain some units that discharge between 30 and 500 ms prior to saccades toward a given area of the visual field; the 'movement field' of that unit. If the animal makes a saccade in the direction of the movement field, but the saccade stops short of the border of the movement field or extends beyond the movement field, the unit does not fire (Figure 5.6). The responses do not depend on proprioceptive feed-back from the extraocular muscles because the movement related activity precedes EMG activity in the eye muscles (Figure 5.7). Many of the

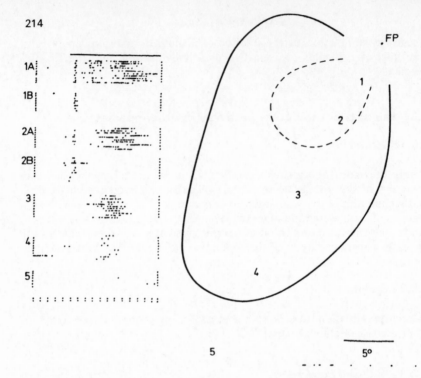

Figure 5.6 Cell with a visual receptive field, outlined by dashed line and a movement field, outlined by solid line. As in Figure 5.4, each dot represents a spike. Each line of dots in 1A, 2A, 3, 4 and 5 represents a response of the unit preceding an eye movement to the location indicated by the number. Each line of dots in 1B and 2B represents the response of the unit to a presentation of light spot, unaccompanied by eye movement, at the location indicated by the number. (From Wurtz and Goldberg[96], Figure 7, by courtesy of *J. Neurophysiol.* and American Physiol. Society.)

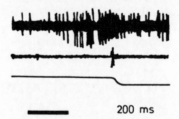

200 ms

Figure 5.7 Relation of cell discharge (upper trace), lateral rectus electromyogram (middle trace) and electrooculogram (lower trace) associated with a 20 degree horizontal saccade from left to right. Note the cell discharge before the lateral rectus activity and before eye movement. (From Wurtz and Goldberg[96], Figure 3, by courtesy of *J. Neurophysiology* and American Physiol. Society.)

units discharging prior to eye movements, particularly the most superficial ones, also have visual receptive fields. For most of these units the visual receptive fields and the movement fields are in the same portion of the visual field, but are not identical (Figure 5.6). Sometimes the visual receptive field is larger; sometimes the movement field is larger. Thus, the colliculus contains a topographic map of movement fields as well as a topograhic map of sensory receptive fields.

The sufficient condition for the firing of these units is a saccade that ends in the movement field of the unit. It does not matter whether the saccade is evoked by a visual stimulus, is a spontaneous eye movement in the dark, or is a saccade made during vestibular or optokinetic nystagmus. In contrast, the visual cortex does not contain units that fire in relation to eye movements. The response of a cortical unit to rapid eye movements is always similar to its response to rapid stimulus movement in front of a stationary eye[97].

The relationship between the discharge of these units and smooth pursuit eye movements is less clear. Wurtz and Goldberg[96] state that collicular units do not fire during smooth pursuit movements slower than 10 degrees per second. The units occasionally discharge during rapid pursuit movements, but these discharges always precede corrective saccades. Schiller and Koerner[60] state that units with receptive fields less than 5 degrees from the fovea respond both during smooth pursuit and before small saccades. Their illustration of this phenomenon, however, suggests that the high frequency bursts of these units usually occur just prior to corrective saccades.

5.7.2 Cats[98]

Straschill and Hoffmann[98] have studied eye movement related activity in the cat superior colliculus using the encephale isolé preparation. Their results are difficult to compare with the primate results or to integrate with other information about the cat colliculus because the size and direction of the eye movements are not described in detail and are not related to the units' visual receptive field. Nor are these units anatomically located within the colliculus. Twenty-four per cent of the units respond to visual stimuli but do not alter their firing in conjunction with eye movements. The activity of 13% of the cells is suppressed in synchrony with eye movements. Fifty-three per cent require a retinal image moving in a given direction. This requirement can be met by moving the stimulus in that direction or by an eye movement in the opposite direction. The firing of these units does not precede eye movements. Ten per cent of the units appear to be similar to those described by the primate investigators in that they respond in synchrony with eye movement in both light and dark, and some discharge prior to eye movements.

5.7.3 Interpretation

The existence of collicular units with visual receptive fields and movement fields in the same region of the visual field provides further evidence that the colliculus in involved is using visual information to influence motor responses.

We cannot determine from the properties of these cells whether activity of collicular cells can initiate eye movements or whether the colliculus is essential for the performance of eye movements or any other visual task. The experimental results bearing on these two questions will be discussed in the next sections.

5.8 ELECTRICAL STIMULATION OF THE SUPERIOR COLLICULUS

Eye movements can be evoked by stimulation of many areas of the brain. Among these are the visual cortex, frontal eye fields, superior colliculus and, of course, the oculomotor nuclei[5]. Some inferences about the role of each of these structures in the control of eye movements can be made by comparing the eye movements evoked by stimulating them electrically. Unfortunately, detailed comparisons are available only in the primate. The primate is probably the animal of choice for these studies. The alert primate can be held with his head rigidly restrained and eye movements evoked by visual stimulation and electrical stimulation can be studied quantitatively.

Since most of the earlier qualitative work was performed on cats, the effects of electrical stimulation of the cat colliculus will be discussed first.

5.8.1 Cats

Apter[99] provided the first evidence that the size and direction of eye movements evoked by collicular stimulation was related to the topographic map of the visual field of the colliculus. She put a crystal of strychnine on the colliculus and found that subsequent photic stimulation caused conjugate eye movements towards the portion of the visual field represented on the strychninised portion of the colliculus. It is not clear from Apter's experiments whether or not these movements were 'goal directed'; that is, whether they brought the eyes to a specific position in the orbit. Syka and Radil-Weiss[100] and Straschill and Rieger (described by Schiller[63]) have obtained similar results with electrical stimulation. Syka and Radil-Weiss add that the size of the eye movement evoked by electrical stimulation depends on stimulus duration and Straschill and Rieger have found goal-directed eye movements. Schiller[63], however, believes that unless the evoked eye movements are very large, their size and direction depend on the location of the stimulating electrode and not on the initial position of the eyes in the head or on stimulus parameters. Thus rostral stimuli evoke small contralateral eye movements, and caudal stimuli evoke large ones. Medial stimuli evoke eye movements with an upward component and lateral stimuli evoke eye movements with a downward component (cf. Straschill's results described by Schiller[63]).

The movements produced by electrical stimulation of unrestrained cats are remarkably similar to natural orientating movements. Weak stimuli cause movements of the eyes and pinnae[78, 101]. The size and direction of both eye and pinna movements again depends on the stimulation site. Rostral stimulation causes both ears to turn forward. Stimulation in the colliculus causes the ipsilateral ear to turn forward and the contralateral ear to turn backward. Caudal stimulation causes only backward turning of the contralateral ear. The effect of electrode location of pinnae movement is consistent with the notion that there is a map of the auditory field as well as a map of the visual field on the colliculus and that the colliculus has a role in orientation to auditory stimuli.

As the stimulus intensity is increased, the cat makes contralateral movements of his head, body and limbs. He may even turn completely around. Surprisingly, the ability of collicular stimulation to evoke movement does not depend upon the integrity of the cortico-tectal pathway. Schaeffer[78] has obtained these movements in decorticate cats.

The effects of tectal stimulation on cat neck motoneurones can be predicted from the behavioural effects of collicular stimulation. Electrical stimulation of the cat colliculus causes depolarising postsynaptic potentials in the contralateral flexor motoneurones and hyperpolarising postsynaptic potentials in ipsilateral flexor motoneurones[51]. This pattern of motoneurone activation would cause contralateral turning of the head. Tectal output probably reaches neck motoneurones via the tecto-reticular pathway since cutting the tectospinal tract has no effect on the postsynaptic potentials.

5.8.2 Rabbits[78]

Electrical stimulation of the rostral portion of the rabbit colliculus causes ipsilateral rather than contralateral eye and head movements. Since the rabbit's eyes are placed laterally, he must move his eye ipsilaterally in order to move the centre of his retina toward the rostral visual field. Caudal stimulation causes contralateral movements and such movements would bring the centre of his eye into the caudal visual field. Thus, these are just the movements required to bring the centre of the contralateral eye into the portion of the visual field that is mapped on the stimulated portion of the colliculus.

5.8.3 Primates[64,102,103]

Conjugate eye movements are evoked by electrical stimulation in all layers of the primate superior colliculus, but the threshold current decreases dramatically to 1-9 µA as the electrode enters the deep grey and white layers. These layers contain the cells that fire prior to eye movement and the axons that provide the collicular efferents to the brain stem. As in the cat and rabbit, electrical stimulation evokes saccades to the portion of the visual field containing the receptive fields (superficial layers) or the movement fields (deep layers) of the stimulated cells. These movements are clearly not goal directed. Rather the size and direction of movement evoked by stimulation

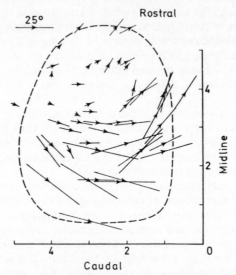

Figure 5.8 Motor map of the colliculus showing the size and direction of saccades elicited by electrical stimulation at different collicular locations. (From Robinson[102], Figure 4, by courtesy of *Vision Res.* and Pergamon Press.)

of a particular site is constant regardless of the initial position of the eye in the orbit (Figure 5.8.)

Once threshold is reached, increasing the frequency of pulses in the stimulus train or slightly increasing the duration of the train does not change the evoked eye movement. Increases in stimulus current cause slight decreases in saccade latency but have no other effects. If the length of the stimulus train is very long, a second saccade occurs. This saccade has the same amplitude and direction as the first. Continuing the stimulus eventually evokes a third saccade and so on. The number of saccades evoked by very long stimulus trains is limited only by the range of movement of the eyeball.

Electrical stimulation of two collicular points simultaneously[102] does not mimic the presentation of two visual targets for saccades. If the two visual targets are presented simultaneously, the eye saccades to one or the other. If two collicular points are stimulated at once, the resulting saccade is the mean of the saccades that would have been evoked by either stimulus presented alone. Thus stimulating a rostral and a caudal site simultaneously causes a smaller saccade than does stimulating the caudal site alone.

If two visual targets for saccades are presented to humans in rapid succession, there is a delay of about 200 ms between the end of the saccade toward the first target and the beginning of saccade toward the second target[104]. An identical experiment has not been performed on monkeys. A similar refractory period results if two collicular sites on the same side of the brain are stimulated sequentially; the latency of the second saccade is increased[102]. If, however, the two stimulated points are on opposite sides of the brain, causing saccades in opposite directions, the two saccades occur independently, unless the time between the two stimuli is so small that the saccades interfere with each other mechanically. Therefore, the refractory period between two visually controlled saccades is not generated in the colliculus or in structures between the colliculus and the oculomotor nuclei.

The eye movements evoked by electrical stimulation of the colliculus are rather similar to those evoked by electrical stimulation of the frontal eye fields[105] and visual cortex, although thresholds are smallest in the colliculus (1–9 μA in deep colliculus, 40–1500 μA in frontal eye fields and 200–2000 μA in visual cortex)[63]. Electrical stimulation of each of these areas causes eye movements whose size and direction are independent of the initial position of the eye. The eye movements evoked by visual cortex stimulation may be mediated through the superior colliculus since they are abolished by collicular ablation. In contrast, eye movements evoked by frontal eye field stimulation are probably not mediated by the colliculus. These movements are not abolished by collicular ablation[63]. The latency from stimulation of the frontal eye fields to eye movements is shorter than the latency from collicular stimulation to eye movements. Although the activity of single units in the frontal eye fields is related to eye movements, these units do not discharge prior to eye movements[106]. Hence they are probably not involved in the *initiation* of normal eye movements.

Eye movements initiated by stimulation of the abducens nucleus are quite different from those evoked by collicular stimulation[63, 103]. In the abducens nucleus increasing either the frequency or length of the stimulus train increases the size of the evoked saccade. Perhaps higher frequencies stimulate higher threshold motoneurones while longer trains enable the lateral rectus muscle to develop more tension. In contrast, the size of the saccades evoked by collicular stimulation can be increased only by moving the electrode caudally. This suggests that caudal collicular cells provide input to more abducens neurones and/or more prolonged input to abducens neurones than do rostral collicular cells.

Electrical stimulation can never mimic the natural pattern of cell firing. Nevertheless, such movements are elicited with very little current by stimulation of cells discharging prior to eye movements. The elicited movements are very similar to normal orientating movements and they always serve to bring the portion of the visual field projecting to the stimulation site onto the area of central vision. These results strongly support the notion that activity in collicular cells can initiate orientating movements of the head and eyes.

5.9 EFFECTS OF COLLICULAR LESIONS

Although lesion studies are notoriously difficult to interpret, some effects of collicular lesions are strikingly different from the effects of lesions of other portions of the visual system. For this reason, such studies provide considerable insight into the function of the colliculus in normal animals. Most of the lesion studies on subprimates have dealt with the role of the colliculus in visually guided behaviour and pattern perception, but have not made careful observations of effects on eye movements. In primates restrained in primate chairs, the effects of collicular lesions on eye movements can be studied in some detail. Such studies are, however, just beginning and detailed descriptions of the effects of collicular lesions on a wide variety of tasks requiring eye movement and visual attention are not yet available.

5.9.1 Effects of collicular lesions on orientation to visual, auditory and somatic stimuli[107-109]

Immediately following a unilateral collicular lesion, cats ignore stimuli presented to the contralateral visual field, they fail to follow stimuli moved from the ipsilateral to the contralateral field and they circle ipsiversively. Although they respond to clicks on both sides of the body, the contralateral pinnae is not mobile to sound and they do not reliably search for the origin of contralateral sounds. Similarly, the response to touch is decreased over the entire contralateral side of the body. These defects decrease somewhat with time. One month after the lesion, the animals can follow slowly moving objects in the contralateral visual field within 30 degrees of the midline. They still do not respond to fast moving objects in the contralateral field or to any objects in the contralateral field more than 30 degrees from the midline. Presenting two visual stimuli on opposite sides of the midline always results in a response to the ipsilateral stimulus. Responses to contralateral sound and touch also improve with time, but never become entirely normal.

Unilateral lesions of the brachium of the superior colliculus, leaving the colliculus itself intact, result in the visual neglect symptoms but not the circling toward the ipsilateral side. Sprague and Meikle[109] interpret this to mean that the sensory deficits may be mediated by ascending pathways while the motor deficits are mediated by descending pathways.

Following bilateral lesions of the superior colliculus, cats initially appear to be blind and respond very sluggishly to auditory and tactile stimuli. They gradually recover their ability to respond to slowly moving objects, but cannot follow rapidly moving objects nor can they lift their gaze above the horizontal. The response to tactile and auditory stimuli improves with time, but the response to tactile stimuli remains abnormal in the hind limbs, and the animals never orientate to auditory stimuli above their heads.

In contrast, lesions of area 17 in the cat produce no obvious deficits in visually guided behaviour[103]. Lesions including areas 17, 18 and 19 result in relatively mild deficits; that is, the animals are somewhat moie attentive to ipsilateral than to contralateral visual stimuli. If the cortical lesions are extended to include the middle and posterior suprasylvian gyri as well as the lateral and postlateral gyri, the animals become markedly inattentive to contralateral visual stimuli.

Ablation of the colliculus in hamster[111, 112], tree shrew[113] and rat[114] also causes deficits in visually guided behaviour. In tree shrew[113], lesions of the deep collicular layers, those layers providing descending output to the brain stem and reticulospinal tract, cause the animals to sit motionless in their cages and show no visually guided behaviour. In contrast, lesions of the superficial layers cause some deficits in pattern vision (Section 5.9.2) but do not cause motor deficits.

A single study on the effect of collicular lesions in rats[113] also demonstrates the role of this structure in visual motor coordination. Intact rats are trained on a jumping stand surrounded by one dark and five light boxes. Their task is to jump into the dark box. Following collicular lesions, the animals can still jump from the stand but do not perform the task. If the apparatus is changed so that the floor from the platform to each box is continuous, the animals walk carefully around the floor, look into each box and enter the dark one.

The effects of collicular lesions on visually guided behaviour in monkeys are variable. Denny-Brown[114] reports that monkeys with complete bilateral collicular lesions appear virtually blind immediately after the lesion and remain unresponsive to most visual stimuli for many weeks. The extent of recovery varies tremendously with the extent of the lesion. Anderson and Symmes[115], in contrast, report severe deficits, including apparent blindness, immediately after the lesion, but a return to relatively normal behaviour within a week. The monkeys have a tendency to make somewhat fewer eye movements while exploring their cages, but this disappears gradually over several weeks.

5.9.2   Effects of collicular lesions on pattern discrimination

In cat bilateral collicular lesions do not impair the re-learning of preoperatively learned pattern discriminations, but do impair the animal's ability to orientate to the correct stimulus at some distance from it. The pattern discrimination stimuli are usually mounted on doors and the animal's task is to push the door containing the correct stimulus. If the two doors are separated by a barrier so that the animal must choose the correct stimulus at a distance, collicular lesions greatly increase the number of times the animal enters the incorrect alley[116]. If, on the other hand, there is no barrier between the stimuli, and the animal can walk back and forth from one stimulus to the other, collicular lesions do not impair his ability to choose the correct door[117].

Schneider[110, 111] tested directly the hypothesis that undercutting the superior colliculus impairs the ability of the golden hamster to orientate to visual stimuli, but does not impair his ability to discriminate between patterns. (Undercutting the colliculus severs all of its descending connections, but leaves the colliculus itself intact.) He used an apparatus in which the correct and incorrect stimuli were separated by a barrier, but he allowed animals to correct their errors if they entered the incorrect alley. He counted both the number of times the animals entered the incorrect alley and the number of times they pushed the door containing the incorrect pattern. He found that as normal animals learn the pattern discrimination they stop entering the incorrect alley and pushing the incorrect door simultaneously. The animals with undercut colliculi, however, continue to enter the incorrect alley but then correct their errors. They made no more door-pushing errors than did normal hamsters. (Schneider also devised a control experiment to be certain that the animal's inability to choose the correct stimulus at a distance was not the result of myopia.)

Colliculectomised monkeys restrained in primate chairs have no difficulty in relearning preoperatively learned pattern, colour and flicker discriminations. In contrast, they have great difficulty in relearning to discriminate between rates of movement of a visual target, although they discriminate readily between a stationary and a moving target. Even this deficit, however, disappears in time and the monkeys eventually relearn the task[115]. Perhaps the collicular cells responsive to specific rates of stimulus movement can be used to make this discrimination, but the monkey has alternative methods of performing the task when this one is not available.

Although collicular lesions do not impair the ability of cats to relearn preoperatively learned pattern discrimination, they greatly increase the difficulty of learning new pattern discriminations postoperatively. Sprague and his colleagues[107] demonstrated this effect in split-brain cats with the left colliculus removed. In these animals the left eye projects only to the left side of the brain and the right eye only to the right side of the brain. By covering one eye, each side of the brain can be trained independently, the intact right brain of each animal being a control for the operated left brain. Unfortunately, most animals were trained only postoperatively. While some animals demonstrated the ability to relearn preoperatively learned discriminations and others demonstrated the inability of the lesioned side of the brain to learn new discriminations postoperatively, no single animal demonstrated both effects. In spite of this difficulty, the mass of data obtained from a large number of animals trained on many different pattern discriminations is quite convincing.

Anderson and Williamson[118] used animals with bilateral collicular lesions to demonstrate a similar effect. Animals taught a pattern discrimination before collicular lesions relearned the task easily postoperatively. Animals trained only postoperatively learned the task with great difficulty or were completely unable to learn it.

In contrast, cortical lesions restricted to area 17 have no effect on the performance of preoperatively learned discriminations or on the learning of new discriminations postoperatively[107]. Thus, the role of the colliculus in pattern discrimination learning does not depend on the input the colliculus receives from area 17[79].

The inability of colliculectomised animals to learn new pattern discriminations suggests that these animals have difficulty in making rapid changes in visual orientation and attention. Only by looking back and forth between the two stimuli can the animal determine what features distinguish the positive from the negative stimulus. If the animal cannot rapidly change the portion of the visual field he is attending to, he will have difficulty in learning new pattern discriminations. Preoperatively learned discrimination should, however, be much easier because the animal has already learned what features distinguish the positive from the negative stimulus. This hypothesis might be tested by a pattern discrimination task in which the stimuli were presented sequentially in the same location rather than simultaneously in different locations. Such a task would not force the animal to make rapid changes in fixation. With this type of training procedure, colliculectomised and normal animals should learn new pattern discriminations equally well.

5.9.3 Effects of collicular lesions on eye movement

Pasik, Pasik and Bender[119] report that once colliculectomised animals recover from surgery they are able to make eye movements in all directions. At first optokinetic nystagmus is slower than normal, but it is qualitatively normal 10 days after surgery. Possible quantitative effects of collicular ablation on nystagmus have not been examined, and we do not know, for example, if the relation between stimulus velocity and eye velocity is changed, if threshold velocity is changed or if threshold contrast is changed.

Denny-Brown[114] has, however, reported much more profound deficits in eye movements. He suggests that recovery of optokinetic nystagmus occurs in some but not all animals. The discrepancies between these reports is probably due to variations in the size of the lesions. Denny-Brown's lesions were extremely large and probably invaded the inferior colliculus, pretectum and central grey. On the other hand, the lesions illustrated by Pasik, Pasik and Bender may not be complete and clearly do not invade the pretectum.

Wurtz and Goldberg[120] have made a quantitative study of the effect of collicular lesions on voluntary saccades. They train animals to fixate a light in the visual field and to saccade to a new fixation point when the first fixation light goes off and a new one goes on. Following electrolytic lesions of the colliculus, eye movements observed grossly are quite normal. The latency between the appearance of a new fixation point and the initiation of the saccade has, however, increased by 150–300 ms. The speed and accuracy of the saccade are not affected. By the second day after the lesion only saccades to the portion of the visual field represented by the lesioned area of the colliculus are altered. Saccades to other portions of the visual field are normal in all respects.

Wurtz and Goldberg wondered whether the small deficit might be due to the small size of the lesion. When they made large lesions involving almost the entire superior colliculus, they found an increase in the latency of saccades to all points in the contralateral visual field but saccades to the ipsilateral visual field remain normal. Increases in saccade latency decrease with time and disappear completely 1–7 weeks after the lesion. The reason for the recovery is unknown.

These results contrast dramatically with a brief report of Schiller's[63, 103] on the effects of collicular ablation. He states that the ablation of the superior colliculus in primates results in persistent eye movement deficits in some, but not all, animals. Differences in lesion size might account for the variability and for the disagreements between laboratories, but it is difficult to propose explanations until a more complete report is published.

5.10 SUMMARY AND CONCLUSIONS

Stimulation and lesion studies performed before 1965 suggested that the superior colliculus is somehow involved in the control of eye movements.

In 1965, Sprague and Meikle[109] published a detailed neurological study of the effect of collicular ablation in cats. They found that after ablation of the superior colliculus cats could make eye movements in all directions but were curiously inattentive to auditory and somatic stimuli as well as to visual stimuli. If an animal fails to orientate to a stimulus, he may be completely unable to move the retinal image of the stimulus onto the fovea and keep it there. That is, the colliculus may be required for 'foveation'. This is Schiller's[103] view and is consistent with his finding that at least some colliculectomised animals are afflicted with persistent eye movement deficits. On the other hand, failure to orientate to a stimulus may merely reflect an inability to shift attention from one area of the visual field to another. This is the view of Wurtz and Goldberg[120] and is consistent with their finding that animals with colliculus lesions 'can acquire the target perfectly, but only take longer to start'. Clearly, a resolution of the disagreements about the effects of collicular lesions is a prerequisite to resolving the more general disagreement on the function of the colliculus.

The nature of the sensory receptive fields and the movement fields of collicular cells probably favours the attention shift hypothesis. The visual receptive fields of collicular cells (especially those in the deep layers that provide descending output) are much larger than the visual receptive fields of cortical cells. Thus the visual cortex would seem to be better suited than the colliculus for precise stimulus localisation. Many deep layer collicular cells respond to auditory and/or somatic stimuli as well as to visual stimuli. Although the auditory and visual receptive fields of these units are located in the same portion of the sensory field, such units are unlikely to provide precise information about auditory stimulus location, because the relation between an animal's auditory field and its visual field changes as the animal moves its eyes in its head. The movement fields of deep collicular units are too large to provide fine control of fixation. The smallest movement fields are 3–4 degrees in diameter, while the saccades that an animal uses to acquire visual targets located 10 degrees from the fovea have a standard deviation of only 1.6 degrees[103].

The ability of colliculectomised animals to relearn preoperatively learned pattern discriminations and their difficulty in learning new pattern discriminations provides another weak argument in favour of the attention shift notion. The animals have not lost the ability to fixate. In order to perform preoperatively learned pattern discriminations, they must fixate each pattern in order to determine whether it is the positive or the negative pattern. In contrast, the rapid alternations in attention and fixation that must be required to learn new discriminations seem to be very difficult for these animals.

The nature of the retinotopic map on the colliculus is not particularly consistent with either notion. If the colliculus were required for the acquisition of visual targets in the periphery of the visual field or for shifts of attention to another area of the visual field, one would not expect the map of the central area of vision to be magnified at the expense of the map of the visual periphery.

On the other hand, the effects of electrical stimulation favour the foveation hypothesis. For any given stimulus location saccades evoked by repeated stimuli vary very little in size and direction. The foveation hypothesis is also supported by the fact that the movement fields are tuned; cells fire more vigorously prior to saccades that will reach the centre of the field than prior to saccades that will terminate on the edge of field[103]. Thus many tuned units working together might provide more precise specification of an eye movement than any single unit can do on its own.

In fact, we do not really have sufficient information to distinguish between the two hypotheses; that is, we do not know the exact role of the colliculus in the control of eye movements or other orientating responses. Although animals can make eye movements in the absence of the colliculus, the polymodal sensory receptive fields of these cells, the existence of cells discharging before eye movements, the effects of electrical stimulation and the effects of ablation all indicate that the colliculus is involved in motor responses to sensory stimuli. We cannot, however, specifiy whether the colliculus is required for the rapid initiation of orienting movements, for the fine control of such movements, or for other aspects of sensorimotor coordination that have not yet been studied. In addition, we do not know that the colliculus has the same functions in all species. The interspecies variations in the incidence of directionally selective units and apparent variations in the role of the cortico-collicular pathway suggest that it doesn't. Further elucidation of collicular function requires studies of collicular cell activity during a wide variety of tasks requiring sensorimotor coordination and studies of the effects of collicular lesions on these tasks.

Note added on proof

Hoffmann[124] has recently published a detailed study of the retinal and cortical inputs to the colliculus. He found that 80 per cent of the Y-cells in the lateral geniculate nucleus can be activated from the colliculus with short latencies (less than 2.0 ms). This result shows that the axons of many Y-retinal ganglion cells bifurcate, sending branches to both colliculus and geniculate. Cortical cells projecting to the colliculus are also driven by Y-geniculate cells. (Y-geniculate cells receive their input from Y-retinal ganglion cells.) Some collicular cells receive both direct retinal input and cortical input via the Y-system.

References

1. Kuffler, S. W. (1953). Discharge patterns and functional organisation of mammalian retina. *J. Neurophysiol.*, **16**, 37–68
2. Hubel, D. H. and Wiesel, T. N. (1961.) Integrative action in the cat's lateral geniculate body. *J. Physiol.*, **155**, 385–398
3. Hubel, D. H. and Wiesel, T. N. (1962). Receptive fields, binocular interaction and functional architecture in the cat's visual cortex. *J. Physiol.*, **160**, 106–154
4. Hubel, D. H. and Wiesel, T. N. (1965). Receptive fields and functional architecture in two non-striate areas (18 and 19) of the cat. *J. Neurophysiol.*, **28**, 229–289
5. Whitteridge, D. (1960). Central control of eye movements. *Handbook of Physiology, Section 1: Neurophysiology*, 1089–1109 (J. Field, editor) (Washington, D.C.: American Physiological Soc.)
6. Meikle, T. H. and Sprague, J. M. (1964). The neural organisation of the visual pathways in the cat. *Int. Rev. Neurobiol.*, **6**, 149–189

7. Lund, R. D. (1969). Synaptic patterns of the superficial layers of the superior colliculus of the rat. *J. Comp. Neurol.*, **135**, 179–208

8. Lund, R. D. (1972). Anatomic studies on the superior colliculus. *Invest. Opthal.*, **11**, 434–440

9. Hedreen, J. (1969). Patterns of axon terminal degeneration seen after optic nerve section in cats. *Anat. Rec.*, **163**, 198

10. Sterling, P. (1971). Receptive fields and synaptic organisation of the superficial grey layer of the cat superior colliculus. *Vision Res., Suppl.* **3**, 309–328

11. Hendrickson, A., Wilson, M. E. and Toyne, M. J. (1970). The distribution of optic nerve fibers in *Macaca mulatta*. *Brain Res.*, **23**, 425–427

12. Lund, R. D. (1972). Synaptic patterns in the superficial layers of the superior colliculus of the monkey, *Macaca mulatta*. *Exp. Brain Res.*, **15**, 194–211

13. Wilson, M. E. and Toyne, M. J. (1970). Retino-tectal and cortico-tectal projections in *Macaca mulatta*. *Brain Res.*, **24**, 395–406

14. Sefton, A. J. (1968). The innervation of the lateral geniculate nucleus and anterior colliculus of the rat. *Vis. Res.*, **8**, 867–881

15. Hayashi, Y., Sumitomo, I. and Iwama, K. (1967). Activation of lateral geniculate neurons by electrical stimulation of superior colliculus in cats. *Jap. J. Physiol.*, **17**, 638–651

16. Hoffman, K.-P. (1972). The retinal input to the superior colliculus in the cat. *Invest. Opthal.*, **11**, 467–472

17. Michael, C. R. (1972). Visual receptive fields of single neurons in superior colliculus of the ground squirrel. *J. Neurophysiol.*, **35**, 815–832

18. Lund, R. D. and Cunningham, T. J. (1972). Aspects of synaptic and laminar organisation of the mammalian lateral geniculate body. *Invest. Opthal.*, **11**, 291–301

19. Kuypers, H. G. J. M. and Lawrence, D. G. (1967). Cortical projections to the red nucleus and the brain stem in the rhesus monkey. *Brain Res.*, **42**, 151–188

20. Garey, L. J., Jones, E. G. and Powell, T. P. S. (1968). Interrelationships of striate and extra-striate cortex with the primary relay sites of the visual pathway. *J. Neurol. Neurosurg. Psychiat.*, **31**, 135–157

21. Sprague, J. M. (1963). Corticofugal projections to the superior colliculus in the cat. *Anat. Rec.*, **145**, 288

22. Apter, J. T. (1945). Projection of the retina on superior colliculus of cats. *J. Neurophysiol.*, **8**, 123–134

23. Feldon, S., Feldon, P. and Kruger, L. (1970). Topography of the retinal projection upon the superior colliculus of the cat. *Vision Res.*, **10**, 135–143

24. Cynader, M. and Berman, N. (1972). Receptive-field organisation of monkey superior colliculus. *J. Neurophysiol.*, **35**, 187–201

25. Siminoff, R., Schwassmann, H. O. and Kruger, L. (1966). An electrophysiological study of the visual projection to the superior colliculus of the rat. *J. Comp. Neurol.*, **127**, 435–444

26. Lane, R. H., Allman, J. M. and Kass, J. H. (1971). Representation of the visual field in the superior colliculus of the owl monkey (Aotus trivirgatus) *Fed. Proc.*, **30**, 615

27. Kadoya, S., Wolin, L. R. and Massopust, L. C. Jr. (1971). Photically evoked unit activity in the tectum opticum of the squirrel monkey. *J. Comp. Neurol.*, **142**, 495–508

28. Berman, N. and Cynader, M. (1972). Comparison of receptive field organisation of the superior colliculus in Siamese and normal cats. *J. Physiol.*, **224**, 363–389

29. Stone, J. (1966). The naso-temporal division of the cat's retina. *J. Comp. Neurol.*, **126**, 585–600

30. Michael, C. R. (1972). Functional organisation of cells in superior colliculus of the ground squirrel. *J. Neurophysiol.*, **35**, 833–846

31. Lane, R. H., Allman, J. M. and Kaas, J. H. (1971). Representation of the visual field in the superior colliculus of the grey squirrel (*Sciurus carolinesis*) and the tree shrew (*Tupaia glis*). *Brain Res.*, **26**, 277–292

32. Lund, R. D. (1965). Uncrossed visual pathways of hooded and albino rats. *Science*, **149**, 1506

33. Wickelgren, B. G. and Sterling, P. (1969). Influence of visual cortex on receptive fields in the superior colliculus of the cat. *J. Neurophysiol.*, **32**, 16–23

34. Moore, R. Y. and Goldberg, J. M. (1966). Projections of the inferior colliculus in the monkey. *Exp. Neurol.*, **14**, 429–438

35. Moore, R. Y. and Goldberg, J. M. (1963). Ascending projections of the inferior colliculus in the cat. *J. Comp. Neurol.*, **121**, 109–135
36. Powell, E. W. and Hatton, J. B. (1969). Projections of inferior colliculus in cat. *J. Comp. Neurol.*, **136**, 183–192
37. Syka, J. and Straschill, M. (1970). Activation of superior colliculus neurons and motor responses after electrical stimulation of the inferior colliculus. *Exp. Neurol.*, **28**, 384–392
38. Stewart, W. A. and King, R. B. (1963). Fiber projections from the nucleus caudatus of the spinal trigeminal nucleus. *J. Comp. Neurol.*, **121**, 271–295
39. Nauta, W. J. H. and Kuypers, H. G. J. M. (1958). Some ascending pathways in the brain stem reticular formation. *Reticular Formation of the Brain*, 3–30 (H. H. Jasper, L. D. Proctor, R. S. Knighton, W. C. Nashay, and R. T. Costello, editors) (Boston: Little, Brown)
40. Cooper, S., Daniel, P. M. and Whitteridge, D. (1955). Muscle spindles and other sensory endings in the extrinsic eye muscles: the physiology and the anatomy of these receptors and of their connections with the brain stem. *Brain*, **78**, 564–583
41. Fillenz, M. (1955). Responses in the brain stem of the cat to stretch of extrinsic ocular muscles. *J. Physiol.*, **128**, 182–199
42. Astruc, J. (1971). Corticofugal connections of area 8 (frontal eye field) in *Macaca mulatta*. *Brain Res.*, **33**, 241–256
43. Altman, J. and Carpenter, M. B. (1961). Fiber projections of the superior colliculus in the cat. *J. Comp. Neurol.*, **116**, 157–177
44. Graybiel, A. M. (1972). Some extrageniculate visual pathways in the cat. *Invest. Opthal.*, **11**, 322–332
45. Graybiel, A. M. and Nauta, W. J. H. (1971). Some projections of superior colliculus and visual cortex upon the posterior thalamus in the cat. *Anat. Rec.*, **169**, 328
46. Mathers, L. H. (1971). Tectal projection to the posterior thalamus of the squirrel monkey. *Brain Res.*, **35**, 295–298
47. Myers, R. E. (1963). Projections of superior colliculus in the monkey. *Anat. Rec.*, **145**, 264
48. Carpenter, M. B. (1971). Central oculomotor pathways. *The Control of Eye Movements*, 66–103 (P. Bach-y-Rita, C. C. Collins and J. E. Hyde, editors) (New York: Academic Press)
49. Petras, J. M. (1967). Cortical, tectal and tegmental fiber connections in the spinal cord of the cat. *Brain Res.*, **6**, 275–324
50. Nyberg-Hansen, R. (1964). The location and termination of tectospinal fibers in the cat. *Exp. Neurol.*, **9**, 212–227
51. Anderson, M. E., Yoshida, M. and Wilson, V. J. (1971). Influence of superior colliculus on cat neck motoneurons. *J. Neurophysiol.*, **34**, 898–907
52. McIlwain, J. T. and Buser, P. (1968). Receptive fields of single cells in the cat's superior colliculus. *Exp. Brain Res.*, **5**, 314–325
53. Stein, B. E. and Arigbede, M. O. (1972). A parametric study of movement detection properties of neurons in the cat's superior colliculus. *Brain Res.*, **45**, 437–454
54. Straschill, M. and Taghavy, H. (1967). Neuronale reactionem im tectum opticum der katze aug bewegte und stationäre lichtreize. *Exp. Brain Res.*, **3**, 353–367
55. Sterling, P. and Wickelgren, B. G. (1969). Visual receptive fields in the superior colliculus of the cat. *J. Neurophysiol.*, **32**, 1–15
56. Sprague, J. M., Marchiafava, P. L. and Rizzolatti, G. (1968). Unit responses to visual stimuli in the superior colliculus of the unanesthetised, mid-pontine cat. *Arch. Ital. Biol.*, **106**, 169–193
57. Straschill, M. and Hoffman, K-P. (1969). Functional aspects of localisation in the cat's tectum opticum. *Brain Res.*, **13**, 274–283
58. Gordon, B. (1972). The superior colliculus of the brain. *Sci. Amer.*, **227**, No. 6, 72–82
59. Ramon Cajal, S. (1955). *Histologie du Systeme Nerveux de L'homme et des Vertébres*, (Madrid: Sonsejo superior de investigaciones cientificas)
60. Schiller, P. H. and Koerner, F. (1971). Discharge characteristics of single units in superior colliculus of the alert rhesus monkey. *J. Neurophysiol.*, **34**, 920–936
61. Goldberg, M. E. and Wurtz, R. H. (1972). Activity of superior colliculus in behaving monkey. I. Visual receptive fields of single neurons. *J. Neurophysiol.*, **35**, 542–596

62. Humphrey, N. K. (1968). Responses to visual stimuli of units in the superior colliculus of rats and monkeys. *Exp. Neurol.*, **20**, 229–289

63. Schiller, P. H. (1972). The role of the monkey superior colliculus in eye movement and vision. *Invest. Opthal.*, **11**, 451–459

64. Goldberg, M. E. and Wurtz, R. H. (1972). Activity of superior colliculus in behaving monkey. II. The effect of attention on neuronal responses. *J. Neurophysiol.*, **35**, 560–574

65. Updyke, B. V. (1973). *Response Characteristics of Neurons in the Superior Colliculus of Cebus Monkey*, Unpublished Ph.D. dissertation, University of Oregon

66. Kadoya, S., Massopust, L. C. Jr. and Wolin, L. R. (1971). Striate cortex-superior colliculus projection in squirrel monkey. *Exp. Neurol.*, **32**, 98–110

67. Bell, C., Sierra, G., Buendia, N. and Segundo, J. P. (1964). Sensory properties of neurons in the mesencephalic reticular formation. *J. Neurophysiol.*, **27**, 961–987

68. Gordon, B. (1973). Receptive fields in deep layers of cat superior colliculus. *J. Neurophysiol.*, **36**, 157–178

69. Stein, B. E. and Arigbede, M. O. (1972). Unimodal and multimodal response properties of neurons in the cat's superior colliculus. *Exp. Neurol.*, **36**, 179–196

70. Wickelgren, B. G. (1971). Superior colliculus: Some receptive field properties of biomodally responsive cells. *Science*, **173**, 69–72

71. Syka, J. and Straschill, M. (1970). Activation of superior colliculus neurons and motor responses after electrical stimulation of the inferior colliculus. *Exp. Neurol.*, **28**, 384–392

72. Groves, P. M. and Thompson, R. F. (1970). Habituation: A dual-process theory. *Psychol. Rev.*, **77**, 419–450

73. Jassik-Gerschenfeld, D. (1965). Somesthetic and visual responses of superior colliculus neurones. *Nature (London)*, **208**, 898–900

74. Barlow, H. B., Hill, R. M. and Levick, W. R. (1964). Retinal ganglion cells responding selectively to direction and speed of image motion in the rabbit. *J. Physiol.*, **173**, 377–407

75. Horn, G. and Hill, R. M. (1966). Effect of removing the neocortex on the response to repeated sensory stimulation of neurones in the mid-brain. *Nature (London)*, **211**, 754–755

76. Horn, G. and Hill, R. M. (1966). Responsiveness to sensory stimulation of units in the superior colliculus and subjacent tectotegmental regions of the rabbit. *Exp. Neurol.*, **14**, 199–223

77. Masland, R. H., Chow, K. L. and Stewart, D. L. (1971). Receptive-field characteristics of superior colliculus neurons in the rabbit. *J. Neurophysiol.*, **34**, 148–156

78. Schaefer, K. P. (1970). Unit analysis and electrical stimulation in optic tectum of rabbits and cats. *Brain Behav. Evol.*, **3**, 222–240

79. Palmer, L. A., Rosenquist, A. C. and Sprague, J. M. Corticotectal systems in the cat: Their structure and function. *Corticothalamic Projections and Sensorimotor Activities* (T. L. Frigyesi, E. Rinik and M. D. Yahr, editors) (Raven Press) (in press)

80. Hayashi, Y. (1969). Recurrent collateral inhibition of visual cortical cells projecting to superior colliculus in cats. *Vision Res.*, **9**, 1367–1380

81. Hoffman, K.-P. and Straschill, M. (1971). Influences of cortico-tectal and intertectal connections on visual responses in the cat's superior colliculus. *Exp. Brain. Res.*, **12**, 120–131

82. McIlwain, J. T. and Fields, H. L. (1970). Superior colliculus: Single unit responses to stimulation of visual cortex in the cat. *Science*, **170**, 1426–1428

83. McIlwain, J. T. and Fields, H. L. (1971). Interactions of cortical and retinal projections on single neurons of the cat's superior colliculus. *J. Neurophysiol.*, **34**, 763–772

84. Rosenquist, A. C. and Palmer, L. A. (1971). Visual receptive field properties of cells of the superior colliculus after cortical lesions in the cat. *Exp. Neurol.*, **33**, 629–652

85. Rizzolatti, G., Tradardi, V. and Camarda, R. (1970). Unit responses to visual stimuli in the cat's superior colliculus after removal of the visual cortex. *Brain Res.*, **24**, 336–339

86. Spinelli, D. N., Starr, A. and Barrett, T. W. (1968). Auditory specificity in unit recordings from cat's visual cortex. *Exp. Neurol.*, **22**, 75–84

87. Jassik-Gerschenfeld, D. (1966). Activity of somatic origin evoked in the superior colliculus of the cat. *Exp. Neurol.*, **16**, 104–118

88. Wickelgren, B. G. and Sterling, P. (1969). Effect on the superior colliculus of cortical removal in visually deprived cats. *Nature (London)*, **224**, 1032–1033

89. Sterling, P. and Wickelgren, B. G. (1970). Function of the projection from the visual cortex to the superior colliculus. *Brain. Behav. Evol.*, **3**, 210–218

90. Wickelgren-Gordon, B. (1972). Some effects of visual deprivation on the cat superior colliculus. *Invest. Opthal.*, **11**, 460–466

91. Altman, J. A. (1968). Are there neurons detecting direction of sound source motion? *Exp. Neurol.*, **22**, 13–25

92. Benevento, L. A. and Coleman, P. D. (1970). Responses of single cells in cat inferior colliculus to binaural click stimuli: Combinations of intensity levels, time differences and intensity differences. *Brain Res.*, **17**, 387–405

93. Rose, J. E., Gross, N. B., Geisler, D. C. and Hind, J. E. (1966). Some neural mechanisms in the inferior colliculus of the cat which may be relevant to localisation of sound source. *J. Neurophysiol.*, **29**, 288–314

94. Stillman, R. D. (1972). Responses of high-frequency inferior colliculus neurons to interaural intensity differences. *Exp. Neurol.*, **36**, 118–126

95. Wurtz, R. H. and Goldberg, M. E. (1971). Superior colliculus cell responses related to eye movements in awake monkeys. *Science*, **171**, 82–84

96. Wurtz, R. H. and Goldberg, M. E. (1972). Activity of superior colliculus in behaving monkey. III. Cells discharging before eye movements. *J. Neurophysiol.*, **35**, 575–586

97. Wurtz, R. H. (1969). Comparison of effects of eye movements and stimulus movements on striate cortex neurons of the monkey. *J. Neurophysiol.*, **42**, 987–994

98. Straschill, M. and Hoffman, K-P. (1970). Activity of movement sensitive neurons of the cat's tectum opticum during spontaneous eye movements. *Exp. Brain Res.*, **11**, 318–326

99. Apter, J. (1945). Eye movements following strychninisation of the superior colliculus of cats. *J. Neurophysiol.*, **9**, 73–86

100. Syka, J. and Radil-Weiss, T. (1971). Electrical stimulation of the tectum in freely moving cats. *Brain Res.*, **28**, 567–572

101. Hess, W. R. (1954) *Diencephalon: Autonomic and Extrapyramidal Function*, 73 (New York: Grune and Stratton)

102. Robinson, D. A. (1972). Eye movements evoked by collicular stimulation in the alert monkey. *Vision Res.*, **12**, 1795–1808

103. Schiller, P. H. and Stryker, M. (1972). Single unit recording and stimulation in the superior colliculus of the alert rhesus monkey. *J. Neurophysiol.*, **35**, 915–924

104. Westheimer, G. (1954). Mechanism of saccadic eye movements. *Arch. Opthal.* **52**, 710–724

105. Robinson, D. A. and Fuchs, A. F. (1969). Eye movements evoked by stimulation of frontal eye fields. *J. Neurophysiol.*, **32**, 637–648

106. Bizzi, E. (1968). Discharge of frontal eye field neurons during saccadic and following eye movements in unanesthetised monkeys. *Exp. Brain Res.*, **6**, 69–80

107. Berlucci, G., Sprague, J. M., Levy, J. and DiBernardino, A. C. (1972). *Pretectum* and superior colliculus in visually guided behaviour and in flux and form discrimination in the cat. *J. Comp. Physiol., Psychol. Monograph.*, **78**, 123–172

108. Sprague, J. M. (1966). Visual, acoustic and somesthetic deficits in the cat after cortical and midbrain lesions. *The Thalamus*, 391–417 (D. P. Purpura and M. Yahr, editors) (Columbia University Press)

109. Sprague, J. M. and Meikle, T. H. Jr. (1965). The role of the superior colliculus in visually guided behaviour. *Exp. Neurol.*. **11**, 115–146

110. Schneider, G. E. (1967). Contrasting visumotor functions of tectum and cortex in the golden hamster. *Psychol. Forschung.*, **31**, 52–62

111. Schneider, G. E. (1969). Two visual systems: Brain mechanisms for localisation and discrimination are dissociated by tectal and cortical lesions. *Science*, **163**, 895–902

112. Casagrande, V. A., Harting, J. K., Hall, W. C. and Diamond, I. T. (1972). Superior colliculus of the tree shrew: A structural and functional subdivision into superficial and deep layers. *Science*, **177**, 444–447

113. Barnes, P. J., Smith, L. M. and Latto, R. M. (1970). Orientation to visual stimuli and the superior colliculus in the rat. *J. Exp. Psychol.*, **22**, 239–247

114. Denny-Brown, D. (1962). The midbrain and motor integration. *Proc. Roy. Soc. Med.*, **55**, 527–538

115. Anderson, K. V. and Symmes, D. (1969). The superior colliculus and higher visual functions in the monkey. *Brain Res.*, **13**, 37–52

116. Blake, L. (1959). The effect of lesions of the superior colliculus on brightness and pattern discrimination in the cat. *J. Comp. Physiol. Psychol.*, **52**, 272–278

117. Myers, R. E. (1964). Visual deficits after lesion of brain stem tegmentum in cats. *Arch. Neurol.*, **11**, 73–90

118. Anderson, K. V. and Williamson, M. R. (1971). Visual pattern discrimination in cats after removal of the superior colliculi. *Psychon. Sci.*, **24**, 125–127

119. Pasik, T., Pasik, P. and Bender, M. B. (1966). The superior colliculi and eye movements. *Arch. Neurol.*, **15**, 420–436

120. Wurtz, R. H. and Goldberg, M. E. (1972). Activity of superior colliculus in behaving monkey. IV. Effects of lesions on eye movements. *J. Neurophysiol.*, **35**, 587–596

121. Paula-Barbosa, M. M. and Sousa-Pinto, A. (1973). Auditory cortical projections to the superior colliculus in the cat. *Brain Res.*, **50**, 47–61

122. Diamond, I. T., Jones, E. G. and Powell, T. P. S. (1969). The projection of the auditory cortex upon the diencephalon and brain stem in the cat. *Brain Res.*, **15**, 305–340

123. Sterling, P. (1973). Quantitative mapping with the electron microscope: retinal terminals in the superior colliculus. *Brain Res.*, **54**, 347–354

124. Hoffmann, K.-P. (1973). Conduction velocity in pathways from retina to superior colliculus in the cat: a correlation with receptive-field properties. *J. Neurophysiol*, **36**, 409–424

6
Aspects of the Recovery Processes in Nerve

P. DE WEER
Washington University School of Medicine, St Louis, Missouri

6.1 INTRODUCTION 232

6.2 THE DISSIPATION OF IONIC GRADIENTS 233
    6.2.1 *Passive fluxes in the resting nerve* 234
    6.2.2 *Ion movements during stimulation* 235

6.3 OXYGEN CONSUMPTION 235

6.4 ION TRANSPORT BY THE SODIUM PUMP 236
    6.4.1 *General properties of the sodium pump in animal cells* 236
    6.4.2 *Density of pumping sites on the cell membrane* 237
    6.4.3 *Energy source for the sodium pump* 237
        6.4.3.1 *Selectivity* 237
        6.4.3.2 *Affinity* 238
        6.4.3.3 *Operational definition of active transport* 239
    6.4.4 *Effect of ions on the sodium pump* 240
        6.4.4.1 *External sodium and potassium* 240
        6.4.4.2 *Internal sodium and potassium* 242
        6.4.4.3 *Stoichiometry of the sodium pump* 243
    6.4.5 *Effect of ADP* 247
    6.4.6 *Effect of metabolism on the sodium pump* 249

6.5 ELECTROGENIC OPERATION OF THE SODIUM PUMP 250
    6.5.1 *Evidence and criteria for electrogenic pumping in nervous tissue* 251
        6.5.1.1 *Post-tetanic hyperpolarisation* 252
        6.5.1.2 *Hyperpolarisation after injection of sodium ions into neurones* 255

6.5.2   *Effect of the sodium pump on the membrane potential of*
        resting nerve   255
        6.5.2.1   *Effect of temperature on resting potential*   256
        6.5.2.2   *Contribution of the electrogenic pump to the steady-*
                  state resting potential   257
6.5.3   *Effect of membrane potential on the sodium pump*   258
6.5.4   *Physiological role of the electrogenic sodium pump*   261

6.6   EFFECT OF NERVOUS ACTIVITY ON METABOLISM   262

6.7   CONCLUSION   267

ACKNOWLEDGEMENTS   267

6.1   INTRODUCTION

The membrane of nerve cells, like that of most animal cells, separates two aqueous phases of rather different ionic composition. The intracellular phase is at a more negative potential, and has higher potassium and lower chloride and sodium concentrations than the extracellular phase. Furthermore, intracellular concentrations of such divalent cations as magnesium and especially calcium are kept at low levels. None of the ions mentioned is distributed according to purely physical principles (i.e. they are not in Gibbs–Donnan equilibrium), yet the cell membrane is to a greater or lesser degree permeable to all of them. Such non-equilibrium distribution of ions between cell interior and exterior, in the face of demonstrated membrane permeability, requires the intervention of energy-consuming processes, or 'pumps', capable of transporting ions against electrochemical gradients across the membrane. The best studied of these mechanisms is the sodium–potassium pump, i.e. a single membrane-bound agent which actively extrudes sodium ions from, and accumulates potassium ions into, the cell interior at the expense of metabolic energy (ATP).

Underlying the action potential in excitable membranes is a sequence of voltage- and time-dependent permeability changes which results in an influx of sodium ions and an efflux of potassium ions[1]. Owing to this dissipation of electrochemical ion gradients, nervous activity will impose an extra load on the Na^+–K^+ pump machinery. If the cell is to continue to conduct action potentials for any length of time, then it should also possess regulatory mechanisms capable of responding to the extra load by increased pumping activity and increased metabolism.

The purpose of the present paper is to review some selected aspects of these regulatory mechanisms. There are two main issues: (a) the sodium pump itself, and how it is affected by ions and adenine nucleotides; and (b) the supply of energy (ATP) by the cell's metabolism in response to extra loads imposed by, for example, repetitive firing. Although our information remains very sketchy in several respects, a qualitatively coherent picture is emerging from studies on many different preparations: the sodium pump usually transports more sodium out of, than potassium ions into, the cell. Such non-neutral, or 'electrogenic', pumping may (at least in some cells) contribute a sizeable fraction of the normal resting potential, and play a significant role in certain cell functions. Sodium ions entering (and potassium ions leaving) during the conduction of action potentials, stimulate the Na/K transport mechanism, with resulting changes in ATP, ADP, AMP, phosphate and phosphagen concentrations. These changes in turn trigger a complex array of metabolic regulatory mechanisms. Furthermore, calcium ions which enter the cell during nervous activity may also play a vital role in regulatory mechanisms, both electrophysiological and metabolic.

As for the operation of the sodium pump we still do not have a completely satisfactory description of its kinetics with respect to substrates and products (ions and nucleotides), let alone a sensible description of the events at the molecular level. To the extent that the kinetic description is a prerequisite for a molecular understanding, no effort should be spared in obtaining accurate kinetic formulations of the sodium pump and other recovery mechanisms. It would seem that large cell preparations such as the squid giant axon and certain mollusc neurones offer the best prospects for modifying and/or monitoring the many electric, ionic and metabolic parameters which affect the sodium pump. Small cells, on the other hand, may be best suited for the study of metabolic regulatory mechanisms.

6.2 THE DISSIPATION OF IONIC GRADIENTS

Assuming that all unmyelinated nerve cells have similar properties and permit exchange of a rather standard quantity of sodium and potassium per unit area during each action potential, it is clear that the ultimate expenditure of recovery energy, per action potential, will be independent of the area: volume ratio of any particular cell. In small cells, excursion from steady-state conditions will be larger and time constants for recovery shorter than in large nerves. The events will be the same, but they will occur on a shorter time scale in the smaller nerves. If one makes the not unreasonable assumptions of comparable passive sodium leakage fluxes across nerve membranes, comparable ion fluxes per unit area and per impulse regardless of cell size, and comparable properties of the sodium pumping mechanism, one would expect the following rough correlation to hold:

$$\text{Density of pump sites} = a + b \cdot (\text{average firing frequency})$$

This expression reflects the necessity for a minimum number of pump sites to compensate for the gradient energy dissipation (due to passive leakage) which occurs even in the resting state (a), as well as for an additional number of pump sites determined by (b) the maximum average firing frequency which the nerve should be capable of sustaining over prolonged periods of time while performing its normal function in the organism.

6.2.1 Passive fluxes in the resting nerve

The load imposed on resting metabolism by passive leakage of ions down their electrochemical gradients is probably mostly derived from passive sodium entry into the cell. Sodium is the one major ionic constituent of cell systems whose distribution is very far from equilibrium. Passive distribution of sodium would require a cell membrane potential of about $+50$ mV or higher, whereas typical resting potentials are of the order of -50 to -90 mV. Hence sodium ions have a strong tendency to diffuse into the cell, and very little tendency to leak out passively. This statement can be formally expressed by the 'flux–ratio equation' of Ussing[2]: (outflux/influx) $= (C_i/C_0)\exp(E_m F/RT)$ (for a monovalent cation). Applying the flux-ratio equation to nerve cells it is found that passive sodium influx must exceed passive sodium efflux by a factor of about 50. Hence, unidirectional sodium influx (measured with radioactive isotopes) is often equated with net passive sodium influx, which is the parameter of interest in calculating the resting load on the sodium pump. It should be realised that unidirectional (isotopic) influx can only place an upper limit on net influx, due to the fact that part of it may actually take place through so-called 'exchange diffusion' mechanisms which do not result in net transport. Resting sodium influxes of the same order of magnitude have been found in large nerve fibres from a number of different species (in pmol $cm^{-2} s^{-1}$): 61 and 32 for *Sepia officinalis* axons[3, 4]; 40 for intact *Loligo pealei* axons[5]; 57 to 71 for internally dialysed ones[6, 7]; 52 for intact *Dosidicus gigas* axons[8] and 40–65 for internally perfused ones[9]; and 28 for *Loligo forbesi* axons[10]. *Homarus americanus* gave a somewhat lower value of 5 pmol $cm^{-2} s^{-1}$ [11] and substantially higher fluxes (148 pmol) were found for the axons of the tropical squid *Doryteuthis plei*, which normally lives in rather warm waters[12, 13]. Estimates for passive resting sodium influx have also been made for molluscan nerve bodies, and put at 15 pmol $cm^{-2} s^{-1}$ in the case of *Aplysia*[14] and at 25 for land snail (*Helix aspersa*) neurones[15].

The two other major inorganic ions present in nerve cells, potassium and chloride, are distributed near electrochemical equilibrium. This implies that the ratio (passive influx):(passive outflux) for these ions will be near unity and that determination of net passive entry or efflux may be quite difficult indeed. The statement made above that sodium influx is 'probably' responsible for the majority of pumping energy expenditure in the resting cell partly reflects the fact that it has not been possible to determine net passive movement of the other major ions with the same accuracy as that of sodium flux. Some of the minor constituents are also obviously not passively distributed: magnesium[274] and calcium are subject to extrusion from the cell, and so are hydrogen ions[275]. We will briefly mention calcium because it has been investigated in greater detail (see recent reviews[16, 27, 62, 77]) and because of its possible role in regulatory mechanisms. Resting calcium influx into squid giant axons is 1 to 2 orders of magnitude smaller than sodium influx; ranges of 0.04–0.6 pmol $cm^{-2} s^{-1}$ have been reported[17, 18]. Total intracellular calcium concentration is about 500 μM [19, 20] of which only about 0.3 μM is ionised[21], while the bulk is located in a separate compartment[22], probably the mitochondria[20]. The energy expenditure required for the maintenance of a steady state with respect to intracellular calcium is probably trivial compared with other demands on metabolism, and in any event it now seems that most of the calcium expulsion from squid axon may be achieved solely at the expense of sodium ions entering the cell down their electrochemical gradient (perhaps aided by potassium ions leaving the cell down their own gradient), without consumption of ATP[20, 23].

6.2.2. Ion movements during stimulation

During every action potential a number of sodium ions enter the cell and an approximately equal number of potassium ions leave it. Net movements are about three times larger than the minimum required to charge and discharge the membrane capacitor to the peak of the action potential and back. For the giant axon of the squid, *Loligo forbesi*, net entry of sodium has been estimated to be 3.5 and potassium loss, 3.0 pmol cm^{-2} impulse^{-1} [24]. In *Sepia* axons the values were 3.8 and 3.6 pmol cm^{-2} impulse^{-1}, respectively[24]. Somewhat higher net movements were found for *Homarus* nerves: 5.2 pmol cm^{-2} impulse^{-1} for sodium entry and 4.1 for potassium loss[11]. Net potassium loss due to electrical activity has been measured in a few other preparations: *Carcinus* nerve, 1.7 pmol cm^{-2} impulse^{-1} [25] or a little higher[3]; *Loligo pealei*, 3.7 pmol cm^{-2} impulse^{-1} at 24°C[26]. Rabbit vagus nerve gave an unusually low value for potassium loss: 1 pmol cm^{-2} impulse^{-1} [27], which is barely enough to recharge the membrane capacity during a normal-size (110 mV) action potential. A number of uncertainties (actual size of the action potential; precise surface:volume ratio) make this last figure less reliable than the others, however.

It has been known for some time that a very minute quantity of calcium ions enters the squid axon with every impulse[17]; in normal sea-water this quantity is of the order of 16×10^{-15} mol cm^{-2} impulse^{-1}. A recent investigation by Baker, Hodgkin and Ridgway[21] has indicated that at least part of this calcium probably enters through the sodium channels. Little is known about the magnitude of calcium influx in other nerves in physiological circumstances, but several neurones are known where calcium ions can carry a sizeable fraction of the action potential current[28-32, 269]. Even though the quantity of calcium involved in the action potential of many nerve cells constitutes a negligible drain on the energy stores, this ion plays a central role in many physiologically important mechanisms (transmitter release, changes in membrane excitability and permeability, regulation of glycolytic pathways, etc.).

6.3 OXYGEN CONSUMPTION

Ionic gradients dissipated during nervous activity must be replenished at the expense of metabolic energy. Nervous tissue seems to rely mostly on respiration for restoration of energy (ATP) stores; the sensitivity of the brain to anoxia is well known, and preparations like the squid giant axon[34] or crab nerves[35] lose most of their ATP reserve after exposure to cyanide. Well over 40 years ago Fenn[36], as well as Gerard[37] and Meyerhof[38] showed that electrical stimulation of frog sciatic and crab nerve increased oxygen consumption by these tissues. Similar observations have been made by others on nerve trunks[35, 39-44], both myelinated and unmyelinated, as well as on single axons[45]. Increased oxygen consumption by electrically stimulated brain cortex tissue slices is also well documented[46].

The view that this extra oxygen consumption by stimulated nerve fibres reflects, for the most part, extra work performed by the sodium pump in restoring the ionic gradients dissipated during electrical activity, is supported by the following observations: (a) replacement of sodium ions in the bathing solution within lithium ions (which will sustain action potentials but are a poor substrate for the sodium pump) abolishes the extra respiration[35, 40, 43]; (b) ouabain, an inhibitor of the sodium pump in nerve[47] and other cells, reduces or abolishes the post-stimulation oxygen consumption[42-44]; and (c) extracellular potassium and other (Tl^+, Li^+, Rb^+, Cs^+, NH_4^+) monovalent cations stimulate both the sodium pump and oxygen consumption of resting and stimulated tissues with similar kinetics[42, 44]. Comparisons have also been made between the quantity of extra oxygen consumed and the magnitude of the net ion movements during electrical activity. Connelly[41] calculated an $Na:O_2$ ratio (extra sodium lost:extra oxygen consumed) of 5.2 for myelinated nerve; Ritchie's calculated $K:O_2$ ratio for non-myelinated nerve fibres of rabbit vagus was 4.4–5.6[43]. These values are similar to those calculated for brain[46] or kidney[48] cortex slices, but rather smaller than the values of 12–20 suggested for crab (*Maia, Libinia*) nerve[42], and smaller than the $Na:O_2$ ratio of about 20 found in short-circuited frog skins[49, 50]. This disparity may be due to several factors: (a) technical difficulties in estimating net ion fluxes in very small nerve fibres or tissue slices; (b) active transport of sodium and potassium may not proceed with equal efficiency (or rather— with equal $Na:\sim P$ stoichiometry) in different tissues; or (c) perhaps in some tissues post-stimulation energy is expended in processes other than just the replenishment of dissipated sodium and potassium gradients, for example: membrane repair, restoration of other ionic gradients (calcium?), or, in the case of brain cortex, resynthesis or re-accumulation of chemical transmitters.

6.4 ION TRANSPORT BY THE SODIUM PUMP

6.4.1 General properties of the sodium pump in animal cells

The evidence is now overwhelming that outward sodium and inward potassium transport is carried out by a single membrane-bound agent variously called the 'Na/K pump' or briefly the 'sodium pump', for which the energy is derived from the hydrolysis of ATP. The 'pump' is identical to, or intimately associated with, a membrane-bound enzyme first described by Skou[51] and commonly referred to as the 'Na–K ATPase'. The properties of this Na–K ATPase have been abundantly reviewed[52-55] and only the salient properties of the currently most widely accepted[56, 57] (though by no means unchallenged[58]) scheme will be summarised here.

It is postulated that the Na–K ATPase enzyme hydrolyses ATP through a series of intermediate steps involving, first, Na^+-catalysed phosphorylation of the enzyme, presumably associated with outward movement of Na^+; then an irreversible conformational change which requires millimolar amounts of Mg^{2+}; finally, a dephosphorylation step catalysed by potassiumions, presumably concomitant with inward K^+ translocation:

$$E + ATP \xrightleftharpoons{Na^+} E_1 \sim P + ADP \tag{6.1}$$

$$E_1 \sim P \xrightarrow{Mg^{2+}} E_2 - P \tag{6.2}$$

$$E_2 - P + H_2O \xrightarrow{K^+} E + P_i \tag{6.3}$$

Sodium activates the ATPase from the inside of the cell, and potassium from the outside. It is generally understood that the activating ions are also the ones being transported, but this is not necessarily the case, and models with independent 'activating' and 'transport' sites have indeed been proposed[77]. It should be noted in this connection that a 'catalyst transported' pump model built on the above principle must necessarily pump sodium and potassium ions *sequentially*, whereas a 'catalyst-not-transported' model could conceivably transport both ions *simultaneously* in opposite directions.

6.4.2 Density of pumping sites on the cell membrane

The extreme affinity of ouabain for the sodium pump of many animal cells ($K_m \approx 10^{-8}$ to 10^{-7} M) and the recent availability of radioactively labelled ouabain has provided estimates of the total number of sodium pump sites per cell or per unit membrane area. Pump site density seems to vary considerably between cell types: from about 100 to 200 per cell in erythrocytes[59, 60] (or even fewer than 10 per cell in low-potassium sheep erythrocytes[61]) to perhaps one million per cell in HeLa cells[62], i.e. a variation in density of more than three orders of magnitude. Application of the ouabain-binding method to nerve cells has led to estimates of about 750 pump sites per μm^2 in mammalian C fibres[63], apparently about the same density in guinea-pig brain[63, 64], and about 1000 sites μm^{-2} for squid axon[65]. Knowing pump density as well as the magnitude of the pumped ion flux for a given cell, one can calculate the turnover number of ions transported per pump per unit time. When corrected for the effect of temperature, the various estimates for the number of cations transported per site per second in the cells mentioned, including erythrocytes, average a few hundred per second at 37°C; this compares well with the turnover numbers found for the Na–K ATPase isolated from various sources.

6.4.3 Energy source for the sodium pump

6.4.3.1 Selectivity

There is little doubt that ATP is the immediate fuel for the sodium pump. The early finding by the Cambridge group[66] that sodium extrusion could be restored in squid axons poisoned with cyanide, by injection of ATP, phosphoenolpyruvate or phosphoarginine (the phosphagen of invertebrates) had left the question unresolved as to whether the last two compounds were active *per se* or merely replenished ATP through their respective kinase reactions. However, the newer techniques of internal perfusion[67, 68] and internal dialysis[6], which allow removal of all low-molecular weight substances from the cell interior, have eliminated the above ambiguity. Thus Brinley and Mullins[7] found that of several potential phosphate donor substances tested (acetyl phosphate, phosphoenolpyruvate, glyceraldehyde-3-phosphate, phosphoarginine, guanosine-, cytidine-, uridine-, deoxyadenosine- and adenosine-5'-triphosphate and adenosine-5'-di- and monophosphate), only ATP and to a lesser extent deoxy-ATP were capable of supporting active sodium extrusion by the squid giant axon. The same substances were also the only ones able to support active K influx[69], suggesting that an adenine moiety is essential for enzymatic activity. This finding raises the interesting problem as to why substances like acetylphosphate and *p*-nitrophenyl-phosphate are capable of phosphorylating the Na–K ATPase enzyme in the same location as does ATP[70-72], yet cannot serve as an energy source for active transport[7, 69, 74]. To account for this apparent discrepancy, Bond *et al.*[72] have proposed that ATP must be present at *two* sites on the ATPase enzyme: one, a phosphorylating site (also accessible to other phosphate donors) and the other, a catalytic site highly specific for ATP or d-ATP. A multi-site ATPase would be compatible with the sigmoid kinetics (with respect to [ATP]) observed with isolated Na–K ATPase[75, 76].

6.4.3.2 Affinity

Using the technique of internal dialysis in squid giant axon, Brinley and Mullins[7] were able to vary $[ATP]_i$ from 1 µM to 10 mM in order to study its effect on active sodium efflux. Although the kinetics are not simple (the curve does not follow Michaelis–Menten kinetics and shows no clear tendency to saturate at high [ATP] levels), the most striking feature is that $[ATP]_i$ must be reduced 50-fold (from 5 mM to 100 µM) to reduce active sodium efflux by one-half, and perhaps 1000-fold to achieve 90% inhibition of active sodium efflux. In addition, a most curious (and thus far unexplained) effect of strophanthidin on sodium efflux was found at *very low* $[ATP]_i$ levels: unlike what is seen at normal or moderately reduced levels, the cardioactive steroid *enhances* sodium efflux. As shown in Figure 6.1 taken from Mullins[77], the effect of the drug was to bring sodium efflux to a standard value independent of $[ATP]_i$. The nature of this strophanthidin-induced sodium efflux is not clear. It cannot result from increased passive permeability since the simultaneously observed sodium *influx* is much smaller than would be expected from the flux ratio equation. A number of possibilities remain: (a) the drug-induced efflux of sodium is active, and driven by the residual ATP (1–2 µM) present in thoroughly dialysed axons. In order to be independent of [ATP] at concentrations higher than 1 µM, this 'pump' should have a K_m for ATP of well below 1 µM (such a high affinity for ATP $K_m \approx 10^{-7}$ M, is indeed displayed by isolated Na–K ATPase preparations[78, 79]); or (b) the drug-induced sodium efflux represents the appearance of a Na:Na exchange process, possibly occurring through the pump mechanism.

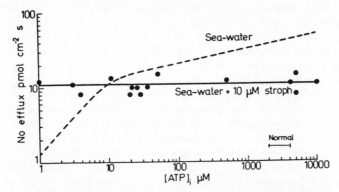

Figure 6.1 Effect of internal [ATP] and external strophanthidin on sodium efflux from internally dialysed squid giant axons. [Na]$_i$ was 80 mM. [ATP]$_i$ was varied over a 10 000-fold range. The broken line represents sodium efflux into normal sea-water (the experimental points—about eighty—are omitted for clarity). The solid line and experimental points represent sodium efflux into sea-water containing 10 μM strophanthidin. Note that at very low [ATP]$_i$, strophanthidin stimulates sodium efflux. (From Mullins[77], by courtesy of North-Holland Pub. Co.)

The difficulty with this view is that it would require a drug-induced Na influx as well as dependence of sodium efflux on external sodium, neither of which has been observed experimentally; or (c) the strophanthidin-induced uphill sodium efflux is driven by the movement of some ion other than sodium down its own electrochemical gradient; candidates are: calcium or magnesium influx, or less likely, potassium efflux.

The main reason for dwelling on the baffling topic of strophanthidin-induced sodium efflux is that it renders some operational definitions of active sodium transport ambiguous.

6.4.3.3 Operational definition of active transport

Thermodynamically uphill movement of an ion is sufficient condition for this movement to be defined as 'active'. However, it may be more practical to define active transport of an ion or molecule as any movement obligatorily linked to the dissipation of an energy source other than its own (electro) chemical gradient. In this framework, uphill movement is not a necessary condition since active transport can conceivably take place against, without, or down an electrochemical gradient. Operationally, there are at least two ways to demonstrate and measure the magnitude of active transport of a given ion or molecule: first, it may be possible to eliminate the energy source for the transport under study (leaving all other conditions unchanged) and second, it may be possible to inhibit the molecular mechanism underlying the transport by means of a suitable specific inhibitor. Certainly, research on the sodium-potassium pump could not have progressed to its present state without the availability of the cardioactive steroids (ouabain, strophanthidin, etc.), with their highly specific blocking action on the sodium pump. Further progress in the understanding of the sodium pump will depend increasingly on quantitative experiments. For example, several lines of evidence indicate that about three sodium ions are expelled and about two potassium ions taken up per molecule of ATP hydrolysed by the pump. It is important to determine whether these ratios hold universally for all cells, whether they are exact and rigidly fixed, or approximate and variable depending on circumstances. Such knowledge is an absolute prerequisite to any kind of detailed model-making. In view of their importance for future research, the limitations of presently available research tools should be clearly appreciated.

A first limitation in one's ability to gauge accurately the magnitude of a given active flux results from the extreme affinity of the sodium pump for its fuel source, ATP. In tissues which rely on respiration for their energy supply, complete interruption of respiratory pathways (through anoxia or exposure to CN^-) will reduce $[ATP]_i$ to very low levels (less than 1% in squid axon, for example). This very low level of ATP (10–50 µM) may escape detection by ordinary analytical methods, yet it is sufficient to activate the sodium pump significantly (5–20%). (On the other hand, calcium ions released from the mitochondria during CN^- poisoning may perhaps contribute to the inhibition of the sodium pump.) At any rate, using inhibition by cyanide as a test, one may underestimate active fluxes by 5–20%. The second more frequently used test involves application of ouabain or another cardioactive steroid to the preparation. Here again, active sodium efflux may be underestimated by 10–20% due to the peculiar effect of such drugs on sodium efflux described in the previous section. In addition, ambiguities may arise from the fact that under certain circumstances which will be described later, part of the ouabain-sensitive sodium efflux may merely represent sodium-for-sodium exchange taking place through the pump machinery.

6.4.4   Effect of ions on the sodium pump

6.4.4.1   External sodium and potassium

The dependence of active sodium efflux on external potassium ions is well known[80-82] and constituted, in fact, the first indication that active transport of both ions was somehow linked. That this stimulation of sodium efflux by external potassium ions is probably of physiological significance is suggested by the fact that in most instances the $[K]_o$ which half-maximally stimulates sodium efflux is in the physiological range[4, 10, 35, 42, 83-91]. The stimulatory effect of $[K]_o$ is strongly dependent on the external sodium concentration: it is larger in the absence than in the presence of sodium ions[10, 42, 85, 89]. The general picture which has emerged from the quoted findings is that in the presence of normal sodium concentrations the curve relating ouabain-sensitive sodium efflux to external potassium increases along a sigmoid curve[10, 86, 88, 89, 91-93]. In media containing subnormal sodium concentrations, $[K]_o$ for half-maximal stimulation becomes smaller as $[Na]_o$

is reduced, and the sigmoid activation curve tends towards a Michaelis–Menten hyperbola with a low K_m and a V_{max} similar to that obtained in solutions containing normal sodium concentrations[10, 89, 94] (Figure 6.2). These findings can be interpreted, among other models, by assuming that activation of sodium efflux by external potassium requires K_o binding to at least two sites, and that Na_o competes for these same sites without being an effective catalyst. From Figure 6.2 it is obvious that under many circumstances removal of external sodium will have a stimulatory effect on active sodium efflux.

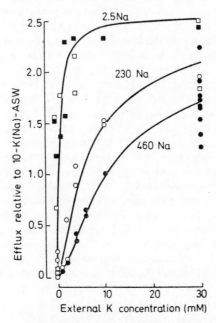

Figure 6.2 Ouabain-sensitive sodium efflux from squid giant axon as a function of the external potassium and sodium concentrations. Efflux is expressed relative to that in normal sea-water containing 10 mM K$^+$ and 460 mM Na$^+$. (From Baker *et al.*[10], by courtesy of Cambridge University Press.)

Ouabain-sensitive potassium influx, too, is influenced by [Na]$_o$ as well as [K]$_o$. In red blood cells, the kinetics of activation of potassium uptake by external cations are very similar to those of sodium efflux: K_o stimulates K influx along a sigmoid curve in the presence of high [Na]$_o$[86, 92, 94, 95, 104]; upon lowering [Na]$_o$ the activation curve shifts to lower concentrations and becomes more hyperbolic in character[94, 95, 104]. Similar observations were made in the case of rubidium uptake by erythrocytes[96, 97]. The data for squid giant axon are somewhat conflicting: Baker *et al.*[10] find a ouabain-sensitive K influx curve (*v.* [K]$_o$ in normal sea-water) which is similar in shape to the sigmoid Na efflux curve discussed above, while Mullins and Brinley[69] report a *linear* increase of ATP-dependent K influx with increasing $[K]_o$, independent of external sodium concentration. The reason for this discrepancy is not clear.

6.4.4.2 Internal sodium and potassium

Active sodium efflux from muscle cells is an S-shaped function of $[Na]_i$[98-102] and is about half-maximal at internal sodium concentrations of about 20 mM. Sodium extrusion from erythrocytes follows similar kinetics[87, 103-105]. Such non-linear kinetics are not altogether surprising in light of other evidence indicating that about three sodium ions seem to be transported for every ATP molecule hydrolysed. In squid axon, however, sodium efflux varies *linearly* with internal sodium concentration[7, 18, 106-108]. Using the internal dialysis[6] technique, Brinley and Mullins[7] varied $[Na]_i$ over a wide range (2–240 mM) and found sodium efflux to be linearly related to $[Na]_i$. The only other nerve tissues where sodium extrusion as a function of $[Na]_i$ has been investigated in any detail are mammalian non-myelinated fibres and snail neurones. Rang and Ritchie[90] found that the post-tetanic hyperpolarisation of rabbit cervical vagus declined exponentially over most of its time course, suggesting that the rate of sodium extrusion was a linear function of concentration. (This evidence is admittedly indirect and its interpretation rests on the assumption that membrane conductance, extracellular potassium levels, and Na : K coupling ratio remain constant throughout. In addition, Rang and Ritchie observed deviations from linearity at the high and low ends of the curve.) In the case of snail (*Helix aspersa*) neurones, Thomas[15, 109] found that intracellular sodium ion activity, measured with sodium-sensitive glass electrodes, declined exponentially after an iontophoretic injection of Na^+, again suggesting that sodium extrusion is proportional to $[Na]_i$. Removal of Na_o also led to an exponential decline of $[Na]_i$ to a new steady state, indicating that even at very low $[Na]_i$ levels (a few mM) where non–linearity would be most conspicuous if it were present, sodium extrusion seems to depend *linearly* on its intracellular concentration (a somewhat puzzling observation of Thomas[15] was that sodium efflux was insensitive to $[Na^+]_i$ below a very low (1 mM) threshold; possibly a slight systematic error was present in the Na^+ activity measuring arrangement). Kostyuk *et al.*[110], working on *Helix pomatia* neurones, also found that sodium efflux (measured as an electrogenic current) declined exponentially after iontophoretic injection of sodium ions.

If sodium efflux and potassium influx are indeed coupled, then one would expect active K influx to depend on $[Na^+]_i$ in a fashion analogous to the dependence of sodium efflux on external potassium concentration. In squid axon, active K uptake is clearly not a linear function of $[Na^+]_i$. Data obtained by Mullins and Brinley[69] suggest that internal sodium ions stimulate K influx half-maximally at about 30 mM. Combined with the fact that sodium efflux increases *linearly* with $[Na^+]_i$, this finding inevitably suggests that the Na : K coupling ratio (sodium ions transported outward per potassium ion transported inward) cannot remain constant under all experimental conditions.

This point will be discussed again below. (See Section 6.4.4.3.)

Other intracellular inorganic ions which might have a direct effect on the sodium-potassium pump include magnesium, calcium, and phosphate ions, but whether these ions play a role in the physiological control of pumping mechanisms is not known. Magnesium is a known co-factor in the Na–K ATPase[51], and could therefore conceivably regulate sodium pumping if its concentration were limiting enough. Free magnesium concentration in erythrocytes has been estimated[111] at 0.13 mM, i.e. low enough to leave an appreciable fraction of intracellular ATP in the free form. In squid giant axon, on the other hand, the free magnesium concentration amounts to 2–3 mM[112] or perhaps even higher (De Weer and Lowe, unpublished). While it is known that excessive levels of free intracellular magnesium have an inhibitory effect on sodium efflux from squid axon[91], it seems unlikely, in view of the wide concentration fluctuations required, that this cell would use the magnesium ion level as a regulator for the sodium pump. The same probably holds true for inorganic phosphate, which is known to inhibit pump-mediated sodium efflux[91, 113] as well as isolated Na–K ATPase preparations[114], but only in concentrations which are not very likely to occur under physiological circumstances.

6.4.4.3 Stoichiometry of the sodium pump

It now seems certain that the sodium pump normally extrudes more sodium ions into, than it takes up potassium ions from the extracellular fluid, i.e. the pump works in 'electrogenic' fashion. It is also clear that more than one sodium ion and probably more than one potassium ion are transported for every molecule of ATP hydrolysed. What is not so certain is whether these unequal stoichiometries are fixed by the very nature of the transport mechanism, or whether they are, in fact, variable according to the experimental conditions or the physiological needs of the cell. Further understanding of the transport mechanism in molecular terms will require more accurate descriptions of the quantitative relationships between Na, K and ATP in the sodium pump. It is probably fair to say that the most accurate data so far have been obtained on erythrocytes. Data obtained in other tissues are often interpreted with reference to the 'ideal' 3Na:2K:1ATP ratio, and corrected upward or downward accordingly.

(a) *Coupling of sodium and potassium fluxes*—The first estimates for the Na:K transport ratio in erythrocytes were rather scattered; values from 2:1[115] to 1:1[83, 116-118] were reported. The value of 3:2 first reported by Post and Jolly[119] and confirmed again 10 years later[120] seems to be the most quoted figure. It was obtained from net cardioactive steroid-sensitive flux measurements over a rather wide range of sodium and potassium concentrations. Garrahan and Glynn[121], making simultaneous measurements of ^{24}Na loss and ^{42}K uptake in red cells from identical batches, found Na:K active transport ratios of 1.20 ± 0.01 and 1.35 ± 0.01 in two very similar experiments. However, the Na/K pump machinery of erythrocytes is known to engage not only in Na:K exchange, but in Na:Na and K:K exchange as well. Incomplete correction for one or the other of these spurious exchanges will affect the apparent coupling ratio. Thus, when Garrahan and Glynn[121] corrected the second of their quoted experiments for ouabain-sensitive $K:K$ exchange which might have taken place, the apparent $Na:K$ coupling ratio was revised from 1.35 to 1.84 ± 0.06. This illustrates that even when the data are obtained with great care, their interpretation (corrections, etc.) is likely to be a difficult problem. Furthermore, it should be emphasised that all the studies mentioned above rely on cardioactive drugs for the operational definition of 'active' fluxes, and that this criterion itself may be less than ideal since ouabain-insensitive fluxes may not be purely passive[7, 77, 122].

Early tracer experiments[4] on the giant axon of cuttlefish showed that pumped sodium efflux exceeds pumped potassium influx by a factor of about $3:2$ or $2:1$[107]. Caldwell et al.[66] found that when phosphoarginine was injected into a CN-poisoned axon of Loligo forbesi, it promoted the active extrusion of 2 or 3 Na ions for every K ion actively taken up. Sjodin and Beaugé[107, 108] working on L. pealei axons determined the magnitude of active sodium efflux and active potassium influx, operationally defined by their respective sensitivity to cyanide poisoning. Cyanide poisoning inhibited about 75% of both total sodium efflux and total potassium influx. There are several difficulties in translating these figures into absolute fluxes (mainly due to the fact that these cells are not in steady state but gain sodium during the experiment) and depending on whether they apply corrections to their data or not, the authors find an $Na:K$ coupling ratio of 2.0–2.7. They also argue that at low $[Na]_i$ concentrations (i.e. about 20 mM) the coupling ratio may be closer to unity. In a more recent investigation on L. forbesi axons by Baker et al.[10], it was found again that active sodium efflux (defined as the ouabain-sensitive fraction) exceeded active K uptake (defined in the same way) by a factor of about $2:1$. After considering several possible sources of error (dilution of labelled K by potassium leaking out into the space immediately external to the axolemma, and possibly $Na:Na$ and $K:K$ exchanges taking place through the pump) the authors thought that the ratio might be reduced somewhat toward the $3:2$ value commonly found for erythrocytes but that a $1:1$ ratio was unlikely.

A more detailed investigation by Mullins and Brinley[69] of active sodium and potassium fluxes in internally dialysed squid giant axons has raised the possibility that $Na:K$ coupling might not be constant. As mentioned already, they found that active K uptake increased linearly with $[K]_o$, whereas activation of Na efflux by K_o displays saturation kinetics. Conversely, Na_i stimulates sodium efflux in linear fashion, but K influx in curvilinear fashion. Even granting that interpretation of these flux data may be complicated by the possible occurrence of $Na:Na$ and $K:K$ exchange through the pump, such kinetics are clearly hard to reconcile with a constant $Na:K$ ratio. Figure 6.3 shows how the ratio between ATP-dependent Na efflux and ATP-dependent K influx in squid axon varies from $1:1$ (or perhaps even less) at very low $[Na]_i$ to $3:1$ or larger at very high $[Na]_i$.

A variable $Na:K$ coupling ratio has also been proposed from time to time for active transport in frog skeletal muscle[123-126] but the relationships between active, passive and exchange diffusion fluxes in this tissue are quite complex[127-130] and it does not seem likely that reliable estimates of active $Na:K$ transport ratios will be easily obtained.

Several authors have proposed values for $Na:K$ transport ratios in single neurones, but these have usually been obtained by rather indirect means and can only be regarded as approximate. For example, Nakajima and Taka-hashi[131] observed long lasting post-tetanic hyperpolarisations in the crayfish stretch receptor neurone, which were convincingly interpreted as due to the operation of an electrogenic sodium pump. From the number of impulses during the tetanus and the electrical capacity of the neurone membrane, and assuming that the quantity of sodium gained during each impulse is 2–3 times the amount needed to charge this capacity, they computed the total Na^+ to be expelled from the cell by the sodium pump during recovery after the tetanus. Dividing the time-integrated hyperpolarisation by the membrane resistance they found that the actual charge expelled during recovery was

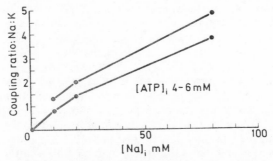

Figure 6.3 Coupling ratio between active sodium and potassium fluxes in internally dialysed squid giant axons as a function of internal sodium concentration. The lower curve is calculated on the assumption that all ATP-dependent K influx is coupled to ATP-dependent sodium efflux. In the upper curve the ATP-dependent K influx value has been corrected for a small component which may be Na_i-independent. (From Mullins and Brinley[69], by courtesy of The Rockefeller Institute Press.)

only 20–30% of the extra sodium gained, suggesting an Na:K coupling ratio of 5:4 to 4:3. Such calculations (with comparable results) were also made for iontophoretically injected sodium, which also produces electrogenic hyperpolarisations in these cells. Similar experiments were performed on *Helix pomatia* neurones by Kostyuk[132] who found that 30% of the Na^+ was expelled electrogenically, and on the so-called follower cells of lobster cardiac ganglion by Livengood and Kusano[133], who found 34% of the injected sodium to be ejected electrogenically, suggesting an Na:K ratio of 3:2. Going one step further towards reducing the number of assumptions and experimental variables in the above calculations, Thomas[109] measured the current necessary for clamping *Helix aspersa* neurones at resting potential during and after iontophoretic injection of a certain amount of sodium acetate. From the discrepancy between the amount of sodium injected and the actual charge transferred across the cell membrane, a ratio of 4:3 to 3:2 between pumped sodium and pumped potassium (presumably) could be computed. Clamping does not eliminate all problems, however. The injected sodium must be accompanied by an anion (acetate, citrate, etc.) and this may lead to diffusion potentials for which the clamp circuitry will compensate by passing currents unrelated to pumping. An additional assumption common to the papers quoted above is that the amount of iontophoretically injected sodium can be accurately determined from the current passed through the iontophoretic electrodes. While it is true that the use of high (3 M) salt concentrations inside the injection electrodes will result in most of the current being carried by cations leaving the anode and by anions leaving the cathode, accurate quantification is a difficult matter complicated by such consider-ations as passive diffusion, bulk flow, electro-osmosis, etc.[134-136]. Before this method is used in more quantitative work, e.g. to elucidate the *exact* Na:K coupling ratio in single cells, it should probably be subjected to a very thorough evaluation and calibration[135]. Using high specific activity isotopes together with low-background counting equipment this may be barely feasible. One important question which could be resolved with present techniques (i.e. without accurate absolute calibration) is whether the Na:K coupling ratio is *variable* depending on circumstances.

In all attempts at determining Na:K pump ratios in nerves quoted so far the authors (except Mullins and Brinley[69]) implicitly assumed that this ratio was fixed. In a few instances it has been suggested that the data might be more easily explained if the Na:K coupling ratio were variable. Rang and Ritchie[90] found that the ions Tl^+, K^+, Rb^+, Cs^+, Li^+ did not have the same relative potency in stimulating post-tetanic hyperpolarisation (a measure of electrogenicity) in rabbit vagus nerves as they had in stimulating post-tetanic oxygen consumption (a measure of sodium transport). Among other possi-bilities they suggested that this observation could be explained by assuming different Na:K, Na:Tl, etc. ratios in the operation of the pump. Baylor and Nicholls[137] found that, during post-tetanic hyperpolarisation in leech sensory neurones, raising the external potassium ion concentration had a more pronounced depolarising effect than before the tetanus. They suggested as one possible explanation that the Na:K coupling ratio of the hyperpolarising electrogenic sodium pump might be variable; that is: increasing external potassium would stimulate K^+ uptake more than it stimulates Na^+ efflux, thus reducing the pump's electrogenicity. More recent evidence from the same laboratory, however[138], suggests that this particular effect may be due to a calcium-induced increase in potassium conductance of the cell membrane. The only strong indication apart from the work of Mullins and Brinley[69], that the Na:K transport coupling ratio might be variable has come from the work of Kostyuk et al.[110] on giant neurones of *Helix pomatia*. Using a voltage-clamp method similar to that of Thomas[109], these authors found that the fraction (post-sodium injection charge transfer)/(quantity of sodium injected) was quite variable from neurone to neurone, ranging from as low as 1.5% to 70%. It was also claimed that the fraction of injected sodium extruded in uncoupled fashion increased with the size of the injected load (as if injected sodium stimulates sodium efflux more than it does potassium uptake). If these findings are confirmed they would certainly constitute strong evidence that Na:K coupling stoichiometry in nerve is not rigidly fixed but flexible depending on circumstances. Such a mechanism would evidently put very severe and interesting constraints on any molecular model for the sodium pump.

(b) *Coupling of ion transport to ATP hydrolysis*—The ratio (ions transported):(ATP hydrolysed) has been repeatedly determined in erythrocytes. Agreement seems best on the ouabain-sensitive Na:ATP ratio, the reported values being 3.1 ± 0.1[139] in non-glycolysing and 3.2 ± 0.2[140] in glycolysing erythrocytes, and 2.91 ± 0.15 in resealed ghosts[121]. For the K:ATP ratio in erythrocytes, values of 2.4 ± 0.1[139], 2.5 ± 0.1[140] and 2.05 ± 0.24[141] have been reported.

The determination of Na:ATP ratios in skeletal muscle presents formidable problems on account of the large phosphagen stores and energetic glycolytic system which this tissue possesses. Using various inhibitors to minimise replenishment of ATP stores from phosphocreatine or through glycolysis or respiration, Dydynska and Harris[142] computed a ratio of 2.5 for the number of Na^+ ions extruded from sodium-loaded frog sartorius and semitendinosus muscles per $\sim$P bond hydrolysed. This figure was later revised to approximately 3.0 when correction was made for some unexpected $\sim$P losses through other pathways[143].

Estimates for Na:$\sim$P ratios in nerve have only been obtained by indirect measurements. In the walking-leg nerve of crabs, Baker[35] arrived at a figure of 2.7 to 4.0 (which compares well with the value of 2.6 ± 0.16 computed from stimulation-induced Na uptake and oxygen consumption figures[42]) using the following considerations: (a) net sodium influx after blocking the pump represents the magnitude of the pump flux, and (b) ouabain-sensitive increase in P_i levels after CN poisoning represents $\sim$P hydrolysis by the sodium pump. About 75% of the $\sim$P breakdown in crab nerve could be ascribed to the operation of the pump. In squid giant axon, with its much smaller surface:volume ratio, the fraction of total $\sim$P breakdown ascribable to the sodium pump was only about 20–25%[144]. Using this figure, Baker and Shaw[144] computed an Na:$\sim$P ratio of about 3 for squid axon. For internally dialysed squid axons (which probably do not produce endogenous ATP), Mullins and Brinley[145] computed in a rather indirect manner an Na:$\sim$P ratio of about 3.

In conclusion, it would appear that the Na:K:ATP stoichiometry in sodium-potassium pumping is far from accurately known. The best evidence, especially in erythrocytes, seems to indicate an Na:$\sim$P ratio of 31; still, more accurate evidence from other tissues, especially nerve, is needed before this figure can be generalised. The other ratios (K:$\sim$P and Na:K) seem to fluctuate much more widely. This undoubtedly reflects the greater difficulty involved in measuring active K fluxes in the presence of large passive components. Nevertheless, the few indications[69, 110] that Na:K ratios might be genuinely variable, should be taken very seriously in view of the profound implications that this finding would have with regard to the kinetics and molecular mechanism of the sodium pump.

6.4.5 Effect of ADP

A striking observation made by the Cambridge group[34, 36, 146] during their experiments on the restoration of the Na/K pump of CN-poisoned squid axons by micro-injection of energy-rich phosphate compounds was that, when sodium efflux was reactivated by ATP, it no longer displayed its characteristic[4] dependence on external potassium; nor did injections of ATP restore active K influx. Phosphoarginine (ArgP), on the other hand, restored K_o-dependent sodium efflux as well as active potassium uptake. Related to these observations was the following: upon exposure to cyanide, the squid axon first loses its phosphoarginine before it loses its ATP; concomitant with the disappearance of ArgP one witnesses the loss of K_o-dependency of sodium efflux. Two possible explanations were offered for these observations[1, 34, 66, 146, 148]: either ArgP plays a role in active K transport, or a high ATP:ADP ratio (maintained through the phosphokinase reaction ArgP + ADP $\rightleftharpoons$ ATP + Arg) is required for sodium efflux to be dependent on external potassium. The question was later resolved in favour of the second alternative[91, 113, 145, 149, 150]: any procedure which increases intracellular [ADP] renders the pump mediated (ouabain-sensitive) sodium efflux less dependent on external potassium. At the same time, this sodium efflux develops a requirement for external sodium[10, 91, 146], suggesting that instead of Na:K linked transport, Na:Na *exchange* is now taking place through the pump machinery. The sodium pump of erythrocytes, too, can engage in Na:Na exchange[95, 151-155]. The view that this Na:Na exchange is indeed taking place through the pump machinery is strongly supported by the following observations: (a) it requires the presence of ATP and (b) is inhibited by cardioactive steroids; (c) the only nucleotide which will support Na:Na exchange is ATP[154] and (d) the magnitudes of Na:Na exchange and Na:K exchange are inversely related in the sense that, all other things being equal, when more Na:Na exchange is taking place through the pump, less Na:K exchange occurs at the same time[152]. Earlier investigations on squid axons[146] had left the question open as to whether inorganic phosphate as well as ADP were necessary for the pump to engage in Na:Na exchange. From the work on resealed erythrocyte ghosts it appeared[152] that high intracellular P_i levels were at least as effective as ADP in switching the sodium pump from the normal Na:K exchanging mode of operation to an Na:Na exchanging one. The idea emerged that the condition necessary for the pump to engage in Na:Na exchange was the presence of a much reduced intracellular $[ATP]:[ADP][P_i]$ ratio[10, 152] (which is a measure of the free energy available from the hydrolysis of ATP), and Caldwell[66, 148, 156] has proposed a model for the sodium pump in which the relative magnitudes of Na:Na and Na:K exchange are sensitive to the free energy produced by hydrolysis of ATP. More recent experiments performed on squid giant axon specifically to distinguish between the effects of ADP and P_i have shown[91, 113] that only ADP shifts the pump's behaviour toward Na:Na exchange. In erythrocytes, Na:Na exchange is also strongly dependent on the intracellular ADP level[154], but the exact role of inorganic phosphate in the phenomenon has not been resolved.

The available evidence indicates that, when exposed to elevated [ADP] levels, the sodium pump engages in Na:Na exchange. An important characteristic of this behaviour is that, while it requires ATP, it apparently does not consume it[121]. A detailed discussion of possible models to account for this behaviour is outside the scope of this review, but it is obvious that a more complete understanding of this peculiar phenomenon will throw additional light on the molecular mechanisms in the operation of the pump. An attractive hypothesis in this regard can be based on the proposed reaction scheme (Section 6.4.1) for the multi-step hydrolysis of ATP by the Na–K ATPase. The first step in the proposed reaction involves reversible phosphorylation of the enzyme by ATP in the presence of sodium ions:

$$E + ATP \rightleftharpoons E.ATP \underset{}{\overset{Na^+}{\rightleftharpoons}} E_1 \sim P.ADP \rightleftharpoons E_1 \sim P + ADP$$

It is tempting to suggest that the (Na^+ requiring) transphosphorylation reaction between ATP and E on the one hand, and the transmembrane Na^+ translocation on the other hand, are one and the same reaction. If [ADP] is kept at very low levels by the cell metabolism, then sodium translocation in one direction would normally far exceed translocation in the other direction, and this ratio would become smaller with increasing [ADP] levels. This scheme is too simple, however, since it does not account for the fact that the antibiotic oligomycin inhibits Na:Na exchange while stimulating (^{14}C)ADP-ATP exchange. Rather than speculate about detailed mechanisms, it might be more profitable to consider possible physiological implications of the described behaviour of the sodium pump.

6.4.6 Effect of metabolism on the sodium pump

Very little is known about possible physiological effects of metabolism in regulating the operation of the sodium pump in nerves. Complete interruption of ATP synthesis will admittedly ultimately result in the depletion of ion gradients and blockage of impulse conduction, but living cells probably have little use for such coarse regulatory mechanisms. The question arises whether it is, in fact, possible to exert fine regulatory control on the sodium pump (and ultimately, on the behaviour of single nerves and nerve networks) via the metabolic condition of the cell. The discussion which follows intends to show that such fine regulation may indeed be possible.

Discussions of the effect of metabolism on pumping are usually held solely in terms of ATP concentrations. Yet the affinity of the sodium pump for ATP is sufficiently high (Section 6.4.3.2) that inordinately wide variations in [ATP] would presumably be required in order to affect sodium efflux to any appreciable extent. Regulation of pumping activity via changes in ATP concentration would be a very inefficient mechanism indeed. Instead, it may be suggested that the intracellular levels of P_i and ADP could serve as regulators. The inhibitory effect of P_i on the sodium pump (Section 6.4.4.2) may not be sufficiently strong to have great physiological significance. ADP, on the other hand, can dramatically alter the behaviour of the sodium pump, in such a way as to render it inefficient for net transport (Na:K exchange being replaced by Na:Na shuttling). Typical cells probably have a normal ATP: ADP concentration ratio of about 10:1 or even higher[158]. Trivial changes in ATP concentration may well be accompanied by a substantial variation in ADP level, resulting in an appreciable alteration in ATP:ADP ratio. Hence agents which alter the metabolic state of a cell (e.g. hormones), could exert control over the sodium pump's behaviour via the ATP:ADP ratio. Small cells which probably devote a considerable fraction of their energy expenditure to ion pumping, might be most susceptible to such control. In the case of nerves, a very high surface-to-volume ratio would make the electrical behaviour of the cell almost instantaneously dependent on the behaviour of the sodium pump.

Himsworth[157] has suggested the existence of a glucose chemoreceptor in the lateral hypothalamus, responsible for the adrenaline release from the adrenal medulla in response to hypoglycaemia. Conceivably, the chemoreceptor might have its ADP level raised due to relative lack of glucose; the sodium pump would partially switch to Na:Na exchange, and the resulting depolarisation might trigger the generation of impulses. The carotid body chemoreceptor senses oxygen tension and fires when PO_2 is lowered. In most cells including squid axon[263] oxygen tension must be reduced to extremely low levels to affect mitochondrial electron transport and hence ATP generation, but Mills and Jöbsis[159] found that in the carotid body, cytochrome a_3 reduction is much more sensitive to a fall in PO_2 than in other tissues, so that ATP:ADP ratios in the carotid body may be unusually sensitive to PO_2 levels. In spite of this finding, Mills and Jöbsis do not espouse the view[160] that impulse generation is mediated via oxidative phosphorylation or ATP levels, mainly because firing frequency and cytochrome reduction during nitrogen anoxia increase practically simultaneously without any phase shift. Biscoe[161], however, has proposed the unconventional[162] theory that the chemoreceptor proper is made up of extremely fine (0.1 μm) nerve endings where, because of the high surface-to-volume ratio, there would be an almost instantaneous effect (a) of ATP production on pumping rate and (b) of pumping rate on membrane potential and hence on firing frequency.

These then are two instances where switching the pump from Na:K exchange to Na:Na shuttling under the influence of ADP, and without the need for large variations in ATP concentration, might conceivably play a regulatory role in physiological processes.

6.5 ELECTROGENIC OPERATION OF THE SODIUM PUMP

As originally proposed by Dean[163] the sodium pump was an electrogenic mechanism capable of extruding sodium ions only. The subsequent finding that sodium extrusion from muscle, nerve and erythrocytes depended on the presence of external potassium (see Section 6.4.4.1) made it seem more likely that Na and K transport were somehow coupled, and several sodium-potassium transport models with a 1:1 coupling ratio were proposed. At the same time, however, evidence from experiments with radioactive isotopes began to indicate that active sodium efflux exceeded active potassium uptake in many cells, and electrical measurements confirmed the occurrence of net charge transfer due to the operation of the Na/K pump. At the present time, electrogenic sodium pumping has been demonstrated or strongly implied in nearly every major cell type (including squid axon[164]) where active transport is known to occur. The current resurgence of interest in the electrogenic nature of the sodium pump is attested to by the recent appearance of no fewer than four reviews[165-168] and a monograph[169] on the topic. The present discussion will be limited to some selected aspects and unresolved problems of electrogenic pumping. For a perceptive account of the development of ideas on electrogenic sodium pumping the reader is referred to the review by Thomas[168].

6.5.1 Evidence and criteria for electrogenic pumping in nervous tissue

Although the earliest isotope flux data obtained from experiments on giant nerves and red blood cells more often than not indicated a disparity between the magnitudes of active sodium and potassium fluxes, probably the first convincing direct evidence that the sodium pump indeed produces a net current flow, came from electrical potential measurements on frog skeletal muscle. Thus, Kernan[170] found that when sodium-loaded frog sartorii were actively extruding sodium, their membrane potential became more negative than the calculated potassium equilibrium potential given by

$$E_K = RT(F)^{-1} \ln([K]_o/[K]_i)$$

indicating that the membrane potential difference was set by something other than a potassium diffusion potential. Kernan suggested a non–neutral sodium pump as the cause for this hyperpolarisation. It is interesting to note that 10 years earlier Stephenson[171] may have observed the same phenomenon, but did not give it[172] the interpretation that Kernan did. Keynes and co-workers[123, 173] confirmed these findings and showed in addition (a) that inhibition of the pump (e.g. by ouabain) abolished the recovery hyperpolarisation, and (b) that potassium uptake must at least in part be chemically (as opposed to electrically) coupled to Na uptake, for muscles were shown to gain K even when the membrane potential was kept more positive than E_K during recovery. Other studies on the same preparation[124, 126, 174-176] confirmed the idea that the sodium pump could generate a net outward current across the membrane. In all papers except the one by Mullins and Noda[174], this conclusion was reached from the observation that E_m of frog skeletal muscle could be considerably more negative than the calculated value of E_K during recovery from sodium loading. Adrian and Slayman[126] also compared rubidium movements and potassium movements in muscles recovering from sodium loading. From the value of the rubidium permeability it appeared that the potential difference across the membrane could have accounted for only 10% of the rubidium influx, suggesting that 90% of the Rb uptake was chemically coupled to sodium extrusion. Since potassium ions are much more permeant than Rb^+, it was concluded that much more than 10% of the K influx could have been driven by the observed membrane potential difference, although for technical reasons it was impossible to set an upper limit to that fraction.

Initial evidence that the sodium pump of nervous tissue was also capable of contributing to the membrane potential was obtained, as in frog muscle, on preparations where pumping had been enhanced by prior loading of the cell interior with sodium. In many cases this loading was achieved 'physiologically', i.e. by subjecting the preparation to repeated stimulation; in larger neurones the technique of intracellular sodium injection (mechanical or iontophoretic) has often been applied.

6.5.1.1 Post-tetanic hyperpolarisation

Ritchie and Straub[177] demonstrated that post-tetanic hyperpolarisation in non-myelinated fibres is due to the operation of the sodium pump (stimulated by the sodium ions entering during every action potential). They considered electrogenic pumping as a possible direct contributor to the membrane potential but rejected this idea because there was at the time very little other evidence for electrogenic pumping in nerve. Instead, potassium depletion (by a neutral Na:K pump) of the extracellular space was suggested as the cause of the hyperpolarisation. Connelly[40], however, noticed in similar experiments on frog nerves that sometimes the membrane potential underwent hyperpolarisation during the tetanus (when clearly the extracellular space could not be depleted of potassium) and concluded therefore, that, post-tetanic hyperpolarisation was due to the electrogenic operation of the sodium pump. This view was later confirmed by others[90, 178, 179]. The best proof for the existence of K_o-stimulated electrogenic sodium pumping during post-tetanic hyperpolarisation in mammalian C fibres was provided by the work of Rang and Ritchie[90], who demonstrated that, after the short-lived post-tetanic hyperpolarisation following stimulation in K-free Ringer's has subsided (presumably when the K^+ ions which emerged from the nerve during stimulation have diffused away or been pumped back in), readmission of external K^+ *hyper*polarises the membrane, and that ouabain prevents this hyperpolarisation.

Hyperpolarisation upon raising $[K]_o$ is most economically accounted for by invoking an electrogenic sodium pump which is stimulated by external potassium, and indeed this criterion has been used as part of the argument for the occurrence of electrogenic sodium pumping in other nervous tissues such as molluscan neurones (*Aplysia*[14, 180, 181], *Helix*[182] and *Anisodoris*[183]), crayfish stretch receptors[131, 223], and mammalian cervical[184] and lobster cardiac ganglia[133]. Additional criteria used in assessing the role of sodium pumping in the post-tetanic hyperpolarisation are the lack of hyperpolarising response when the preparation was stimulated in sodium-free lithium solutions and, of course, the lack of response at low temperatures, or in the presence of ouabain or cyanide.

Further instances where electrogenic sodium pumping has been implicated in post-tetanic hyperpolarisation include leech sensory neurones[137, 138,185] and cat spinal neurones[186]. Finally a phenomenon which, in principle, resembles post-tetanic hyperpolarisation should be mentioned. Koike *et al.*[187] and Brown and Lisman[188] demonstrated in barnacle and *Limulus* photoreceptors, respectively, a post-illumination hyperpolarisation which was abolished by ouabain or the absence of external potassium, and reduced if the receptor was illuminated in sodium-free sea-water. They suggested that sodium ions enter during illumination and subsequently stimulate an electrogenic pump, and supported this by injecting sodium to produce a ouabain-sensitive hyperpolarisation.

Long-lasting post-tetanic hyperpolarisations (PTH) should not automatically be equated with electrogenic pumping, however, without a careful consideration of other alternatives. Meves[189], studying such potentials in frog Ranvier node, concluded that they were due (like the well-known 'undershoot' of the action potential) to increased potassium conductance. Gage and Hubbard[190, 191] working on rat phrenic nerve terminals (where, because of their small size, membrane potential was indirectly inferred from variations in excitability), found little effect of pump inhibitors on post-tetanic reduction of excitability, whereas K_o reduction strongly reduced excitability. They concluded that post-tetanic hyperpolarisation was due to an increase in potassium conductance. More recently, Connor and Stevens[192] have cited

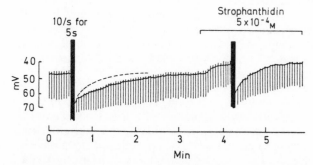

Figure 6.4 Effect of strophanthidin on post-tetanic hyperpolarisation in a sensory neurone (type N) of the leech. A control train of impulses was given at 10 s⁻¹ for 5 s. After exposure to strophanthidin, recovery from the hyperpolarisation following an identical train of impulses was faster, but only slightly so. (For comparison, the time course of this recovery has been superimposed, as a dashed line, on the control recovery.) Note the slight depolarisation upon addition of strophanthidin. (From Jansen and Nicholls[138], by courtesy of the Physiological Society, London.)

preliminary data indicating an increased, slowly decaying, potassium conductance after a train of impulses in *Anisodoris* and *Archidoris* neurones. Meunier[193] has concluded that in *Aplysia* neurons (which definitely do possess an electrogenic sodium pump[180, 181]) post-tetanic hyperpolarisation does *not* result so much from the increased activity of such a pump as from a post-tetanic increase in potassium conductance (membrane resistance was decreased; lowering K_o increased PTH; a reversal potential close to E_K was found). The same phenomenon has been studied in greater detail by Junge[194] and Brodwick and Junge[195] who passed depolarising currents through *Tritonia* and *Aplysia* neurones and observed a 'post-stimulus hyperpolarisation'. This hyperpolarisation (concomitant with a conductance increase) persisted under a variety of conditions where an electrogenic sodium pump was unlikely to operate; it also had a reversal potential. The reversal potential varied with $[K]_o$ and not with $[Na]_o$ or $[Cl]_o$. The conclusion, again, was that the hyperpolarisation resulted from an increase in potassium conductance.

Similar observations were made by Jansen and Nicholls[138] on leech sensory neurones, where previous experiments[137] had demonstrated the role of electrogenic pumping in PTH. In their more recent experiments these authors confirmed the existence of electrogenic pumping, using iontophoretic Na^+ injection to produce strophanthidin-sensitive hyperpolarisation. In addition, they noted that PTH was associated with increased membrane conductance, and that in low $[K]_o$ the hyperpolarisation became more pronounced. Thus, the PTH had at least two components: one due to electrogenic pumping and another due to increased potassium conductance.

It now seems possible that many, if not all, of the increased potassium conductance phenomena mentioned above are mediated via an increase in intracellular free calcium concentration. A calcium-dependent potassium permeability has been exhaustively documented in erythrocytes[196-203] and may also exist in liver cells[204]. To be effective in erythrocytes, Ca^{2+} must be present intracellularly[202]. Meech[205-206], has pressure-injected *Aplysia* neurones with small amounts of $CaCl_2$ and described a resulting long-lasting hyperpolarisation which was shown to be due to a specific increase of membrane permeability to potassium ions. Godfraind et al.[207, 208] have described a dinitrophenol-induced hyperpolarisation in cortical neurones of the cat, which exhibited a reversal potential compatible with E_K and was accompanied by a decrease in membrane resistance. Godfraind et al. concluded that the DNP-induced hyperpolarisation resulted from an elevated potassium conductance, and suggested that this conductance might have been mediated via Ca^{2+} released from the mitochondria as a result of the uncoupling of oxidative phosphorylation. Subsequent work by Krnjevic's group[209, 210] has confirmed this suggestion: iontophoretic injection of Ca^{2+} into cat spinal motoneurones brought about a fall in excitability and membrane resistance, and often a hyperpolarisation. The reversal potential for the effect of Ca^{2+} injection was 15–20 mV more negative than resting potential, and clearly not related to E_{Cl}. The conclusion was that the fall in membrane resistance was mainly due to an increase in potassium conductance. No detailed investigation of electrophysiological effects of Ca^{2+} in squid giant axon has been reported, but Hodgkin and Keynes have mentioned[106] that injection of 12 mM $CaCl_2$ blocked action potentials. Most recently, strong evidence for a $[Ca^{2+}]_i$-induced potassium conductance has come from the work of Jansen and Nicholls on leech sensory neurones mentioned earlier[138]. The portion of the PTH which results from an increase in g_K was found to be very sensitive to external Ca^{2+}. Calcium ions had to be present in the medium *during the tetanus* for the post-tetanic increase in g_K to occur; high Ca^{2+} levels in the medium augmented both the magnitude of the post-tetanic g_K increase and the time constant for its recovery, suggesting that calcium ions entering during activity are responsible for the conductance increase, and that removal of Ca^{2+} from the cell brings g_K down to its original level. Unfortunately, the authors did not succeed in injecting calcium ions directly into the neurones to confirm this attractive hypothesis.

It should be kept in mind, however, that the evidence linking increased potassium conductance to increased $[Ca^{2+}]_i$, is largely circumstantial. Most cells possess very effective sequestration mechanisms (sarcoplasmic reticulum, mitochondria) which will rapidly remove calcium ions from the cytoplasm. In the case of mitochondria, this sequestration is in exchange for protons, and it is therefore possible that some of the phenomena ascribed to elevated $[Ca^{2+}]_i$ may, instead, result from a lowered intracellular pH.

6.5.1.2 Hyperpolarisation after injection of sodium ions into neurones

Larger neurones often allow impalement by several micro-electrodes, one or two of which can then be used to inject salt solutions, either by simple diffusion out of a low resistance electrode, or with the application of pressure, or iontophoretically by passing a current between the injecting electrode and another one inside or outside the cell. In a very early application of this technique, Coombs et al.[211] observed that after electrophoretic injection of sodium ions into mammalian motoneurones the membrane potential fell by about 10 mV, returned in about 5 min and then often increased beyond its original value. An electrogenic sodium pump was suggested as the cause for this hyperpolarisation, but the nature of the preparation probably prevented the application of more satisfactory criteria.

Several authors have reported that injecting sodium ions into snail neurones produces a hyperpolarisation[109, 110, 132, 182, 212, 213] which can be prevented[109, 110, 132, 182, 213] by ouabain or lack of potassium. Thomas[109] has refined such experiments considerably by introducing into the cell an additional current-passing electrode by means of which the membrane potential can be clamped at its resting value before, during and after sodium injection (see Section 6.4.4.3(a)). The current necessary for maintaining the membrane at resting potential after the cell has been injected with sodium, is a measure of the net charge translocated by the electrogenic sodium pump across the membrane in response to the sodium load. Thomas' technique also constitutes the most unambiguous criterion so far for defining electrogenic transport. As already pointed out, however, it is not without problems: injected sodium ions must be accompanied by an anion, and depending on the nature of the latter, more or less strong diffusion potentials may arise for which the clamping circuitry will compensate by passing currents unrelated to transport.

Other preparations where an ouabain-sensitive hyperpolarisation after injection of sodium has been described include crayfish stretch receptor neurones[131]; Aplysia neurones[181]; barnacle[187] and Limulus[188] photoreceptor cells; lobster cardiac ganglion cells[133] and leech sensory neurones[138].

6.5.2 Effect of the sodium pump on the membrane potential of resting nerve

Considering the extensive evidence that, during recovery from physiological or artificial sodium loading, the sodium pump of many nerve cells operates in electrogenic fashion, it is natural to inquire whether an electrogenic pump contributes to the resting membrane potential as well. If only electroneutral pumps operate to generate a dissimilar ion distribution across the cell membrane, the membrane potential will be closely approximated by the following equation:

$$E_m = \frac{RT}{F} \ln \frac{P_K[K]_o + P_{Na}[Na]_o + P_{Cl}[Cl]_i}{P_K[K]_i + P_{Na}[Na]_i + P_{Cl}[Cl]_o} \qquad (6.4)$$

which is usually[214, 215], though not necessarily[174], derived from the assumption of a constant electric field across the membrane.

6.5.2.1 Effect of temperature on resting potential

All other things being equal, raising the temperature by 10°C should, according to equation (6.4), increase the membrane potential by about 3–4%, yet in many preparations the effect of temperature on membrane potential is much larger than expected. In lobster nerve, for example[216, 217], the membrane potential change is about twice that predicted from equation (6.4). Senft[217] showed that adding ouabain to the medium reduces the potential change to the theoretical one, and suggested that the temperature-sensitive component of the membrane potential was produced by an electrogenic sodium pump.

The membrane potential of *Aplysia* neurones similarly is very sensitive to temperature[14, 180]. Carpenter and Alving[180], in experiments analogous to those of Kernan[170] on sodium-loaded frog sartorius muscles, found that warming of *Aplysia* neurones previously kept in the cold resulted in a rapid increase of membrane potential to about 10 mV beyond E_K (determined from the afterpotential after spike conduction); this hyperpolarisation was abolished by ouabain or lack of potassium, and was not accompanied by a change in conductance. Hyperpolarisation beyond E_K clearly indicates that the cell is not in a steady state, for no cell can have E_m indefinitely more negative than E_K unless it possesses an *outward*-going potassium pump, which is unlikely. In more recent experiments Carpenter[14] kept *Aplysia* neurones at 25°C, then suddenly cooled them to 5°C, and found depolarisations averaging 15 mV; in the presence of ouabain, cooling produced a 7 mV *hyper*polarisation. Taken together, and assuming ouabain does not affect permeabilities, these data would indicate a steady-state electrogenic pump component of about 22 mV, i.e. a large contribution indeed. Hyperpolarisation upon cooling in the presence of ouabain indicates that the $P_{Na} : P_K$ ratio decreases in the cold. Such differential effects of temperature on permeabilities have been described in other nerves including squid giant axon (*Dosidicus*)[218] and nerve cell body (*Loligo*)[219], and giant neurones of another marine mollusc, *Anisodoris*[220], as well as in barnacle muscle fibres[221,278]. In the muscle fibre, as opposed to the other examples, the $P_{Na} : P_K$ ratio increased upon cooling. Carpenter[219], comparing the effect of temperature on membrane potential in the presence or absence of strophanthidin, concluded that the sodium pump contributed about 15 mV (and sometimes more) to the resting potential of *Loligo pealei* stellar ganglion neurones. It is possible, however, that these cells contained higher than normal sodium levels, for they were apparently kept in the cold prior to the experiment. It is clearly difficult to draw unambiguous conclusions about the magnitude of the electrogenic pump's contribution to the steady state resting potential from 'temperature-jump' experiments, unless very careful allowance is made for (a) sodium loading at low temperatures and (b) differential ion permeability changes induced by temperature variations.

6.5.2.2 Contribution of the electrogenic pump to the steady-state resting potential

Mullins and Noda[174] have derived an equation for the membrane potential in the presence of electrogenic pumping, which is valid only in the *steady state*. If sodium and potassium are the only important ions being actively transported, then it can be shown that the membrane potential is given by equation:

$$E_m = \frac{RT}{F} \ln \frac{r\, P_K[K]_o + P_{Na}[Na]_o}{r\, P_K[K]_i + P_{Na}[Na]_i} \qquad (6.5)$$

where r is the Na:K transport coupling ratio. If one were suddenly to arrest the pump (e.g. with ouabain) in a cell in steady state, then equation (6.5) will no longer apply but equation (6.4) will be valid. Hence the contribution of the electrogenic sodium pump to the resting potential is given by the difference between equations (6.4) and (6.5), or (since the terms $P_{Na}[Na]_i$ in the denominators are negligible):

$$E_{pump} = \frac{RT}{F} \ln \left[\frac{1}{r} \cdot \frac{r P_K[K]_o + P_{Na}[Na]_o}{P_K[K]_o + P_{Na}[Na]_o + P_{Cl}[Cl]_i} \cdot \left(1 + \frac{P_{Cl}[Cl]_o}{P_K[K]_i} \right) \right] (6.6)$$

Asher (see Thomas[168]) has pointed out that the maximum value which equation (6.6) can acquire (e.g. low P_{Cl} and relatively high P_{Na}) is equal to $RT(F)^{-1}\ln(r)^{-1}$ or 10 mV for a coupling ratio of 3:2. It is worth noting that if P_{Cl} is negligible, the magnitude of the electrogenic pump contribution to the steady state resting potential depends only on the Na:K coupling ratio (r) and on the $P_{Na}:P_K$ permeability *ratio, regardless of total membrane conductance*. This is not surprising for the magnitude of the pump current will be determined in the steady state by the magnitude of sodium influx. Influx, in turn, depends on sodium permeability. So that, at a given $P_{Na}:P_K$ ratio, increased membrane conductance (a) reduces the IR voltage drop for a given pump current, but (b) also increases the intensity of the pump current.

Most values published so far for truly steady state contributions to the resting potential seem to lie well within the limit set for 3:2 coupling by the Mullins–Noda equation. Of the few exceptions: 22 mV for *Aplysia* neurones[14], 15 mV for *Anisodoris* neurones[222] and 15 mV for squid stellar ganglion[219], the last two may have been sodium loaded due to storage in the cold for some time before the experiment. In the former, care was taken to avoid loading, so that the question arises as to whether the coupling ratio might significantly exceed 3:2 in this case. Of other neurones tested for depolarisation upon stopping the pump, the pump contributions were reported to be 2–3 mV for *Helix* neurones[15, 109, 182], 'over 10 mV' for crayfish stretch receptor neurones[223] and 5 mV for leech sensory neurones[137, 138]. Barnacle[187] and

Limulus[188] photoreceptors in the steady state also depolarise upon exposure to ouabain, the former by about 6 mV. So far the only value reported for a nerve fibre in the steady state is that for the squid giant axon, where a 1.4 mV depolarisation upon exposure to strophanthidin was found[164].

6.5.3 Effect of membrane potential on the sodium pump

Elementary thermodynamic considerations show that, if the pump contributes to the resting potential by producing a net current, it should itself be affected by the membrane potential. Rapoport[224] has pointed out that a voltage-sensitive electrogenic pump would behave operationally like a conductance. For example, a 3:2 (i.e. hyperpolarising) Na/K pump might be expected to slow down when the membrane is artificially hyperpolarised. This would result in the apparent membrane conductance being larger in the presence of electrogenic pumping than in its absence. There are several difficulties with such theoretical predictions (conductance change, pumped flux dependence on membrane potential, etc.): although they may exist in principle, they could be undetectable in practice, either because of their small magnitude, or because they are obscured by other effects. For example, Geduldig[225] has found that the membrane conductance of frog skeletal muscle increases upon arresting the sodium pump with ouabain. This conductance increase evidently obscures any 'apparent' conductance due to the operation of an electrogenic pump, as described above. Also Rapoport[224] assumes that the velocity of the pumping mechanism is proportional to the driving force (i.e. the free energy available from ATP hydrolysis minus the energy required for translocating $3 Na^+$ and $2 K^+$ against their respective electrochemical gradients). This is, of course, not how enzymes function unless they operate very near equilibrium or at very low levels of saturation, neither of which is likely in the case of the sodium pump. To use a simple analogy: the velocity of hydrolysis of urea by urease is practically independent of the urea concentration (which is a measure of the driving force), provided this concentration is well over the K_m of the enzyme. Under these conditions the urease reaction is a 'constant ammonia generator' with high internal impedance. As will be discussed below, the electrogenic Na/K pump, when fuelled *in vivo* by a saturating ATP concentration, with ADP and P_i kept at very low levels by cellular metabolism, should probably be considered as a constant current generator operating rather far away from equilibrium and rather unaffected by changes in driving force. The sodium–potassium pump, in this view, is equivalent to a battery with high electromotive force and high internal impedance. Speculation is not very profitable at the present time, however. Existing data on this question are to some extent conflicting, and it is clear that more research is needed on the thermodynamics of the electrogenic sodium–potassium pump. The evidence so far, however, would seem to suggest that the sodium pump is rather insensitive to membrane potential.

Probably the earliest observation on the effect of membrane potential on active sodium efflux was made by Hodgkin and Keynes[4] in *Sepia* axons. Hyperpolarisation by 10–30 mV had no effect on sodium efflux. Brinley and

Mullins[226, 227] have extended similar observations on squid giant axon over a much wider membrane potential range with again, very little evidence for any effect of membrane potential on sodium efflux. The failure to find a reversal potential for the long-lasting post-tetanic hyperpolarisations found in crayfish stretch receptor[131] and cat spinal neurones[186] has, in fact, been used as one argument for ascribing these hyperpolarisations to the operation of an electrogenic pump. The implication, of course, as pointed out by Nakajima and Takahashi[131], is that the electrogenic pump behaves like a constant current generator. Meunier and Tauc[181] have also reported that in *Aplysia* neurones, hyperpolarisation does not affect the electrogenic pump current. Research on the effect of membrane potential on the sodium pump of snail neurones has been reported by two laboratories. Thomas[15], measuring $[Na]_i$ with sodium-sensitive glass electrodes, found that *Helix aspersa* neurones were quite capable of net sodium extrusion when the cell membrane was hyperpolarised by as much as 100 mV, indicating that the sodium pump was not blocked by such hyperpolarisations. Unfortunately, the actual pump rate could not easily be compared with that found at normal potentials, so that a partial inhibition of sodium efflux rate by large hyperpolarisations cannot be excluded. Also, even though Thomas' experiments show that net sodium extrusion still takes place under strong hyperpolarisation, they do not indicate that it is necessarily electrogenic. However, when $[Na]_i$ was reduced to very low levels (where the energy required for sodium extrusion is larger than normal), the pump was still clearly operating in electrogenic fashion. The only evidence to date for a definite effect of cell membrane potential on the activity of the Na/K pump has been put forward by the Russian group of Kostyuk *et al.*[110, 228]. These authors, using Thomas' voltage clamp technique on *Helix pomatia* neurones, found that injection of sodium acetate into the cells resulted in an apparent conductance increase which prevented by ouabain, suggesting the existence of an electrogenic sodium pump whose current output is reduced by hyperpolarisation. That this apparent conductance change does not result from an alteration of the cell's passive permeability properties was inferred from the fact that the two current–voltage curves (before and after sodium injection, or with and without ouabain) merge, rather than cross, at strongly hyperpolarised membrane potential values, indicating that the current source simply vanishes under these conditions. Possibly the most interesting finding in this study was that, whereas pump current was seemingly voltage-dependent, sodium extrusion (as already found by Thomas[15]) was not. This led the authors to suggest that active K^+ uptake increases with increasing hyperpolarisation; in other words, that the Na:K coupling ratio is variable and approaches unity as the membrane potential is raised. Additional evidence in favour of variable Na:K ratios was that the ratio (pump current): (sodium efflux) varied from neurone to neurone, as well as, for a given neurone, with the quantity of sodium injected. This last finding (that the Na:K ratio is larger for larger sodium loads) suggests that $[Na]_i$ stimulates sodium extrusion more than it does potassium uptake. These very interesting findings merit careful consideration since they would constitute, if verified, some of the strongest evidence to date (together with that of Mullins and Brinley[69]) in favour of variable coupling in the Na/K pump. A somewhat disturbing feature of the work of Kostyuk *et al.*[110] is their use of rather large injections of sodium acetate (up to 10–25 µCoulomb per cell). Assuming the dimensions of *Helix pomatia* giant neurones are similar to those of the *Helix aspersa* neurones used by Thomas, one can estimate that a 25 µCoulomb injection may produce an intracellular sodium acetate concentration of roughly 50 mM. This would undoubtedly create acetate diffusion potentials[109] which may well partially mask the electrogenic sodium current. Another puzzling finding reported by Kostyuk *et al.*[110] was that cooling *increased* the pump current and rendered it more resistant to inhibition by hyperpolarisation; this was interpreted on the basis of a model in which potassium transport is more temperature sensitive than sodium transport. These assertions are of such obvious interest that a careful verification is eminently desirable.

The present state of the question of sodium pump dependence on membrane potential can be summarised as follows: pumped *sodium efflux* is probably unaffected by potential[15, 110, 226, 227], but it may be[110, 228] that pump *current* decreases with increasing hyperpolarisation (at least in snail neurones). There are a number of mechanisms by which insensitivity of sodium efflux to membrane potential can be reconciled with the notion of electrogenic pumping: (a) pumped Na efflux is constant, but pumped K influx increases with hyperpolarisation (this is the mechanism favoured by Kostyuk *et al.*[110, 228]); (b) pumped Na efflux is constant, but pumped Na influx increases with hyperpolarisation (available evidence[15, 110, 226, 227] does not favour this model); (c) free energy available from ATP hydrolysis is far in excess of what is required to pump 3 Na^+ outward and 2 K^+ inward, so that 100 mV represents a trivial increase in load compared to the driving force; or (d) the stoichiometry (ions transported):(ATP split) is not a constant 3:1 as currently assumed, but is reduced progressively as the membrane potential increases.

Alternative (c) will be extremely difficult to verify experimentally. In order to calculate the free energy available from ATP hydrolysis *in vivo*, one will need accurate determinations of intracellular concentrations of ATP, ADP and inorganic phosphate, as well as intracellular pH and pMg. In addition, the standard free energy for ATP hydrolysis should, at least in the case of marine organisms, probably be redetermined at the high ionic strengths (≈ 0.5 M) prevailing in these organisms. Making a number of (admittedly less than wholly satisfactory) assumptions, Caldwell and Shirmer[156] have estimated the free energy of ATP hydrolysis in squid giant axon at about 14 kcal mol^{-1}, which is much higher than the 8–9 kcal or so required to extrude three equivalents of sodium ions and absorb two equivalents of potassium ions against the prevailing electrochemical gradients. If Caldwell and Schirmer's high figure can be verified by more direct methods, it would easily account for the lack of membrane potential effect on the sodium pump, since hyperpolarising the membrane to -100 mV would increase the energy required for a 3:2 sodium-potassium exchange by only slightly over 2 kcal $(mol\ ATP)^{-1}$. Conversely, an attempt should be made to determine the free energy for ATP hydrolysis *in vivo* in the case of snail neurones, to verify whether its value precludes a potential sensitive 3:2 pump or not.

The last alternative (a pump where the Na:ATP stoichiometry changes according to demand) is rather unlikely in view of the evidence in favour of a constant $3:1$ ratio in erythrocytes and a few other tissues. However, there is no evidence against it.

6.5.4 Physiological role of the electrogenic sodium pump

The finding that the sodium pump can directly affect membrane potential has stimulated research into its possible role in nerve and muscle physiology. Inevitably a number of functions have been proposed for the electrogenic pump which did not survive subsequent analysis. Thus, stimulation of an electrogenic sodium pump does not seem to be the underlying mechanism of photoreceptor potentials in *Limulus* ventral eye[187] or of slow post-synaptic (transmitter-induced) hyperpolarising potentials in frog sympathetic ganglion cells[229] and in mollusc (snail and *Aplysia*) neurones[230-232]. Evidence to date indicates that physiological activation of electrogenic pumping, apart from metabolic effects, is due solely to changes in the ionic composition of intra- and extracellular fluids (Na_i, K_o), resulting from previous repetitive conduction of action potentials. All proposed physiological roles for the electrogenic pump (so far) reflect this property.

Since hyperpolarisation (by any mechanism including electrogenic pumping) renders nerve membranes less excitable, it is clear that previous activity of a nerve can modify (through post-tetanic hyperpolarisation) its subsequent signalling properties for some time. This phenomenon, of course, can be viewed as an elementary form of memory.

Baylor and Nicholls[137] and Jansen and Nicholls[138] have pointed out that post-activity hyperpolarisation (due to either electrogenic pumping or potassium conductance increase) could play a significant role in nervous integration. The many neurophysiological effects attendant upon hyperpolarisation (alterations of the shape of action potential; rise in threshold, with reduction of firing frequency or eventual conduction block; changes in the amount of transmitter released by presynaptic terminals; changes in amplitude or sign of postsynaptic potentials; conduction block at bifurcations; etc.) obviously will, alone or in combination, profoundly affect the signalling properties of networks of even modest complexity.

Another physiological function in which electrogenic hyperpolarisation has been implicated is sensory adaptation[223, 233]. Sokolove and Cooke[223] have shown that the adaptation (i.e. reduction of firing frequency) of crayfish tonic stretch receptor to a constant stimulating current was affected by a number of manoeuvres known to inhibit sodium pumping, including removal of K_o, application of strophanthidin or cyanide, anoxia, and cooling. They concluded that an electrogenic sodium pump, stimulated by sodium entering during the initial train of impulses, was responsible for the adaptation to lower firing frequencies. When challenged by a steady stimulating current, certain giant neurones of marine molluscs also respond with a train of impulses of decreasing frequency. There is good evidence[192, 195] that in this case the adaptation is due not so much to the activation of an electrogenic pump as to an increase in membrane conductance for potassium, possibly secondary to increased intracellular calcium levels.

The firing frequency of some pacemaker cells may also be regulated by electrogenic pumping. Ayrapetyan[234] has observed that the hyperpolarisation which separates spontaneous bursts of activity in certain giant neurones of the snail can be modified by factors (temperature, strophanthidin, metabolic inhibitors) which affect the sodium pump, and has suggested electrogenic pumping as a way by which metabolism can control the discharge frequency of spontaneously active nerves. A similar conclusion was reached by Romey and Arvanitaki-Chalazonitis[235], who found that the discharge pattern of two types of spontaneously active neurones of *Aplysia* (bursting and constant-frequency) was sensitive to oxygen tension and temperature. Finally, the rhythmic discharge pattern of the cardiac ganglion which determines the heart rate of crustacea has been shown by Livengood *et al.*[133, 236] to be modified by factors which affect the sodium pump, and clear evidence for an electrogenic pump in the 'follower cells' of these ganglia was found[133]. Thus the authors concluded that the electrogenic pump could exert control over the heart rate by modulating the discharge pattern of the cardiac ganglion.

In addition to the 'physiological' roles for electrogenic pumping in nervous integration, sensory adaptation and pacemaker modulation, mentioned above, one might conceive of an electrogenic pump as a safety device against 'catastrophic firing'. Spontaneously firing nerves often do so at frequencies which result in a Na^+ influx well in excess of what the sodium pump can cope with. Were it not for a hyperpolarising electrogenic pump, a spontaneously firing cell would continue to discharge action potentials until its ion gradients were depleted to their limits of usefulness. Such a state of affairs would be undesirable indeed. Of course, any other mechanism which renders the membrane less excitable after a discharge (such as the post-activity potassium conductance increase) would be equally useful in this respect.

6.6 EFFECT OF NERVOUS ACTIVITY ON METABOLISM

How does conduction of action potentials lead to acceleration of the Embden–Meyerhof pathway (glycolysis) and oxygen consumption in nerve? A complete answer to this question should identify all changes in the concentration levels of ionic and metabolic constituents, as well as the temporal relationship between them. This information, combined with a knowledge of the kinetic and regulatory properties of all enzymes involved, would enable one to identify precisely the control mechanisms which allow the nerve to restore the steady state disturbed by the conduction of action potentials. A complete description of this admittedly complicated chain of events has not yet been achieved, although it would seem that with presently available techniques for biochemical micro-analysis[237] it should be possible to assay for all or nearly all Embden–Meyerhof pathway intermediates (and Krebs cycle intermediates as well) in such high surface-to-volume ratio preparations as, for example, mammalian C fibres or Garfish olfactory nerve[238]. The available information includes reasonably complete data (mentioned above) on the initial trigger (influx of sodium and calcium ions, efflux of potassium ions), as well as on the final end-result: consumption of oxygen and carbohydrates and production of carbon dioxide or lactate. The changes in sodium and potassium ion concentrations (at least) activate the sodium/potassium ATPase in a manner which is still far from completely understood. This activation of the sodium pump results in ATP consumption, ADP and P_i production, and perhaps a slight pH change as well (due to the differences between the acid dissociation constants of ATP, ADP and P_i). ADP itself undergoes at least two kinds of reaction: one a dismutation into ATP and AMP through the myokinase reaction; the other a phosphorylation into ATP through a creatine- (arginine-, etc.) phosphokinase reaction. Since all three nucleotides as well as the phosphagens and inorganic phosphate and calcium ions have stimulatory or regulatory effects on one or more steps in the glycolytic and oxidative pathways, there ensues an extremely complex chain of events whose complete elucidation will require a careful assay of all relevant intermediates before and after conduction of a train of impulses. In the case of nerve axons, useful data are available on only one of these metabolic intermediates: reduced NADH (its fluorescence allows it to be conveniently assayed *in vivo*). Interesting preliminary conclusions concerning regulatory mechanisms in stimulated nerve preparations have been drawn from the observation of $NADH/NAD^+$ levels, as well as from comparisons with analogous (and more complete) data in other preparations, but as already stated, a fuller understanding must await a much more thorough investigation of stimulation-induced metabolic changes than is presently available.

Post-stimulation changes in the levels of ATP, ADP, AMP, P_i and phosphocreatine in rabbit vagus nerve have been reported[239-241]. Greengard and Straub[239] found that immediately after a 15 s stimulation at 50 shocks s^{-1} the ATP and phosphocreatine (CrP) levels were 17% below normal and there was some indication that ~P breakdown was accompanied by an equivalent increase in ADP and AMP concentrations. Even conservative calculations make it clear, however, that without ~P regeneration by metabolism, the ATP and CrP energy stores would have been depleted several times over during stimulation, indicating that metabolism does indeed regenerate ATP with very little delay. Montant and Chmouliovsky[240] later showed that, by judicious spacing of two 15 s periods of stimulation, ATP levels could indeed be brought down to as little as 5–10% of the control level. Greengard and Straub[239] also attempted to assay for glucose-6-P, 1,3-diphosphoglycerate, phosphoenolpyruvate, a-ketoglutarate and pyruvate. All but pyruvate were below the detection limit (30 μmol kg^{-1} wet); pyruvate content was about 0.2 mmol kg^{-1} wet, and was unaffected by stimulation. In the nearly 15 years since this work was done, only a few attempts have been made to apply improved analytical methods to the study of metabolic regulation in stimulated nerve trunks. In a more recent investigation by Chmouliovsky et al.[241], the time course of the concentration changes of some important constituents was followed in greater detail. After a 15 s tetanus at 50 shocks s^{-1}, ATP fell and P_i rose (both from a baseline of about 1.8 mM) with rather similar time constants (maximum at 25 s after the tetanus); ADP seemed to rise somewhat more slowly but the (modest) fall in CrP definitely took longer to develop than the other changes, suggesting that perhaps the creatine kinase reaction is of lesser importance in the immediate metabolic response; AMP also rose to about twice its original level. These changes, which result from the operation of the sodium pump, set in motion a sequence of reactions (glycolysis and respiration) designed to restore original conditions. In frog sciatic nerve, Okada and McDougal[270] found no appreciable changes in the levels of high-energy phosphate compounds during high-frequency stimulation in the presence of oxygen. In the absence of more complete data on stimulated nerve trunks, some pertinent information can profitably be gleaned from other preparations.

Lowry and co-workers[242, 243] induced stimulation of glycolysis in mouse brain by complete ischaemia (decapitation) and determined the time course of the change in concentration for all intermediates of the Embden–Meyerhof pathway. The concentrations of glucose, glucose-6-phosphate, are fructose-6-phosphate were reduced below control levels whereas the others were elevated, indicating that control of glycolysis was exerted at the level of phosphofructokinase. In addition, evidence was presented that hexokinase is a control point, and that glycogen phosphorolysis was accelerated. Rolleston and Newsholme[244], working on the premise that, metabolic pathways, those enzymes which catalyse reactions that are apparently far from equilibrium in steady-state conditions must be capable of controlling that pathway, concluded that, in addition to the enzymes mentioned above, pyruvate kinase and possibly glyceraldehyde-3-phosphate dehydrogenase could regulate glycolysis. The mechanism of some of these regulatory operations can itself be extraordinarily complex. For example, the activity of phosphofructokinase is subject to regulation by an impressive list of modifiers[245, 246]: it is inhibited by ATP, and this inhibition is lifted by AMP, P_i, and fructose-6-phosphate; ADP also has a stimulatory action, and so has fructose diphosphate; in addition, inhibition by physiological concentrations of citrate and phosphocreatine has been demonstrated[247, 248]. Evidently all effects of increased sodium pumping (decrease in ATP and CrP, increase in ADP, AMP and P_i) could thus cooperate to stimulate the catalytic activity of phosphofructokinase.

Transition from aerobic to anaerobic conditions in heart muscle also speeds up glycolysis through an almost immediate facilitation of the phosphofructokinase reaction[249]. This facilitation can again be accounted for by the observed changes in nucleotide, phosphagen and inorganic phosphate concentrations: ATP and CrP levels fall, while ADP, AMP and P_i levels rise, the latter two most markedly. Tetanic stimulation of frog skeletal muscle leads to a proportional increase in glycolysis which is due to stimulation of glycogen phosphorylase as well as phosphofructokinase activity[250, 251]. The activation of glycogen phosphorylase was shown[250] to result from the conversion of inactive glycogen phosphorylase b to active phosphorylase a (catalysed by phosphorylase b kinase). Activation occurred not only during contraction, but also during K_o-induced depolarisation or exposure to caffeine (all of which increase intracellular calcium levels). Since it had been shown by Krebs et al.[252] that muscle phosphorylase b kinase activity was increased under certain conditions by Ca^{2+}, Danforth and Helmreich[250] tentatively suggested that calcium ions which enter myoplasm during contraction might also play a role in activating the metabolic machinery necessary for sustaining contraction and restoring the initial state. Unfortunately, the phosphorylase kinase activation by Ca^{2+} described by Krebs and co-workers[252, 253] appears to require rather high Ca^{2+} concentrations, and to be irreversible; these two properties make this particular mechanism a poor candidate for fine physiological control. More recently, several research groups[254, 271-273] have re-examined this important question and described a seemingly different mechanism for the reversible activation of muscle phosphorylase b kinase by very low (10^{-7} M) concentrations of Ca^{2+}. Whatever the precise mechanism, the idea that calcium ions activate the metabolic as well as the actomyosin machinery in contracting muscle seems very attractive indeed. Additional evidence for the regulation of glycolysis in contracting muscle by glycogen phosphorylase and phosphofructokinase has come from a thorough investigation of blowfly flight muscle by Sacktor and co-workers[255, 256] who determined the time course of the concentration changes of well over 30 metabolic and high-energy phosphate intermediates during the enormous (100-fold) increase in glycolytic rate initiated by flight. The changes in phosphoarginine and adenine nucleotides (especially AMP) could account for the activation of phosphofructokinase; the trigger for glycogen phosphorylase was not identified; and there was also some indication that glyceraldehyde-3-phosphate dehydrogenase could serve as a control point. Another instance where a kinetic analysis of the concentration changes of high-energy phosphate compounds and glycolytic intermediates in a preparation subjected to a physiological stimulus has yielded useful information on control mechanisms, is the work of Williamson et al.[257, 258] on the electric organ of Electrophorus electricus. Here again, the principal control sites were identified as glycogen phosphorylase and phosphofructokinase. The phosphocreatine, nucleotide and P_i changes observed (which result from the operation of the sodium pump) could account for the observed activation of phosphofructokinase. The trigger for the observed activation of phosphorylase b kinase was not identified, but by analogy with the mechanism proposed by Danforth and Helmreich[250] for skeletal muscle it was suggested that Ca^{2+} might play a role in this activation.

One metabolic co-factor which occupies a special position in both glycolysis and respiration is the NADH/NAD$^+$ couple. The fact that NADH is fluorescent, whereas NAD$^+$ is not, has been exploited by a number of researchers in attempts to elucidate metabolic control mechanisms in vivo in a variety of tissues including frog and toad muscle[259-261], Electrophorus electroplaque[262], and nerve[263-266]. It is fair to say that if interpretation of NADH fluorometry in terms of metabolic control mechanisms has progressed further in studies on muscle and electric organ than it has in studies on nerve, it is because muscle and electroplaque research has benefited from the knowledge gained independently with enzymatic and micro-analytical procedures. In the case of electric organ of Electrophorus, Aubert et al.[262] interpreted the changes in fluorescence emission observed during periods of recovery from discharge as indicating NAD$^+$ reduction (in the glyceraldehyde-3-P dehydrogenase reaction) due to activation of glycolysis. (Electric organ derives its energy mostly from glycolysis and contains very few mitochondria.) There was an unexpectedly long delay in the onset of NAD$^+$ reduction, which could not be explained solely on the basis of fluorometric techniques, but was later shown by Williamson et al.[257] (using enzymatic analysis) to be due to the slow onset of phosphorylase b kinase activation. In muscle the analysis of fluctuations in NADH fluorescence after contraction is more complicated because both glycolysis and mitochondrial respiration may be stimulated (the former by the factors discussed earlier, the latter by the elevated ADP levels[267]). Since glycolysis produces cytoplasmic NADH whereas respiration produces mitochondrial NAD^+, the fluorescence response to muscle contraction will often be biphasic[260, 261], and its interpretation correspondingly difficult.

The response of nerve NADH fluorescence to stimulation is equally complex[264, 266]. In a thorough investigation of fluorescence changes after stimulation of rabbit vagus nerve, Landowne and Ritchie[265, 266] found several distinct phases in the fluorescence response, whose relative importance was affected by the incubation temperature. The phase of fluorescence increase (most pronounced at high temperatures) was ascribed to NAD^+ reduction due to increased glycolytic flux (it was insensitive to mitochondrial inhibitors) but, remarkably enough, sodium pump inhibition by ouabain had no effect on this glycolysis stimulation, suggesting that the known regulatory effects of nucleotides, inorganic phosphate and phosphocreatine on phosphofructokinase are of secondary importance in this preparation. Since, on the other hand, calcium ions were required in the bathing medium for the stimulation-induced fluorescence increase to occur, it seems possible that in this tissue a major control mechanism for glycolytic flow is the activation of phosphorylase b kinase by calcium ions entering during the nerve impulse. Landowne and Ritchie[265] also observed several phases of fluorescence *decrease*, i.e. NAD^+ production, probably due to mitochondrial respiration. One phase was abolished by ouabain and thus presumably represented ADP-induced respiration; another phase depended on the presence of calcium ions, and may well be due to Ca^{2+} induced mitochondrial respiration (during which Ca^{2+} is taken up by the mitochondria, instead of ATP being generated). A third fraction of the stimulation-induced decrease in fluorescence (insensitive to external calcium or ouabain, but dependent on the presence of extracellular sodium) probably remains unexplained, since the argument offered by Landowne and Ritchie[265] to explain the requirement of this fraction for Na^+, and its persistence in the presence of ouabain, seems unlikely. These authors propose that, even in the presence of ouabain, the first sequence in the operation of the sodium pump (reaction 6.1, Section 6.4.1) can take place before the enzyme comes to a halt. The ADP released in this single 'half-stroke' of the pump would then lead to oxidation of an equivalent amount of mitochondrial NADH. A difficulty with this hypothesis is that rabbit vagus nerve membrane is rather permeable to sodium ions[268], which means that there must be a continuous turnover of the sodium pump, and that all ATPase molecules must be vulnerable to ouabain inhibition without necessarily having to wait for the extra sodium load which accompanies impulse conduction. A test of Landowne and Ritchie's hypothesis would be to verify whether this pump-derived ADP production in the presence of ouabain can indeed be obtained only in the first post-stimulation period, and not in subsequent ones.

From the foregoing discussion it will be evident that further progress in the understanding of metabolic regulation in stimulated nerve cells will require a painstaking biochemical analysis of the time course of all relevant metabolic intermediates in a well-defined preparation. Such an analysis seems possible with presently available techniques.

6.7 CONCLUSION

Nerve stimulation sets in motion an astounding number of regulatory mechanisms designed to restore the initial resting state at the expense of metabolic energy. The well-documented sodium influx and potassium efflux which accompany action potential conduction cause the sodium–potassium pump to be stimulated. The stoichiometry and kinetics of this pump stimulation are complex and still poorly understood, but it appears that the Na/K, pump, under most circumstances, actively extrudes more sodium ions than it absorbs potassium ions (though quite possibly not in fixed proportion), and thus causes a net charge transfer across the membrane in a manner which can be tentatively described as a constant current generator. This electrogenic operation of the sodium pump contributes to the membrane potential at rest as well as during recovery. The transient membrane hyperpolarisation which follows nervous activity is implicated in such physiological functions as integration, sensory adaptation, and pacemaker modulation. Hyperpolarisation may also serve as a safety device against catastrophic repetitive firing. The operation of the sodium pump (the Na–K ATPase) results in a reduction of intracellular ATP and phosphagen concentrations, and a concomitant increase of [ADP] and especially [AMP] and [P_i]. These concentration changes then somehow affect mitochondrial respiration ([ADP]?) as well as glycolysis. It is presumed that phosphofructokinase, being affected by all of the phosphate compounds mentioned, occupies a central position in glycolysis regulation in nerve, as it does in several other tissues which have been studied more thoroughly in this respect. Only direct biochemical analysis of peripheral nerve can assess the relative importance of the various putative regulatory sites in this tissue.

If sodium pumping clearly affects the metabolic state of nerve tissue, the converse may also be true. Indications are that [ADP] affects the behaviour of the Na/K pump in such a way that, at least in certain specialised tissues, variations in oxygen tension or energy supply within the physiological range might control membrane potentials and firing frequency via an effect on the pump.

A third ion besides sodium and potassium, whose movements during spike conduction or membrane depolarisation has attracted a great deal of attention[16], is Ca^{2+}. It has been proposed that calcium entering during the action potential is responsible for the stimulation of glycolytic flux observed after repetitive firing, through its activating effect on the enzyme phosphorylase *b* kinase. Another fascinating aspect of the rise in intracellular calcium concentration after spike conduction is that it appears to enhance the potassium conductance of the cell membrane, thus further contributing to the post-activity hyperpolarisation attributed to the operation of the electrogenic sodium pump.

Acknowledgements

The author gratefully acknowledges the critical comments made on an earlier version of this review by Drs M. P. Blaustein, C. C. Hunt, L. J. Mullins and C. M. Rovainen. The author's research referred to in this paper was supported by grants from the National Institutes of Health.

References

1. Hodgkin, A. L. (1964). *The Conduction of the Nervous Impulse* (Liverpool: Liverpool University Press)
2. Ussing, H. H. (1949). The distinction by means of tracers between active transport and diffusion. The transfer of iodide across the isolated frog skin. *Acta Physiol. Scand.*, **19**, 43
3. Keynes, R. D. (1951). The ionic movements during nervous activity. *J. Physiol. (Lond.)*, **114**, 119
4. Hodgkin, A. L. and Keynes, R. D. (1955). Active transport of cations in giant axons from *Sepia* and *Loligo*. *J. Physiol. (Lond.)*, **128**, 28
5. Brinley, F. J., Jr and Mullins, L. J. (1965). Ion fluxes and transference numbers in squid axons. *J. Neurophysiol.*, **28**, 526
6. Brinley, F. J., Jr. and Mullins, L. J. (1967). Sodium extrusion by internally dialyzed squid axons. *J. Gen. Physiol.*, **50**, 2303
7. Brinley, F. J., Jr. and Mullins, L. J. (1968). Sodium fluxes in internally dialyzed squid axons. *J. Gen. Physiol.*, **52**, 181
8. Canessa-Fischer, M., Zambrano, F. and Rojas, E. (1968). The loss and recovery of the sodium pump in perfused giant axons. *J. Gen. Physiol.*, **51**, 162
9. Rojas, E. and Canessa-Fischer, M. (1968). Sodium movements in perfused squid giant axons. *J. Gen. Physiol.*, **52**, 240
10. Baker, P. F., Blaustein, M. P., Keynes, R. D., Manil, J., Shaw, T. I. and Steinhardt, R. A. (1969). The ouabain-sensitive fluxes of sodium and potassium in squid giant axons. *J. Physiol. (Lond.)*, **200**, 459
11. Brinley, F. J., Jr. (1965). Sodium, potassium, and chloride concentrations and fluxes in the isolated giant axon of *Homarus*. *J. Neurophysiol.*, **28**, 742
12. Villegas, R., Villegas, G. M., Blei, M., Herrera, F. C. and Villegas, J. (1966). Non-electrolyte penetration and sodium fluxes through the axolemma of resting and stimulated medium sized axons of the squid *Doryteuthis plei*. *J. Gen. Physiol.*, **50**, 43
13. Villegas, R., Villegas, G. M., DiPolo, R. and Villegas, J. (1971). Nonelectrolyte permeability, sodium influx, electrical potentials, and axolemma ultrastructure in squid axons of various diameters. *J. Gen. Physiol.*, **57**, 623
14. Carpenter, D. O. (1970). Membrane potential produced directly by the Na^+ pump in *Aplysia* neurons. *Comp. Biochem. Physiol.*, **35**, 371
15. Thomas, R. C. (1972). Intracellular sodium activity and the sodium pump in snail neurones. *J. Physiol. (Lond.)*, **220**, 55
16. Baker, P. F. (1972). Transport and metabolism of calcium ions in nerve. *Progr. Biophys. Mol. Biol.*, **24**, 177
17. Hodgkin, A. L. and Keynes, R. D. (1957). Movements of labelled calcium in squid giant axons. *J. Physiol. (Lond.)*, **138**, 253
18. Baker, P. F., Blaustein, M. P., Hodgkin, A. L. and Steinhardt, R. A. (1969). The influence of calcium on sodium efflux in squid axons. *J. Physiol. (Lond.)*, **200**, 431
19. Keynes, R. D. and Lewis, P. R. (1956). The intracellular calcium contents of some invertebrate nerves. *J. Physiol. (Lond.)*, **134**, 399
20. Blaustein, M. P. and Hodgkin, A. L. (1969). The effect of cyanide on the efflux of calcium from squid axons. *J. Physiol. (Lond.)*, **200**, 497
21. Baker, P. F., Hodgkin, A. L. and Ridgway, E. B. (1971). Depolarization and calcium entry in squid giant axons. *J. Physiol. (Lond.)*, **218**, 709
22. Luxoro, M. and Yanez, E. (1968). Permeability of the giant axon of *Dosidicus gigas* to calcium ions. *J. Gen. Physiol.*, **51**, 115
23. DiPolo, R. (1973). Is the sodium dependent calcium efflux in squid axons ATP dependent? *Biophys. J.*, **13**, 104A
24. Keynes, R. D. and Lewis, P. R. (1951). The sodium and potassium content of cephalopod nerve fibres. *J. Physiol. (Lond.)*, **114**, 151

25. Hodgkin, A. L. and Huxley, A. F. (1947). Potassium leakage from an active nerve fibre. *J. Physiol. (Lond.)*, **106**, 341
26. Shanes, A. M. (1954). Effect of temperature on potassium liberation during nerve activity. *Amer. J. Physiol.*, **177**, 377
27. Keynes, R. D. and Ritchie, J. M. (1965). The movements of labelled ions in mammalian non-myelinated nerve fibres. *J. Physiol. (Lond.)*, **179**, 333
28. Gerasimov, V. D., Kostyuk, P. G. and Maiskii, V. A. (1965). The influence of divalent cations on the electrical characteristics of membranes of giant neurones. *Biophysics*, **10**, 447
29. Meves, H. (1966). Das Aktionspotential der Riesennervenzellen der Weinbergschnecke *Helix pomatia*. *Pflugers Archiv.*, **289**, R10
30. Kerkut, G. A. and Gardner, D. R. (1967). The role of calcium ions in the action potentials of *Helix aspersa neurones*. *Comp. Biochem. Physiol.*, **20**, 147
31. Meves, H. (1968). The ionic requirements for the production of action potentials in *Helix pomatia* neurones. *Pfluegers Archiv.*, **304**, 215
32. Geduldig, D. and Junge, D. (1968). Sodium and calcium components of action potentials in the *Aplysia* giant neurone. *J. Physiol. (Lond.)*, **199**, 347
33. Geduldig, D. and Gruener, R. (1970). Voltage clamp of the *Aplysia* giant neurone: early sodium and calcium currents. *J. Physiol. (Lond.)*, **211**, 217
34. Caldwell, P. C. (1960). The phosphorus metabolism of squid axons and its relationship to the active transport of sodium. *J. Physiol. (Lond.)*, **152**, 545
35. Baker, P. F. (1965). Phosphorus metabolism of intact crab nerve and its relation to the active transport of ions. *J. Physiol. (Lond.)*, **180**, 383
36. Fenn, W. O. (1927). The oxygen consumption of frog nerve during stimulation. *J. Gen. Physiol.*, **10**, 767
37. Gerard, R. W. (1927). Studies on nerve metabolism. II. Respiration in oxygen and nitrogen. *Amer. J. Physiol.*, **82**, 381
38. Meyerhof, O. and Schultz, W. (1929). Ueber die Atmung des marklosen Nerven. *Biochem. Z.*, **206**, 158
39. Brink, F., Bronk, D. W., Carlson, F. D. and Connelly, C. M. (1952). The oxygen uptake of active axons. *Cold Spring Harb. Symp. Quant. Biol.*, **17**, 53
40. Connelly, C. M. (1959). Recovery processes and metabolism of nerve. *Rev. Mod. Phys.*, **31**, 475
41. Connelly, C. M. (1962). Metabolic and electrochemical events associated with recovery from activity. *Proc. XXII int. Congr. Physiol.*, **1**, 600
42. Baker, P. F. and Connelly, C. M. (1966). Some properties of the external activation site of the sodium pump in crab nerve. *J. Physiol. (Lond.)*, **185**, 270
43. Ritchie, J. M. (1967). The oxygen consumption of mammalian non-myelinated nerve fibres at rest and during activity. *J. Physiol. (Lond.)*, **188**, 309
44. Rang, H. P. and Ritchie, J. M. (1968). The dependence on external cations of the oxygen consumption of mammalian non-myelinated fibres at rest and during activity. *J. Physiol. (Lond.)*, **196**, 163
45. Connelly, C. M. and Cranefield, P. F. (1953). *Proc. XIX int. Congr. Physiol.* The oxygen consumption of the stellar nerve of the squid (*Loligo Pealiei*). 276 (1953: Montreal)
46. McIlwain, H. and Joanny, P. (1963). Characteristics required in electrical pulses of rectangular time-voltage relationships for metabolic change and ion movement in mammalian cerebral tissues. *J. Neurochem.*, **10**, 313
47. Caldwell, P. C. and Keynes, R. D. (1959). The effect of ouabain on the efflux of sodium from a squid giant axon. *J. Physiol. (Lond.)*, **148**, 8P
48. Whittam, R. and Willis, J. S. (1963). Ion movements and oxygen consumption in kidney cortex slices. *J. Physiol. (Lond.)*, **168**, 158
49. Zerahn, K. (1956). Oxygen consumption and active sodium transport in the isolated frog skin. *Acta Physiol. Scand.*, **36**, 300
50. Vieira, F. L., Caplan, S. R. and Essig, A. (1972). Energetics of sodium transport in frog skin. I. Oxygen consumption in the short-circuited state. *J. Gen. Physiol.*, **59**, 60
51. Skou, J. C. (1957). The influence of some cations on an adenosine triphosphatase from peripheral nerves. *Biochim. Biophys. Acta*, **23**, 394
52. Albers, R. W. (1967). Biochemical aspects of active transport. *Ann. Rev. Biochem.*, **36**, 727

53. Glynn, I. M. (1968). Membrane adenosine triphosphatase and cation transport. *Brit. Med. Bull.*, **24**, 165
54. Whittam, R. and Wheeler, K. P. (1970). Transport across cell membranes. *Ann. Rev. Physiol.*, **32**, 21
55. Caldwell, P. C. (1969). Energy relationships and the active transport of ions, in *Current Topics in Bioenergetics* (D. R. Sanadi, editor), Vol. 3, 251 (New York: Academic Press)
56. Fahn, S., Koval, G. J. and Albers, R. W. (1966). Sodium-potassium-activated adenosine triphosphatase of *Electrophorus* electric organ. *J. Biol. Chem.* **241**, 1882
57. Post, R. L., Kume, S., Tobin, T., Orcutt, B. and Sen, A. K. (1969). Flexibility of an active center in sodium-plus-potassium adenosine triphosphatase. *J. Gen. Physiol.*, **54**, 306s
58. Skou, J. C. (1971). The role of the phosphorylated intermediate in the reaction of the $(Na^+ + K^+)$-activated enzyme system, in *Membrane Bound Enzymes* (G. Porcellati and F. di Jeso, editors), Vol. 14 of *Advances in Experimental Medicine and Biology*, 175 (New York: Plenum Press)
59. Hoffman, J. F. (1969). The interaction between tritiated ouabain and the Na–K pump in red blood cells. *J. Gen. Physiol.*, **54**, 343
60. Ellory, J. C. and Keynes, R. D. (1969). Binding of tritiated digoxin to human red cell ghosts. *Nature (London)*, **221**, 776
61. Dunham, P. B. and Hoffman, J. F. (1971). Active cation transport and ouabain binding in high potassium and low potassium red blood cells of sheep. *J. Gen. Physiol.*, **58**, 94
62. Baker, P. F. and Willis, J. S. (1972). Binding of the cardiac glycoside ouabain to intact cells. *J. Physiol. (Lond.)*, **224**, 441
63. Landowne, D. and Ritchie, J. M. (1970). The binding of tritiated ouabain to mammalian non–myelinated nerve fibres. *J. Physiol. (Lond.)*, **207**, 529
64. Baker, P. F. and Willis, J. S. (1969). On the number of sodium pumping sites in cell membranes. *Biochim. Biophys. Acta*, **183**, 646
65. Baker, P. F. and Willis, J. S. (1972). Inhibition of the sodium pump in squid axons by cardiac glycosides: dependence on extracellular ions and metabolism. *J. Physiol. (Lond.)*, **224**, 463
66. Caldwell, P. C., Hodgkin, A. L., Keynes, R. D. and Shaw, T. I. (!960). The effect of injecting 'energy rich' phosphate compounds on the active transport of ions in the giant axons of *Loligo. J. Physiol. (Lond.)*, **152**, 561
67. Baker, P. F., Hodgkin, A. L. and Shaw, T. I. (1962). Replacement of the axoplasm of giant nerve fibres with artificial solutions. *J. Physiol. (Lond.)*, **164**, 330
68. Oikawa, T., Spyropoulos, C. S., Tasaki, I. and Teorell, T. (1961). Methods for perfusing the giant axon of *Loligo pealii. Acta Physiol. Scand.*, **52**, 195
69. Mullins, L. J. and Brinley, F. J., Jr. (1969). Potassium fluxes in dialyzed squid axons. *J. Gen. Physiol.*, **53**, 704
70. Bond, G. H., Bader, H. and Post, R. L. (1966). Acetyl phosphate as substrate for $(Na^+ + K^+)$-ATPase. *Fed. Proc.*, **25**, 567(A)
71. Israel, Y. and Titus, E. (1967). A comparison of microsomal $(Na^+ + K^+)$-ATPase with K^+-acetylphosphatase. *Biochim. Biophys. Acta*, **139**, 450
72. Bond, G. H., Bader, H. and Post, R. L. (1971). Acetyl phosphate as a substitute for ATP in $(Na^+ + K^+)$-dependent ATPase. *Biochim. Biophys. Acta*, **241**, 57
73. Robinson, J. D. (1971). K^+-stimulated incorporation of ^{32}P from nitrophenyl phosphate into a $(Na^+ + K^+)$-activated ATPase preparation. *Biochem. Biophys. Res. Comm.*, **42**, 880
74. Garrahan, P. J. and Rega, A. F. (1972). Potassium activated phosphatase from human red blood cells. The effects of p-nitrophenylphosphate on cation fluxes. *J. Physiol. (Lond.)*, **223**, 595
75. Squires, R. F. (1965). On the interactions of Na^+, K^+, Mg^{++} and ATP with the Na^+ plus K^+ activated ATPase from rat brain. *Biochem. Biophys. Res. Comm.*, **19**, 27
76. Robinson, J. D. Kinetic studies on a brain microsomal adenosine triphosphatase. Evidence suggesting conformational changes. *Biochemistry*, **6**, 2350
77. Mullins, L. J. (1972). Active transport of Na^+ and K^+ across the squid axon membrane, in: *The Role of Membranes in Secretory Processes*, 182 (L. Bolis, editor) (Amsterdam: North-Holland)

78. Nørby, J. G. and Jensen, J. (1971). Binding of ATP to brain microsomal ATPase. Determination of the ATP-binding capacity and the dissociation constant of the enzyme-ATP complex as a function of K^+ concentration. *Biochim. Biophys. Acta*, **233**, 104

79. Hegyvary, C. and Post, R. L. (1971). Binding of adenosine triphosphate to sodium and potassium ion-stimulated adenosine triphosphatase. *J. Biol. Chem.*, **246**, 5234

80. Harris, E. J. and Maizels, M. (1951). The permeability of human erythrocytes to sodium. *J. Physiol. (Lond.)*, **113**, 506

81. Hodgkin, A. L. and Keynes, R. D. (1953). Sodium extrusion and potassium absorption in *Sepia* axons. *J. Physiol. (Lond.)*, **120**, 46P

82. Keynes, R. D. (1954). The ionic fluxes in frog muscle. *Proc. Roy. Soc. (Lond.)*, *B*, **142**, 359

83. Glynn, I. M. (1956). Sodium and potassium movements in human red cells. *J. Physiol. (Lond.)*, **134**, 278

84. Glynn, I. M. (1957). The ionic permeability of the red cell membrane. *Progr. Biophys.*, **8**, 242

85. Post, R. L., Merritt, C. R., Kinsolving, C. R. and Albright, C. D. (1960). Membrane adenosine triphosphatase as a participant in the active transport of sodium and potassium in the human erythrocyte. *J. Biol. Chem.*, **235**, 1796

86. Sachs, J. R. and Welt, L. G. (1967). The concentration dependence of active potassium transport in the human red blood cell. *J. Clin. Invest.*, **46**, 65

87. Sachs, J. R. (1970). Sodium movements in the human red blood cell. *J. Gen. Physiol.*, **56**, 322

88. Sjodin, R. A. and Beaugé, L. A. (1968). Strophanthidin-sensitive components of potassium and sodium movements in skeletal muscle as influenced by the internal sodium concentration. *J. Gen. Physiol.*, **52**, 389

89. Sjodin, R. A. (1971). The kinetics of sodium extrusion in striated muscle as functions of the external sodium and potassium ion concentrations. *J. Gen. Physiol.*, **57**, 164

90. Rang, H. P. and Ritchie, J. M. (1968). On the electrogenic sodium pump in mammalian non–myelinated nerve fibres and its activation by various external cations. *J. Physiol. (Lond.)*, **196**, 183

91. De Weer, P. (1970). Effects of intracellular adenosine-5'-diphosphate and orthophosphate on the sensitivity of sodium efflux from squid axon to external sodium and potassium. *J. Gen. Physiol.*, **56**, 583

92. Hoffman, J. F. (1962). Properties of the active cation transport in rat red blood cells. *Fed. Proc.*, **21**, 145A

93. Hoffman, J. F. (1966). The red cell membrane and the transport of sodium and potassium. *Amer. J. Med.*, **40**, 666

94. Priestland, R. N. and Whittam, R. (1968). The influence of external sodium ions on the sodium pump in erythrocytes. *Biochem. J.*, **109**, 369

95. Garrahan, P. J. and Glynn, I. M. (1967). The sensitivity of the sodium pump to external sodium. *J. Physiol. (Lond.)*, **192**, 175

96. Beaugé, L. A. and Ortiz, O. (1971). Sodium and rubidium fluxes in rat red blood cells. *J. Physiol. (Lond.)*, **218**, 533

97. Beaugé, L. A. and Adragna, N. (1971). The kinetics of ouabain inhibition and the partition of rubidium influx in human red blood cells. *J. Gen. Physiol.*, **57**, 576

98. Keynes, R. D. and Swan, R. C. (1959). The effect of external sodium concentration on the sodium fluxes in frog skeletal muscle. *J. Physiol. (Lond.)*, **147**, 591

99. Mullins, L. J. and Frumento, A. S. (1963). The concentration dependence of sodium efflux from muscle. *J. Gen. Physiol.*, **46**, 629

100. Harris, E. J. (1965). The dependence of efflux of sodium from frog muscle on internal sodium and external potassium. *J. Physiol. (Lond.)*, **177**, 355

101. Carmeliet, E. E. (1964). Influence of lithium ions on the transmembrane potential and cation content of cardiac cells. *J. Gen. Physiol.*, **47**, 501

102. Brinley, F. J., Jr. (1968). Sodium and potassium fluxes in isolated barnacle muscle fibres. *J. Gen. Physiol.*, **51**, 445

103. Maizels, M. (1968). Effect of sodium content on sodium efflux from human red cells suspended in sodium-free media containing potassium, rubidium, caesium or lithium chloride. *J. Physiol. (Lond.)*, **195**, 657

104. Hoffman, P. G. and Tosteson, D. C. (1971). Active sodium and potassium transport in high potassium and low potassium sheep red cells. *J. Gen. Physiol.*, **58**, 438

105. Garay, R. P. and Garrahan, P. J. (1973). The interaction of sodium and potassium with the sodium pump in red cells. *J. Physiol. (Lond.)*, **231**, 297
106. Hodgkin, A. L. and Keynes, R. D. (1956). Experiments on the injection of substances into squid giant axons by means of a microsyringe. *J. Physiol. (Lond.)*, **131**, 592
107. Sjodin, R. A. and Beaugé, L. A. (1967). The ion selectivity and concentration dependence of cation coupled active sodium transport in squid giant axons. *Curr. Mod. Biol.*, **1**, 105
108. Sjodin, R. A. and Beaugé, L. A. (1968). Coupling and selectivity of sodium and potassium transport in squid giant axons. *J. Gen. Physiol.*, **51**, 152
109. Thomas, R. C. (1969). Membrane current and intracellular sodium changes in a snail neurone during extrusion of injected sodium. *J. Physiol. (Lond.)*, **201**, 495
110. Kostyuk, P. G., Krishtal, O. A. and Pidoplichko, V. I. (1972). Potential dependent membrane current during the active transport of ions in snail neurones. *J. Physiol. (Lond.)*, **226**, 373
111. Rose, I. A. (1968). The state of magnesium in cells as estimated from the adenylate kinase equilibrium. *Proc. Nat. Acad. Sci.*, **61**, 1079
112. Baker, P. F. and Crawford, A. C. (1972). Mobility and transport of magnesium in squid giant axons. *J. Physiol. (Lond.)*, **227**, 855
113. De Weer, P. (1970). Effects of intracellular ADP and P_i on the sodium pump of squid giant axon. *Nature (London)*, **226**, 1251
114. Hexum, T., Samson, F. E., Jr. and Himes, R. H. (1970). Kinetic studies of membrane $(Na^+-K^+-Mg^{2+})$-ATPase. *Biochim. Biophys. Acta*, **212**, 322
115. Harris, E. J. (1954). Linkage of K and Na active transport in human erythrocytes, in *Active Transport and Secretion*, 228 (R. Brown and J. F. Danielli, editors) (Cambridge: Cambridge University Press)
116. Gill, T. J. and Solomon, A. K. (1959). Effect of ouabain on sodium flux in human red cells. *Nature (London)*, **183**, 1128
117. McConaghey, P. D. and Maizels, M. (1962). Cation exchanges of lactose-treated human red cells. *J. Physiol. (Lond.)*, **162**, 485
118. Tosteson, D. C. and Hoffman, J. F. (1960). Regulation of cell volume by active cation transport in high and low potassium sheep red cells. *J. Gen. Physiol.*, **44**, 169
119. Post, R. L. and Jolly, P. C. (1957). The linkage of sodium, potassium and ammonium active transport across the human erythrocyte membrane. *Biochim. Biophys. Acta*, **25**, 118
120. Post, R. L., Albright, C. D. and Dayani, K. (1967). Resolution of pump and leak components of sodium and potassium ion transport in human erythrocytes. *J. Gen. Physiol.*, 50, 1201
121. Garrahan, P. J. and Glynn, I. M. (1967). The stoicheiometry of the sodium pump. *J. Physiol. (Lond.)*, **192**, 217
122. Sachs, J. R. (1971). Ouabain-insensitive sodium movements in the human red blood cell. *J. Gen. Physiol.*, **57**, 259
123. Keynes, R. D. and Rybova, R. (1963). The coupling between sodium and potassium fluxes in frog sartorius muscle. *J. Physiol. (Lond.)*, **168**, 58P
124. Mullins, L. J. and Awad, M. Z. (1965). The control of the membrane potential of muscle fibers by the sodium pump. *J. Gen. Physiol.*, **48**, 761
125. Keynes, R. D. (1965). Some further observations on the sodium efflux in frog muscle. *J. Physiol. (Lond.)*, **178**, 305
126. Adrian, R. H. and Slayman, C. L. (1966). Membrane potential and conductance during transport of sodium, potassium and rubidium in frog muscle. *J. Physiol.*, **184**, 970
127. Keynes, R. D. and Steinhardt, R. A. (1968). The components of the sodium efflux in frog muscle. *J. Physiol. (Lond.)*, **198**, 581
128. Horowicz, P., Taylor, J. W. and Waggoner, D. M. (1970). Fractionation of sodium efflux in frog sartorius muscles by strophanthidin and removal of external sodium. *J. Gen. Physiol.*, **55**, 401
129. Sjodin, R. A. and Beaugé, L. A. (1973). An analysis of the leakages of sodium ions into and potassium ions out of striated muscle cells. *J. Gen. Physiol.*, **61**, 222
130. Beaugé, L. A., Medici, A. and Sjodin, R. A. (1973). The influence of external caesium ions on potassium efflux in frog skeletal muscle. *J. Physiol. (Lond.)*, **228**, 1
131. Nakajima, S. and Takahashi, K. (1966). Post-tetanic hyperpolarization and electrogenic Na pump in stretch receptor neurone of crayfish. *J. Physiol. (Lond.)*, **187**, 105

132. Kostyuk, P. G. (1970). Active transport of ions in a nerve cell and its connection with the electrical processes on surface membrane. *Ukr. Biochem. J.*, **43**, 9

133. Livengood, D. R. and Kusano, K. (1972). Evidence for an electrogenic sodium pump in follower cells of the lobster cardiac ganglion. *J. Neurophysiol.*, **35**, 170

134. Coombs, J. S., Eccles, J. C. and Fatt, P. (1955). The specific ionic conductances and the ionic movements across the motoneuronal membrane that produce the inhibitory post-synaptic potential. *J. Physiol. (Lond.)*, **130**, 326

135. Krnjevic, K., Mitchell, J. F. and Szerb, J. S. (1963). Determination of iontophoretic release of acetylcholine from micropipettes. *J. Physiol. (Lond.)*, **165**, 421

136. Curtis, D. R. (1964). Microelectrophoresis, in *Physical Techniques in Biological Research* Vol. V, 144 (W. L. Nastuk, editor) (New York and London: Academic Press)

137. Baylor, D. A. and Nicholls, J. G. (1969). After-effects of nerve impulses on signalling in the central nervous system of the leech. *J. Physiol. (Lond.)*, **203**, 571

138. Jansen, J. K. S. and Nicholls, J. G. (1973). Conductance changes, an electrogenic pump and the hyperpolarisation of leech neurones following impulses. *J. Physiol. (Lond.)*, **229**, 635

139. Sen, A. K. and Post, R. L. (1964). Stoichiometry and localization of adenosine triphosphate-dependent sodium and potassium transport in the erythrocyte. *J. Biol. Chem.*, **239**, 345.

140. Whittam, R. and Ager, M. E. (1965). The connexion between active cation transport and metabolism in erythrocytes. *Biochem. J.*, **97**, 214

141. Gárdos, G. (1964). Connection between membrane adenosine-triphosphatase activity and potassium transport in erythrocyte ghosts. *Experientia*, **20**, 387

142. Dydynska, M. and Harris, E. J. (1966). Consumption of high-energy phosphates during active sodium and potassium interchange in frog muscle. *J. Physiol. (Lond.)*, **182**, 92

143. Harris, E. J. (1967). The stoicheiometry of sodium ion movement from frog muscle. *J. Physiol. (Lond.)*, **193**, 455

144. Baker, P. F. and Shaw, T. I. (1965). A comparison of the phosphorus metabolism of intact squid nerve with that of the isolated axoplasm and sheath. *J. Physoil. (Lond.)*, **180**, 424

145. Mullins, L. J. and Brinley, F. J., Jr. (1967). Some factors influencing sodium extrusion by internally dialyzed squid axons. *J. Gen. Physiol.*, **50**, 2333

146. Caldwell, P. C., Hodgkin, A. L., Keynes, R. D. and Shaw, T. I. (1960). Partial inhibition of the active transport of cations in the giant axons of *Loligo*. *J. Physiol. (Lond.)*, **152**, 591

147. Keynes, R. D. (1960). The effect of complete and partial inhibition of metabolism on active transport in nerve and muscle. *Ciba Foundation Study Group No. V.* Regulation of the Inorganic Ion Content of Cells, 77

148. Caldwell, P. C. (1968). Factors governing movement and distribution of inorganic ions in nerve and muscle. *Physiol. Rev.*, **48**, 1

149. De Weer, P. (1968). Restoration of a potassium-requiring sodium pump in squid giant axons poisoned with CN and depleted of arginine. *Nature (London)*, **219**, 730

150. Baker, P. F., Foster, R. F. Gilbert, D. S. and Shaw, T. I. (1971). Sodium transport by perfused giant axons of *Loligo*. *J. Physiol. (Lond.)*, **219**, 487

151. Garrahan, P. J. and Glynn, I. M. (1967). The behaviour of the sodium pump in red cells in the absence of external potassium. *J. Physiol. (Lond.)*, **192**, 159

152. Garrahan, P. J. and Glynn, I. M. (1967). Factors affecting the relative magnitudes of the sodium:potassium and the sodium:sodium exchanges catalysed by the sodium pump. *J. Physiol. (Lond.)*, **192**, 189

153. Garrahan, P. J. and Glynn, I. M. (1967). The incorporation of inorganic phosphate into adenosine triphosphate by reversal of the sodium pump. *J. Physiol. (Lond.)*, **192**, 237

154. Glynn, I. M. and Hoffman, J. F. (1971). Nucleotide requirements for sodium–sodium exchange catalysed by the sodium pump in human red cells. *J. Physiol. (Lond.)*, **218**, 239

155. Glynn, I. M., Hoffman, J. F. and Lew, V. L. (1971). Some 'partial reactions' of the sodium pump. *Phil. Trans. Roy. Soc. Lond. B*, **262**, 91

156. Caldwell, P. C. and Schirmer, H. (1965). The free energy available to the sodium pump of squid giant axons and changes in the sodium efflux on removal of the extracellular potassium. *J. Physiol. (Lond.)*, **181**, 25P

157. Himsworth, R. L. (1970). Hypothalamic control of adrenaline secretion in response to insufficient glucose. *J. Physiol. (Lond.)*, **206**, 411
158. Slater, E. C. (1969). The oxidative phosphorylation potential, in *Round Table Discussion on the Energy Level and Metabolic Control in Mitochondria* (S. Papa, J. M. Tager, E. Quagliariello and E. C. Slater, editors) (Adriatica Editrice: Bari)
159. Mills, E. and Jöbsis, F. F. (1970). Simultaneous measurement of cytochrome a_3 reduction and chemoreceptor afferent activity in the carotid body. *Nature (London)*, **225**, 1147
160. Krylov, S. S. and Anichkov, S. V. (1968). The effect of metabolic inhibitors on carotid chemoreceptors, *Proceedings of the Waters Foundation Symposium on Arterial Chemoreceptors*, 103 (R. W. Torrance, editor) (Oxford and Edinburgh: Blackwell Scientific Publications)
161. Biscoe, T. J. (1971). Carotid Body: structure and function. *Physiol. Rev.*, **51**, 437
162. Torrance, R. W. (1968). Prolegomena, *Proceedings of the Waters Foundation Symposium on Arterial Chemoreceptors*, 1 (R. W. Torrance, editor) (Oxford and Edinburgh: Blackwell Scientific Publications)
163. Dean, R. B. (1941). Theories of electrolyte equilibrium in muscle. *Biol. Symp.*, **3**, 331
164. De Weer, P. and Geduldig, D. (1973). Electrogenic sodium pump in squid giant axon. *Science*, **179**, 1326
165. Kernan, R. P. (1970). Electrogenic or linked transport, *Membranes and Ion Transport*, Vol. I 395 (E. E. Bittar, editor) (London: Wiley)
166. Koketsu, K. (1971). The electrogenic sodium pump. *Adv. Biophys.*, **2**, 77
167. Ritchie, J. M. (1971). Electrogenic ion pumping in nervous tissue, in *Current Topics in Bioenergetics*, Vol. 4, 327 (D. R. Sanadi, editor) (New York and London: Academic Press)
168. Thomas, R. C. (1972). Electrogenic sodium pump in nerve and muscle cells. *Physiol. Rev.*, **52**, 563
169. Kerkut, G. A. and York, B. (1971). *the Electrogenic Sodium Pump.* (Bristol: Scientechnica)
170. Kernan, R. P. (1962). Membrane potential changes during sodium transport in frog sartorius muscle. *Nature (London)*, **193**, 986
171. Stephenson, W. K. (1953). Membrane potential changes in fibers of the frog sartorius muscle during sodium extrusion and potassium accumulation. *Biol. Bull.*, **105**, 385
172. Stephenson, W. K. (1957). Membrane potential changes and ion movements in the frog sartorius muscle. *J. Cell. Comp. Physiol.*, **50**, 105
173. Cross, S. B., Keynes, R. D. and Rybova, R. (1965). The coupling of sodium efflux and potassium influx in frog muscle. *J. Physiol. (Lond.)*, **181**, 865
174. Mullins, L. J. and Noda, K. (1963). The influence of sodium-free solutions on the membrane potential of frog muscle fibers. *J. Gen. Physiol.*, **47**, 117
175. Frumento, A. S. (1965). Sodium pump: its electrical effects in skeletal muscle. *Science*, **147**, 1442
176. Harris, E. J. and Ochs, S. (1966). Effects of sodium extrusion and local anaesthetics on muscle membrane resistance and potential. *J. Physiol. (Lond.)*, **187**, 5
177. Ritchie, J. M. and Straub, R. W. (1957). The hyperpolarization which follows activity in mammalian non–medullated fibres. *J. Physiol. (Lond.)*, **136**, 80
178. Straub, R. W. (1961). On the mechanism of post-tetanic hyperpolarization in myelinated nerve fibres from the frog. *J. Physiol. (Lond.)*, **159**, 19P
179. Holmes, O. (1962). Effects of pH, changes in potassium concentration and metabolic inhibitors on the after-potentials of mammalian non–medullated nerve fibres. *Arch. Int. Physiol.*, **70**, 211
180. Carpenter, D. O. and Alving, B. O. (1968). A contribution of an electrogenic Na^+ pump to membrane potential in *Aplysia* neurons. *J. Gen. Physiol.*, **52**, 1
181. Meunier, J. M. and Tauc, L. (1970). Participation d'une pompe métabolique au potentiel de repos de neurones d'aplysie. *J. Physiol. (Paris)*, **62**, 192
182. Kerkut, G. A. and Thomas, R. C. (1965). An electrogenic sodium pump in snail nerve cells. *Comp. Biochem. Physiol.*, **14**, 167
183. Gorman, A. L. F. and Marmor, M. F. (1970). Contributions of the sodium pump and ionic gradients to the membrane potential of a molluscan neurone. *J. Physiol. (Lond.)*, **210**, 897
184. Kosterlitz, H. W., Lees, G. M. and Wallis, D. I. (1970). Further evidence for an

electrogenic pump in a mammalian sympathetic ganglion. *Brit. J. Pharmacol.*, **38**, 464P

185. Nicholls, J. G. and Baylor, D. A. (1958). Long-lasting hyperpolarization after activity of neurons in leech central nervous system. *Science*, **162**, 279

186. Kuno, M., Miyahara, J. T. and Weakly, J. N. (1970). Post-tetanic hyperpolarization produced by an electrogenic pump in dorsal spinocerebellar tract neurones of the cat. *J. Physiol. (Lond.)*, **210**, 839

187. Koike, H., Brown, H. M. and Hagiwara, S. (1971). Hyperpolarization of a barnacle photoreceptor membrane following illumination. *J. Gen. Physiol.*, **57**, 723

188. Brown, J. E. and Lisman, J. E. (1972). An electrogenic sodium pump in *Limulus* ventral photoreceptor cells. *J. Gen. Physiol.*, **59**, 720

189. Meves, H. (1961). Die Nachpotentiale isolierten markhaltigen Nervenfasern des Frosches bei tetanischer Reizung. *Pfluegers Archiv.*, **272**, 336

190. Gage, P. W. and Hubbard, J. I. (1964). Ionic changes responsible for post-tetanic hyperpolarization. *Nature (London)*, **203**, 653

191. Gage, P. W. and Hubbard, J. I. (1966). The origin of the post-tetanic hyperpolarization of mammalian motor nerve terminals. *J. Physiol. (Lond.)*, **184**, 335

192. Connor, J. A. and Stevens, C. F. (1971). Prediction of repetitive firing behaviour from voltage clamp data on an isolated neuron soma. *J. Physiol. (Lond.)*, **213**, 31

193. Meunier, J. M. (1971). Activation de la pompe à sodium dans les neurones géants d'aplysie. *J. Physiol. (Paris)*, **63**, 254A

194. Junge, D. (1972). Increased K-conductance as proximate cause of post-stimulus hyperpolarisation in *Tritonia* neurones. *Comp. Biochem. Physiol.*, **42A**, 975

195. Brodwick, M. S. and Junge, D. (1972). Post-stimulus hyperpolarization and slow potassium conductance increase in *Aplysia* giant neurone. *J. Physiol. (Lond.)*, **223**, 549

196. Gárdos, G. (1959). The role of calcium in the potassium permeability of human erythrocytes. *Acta Physiol. Hung.*, **15**, 121

197. Whittam, R. (1968). Control of membrane permeability to potassium in red blood cells. *Nature (London)*, **219**, 610

198. Romero, P. J. and Whittam, R. (1971). The control by internal calcium of membrane permeability to sodium and potassium. *J. Physiol. (Lond.)*, **214**, 481

199. Lew, V. L. (1970). Effect of intracellular calcium on the potassium permeability of human red cells. *J. Physiol. (Lond.)*, **206**, 35P

200. Lew, V. L. (1971). On the ATP dependence of the Ca^{2+}-induced increase in K^+ permeability observed in human red cells. *Biochim. Biophys. Acta*, **233**, 827

201. Lew, V. L. (1971). Effect of ouabain on the Ca^{2+}-dependent increase in K^+ permeability in depleted guinea-pig red cells. *Biochim. Biophys. Acta*, **249**, 236

202. Blum, R. M. and Hoffman, J. F. (1972). Ca-induced K transport in human red cells: localization of the Ca-sensitive site to the inside of the membrane. *Biochem. Biophys. Res. Comm.*, **46**, 1146

203. Kregenow, F. M. and Hoffman, J. F. (1972). Some kinetic and metabolic characteristics of calcium-induced potassium transport in human red cells. *J. Gen. Physiol.*, **60**, 406

204. van Rossum, G. D. V. (1970). Relation of intracellular Ca^{2+} to retention of K^+ by liver slices. *Nature (London)*, **225**, 638

205. Meech, R. W. and Strumwasser, F. (1970). Intracellular calcium injection activates potassium conductance in *Aplysia* nerve cells. *Fed. Proc.*, **29**, 834A

206. Meech, R. (1972). Intracellular calcium injection causes increased potassium conductance in *Aplysia* neurones. *Comp. Biochem. Physiol.*, **42A**, 493

207. Godfraind, J. M., Krnjevic, K. and Pumain, R. (1970). Unexpected features of the action of dinitrophenol on cortical neurones. *Nature (London)*, **228**, 562

208. Godfraind, J. M., Kawamura, H., Krnjevic, K. and Pumain, R. (1971). Actions of dinitrophenol and some other metabolic inhibitors on cortical neurones. *J. Physiol. (Lond.)*, **215**, 199

209. Feltz, A., Krnjevic, K. and Lisiewicz, A. (1972). Intracellular free Ca^{2+} and membrane properties of motoneurones. *Nature New Biol.*, **237**, 179

210. Krnjevic, K. and Lisiewicz, A. (1972). Injections of calcium ions into spinal motoneurones. *J. Physiol. (Lond.)*, **225**, 363

211. Coombs, J. S., Eccles, J. C. and Fatt, P. (1955). The electrical properties of the motoneurone membrane. *J. Physiol. (Lond.)*, **130**, 291

212. Chiarandini, D. J. and Stefani, E. (1967). Two different ionic mechanisms generating the spike 'positive' after potential in molluscan neurons. *J. Gen. Physiol.*, **50**, 1183
213. Moreton, R. B. (1969). An investigation of the electrogenic sodium pump in snail neurones, using the constant-field theory. *J. Exptl. Biol.*, **51**, 181
214. Goldman, D. E. (1943). Potential, impedance and rectification in membranes. *J. Gen. Physiol.*, **27**, 37
215. Hodgkin, A. L. and Katz, B. (1949). The effect of sodium on the electrical activity of the giant axon of the squid. *J. Physiol. (Lond.)*, **108**, 37
216. Dalton, J. C. and Hendrix, D. E. (1962). Effects of temperature on membrane potentials of lobster giant axon. *Amer. J. Physiol.*, **202**, 491
217. Senft, J. P. (1967). Effects of some inhibitors on the temperature-dependent component of resting potential in lobster axon. *J. Gen. Physiol.*, **50**, 1835
218. Latorre, R. and Hidalgo, M. C. (1969). Effect of temperature on resting potential in giant axons of squid. *Nature (London)*, **221**, 962
219. Carpenter, D. O. (1973). Electrogenic sodium pump and high specific resistance in nerve cell bodies of the squid. *Science*, **179**, 1336
220. Gorman, A. L. F. and Marmor, M. F. (1970). Temperature dependence of the sodium–potassium permeability ratio of a molluscan neurone. *J. Physiol. (Lond.)*, **210**, 919
221. DiPolo, R. and Latorre, R. (1972). Effect of temperature on membrane potential and ionic fluxes in intact and dialysed barnacle muscle fibres. *J. Physiol. (Lond.)*, **225**, 255
222. Marmor, M. F. and Gorman, A. L. F. (1970). Membrane potential as the sum of ionic and metabolic components. *Science*, **167**, 65
223. Sokolove, P. G. and Cooke, I. M. (1971). Inhibition of impulse activity in a sensory neuron by an electrogenic pump. *J. Gen. Physiol.*, **57**, 125
224. Rapoport, S. I. (1970). The sodium–potassium exchange pump: relation of metabolism to electrical properties of the cell. I. Theory. *Biophys. J.*, **10**, 246
225. Geduldig, D. (1968). A ouabain-sensitive membrane conductance. *J. Physiol. (Lond.)*, **194**, 521
226. Brinley, F. J., Jr. and Mullins, L. J. (1970). The effect of membrane potential and internal potassium ions on sodium efflux from dialyzed squid axons. *Biophys. J.*, **10**, 9A
227. Brinley, F. J., Jr. and Mullins, L. J. (1971). The fluxes of sodium and potassium across the squid axon membrane under conditions of altered membrane potential. *Fed. Proc.* **30**, 255A
228. Kostyuk, P. G., Krishtal, O. A. and Pidoplichko, V. I. (1972). Electrogenic sodium pump and related conductance changes in the membrane of snail neurons. *Biofisika*, **17**, 1048
229. Libet, B. and Kobayashi, H. (1969). Generation of adrenergic and cholinergic potentials in sympathetic ganglion cells. *Science*, **164**, 1530
230. Kehoe, J. S. and Ascher, P. (1970). Re-evaluation of the synaptic activation of an electrogenic sodium pump. *Nature (London)*, **225**, 820
231. Kunze, D. L. and Brown, A. M. (1971). Internal potassium and chloride activities and the effects of acetylcholine on identifiable *Aplysia* neurones. *Nature (London)*, **229**, 229
232. Kehoe, J. (1972). Ionic mechanisms of a two-component cholinergic inhibition in *Aplysia* neurones. *J. Physiol. (Lond.)*, **225**, 85
233. Nakajima, S. and Onodera, K. (1969). Membrane properties of the stretch receptor neurones of crayfish with particular reference to mechanisms of sensory adaptation. *J. Physiol. (Lond.)*, **200**, 161
234. Ayrapetyan, S. N. (1969). On regulation mechanism of spontaneous activity of snail giant neurons. *Biofisika*, **14**, 866
235. Romey, G. and Arvanitaki-Chalazonitis, A. (1970). Contrôle par la pompe à cations des modes d'activité des neurones identifiables (*Aplysia*). *J. Physiol. (Paris)*, **62**, supp. 1, 210
236. Livengood, D. R., Pencek, T. L. and Kusano, K. (1971). Modulation of the burst discharge rate of the lobster cardiac ganglion by an electrogenic Na$^+$ pump. *Biol. Bull.*, **141**, 396
237. Lowry, O. H. and Passonneau, J. V. (1972). *A Flexible System of Enzymatic Analysis*. (New York and London: Academic Press)
238. Easton, D. E. (1971). Garfish olfactory nerve: easily accessible source of numerous large, homogeneous, nonmyelinated axons. *Science*, **172**, 952
239. Greengard, P. and Straub, R. W. (1959). Effect of frequency of electrical stimulation

on the concentration of intermediary metabolites in mammalian non–myelinated fibres. *J. Physiol. (Lond.)*, **148**, 353

240. Montant, P. and Chmouliovsky, M. (1968). Energy-rich metabolites in stimulated mammalian non–myelinated nerve fibres. *Experientia*, **24**, 782

241. Chmouliovsky, M., Schorderet, M. and Straub, R. W. (1969). Effect of electrical activity on the concentration of phosphorylated metabolites and inorganic phosphate in mammalian non–myelinated nerve fibres. *J. Physiol. (Lond.)*, **202**, 90P

242. Lowry, O. H., Passounneau, J. V., Hasselberger, F. X. and Schulz, D. W. (1964). Effect of ischemia on known substrates and cofactors of the glycolytic pathway in brain. *J. Biol. Chem.*, **239**, 18

243. Lowry, O. H. and Passonneau, J. V. (1964). The relationship between substrates and enzymes of glycolysis in brain. *J. Biol. Chem.*, **239**, 31

244. Rolleston, F. S. and Newsholme, E. A. (1967). Control of glycolysis in cerebral cortex slices. *Biochem. J.*, **104**, 524

245. Passonneau, J. V. and Lowry, O. H. (1962). Phosphofructokinase and the Pasteur effect. *Biochem. Biophys. Res. Commun.*, **7**, 10

246. Lowry, O. H. and Passonneau, J. V. (1966). Kinetic evidence for multiple binding sites on phosphofructokinase. *J. Biol. Chem.*, **241**, 2268

247. Krzanowski, J. and Matchinsky, F. M. (1969). Regulation of phosphofructokinase by phosphocreatine and phosphorylated glycolytic intermediates. *Biochem. Biophys. Res. Commun.*, **34**, 816

248. Kemp, R. G. (1971). Rabbit liver phosphofructokinase. Comparison of some properties with those of muscle phosphofructokinase. *J. Biol. Chem.*, **246**, 245

249. Williamson, J. R. (1966). Glycolytic control mechanisms. II. Kinetics of intermediate changes during the aerobic–anoxic transition in perfused rat heart. *J. Biol. Chem.*, **241**, 5026

250. Danforth, W. H. and Helmreich, D. (1964). Regulation of glycolysis in muscle. I. The conversion of phosphorylase *b* to phosphorylase *a* in frog sartorius muscle. *J. Biol. Chem.*, **239**, 3133

251. Karpatkin, S., Helmreich, E. and Cori, C. F. (1964). Regulation of glycolysis in muscle. II Effect of stimulation and epinephrine in isolated frog sartorius muscle. *J. Biol. Chem.*, **239**, 3139

252. Krebs, E. G., Groves, D. J. and Fisher, E. H. (1959). Factors affecting the activity of muscle phosphorylase *b* kinase. *J. Biol. Chem.*, **234**, 2867

253. Meyer, W. L., Fischer, E. H. and Krebs, E. G. (1964). Activation of skeletal muscle phosphorylase *b* kinase by Ca^{2+}. *Biochemistry*, **3**, 1033

254. Ozawa, E., Hosoi, K. and Ebashi, S. (1967). Reversible stimulation of muscle phosphorylase *b* kinase by low concentrations of calcium ions. *J. Biochem. (Japan)*, **61**, 531

255. Sacktor, B. and Wormser-Shavit, E. (1966). Regulation of metabolism in working muscle *in vivo*. I. Concentrations of some glycolytic, tricarboxylic acid cycle, and amino acid intermediates in insect flight muscle during flight. *J. Biol. Chem.*, **241**, 624

256. Sacktor, B. and Hurlbut, E. C. (1966). Regulation of metabolism in working muscle *in vivo*. II. Concentrations of adenine nucleotides, arginine phosphate, and inorganic phosphate in insect flight muscle during flight. *J. Biol. Chem.*, **241**, 632

257. Williamson, J. R., Cheung, W. Y., Coles, H. S. and Herczeg, B. E. (1967). Glycolytic control mechanisms. IV. Kinetics of glycolytic intermediate changes during electrical discharge and recovery in the main organ of *Electrophorus electricus*. *J. Biol. Chem.*, **242**, 5112

258. Williamson, J. R., Herczeg, B. E., Coles, H. S. and Cheung, W. Y. (1967). Glycolytic control mechanisms. V. Kinetics of high energy phosphate intermediate changes during electrical discharge and recovery in the main organ of *Electrophorus electricus*. *J. Biol. Chem.*, **242**, 5119

259. Chance, B. and Jöbsis, F. (1959). Changes in fluorescence in a frog sartorius muscle following a twitch. *Nature (London)*, **184**, 195

260. Jöbsis, F. J. and Duffield, J. C. (1967). Oxidative and glycolytic recovery metabolism in muscle. Fluorometric observations on their relative contributions. *J. Gen. Physiol.*, **50**, 1009

261. Godfraind-De Becker, A. (1972). Heat production and fluorescence changes of toad sartorius muscle during aerobic recovery after a short tetanus. *J. Physiol. (Lond.)*, **223**, 719

262. Aubert, X., Chance, B. and Keynes, R. D. (1964). Optical studies of biochemical events in the electric organ of *Electrophorus*. *Proc. Roy. Soc. (Lond.)*, *B*, **160**, 211

263. Doane, M. G. (1967). Fluorometric measurement of pyridine nucleotide reduction in the giant axon of the squid. *J. Gen. Physiol.*, **50**, 2603

264. Rodriguez-Estrada, C. (1967). Fluorometric determination of $NADH_2$ levels in dorsal root ganglion following peripheral nerve stimulation. *Brain. Res.*, **6**, 217

265. Landowne, D. and Ritchie, J. M. (1971). Optical studies on the kinetics of the sodium pump in mammalian non–myelinated nerve fibres. *J. Physiol. (Lond.)*, **212**, 483

266. Landowne, D. and Ritchie, J. M. (1971). On the control of glycogenolysis in mammalian nervous tissue by calcium. *J. Physiol. (Lond.)*, **212**, 503

267. Chance, B. and Williams, G. R. (1955). Respiratory enzymes in oxidative phosphorylation. I. Kinetics of oxygen utilization. *J. Biol. Chem.*, **217**, 383

268. Armett, C. T. and Ritchie, J. M. (1963). On the permeability of mammalian non–myelinated fibres to sodium and to lithium ions. *J. Physiol. (Lond.)*, **165**, 130

269. Stinnakre, J. and Tauc, L. (1973). Calcium influx in active *Aplysia* neurones detected by injected aequorin. *Nature New Biol.*, **242**, 113

270. Okada, Y. and McDougal, D. B., Jr. (1971). Physiological and biochemical changes in frog sciatic nerve during anoxia and recovery. *J. Neurochem.*, **18**, 2335

271. Heilmeyer, L. M. G., Jr., Meyer, F., Haschke, R. H. and Fischer, E. H. (1970). Control of phosphorylase activity in a muscle glycogen particle. II. Activation by calcium. *J. Biol. Chem.*, **245**, 6649

272. Brostrom, C. O., Hunkeler, F. L. and Krebs, E. G. (1971). The regulation of skeletal muscle phosphorylase kinase by Ca^{2+}. *J. Biol. Chem.*, **264**, 1961

273. Ozawa, E. (1972). Activation of muscular phosphorylase *b* kinase by a minute amount of Ca ion. *J. Biochem.*, **71**, 321

274. Baker, P. F. and Crawford, A. C. (1972). Mobility and transport of magnesium in squid giant axons. *J. Physiol. (Lond.)*, **227**, 855

275. Caldwell, P. C. (1958). Studies on the internal pH of large muscle and nerve fibres. *J. Physiol. (Lond.)*, **142**, 22

276. Renter, H. (1973). Divalent cations as charge carriers in excitable membranes. *Prog. Biophys. Mol. Biol.*, **26**, 1

277. Bastein, M. P. (1974). The interrelationship between sodium and calcium fluxes across cell membranes. *Ergebn. Physiol.*, **70**, (in press)

278. Fischbarg, J. (1972). Ionic permeability changes as the basis of the thermal dependence of the resting potential in barnacle muscle fibres. *J. Physiol. (Lond.)*, **224**, 149

7
The Physiology of Skeletal Muscle

A. J. BULLER
University of Bristol

7.1	INTRODUCTION	279
7.2	THE MOLECULAR LEVEL	281
7.3	THE MOTOR UNIT	287
7.4	FAST-TWITCH AND SLOW-TWITCH MUSCLES	289
7.5	NEURAL CONTROL OF MUSCLE SPEED	295
7.6	THE MOTOR DISCHARGE PATTERN	297
7.7	THE WHOLE ANIMAL	299
7.8	SUMMARY	300

7.1 INTRODUCTION

It is likely that man has been interested in skeletal muscle since his first realisation that it was these structures which determined both his power and his speed of movement. However, for many hundreds of years the techniques necessary to examine the contractile mechanism in any detail were unavailable to him, and little more than philosophical speculation was possible. A brief, but fascinating account of this period is contained in the first chapters of Dr Dorothy Needham's recent authoritative book, 'Machina Carnis'[94].

While important experimental observations were made during the nineteenth century, the great acceleration in the acquisition of knowledge concerning the contraction process began at the turn of this century when two

279

men, W. M. Fletcher and A. V. Hill, entered the list. It is interesting to
recall that while by today's reckoning the former would be considered a
'biochemist' and the latter a 'physiologist', during the early years of this
century both were to be found working in the Physiological Laboratories
at Cambridge, and both published their results in the *Journal of Physiology*.
To be sure, W. M. Fletcher might have been thought of by his contemporaries
as a physiological chemist, but the dichotomy which was to occur between
biochemistry and physiology had not yet occurred. A succinct statement
of the spirit of the Cambridge Laboratory at this time is to be found in the
Introduction to Sections A and B of A. V. Hill's biographical text 'Trails and
Trials in Physiology'[1]. Fletcher was the older man (he was Hill's tutor when
the latter was an undergraduate at Cambridge) and his work—later in
collaboration with Gowland Hopkins—initiated the unravelling of the
respiratory process in muscle, a problem that occupied muscle biochemists
for many years. Hill's more 'biophysical' investigation of the heat production
of skeletal muscle began in 1910 as a direct result of Fletcher and Hopkins'
work, and its understanding, together with its accompanying mechanical
correlates, was to occupy muscle physiology for many years.

It was perhaps inevitable that, in spite of the simultaneous blossoming
some 65 years ago of a better understanding of both the chemistry and physics
of muscle contraction, the studies of muscle biochemistry and muscle
physiology should drift apart. There were many reasons for the emergence
of biochemistry as a separate scientific discipline, but the establishment of
separate departments of biochemistry inevitably led to some loss of contact
between biochemists and physiologists. Those who had known unity in
earlier days occasionally attempted a reunification (e.g. A. V. Hill's article
'A challenge to biochemists'[2]) but the time was not truly ripe. There was much
to be done by biochemists in seeking the immediate source of energy for contraction, physiologists had much to learn about the mechanical behaviour of
skeletal muscle, and so the two groups were not interdependent. The emergence of the sliding filament hypothesis, now some 20 years old, has concentrated effort at the molecular level and has resulted in biochemists and
biophysicists once more collaborating in an attempt to understand the conformational changes in the contractile proteins which probably represent the
ultimate contractile process. It is perhaps a reflection on scientific methods
that many of those working in this area would no longer consider themselves
either biochemists or physiologists, but rather cellular biologists.

The recent rapid progress in the understanding of events at the cellular
level has completely overshadowed slower progress in the unravelling of the
problems of muscle organisation at the multicellular level, but such progress
is essential if there is to be a full understanding of the coordinated usage of
skeletal muscles in an intact animal.

As an illustration of the biological importance of the multicellular concept
it is worth recalling the elementary fact that in the mammal individual
muscle fibres are organised into motor units. A motor unit consists of a motor
neurone and the group of skeletal muscle fibres which it innervates. The
functional importance of the motor unit is that it behaves in an all-or-none
manner, and therefore represents the minimal unit of either willed or reflex
activity which can occur in the normal animal. The single muscle fibre, far

less the sarcomere, is not a 'functional' unit in terms of the organisation of movement in the intact animal, and even if a full understanding of the events at the molecular level is achieved this, of itself, will give no insight into the manner in which an animal coordinates its muscular efforts.

Alongside the studies of motor unit characteristics has come a better understanding of the total influence the motor neurone brings to bear on the muscle fibres it innervates. The hypothesis of a 'trophic' influence which nerve exerts on muscle (supposedly independent of the passage of motor nerve impulses) has made numerous appearances in the literature over the last hundred years or so. A review of this topic is to be found in 'The Denervated Muscle' edited by Ernst Gutmann[3]. While the final answers to some of the problems in this field remain to be discovered, interest has been re-awakened in the modifications which different innervations can induce in skeletal muscle. Indeed, as a result of work in this field there are now those who believe that some diseases formerly thought to be purely muscular in origin may in fact have a neurogenic basis (see for example 'Disorders of Muscle' edited by John Walton[4]).

At a still higher level of organisation there is a field of study which aims at understanding the integrated and coordinated use of the skeletal musculature of the intact animal. The techniques used are very different from those of either the cellular biologist or the motor unit physiologist. Basically measurements are made of the forces developed and accelerations and velocities attained by various parts of the unrestrained animal. From this information and a knowledge of the sites of origin and insertion of the muscles some understanding of the physiological usage of the skeletal musculature may be obtained. An introduction to this type of work is contained in a small book entitled 'How Man Moves' by Sven Carlsöö[5].

It will be apparent from this introduction that the range of investigations being undertaken in order to obtain a better understanding of the mechanism of skeletal muscle activity is large. Inevitably at any one time one field of endeavour is pre-eminent and others lag in popularity, but knowledge obtained in one area reflects on the others, even though the techniques used to obtain it may vary widely. Too often differences of technique have led to misunderstanding and this is unfortunate, but scientists are as capable of bigotry as any other section of the community.

It is the aim of this review to survey briefly the current concepts of the events occurring at the molecular level during contraction of skeletal muscle then to discuss the organisation of mammalian muscles and the influences brought to bear on them by the motor innervation and finally to note some of the factors affecting the integration of muscle activity in the intact animal. Throughout consideration will be confined to skeletal twitch muscle and the qualitatively different slow tonic muscle (cf. Kuffler and Vaughan Williams[6]) will not be discussed.

7.2 THE MOLECULAR LEVEL

There is an adage, attributed to A. V. Hill, which exhorts the investigator who has selected his problem, to seek the biological preparation which is best suited for the work to be undertaken. This second task is certainly no less demanding than the first. For many years the frog sartorius muscle was the preparation of choice for the muscle physiologist, and it was this preparation which yielded the early important results on heat production. The muscle is thin, and its parallel fibres run from end to end. Both the metabolism and the speed of the muscle's mechanical responses can be greatly reduced by working at 0 °C. It was also from work on this preparation that Hill[7] devised the analogue of muscle illustrated in Figure 7.2.

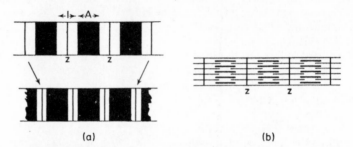

(a)   (b)

Figure 7.1 Diagrammatic representation of the two types of observation which led to the sliding filament hypothesis:
(a) The change in striation spacing observed on stimulation of single muscle fibres.
A = A band = thick (myosin) filaments
I = I band = thin (actin) filaments
Z = Z line (distance between 2 adjacent Z lines is one sarcomere).
The lower diagram shows a moderately contracted fibre. Note the constant width of the A band, but decreased width of each sarcomere.
(b) Diagram of the E.M. appearance of a myofibril. Note the thicker myosin filaments, and the actin filaments extending in either direction from each Z line

It must be recalled that during this period, which lasted from 1910 to 1948, little was known (in a modern sense) of the ultrastructure of the individual muscle fibres. The banded appearance of the fibres was thought to be due to an orderly array of fibrils[8] but the changes which occurred in the banding during contraction were still in dispute. It was in the period 1948–1955 that the observations were made which led to the general acceptance of what is now called the sliding filament hypothesis. The observations were of two kinds. On the one side the ultrastructural details of skeletal muscle were unravelled using ultrathin sectioning and the electron microscope, these observations being made, of necessity, on fixed and therefore dead material (Figure 7.1). In this work H. E. Huxley[9, 10] played a dominant role. On the other side observations were made on relaxed and contracting single living vertebrate muscle fibres[11, 12] and on myofibrils which could be activated by irrigation with adenosinetriphosphate (ATP) solutions[13]. Both these latter sets of experiments showed characteristic reversible changes in the striation spacing during activity. Taken together these two lines of research strongly suggested that the fundamental mechanism in the contractile response was some interaction between the actin and myosin (the filaments identified by the electron microscope) which resulted in a sliding of the actin over the myosin (the change in striation spacing observed during contraction) (Figure 7.1). From the first propounding of this theory to the present time much thought and experimental ingenuity has been lavished on confirming the validity of the hypothesis and exploring the sequence of events which leads to the interaction between the two major myofibrillar proteins. By 1954 the mechanism by which an impulse in the motor nerve fibre led, via the endplate potential, to the propagation of a muscle fibre action potential was well documented[14]. Subsequent work in this field has been delightfully and succinctly described by Bernard Katz in his small book 'Nerve, muscle and synapse'[95]. However, the problem remained as to how the surface electrical wave initiated the mechanical events, the process now known as electromechanical coupling. A. V. Hill[15, 16] had pointed

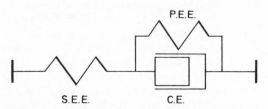

Figure 7.2 Diagrammatic analogue model of muscle.
C.E. = the contractile element, the tension generating actin and myosin.
P.E.E. = parallel elastic element, the connective tissue surrounding each contractile element.
S.E.E. = series elastic element. Note that some of the series element resides in connective tissue and tendon, but some probably exists in the contractile element (see text)

out some years earlier that the rapidity with which the contractile mechanism was switched on precluded the possibility that activity depended on the inward diffusion of some ion from the surface membrane which followed a permeability change accompanying the action potential. Similarly Sten-Knudsen[17] had demonstrated that the current flow resulting from the action potential could not directly act as an adequate stimulus to those myofibrils away from the surface membrane.

Again, as in the work leading to the sliding filament hypothesis, there was a happy concordance of new anatomical and physiological observations. The now classical observations of Porter and Palade[18] described the appearance of the sarcoplasmic reticulum as seen with the electron microscope. A brief review of this and later work has been published by Porter and Clara Franzini-Armstrong[19]. At the same time as Porter and Palade's high resolution electron microscopy was proceeding in America, A. F. Huxley and Taylor[20, 21] and later A. F. Huxley and Straub[22] were exploring the electrical sensitivity of the surface membrane of single muscle fibres between adjacent Z lines. It was originally in A. F. Huxley's mind that the Z line might be the region of inward propagation of an electrical signal which initiated the mechanical events. Indeed, from the work on frog fibres in which A. F. Huxley and Taylor[20] found that contraction could only be obtained following the application of an electrical pulse at the region of the Z line it appeared that this hypothesis was correct. However, subsequent work with crab and lizard fibres[21, 22] revealed that it was the level at which the transverse tubules opened on to the surface of the muscle fibre which was important, irrespective of where these openings occurred in relation to the striation pattern. In the frog the T tubules open to the surface at the level of the Z lines, while in the crab and lizard the openings are approximately at the level of the A/I junction. The E.M. confirmation that the transverse tubule/sarcoplasmic reticulum junctions also occurred at these levels made it very likely that the tubule system was concerned with the inward transmission of the electrical signal.

For some time it appeared probable that the surface action potential led to an inward propagation that was passive, that is, the spread of the electrical signal down the transverse tubule occurred with an intensity that decreased with distance. It seemed that the diameter of the tubules was too small, and the internal resistance therefore too high, to allow of an active process. Indeed it was suggested that skeletal muscle fibres retained the diameter they possessed because their radius corresponded to the maximal distance of passive, but liminal, electrotonic spread. More recent work[23] indicates that sodium channels probably exist in lesser concentration along the walls of the transverse tubules than they do on the surface membrane of the muscle fibres. If this is correct, inward electrical spread will be active along the length of the tubules, and some factor other than the electrical signal must be responsible for maintaining fibre diameter.

Once the mechanism of inward propagation had been established attention was concentrated on the next step of the electromechanical coupling.

From the early experiments of Mines[24] it had appeared likely that calcium ions played some part in the contraction process independent of any function they might serve at the surface membrane. Support for this view grew, and in 1962 Ebashi and Lipmann[25] isolated from muscle homogenates vesicles which possessed the ability to accumulate free calcium ions from their environment. It is demonstrated that ATP was the energy source for the sequestration. Subsequently it was shown by other authors that the vesicles were fragments of disrupted sarcoplasmic reticulum, and later still Winegrad[26] demonstrated outward movement of calcium from within the sarcoplasmic reticulum during muscle contraction.

The use of aequorin (a photoprotein which can be extracted from the luminous jellyfish *Aequorea Forskalea*), as a calcium indicator has recently allowed a very much more detailed examination of the calcium transient that accompanies the contraction process. Again A. V. Hill's advice to find a suitable biological preparation was heeded, and the very large diameter fibres which may be found in the barnacle (*Balanus nubilus*, Darwin) were used. By injecting aequorin into a single muscle fibre it was demonstrated by Ashley and Ridgeway[27] that during rest a very low calcium concentration exists in the environment of the actin and myosin filaments, but that following electrical excitation of the fibre the calcium concentration rises rapidly and this change is accompanied by muscle contraction. The shape of the calcium transient suggests that this ion controls the rate of tension development. The full dynamics of the calcium movement out of, and back into, the sarcoplasmic reticulum remain to be elucidated, but there now seems little doubt that the electrical invasion of the transverse tubules is the trigger event for the calcium release. At the present time it is not clear whether the coupling between the transverse tubule and the sarcoplasmic reticulum is electrical, via a junctional communication, or whether the electrical invasion of the transverse tubule permits a small entry of calcium into the muscle fibre which then acts regeneratively on the sarcoplasmic reticulum leading to the 'calcium transient'.

The site of action of the released calcium varies from species to species. It was originally thought that it was always bound by the actin filaments, but in some species it has been shown by A. G. Szent-Györgyi to be bound to the myosin. Such muscles are called 'myosin-controlled' but they will not be further discussed in this review.

In the common 'actin-controlled' muscles it now seems likely that the calcium ions which are released from the sarcoplasmic reticulum become bound to the troponin which is associated with the protein tropomyosin. Tropomyosin lies in the groove of the actin helix. The calcium-troponin complex induces a conformational change which allows the actin filament to interact with myosin. So long as the troponin sites (probably two per molecule) are occupied by calcium ions, interaction between actin and myosin can continue, but once the re-accumulation of calcium by the S.R. removes calcium, actin/myosin interaction ceases and relaxation occurs.

This brings us finally to the nature of the interaction of the actin and myosin filaments. From the time of the first ultrathin, high-resolution electron-micrographs of skeletal muscle the lateral protuberances from the myosin filaments attracted attention. It now seems certain that it is these projections which 'bridge' the gap between actin and myosin and attach to the actin during muscular contraction.

The inference that it was the formation of bridges between the actin and myosin which accounted for tension development during isometric contraction required that tension development should be proportional to the extent of overlap between the actin and myosin filaments, since only where overlap existed could bridge formation occur. That shortening did not occur in sarcomeres which had been stretched to an extent such that there was no actin/myosin overlap had been demonstrated by Huxley and Peachey[28], but the definitive experiments correlating sarcomere length with isometric tension development were published by Gordon et al. in 1966[29]. These precise and technically delightful experiments demonstrated a truly remarkable correlation between filament overlap and tension development which greatly supported the bridge hypothesis.

Attention was next concentrated on the form of the myosin filaments. H. E. Huxley demonstrated the manner in which myosin molecules aggregated to form myofilaments, and how it came about that the lateral projections were orientated in opposite directions at the two ends of each filament. Subsequent biochemical examination by Lowey et al.[30], confirmed the earlier work of Szent-Györgyi and showed that myosin could be split into light and heavy meromyosin fractions, the latter being capable of further subdivision into a S1 globular part and an S2 linear part. The S1 unit corresponds to the terminal head of a myosin bridge, the S2 to the body of the bridge and the light meromyosin to the backbone structure which, having undergone aggregation with other light meromyosin units, forms the body of myosin filament. That the bridges move during muscle contraction has been demonstrated by x-ray diffraction measurements[31] but it remains unknown exactly how the bridges operate to develop tension or produce sliding. At this point it is pertinent to mention one of the many models of muscle contraction that have been published during the past 20 years.

In 1957, A. F. Huxley in a paper entitled 'Muscle Structure and Theories of Contraction' proposed a mechanism of interaction between actin and myosin which, in principle, has dominated thinking in this field to the present day[32]. If the dates of many of the references to original work quoted above are noted and compared with the date of the A. F. Huxley model, his achievement may be seen to be remarkable. In his model A. F. Huxley proposed that the lateral projections of the myosin filaments were continuously in motion relative to the main body of the myofilament due to thermal agitation. When a projection contacted an active site on an adjacent actin filament, combination occurred. It was suggested that the rate constants for the formation and breaking of bridges depended on the distance of the myosin head from its equilibrium position. Using this model and making certain assumptions concerning the rate constants Huxley was able to explain many of the observed characteristics of muscle and to predict certain others. Although it has undergone several detailed modifications since 1957 the A. F. Huxley model continues to serve a most important role as a modeller's norm, and so far it has been able to 'accommodate' most of the more recently acquired knowledge.

One elaboration of the original hypothesis which is now generally accepted is that the movement imparted to the actin is not due to a linear movement of a fixed lateral (myosin) projection but to a rotation of the globular head of the myosin after it has become attached to the actin[96]. Recently A. F. Huxley and Simmons[33] have suggested that this 'rotation' takes place in a series of discrete steps (probably two) which produce either translatory motion in the actin if the latter is free to move, or tension in the elastic S2 meromyosin unit if relative movement of the actin and myosin is not possible (isometric contraction). This hypothesis is supported by data obtained from rapid length changes imposed on single muscle fibres.

So far nothing has been said of the energy sources for these mechanical events. It is known that the myosin ATPase resides in the headpiece. It is further appreciated that the ATPase activity of the myosin can vary from muscle to muscle and from species to species (see below) and it is assumed that these differences are due to sequence and conformational differences in the protein. The splitting of ATP which is the immediate source of energy for the contractile process occurs after the attachment of myosin to actin and probably only after the second step of a two-stage process[34]. The breaking of the bridge which accompanies ATP splitting renders that bridge free to re-engage at a new actin site providing that the appropriate troponin is still binding calcium.

So concludes the brief survey of the development of our present knowledge concerning the molecular structures and events which underly the contractile process in skeletal muscle. No attempt has been made to compile an exhaustive bibliography, but rather have some key observations been highlighted.

While many points of detail remain to be elucidated a broad picture has emerged of the events which lead to tension development or shortening in each sarcomere following the arrival of the action potential at its surface membrane. When sarcomeres are placed in series (as in a muscle fibre), and muscle fibres are placed in parallel (as in a muscle) it is pertinent to remember that the muscle's maximum velocity of isotonic shortening will be determined by the number of sarcomeres in series, while the muscle's maximum isometric tension development will be determined by the number of sarcomeres in parallel. Such considerations are the essence of the succeeding section.

7.3 THE MOTOR-UNIT

The fundamental observations described in the previous section, with the sole exception of the end-plate potential, were made using direct stimulation of the muscle. The method of application of the stimuli varied from multi-electrode assemblies for the simultaneous 'all over' activation of the frog sartorious muscle to saline filled microelectrodes for the stimulation of single muscle fibres. The use of indirect stimulation—that is, the stimulation of the motor nerve rather than the muscle—introduces the complication that each nerve fibre typically innervates a group of muscle fibres. The number of fibres innervated by a single motor neurone can vary widely (in the cat motor units containing between four and several hundred muscle fibres have been described) but there is no clear understanding as to why such variability exists. It is apparent that the larger the inertial mass of the part to be moved the greater must be the number of active muscle fibres in parallel to produce a given movement, but whether other factors also play a part in determining motor unit size is unknown. The distribution of the fibres within the parent muscle can also vary. It is also of interest to note that while the vast majority of the observations described in the previous section were made on preparations obtained from lower vertebrates or crustacae, those on motor units now to be described were almost uniformly obtained from mammals, in particular cats and rats.

It has been known for many years[35] that denervated mammalian skeletal muscle exhibits an increased sensitivity to its neuromuscular chemical transmitter acetylcholine (A.Ch.). Subsequently it was shown by Ginetzinsky and Shamarina[36] and, in greater detail, by Axelsson and Thesleff[37] that following chronic denervation there is a great increase in the length of each muscle fibre which is sensitive to low concentrations of acetylcholine. In normally innervated muscle fibres the sensitive region is strictly limited to the area of the end plate but 10 days after denervation the entire fibre may exhibit sensitivity. If the motor nerve is permitted to grow back into the muscle, the A.Ch. sensitive area of the reinnervated fibres again shrinks.

In 1962 Diamond and Miledi[38] extended the work of Ginetzinsky and Shamarina[36] on the acetylcholine sensitivity of immediately postnatal mammalian muscle fibres. Whereas the Russian authors had used newborn rabbits Diamond and Miledi used late foetal and early postnatal rats. Both sets of results indicated that before innervation—that is when the developing fibres were at the myotube stage—the fibres were sensitive to acetylcholine along their entire length, but with the arrival of the terminals of the motor nerve axons and the formation of early neuromuscular junctions the A.Ch. sensitivity regressed, ultimately reducing to the adult pattern a few weeks after birth. A somewhat fuller review of this topic has been published elsewhere[39]

It would therefore appear that the 'sculpturing' of motor units, both as regards the number of muscle fibres in each unit and their spatial distribution within the parent muscle is determined at about the time of birth. The problem has recently been studied by Bagust et al.[40], who have demonstrated that poly-neuronal innervation is common in kitten hind-limb muscles within the first 3 days of birth, is less common by 2 weeks of age and is effectively absent by 6 weeks. That polyneuronal innervation is extremely uncommon in adult cat hind-limb muscles had previously been shown by Brown and Matthews[41], Once the excess innervation (which presumably occurs because of the chance multiple innervation of the acetylcholine sensitive myotube) has been shed each individual motoneurone is left innervating a group of muscle fibres. This constitutes the motor unit. Why the muscle fibres shed all but one of their innervations is not known, but it was observed many years ago[42] that once a mammalian motoneurone effectively innervates a muscle fibre it inhibits the formation of additional neuromuscular junctions. This is certainly true in limb muscles, but such behaviour must be carefully distinguished from the *replacement* of neuromuscular junctions suggested by Barker and Ip[43]. It must also be noted that it is artificially possible to induce multiple innervation of mammalian muscle fibres after blocking the motor nerve with local anaes-thetic[44], but this is an abnormal and possibly transient situation.

The subsequent elongation of the individual muscle fibres which accom-panies the growth of the animal is accomplished by the addition of sarco-meres[45,46] and it is interesting to note that mammalian skeletal muscle fibres appear to retain the ability to increase or decrease the number of sarcomeres according to circumstances throughout life[47].

At the time of their first innervation all the limb muscle fibres of any particular mammal are similar in their contractile behaviour. It has been pointed out above that the muscle fibres are organised into motor units about the time of birth, each muscle fibre typically being innervated by only a single motoneurone. Following innervation each motor unit develops a speed of contraction which is determined by its motor innervation, the time taken to reach maturity being about 8 weeks in the rat and cat[48,49].

As a first approximation (but see below) it may be stated that the adult animal of each mammalian species possess a mixture of two types of motor units in their limb musculature. These are known as fast-twitch units and slow-twitch units. It must be stressed that motor units with differing contrac-tion times may occur at other sites in the body, for example the very rapidly contracting motor units of the extrinsic eye muscles[50], but consideration will here be limited to the types found in the limb musculature. In all the species so far studied the slow-twitch motor units have a contraction time that is some three to four times longer than the fast-twitch units, although the absolute values vary widely from species to species (see Figure 7.5). There have been several important studies of motor unit characteristics in recent years[51-54] but possibly two of the more recent, that by Close[55] concerned with the rat, and that by Bagust, Knott, Lewis, Luck and Westerman[56] concerned with the cat, are of special interest. Both of these papers suggested that, as judged by speed of mechanical response, there were probably three and not two types of motor unit in the hind-limb musculature. The third type, intermediate in speed between the well recognised fast-twitch and slow-twitch units, was found to be relatively infrequent, forming only some 5–10 % of the total number of the muscle's motor units. In both papers attempts were made to correlate the three types of unit (characterised by their contractile behaviour) with the histochemical results of other authors, but this topic will not be pursued in this article. The significance of the different units is not known, but Lewis and his colleagues suggested that the three types might (in each species) indicate three different forms of myosin[57]. As will be described later, there is evidence that the type of myosin contained within each muscle fibre is determined by its motor innervation.

While the number of studies of motor units is increasing—and rightly so since, as stressed above, they are the functional units of skeletal muscle activity—there have been many more studies of the contraction characteristics of whole muscles. Muscles are collections of motor units and each muscle takes origin from one site and is inserted into another. The number of motor units and the complexity of their arrangement and alignment within different muscles varies enormously, but the total response of each muscle to stimulation of its motor nerve is the summation of the component motor unit responses.

In many commonly used laboratory mammals such as the mouse, rat, guinea-pig, rabbit and cat, there is a marked tendency to segregate either slow-twitch or fast-twitch motor units into particular anatomical muscles, with the result that muscles are also referred to as slow-twitch and fast-twitch. It should be clear however, that few, if any, muscles are completely homogenous in the characteristics of their motor unit populations, but nearly all limb muscles show a marked predominance of either fast-twitch or slow-twitch units, thereby giving credence to the nomenclature fast-twitch and slow-twitch muscles. In the species listed above the slow-twitch muscles (containing a majority of slow-twitch units) usually appear redder in colour than the fast-twitch muscles. This is generally attributed to a greater concentration of myoglobin[58] and has resulted in the nomenclature red and white muscles. Such terms are entirely justifiable to describe colour, but should not be used interchangeably with the terms slow-twitch and fast-twitch since the correlation between colour and contraction speed is by no means perfect.

7.4 FAST-TWITCH AND SLOW-TWITCH MUSCLES

An anatomical muscle is a complex structure. The rapid progress in our understanding of the interaction between actin and myosin has tended to distract attention from the analogue of muscle proposed by Hill[7], so that we may easily fall into the trap of ignoring the inevitable presence of the series elastic element (Figure 7.2). The events occurring in the contractile machinery can in fact only lead to the development of tension or shortening via the compliant connective tissue and tendon which connects that machinery to the muscle's origin and insertion. When a relaxed muscle is stretched, the

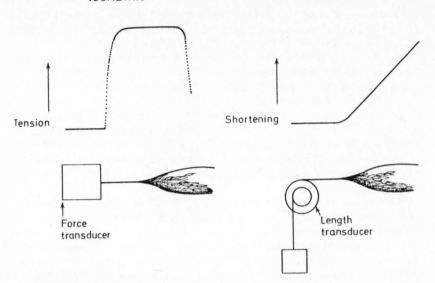

ISOMETRIC ISOTONIC

Tension

Shortening

Force
transducer

Length
transducer

Figure 7.3 Diagrammatic representation of left: isometric recording, right: isotonic recording. During isometric recording the muscle is not permitted to shorten (i.e. the force transducer has a very low compliance), the record shows tension development against time.

During isotonic recording the muscle is permitted to shorten and lift various loads, the record shows shortening against time. For afterloaded recording a stop would be needed on the length transducer (see text)

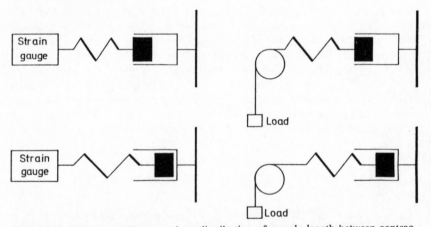

Strain
gauge

Strain
gauge

Load

Load

Figure 7.4 Diagram to illustrate the redistribution of muscle length between contractile element and series elastic element during isometric and isotonic recording.
Left: Isometric recording. Above, relaxed muscle; below, contracted. Note the stretching of the S.E.E. while the total muscle length remains unaltered.
Right: Isotonic recording. Above, muscle just before shortening commences, i.e. at the end of the isometric phase; below, after shortening and lifting load. Note that the S.E.E. is stretched to an extent determined by the load during the isometric phase, but undergoes no further extension during isotonic shortening

change in length is shared between the series elastic element and the connective tissue that is in parallel with the actin and myosin (the parallel elastic element). The (passive) tension that can be measured at the tendon during such stretching is borne by the connective tissue and not by the myofilaments. When the muscle contracts, the parallel elastic element is unloaded and the series elastic element is stretched by an amount which is dependent upon the force which the muscle develops. It is clear that during contraction not all of the series elasticity resides in the tendon, some is certainly located inside the sarcomeres, probably in the S2 segments of the attached myosin molecules[33], but unfortunately this does not mean that the component present in the tendon and other connective tissue can be ignored. Its presence produces small but inevitable differences in the time course of tension development between the muscle's origin and insertion and that which may be inferred to occur (but cannot be directly measured) between the actin and myosin.

Two methods are commonly used to record the contraction of skeletal muscle. They are illustrated diagrammatically in Figures 7.3 and 7.4.

In isometric recording the muscle is caused to contract while being held at constant length (in fact some change in length must occur to operate the force transducer, but this change may be made negligibly small) and the tension developed recorded. During isometric recording the total muscle length is constant, but there is some shortening of the contractile elements with a resultant stretching of the series elastic elements (see Figure 7.4).

In isotonic recording a length transducer is used to measure the extent and velocity of muscle shortening when moving different loads. In *afterloaded* isotonic contractions a stop is used to prevent the muscle from being stretched by heavy loads. Under these conditions the muscle first contracts isometrically until the force developed equals the value of the load (during this phase there will be some stretching of the series elastic element), and then shortens, thereby lifting the load (during this phase there will be no further lengthening of the series elastic element providing the load is kept constant, i.e. inertial effects are negligible). It is apparent that if the load is greater than the isometric tension the muscle can develop, it cannot be moved.

Figure 7.5 illustrates the maximal isometric twitch contractions of the comparable fast-twitch and slow-twitch muscles of a rat and a cat. The factors which are important in obtaining optimal responses have been discussed elsewhere[59], and an excellent general review has recently been published by Close[60]. In both species there is a clear differentiation between the contraction times (T.P. Figure 7.5) of the two muscles, there is also an obvious difference between the contraction times of the two fast-twitch and the two slow-twitch muscles. The significance of this latter observation will be discussed later.

If, instead of applying a single maximal stimulus to the motor nerve as is done to achieve a twitch response, repetitive stimuli are used, summation of the mechanical responses is obtained. If the rate of stimulation is sufficiently high the individual contraction processes cannot be identified and a fused isometric tetanic contraction is obtained, as in the upper recordings of Figure 7.6. It will be noted that the rate of tension development during tetanic stimulation is slower in slow-twitch muscle, and that a tension plateau is not reached. The ratio of the maximum twitch tension to the maximum tetanic

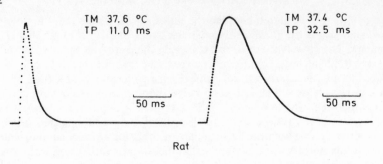

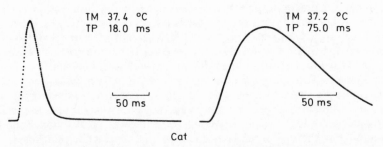

Rat

TM 37.6 °C
TP 11.0 ms
50 ms

TM 37.4 °C
TP 32.5 ms
50 ms

TM 37.4 °C
TP 18.0 ms
50 ms

TM 37.2 °C
TP 75.0 ms
50 ms

Cat

Figure 7.5 Maximal isometric twitch responses from left, the same anatomical fast-twitch muscle (flexor digitorum longus) and right, the same anatomical slow-twitch muscle (soleus) from above, the rat and below, the cat.
TM = Temperature in degrees centigrade.
TP = Time to peak (the time from the start of contraction until the time of peak tension) in milliseconds.
Time bar = 50 ms
   The dotted appearance of this and other records is due to the sampling rate of the digital computer used

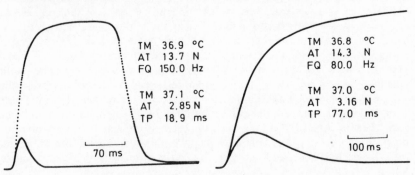

TM 36.9 °C
AT 13.7 N
FQ 150.0 Hz

TM 36.8 °C
AT 14.3 N
FQ 80.0 Hz

TM 37.1 °C
AT 2.85 N
TP 18.9 ms

TM 37.0 °C
AT 3.16 N
TP 77.0 ms

70 ms

100 ms

Figure 7.6 Superimposed maximal isometric twitch and tetanus (recorded at the same gain) from left, a typical cat fast-twitch muscle and right, a typical cat slow-twitch muscle.
TM = Temperature in degrees centigrade.
AT = Active tension (the maximum tension developed during the contraction process) in newtons.
FQ = the frequency of stimulation used to obtain the tetanic contraction in hertz.
TP = Time to peak of the twitch response in milliseconds.
Note the similar twitch : tetanus ratios

tension (the twitch: tetanus ratio) is typically between 0.2 and 0.25 for both types of muscle.

The reason why the tension developed during a tetanus is larger than that developed during a maximum twitch is not fully understood. It is common to suppose that full activation is not achieved during a single twitch, though what this means is also far from clear. It may be that in mammalian muscle at 37 °C insufficient calcium is liberated from the S.R. following a single muscle action potential to saturate the troponin sites. This would mean that less than the maximum number of bridges could form, which in turn would render it impossible for the muscle to produce its maximum (tetanic) tension. Repetitive stimulation, if sufficiently rapid, would lead to a greater concentration of calcium ions in the sarcoplasm and a saturation of all the troponin sites. Tetanic tension would therefore be developed.

In two recent studies Bagust[61] using slow-twitch muscles, and Bagust et al.[56] using fast-twitch muscles have shown that in each type of muscle the twitch:tetanus ratios of the individual motor units are significantly correlated with the contraction times of those units. Their interpretation of these observations is that the motor nerve determines, in some unspecified way, not only the type of myosin in each fibre (see above) but also the extent of the calcium transient. Further experiments are needed to test this intriguing hypothesis.

Figure 7.7 illustrates records of isotonic shortening from a fast-twitch and a slow-twitch muscle of the cat. It may be seen that the heavier the load (P) the lower the velocity of shortening (V). That the relationship between load and shortening velocity is curvilinear was first noted by Fenn and Marsh[62], and this fact has been amply confirmed since that time (see for example Wilkie[63]). The relationship may be adequately fitted by a number of different equations, each of which contains two (or more) arbitrary constants. Of these the best known is that due to Hill[3] which may be expressed as:

$$(P + a)(V + b) = (P_0 + a)b$$

where P = load, V = velocity of shortening, P_0 = maximum isometric tension and, a and b = constants

It must be stressed that no special significance should be attached to the Hill equation, it merely provides a convenient method of expressing and communicating force velocity data.

Different muscles from the same animal, and similar muscles from different animals have various values of isometric tetanic tension. Since a muscle's maximum tetanic tension corresponds to the value of load which the muscle just cannot lift, it is convenient to scale the load axis of a force velocity graph in fractions of the isometric tetanic tension, P_0 (see Figure 7.8). Until comparatively recently, it was customary to scale the velocity axis in muscle lengths per second. However, there was always the possibility of ambiguity over muscle length and fibre length (in many muscles the fibres do not stretch the whole length of the muscle[64]), and Close[48] has introduced the technique of scaling the velocity axis in micrometers per second per sarcomere (see Figure 7.8.). Obviously this method requires a knowledge of the mean number of sarcomeres per muscle fibre, but it allows unambiguous comparisons between different muscles.

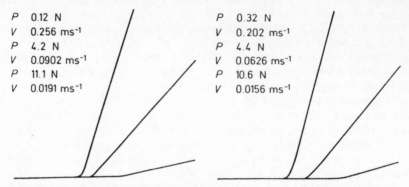

P	0.12 N		P	0.32 N	
V	0.256 ms⁻¹		V	0.202 ms⁻¹	
P	4.2 N		P	4.4 N	
V	0.0902 ms⁻¹		V	0.0626 ms⁻¹	
P	11.1 N		P	10.6 N	
V	0.0191 ms⁻¹		V	0.0156 ms⁻¹	

Figure 7.7 Three superimposed records of isotonic shortening against different loads from left, a typical cat fast-twitch muscle and right, a typical cat slow-twitch muscle. (The system gain is different for the two sets of records).

In each case the uppermost record shows the shortening against the lightest load (0.12 N left and 0.32 N right).

P = Load in newtons
V = Velocity of shortening in ms^{-1}

Note the increased latency before shortening with increasing load. This additional latency is the time taken for the development of isometric tension equal to the load

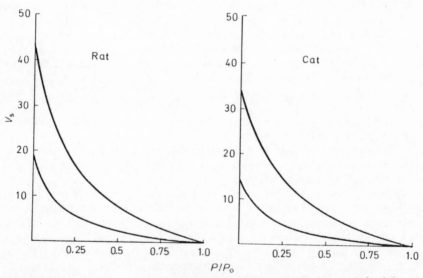

Figure 7.8 Force velocity curves plotted using Hills equation (see text) for left, rat muscles right, cat muscles. In each graph the upper curve represents the results from a fast-twitch muscle and the lower curve the results from a slow-twitch muscle.

Note the greater maximum shortening velocity of each type of rat muscle.

Note also the greater curvature of the force velocity relationship for each type of slow-twitch muscle

Figure 7.8 illustrates typical force velocity curves for a fast-twitch and a slow-twitch muscle from the rat (data from Close[48]) and the cat[65]. As might be expected from the results obtained with isometric recording, the maximum shortening velocity (the velocity at zero load) for each type of muscle is greater in the rat than the cat, and in both species the maximum shortening velocity of fast-twitch muscle is some two and a half times greater than that of slow-twitch muscle.

Further examination of Figure 7.8 will show an additional difference between force velocity curves of slow-twitch and fast-twitch muscles. The curvature (downward convexity) of the former is greater than it is for the latter. The extent of the curvature may be indicated by the ratio $a:P_0$. The value of this ratio is approximately 0.15 for both rat and cat slow-twitch muscles and approximately 0.3 for the two fast-twitch muscles. On theoretical grounds Woledge[66] has suggested that greater curvature, (i.e. a smaller value of $a:P_0$), indicates greater muscle efficiency. This expectation appears to be borne out by recent myothermic measurements on rat muscle[67, 68] which indicate that fast-twitch muscles sacrifice energetic economy for greater speed of shortening. A return to this fact will be made in the final section.

7.5 NEURAL CONTROL OF MUSCLE SPEED

While it has been known for many years that normal mammalian skeletal muscle remains at rest until the contractile mechanism is turned on by the arrival of one or more nerve impulses, it has only recently been appreciated that the motor innervation also exerts a marked influence on the speed of muscle contraction. This fact was brought to light by a chance—and totally unexpected—observation made by J. C. Eccles in 1958[69]. He had performed aseptic operations on one-day-old kittens in which he divided the motor nerves of two hind-limb skeletal muscles on each side and on one side reunited the cut nerve ends, so that self-reinnervation of the muscles occurred, and on the opposite side so sutured the nerves that cross-reinnervation occurred (see Figure 7.9). The primary object of the experiments was to observe whether, following reinnervation, the synaptic connections on to the motoneurones reinnervating the two muscles differed on the two sides. By good fortune Eccles chose to use one fast-twitch muscle and one slow-twitch muscle. At the first terminal experiment some 6 months after the aseptic operations had been performed it was found that there were only slight differences between the synaptic connections on the two sides, but the formerly fast-twitch muscle on the cross-reinnervated side was seen to contract very slowly when its motor nerve was stimulated, and the formerly slow-twitch muscle was noted to contract more rapidly. No such changes were seen in the speed of contraction of the self-reinnervated muscles. The isometric responses of self- and cross-reinnervated fast-twitch and slow-twitch muscles of the cat were therefore examined in some detail[70] and the original observation confirmed. At this time there was little idea as to which part of the contractile machinery had been altered by the changed motor innervation, or how the motor nerves exercised their influence. Since 1960 considerable progress has been achieved in understanding what part of the machinery may be altered by cross-reinnervation. The first important step was taken by Russell Close[71,72] who demonstrated that, in the rat, cross-reinnervation led to marked alterations in the force–velocity characteristics of the muscles, the curve for the cross-reinnervated slow-twitch muscle coming to resemble that of a normal fast-twitch muscle and vice versa. No such changes occurred following self-reinnervation. Close's observations in the rat have now been confirmed in the cat[73]. In 1967 Bárány[74] published a paper drawing attention to the correlation that appeared to exist between the maximum speed of muscle shortening and the ATPase activity of the myosin extracted from the muscle. This observation suggested that the alteration in the force–velocity curves following cross-reinnervation might be due to changes in the ATPase activity of the myosin. Joint work by Bárány and Close[75] showed that this

Reinnervation

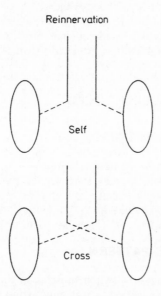

Self

Cross

Figure 7.9 Diagrammatic representation of the two types of reinnervation undertaken by J. C. Eccles (see text). At aseptic operation two motor nerves, one supplying a fast-twitch muscle and one supplying a slow-twitch muscle, were cut on both sides (indicated by the junction of the vertical and dotted lines). In self-reinnervation (upper diagram) the two ends of each cut nerve were then sewn together. In cross-reinnervation (lower diagram) the proximal end of one cut nerve was sewn to the distal end of the other cut nerve, and vice versa. Reinnervation was allowed to occur for 6–12 months before the animals were finally examined

was indeed the case for the rat. Comparable alterations in the myosin ATPase activity of cat muscle following cross-reinnervation was reported by Samaha, Guth and Albers[76], but these authors did not provide any data on force–velocity changes following reinnervation.

Although the changes in the force–velocity characteristics of cross-reinnervated muscle are well documented, and clearly seem to be the result of the production of a new myosin inside the cell, this change, by itself cannot fully explain the alterations which may be seen in the isometric myogram. It was stated above that for a given form of myosin the twitch: tetanus ratio depends upon the extent and time course of activation occurring during a single twitch. In order to explain the twitch:tetanus ratios observed in cross-reinnervation muscles it is necessary to invoke some alteration in activation. It has been suggested that activation is related to the calcium transient, and it had been demonstrated by Sreter and Gergely[77] that the calcium sequesting ability of S.R. isolated from normal fast-twitch and slow-twitch muscle was different. Mommaerts, Buller and Seraydarian[78] accordingly looked at the calcium uptake capacity of S.R. fragments isolated from cross-reinnervated cat muscles. As expected the characteristics had crossed, the S.R. obtained from cross-reinnervated slow-twitch muscle behaving more like normal or self-reinnervated fast-twitch muscle, and vice versa.

From the sum of this work it appears that at least two changes may be produced by cross-reinnervation of mammalian fast-twitch and slow-twitch skeletal muscle. The first is an alteration in the ATPase activity of the myosin, the second an alteration in the extent and time course of activation following a single stimulus. This latter is probably related to the release and reaccumulation of calcium ions by sarcoplasmic reticulum. Close[79] has suggested that the two changes are causally related. However, there does not appear to be a closely-linked relationship since changes in activation often occur on a different time scale from the changes in maximum shortening velocity, and, on occasions, it appears that cross-reinnervation may lead to changes in activation without concomitant changes in the force velocity characteristics[65].

Finally, with regard to cross-reinnervation, it does now seem that the nature and extent of the changes seen following altered innervation depend specifically on the motor nerve used. Reference has been made above to the situation in which no increase in the maximum shortening velocity of cat slow-twitch muscle was observed following apparently entirely satisfactory cross-reinnervation. Similar failure to obtain complete transition has been observed in the rat (A. R. Luff, personal communication). Why these differences occur is as yet unknown, perhaps it is related to the differential re-innervation rates of different motor axons[80], perhaps to the pattern of nerve impulses passing along the motor axons following reinnervation (see below). Further study of the motor unit populations of cross and self-reinnervated muscles is required to answer this question.

7.6 THE MOTOR DISCHARGE PATTERN

While the existence of fast-twitch and slow-twitch muscles in the limbs of mammals has been recognised for over 100 years, it is only within the last 20 years that the motoneurones innervating the two types of muscle have clearly been shown to be different[69, 81]. In particular there is evidence to show that the conduction velocity of the axons of motoneurones innervating slow-twitch muscle conduct more slowly than those of the motoneurones inner-vating fast-twitch muscle, and there is probably a strong correlation between axon conduction velocity and twitch time to peak at the motor unit level[56]. Also the motoneurones innervating slow-twitch muscle typically show a longer afterhyperpolarisation than do those motoneurones innervating fast-twitch muscles[82]. This latter fact probably accounts for the lower maximum impulse discharge rates exhibited by slow-twitch motoneurones.

That slow-twitch muscle had a lower threshold than fast-twitch in the static component of the stretch reflex had been demonstrated by Liddell and Sherrington[83] and Denny-Brown[84]. Granit elaborated their observations and showed that the motoneurones innervating slow-twitch muscle responded to a suitable stretch afferent input by a maintained (tonic) discharge, while the motoneurones innervating fast-twitch muscle typically responded to a similar input by a burst (phasic) discharge. He noted however that phasic motoneurones could be caused to produce a maintained discharge if the drive was sufficiently great.

In 1963 Gerta Vrbová[85] described the electromyogram (E.M.G.) patterns obtained from a fast-twitch and a slow-twitch muscle of the hind limb of normal unanaesthetised rabbits. As anticipated from the earlier work outlined above, the slow-twitch muscle produced a pattern indicating maintained low frequency activity of motor units whether the animal was standing, sitting or moving. The fast-twitch muscle showed bursts of activity corresponding with sudden movements, but no maintained activity. In the same paper Vrbová described a decrease in the E.M.G. activity of the slow-twitch muscle following tenotomy, and in a following paper[86] she suggested that the reduction in the isometric twitch-time observed in the tenotomized slow-twitch muscle was a direct result of the decreased frequency of discharge from the muscle's motoneurones. While it remains possible to criticise the details of some of Gerta Vrbová's experiments, there can be no doubt that these two papers provided the first serious suggestion that the pattern of nerve impulses was a powerful factor in determining the speed of contraction of mammalian skeletal muscle. Subsequently Salmons and Vrbová[87] used an implanted stimulator to provide long-term (up to 6 weeks) low frequency $(10 s^{-1})$ stimulation of fast-twitch muscle and reported slowing of the isometric twitch contraction time of the muscle at the terminal experiment. More recently, Sreter et al.[88], have reported that long-term stimulation of a fast-twitch muscle causes it to produce myosin typical of a slow-twitch muscle, that is, having a low ATPase activity. Al-Amood et al.[89], have shown that long-term stimulation of a fast-twitch muscle leads to a reduction in its maximum velocity of isotonic shortening and a decrease in the value of $a:P_0$, both changes being towards values typically found in slow-twitch muscle.

Putting this information together it is apparent that the pattern of motor nerve impulses reaching the muscle fibres of a motor unit determine the type of myosin produced by those fibres, with consequential effects on the speed of contraction of that motor unit. Whether the long-term pattern of impulses also influences the extent of activation of the fibres following a single stimulus is not yet known, though the twitch : tetanus ratios of the chronically stimulated muscles were typically larger than are found in normal slow-twitch muscles.

At the present time it is still impossible to say if all the changes which may be observed in mammalian muscles following cross-reinnervation are attributable to an altered pattern of activity in the reinnervated muscle fibres. Indeed, as yet, there is no direct evidence that the E.M.G. pattern of either a fast-twitch or a slow-twitch muscle does change following cross-reinnervation, but such information cannot be long delayed. Whether or not it is necessary to invoke a 'trophic' (i.e. non-impulse) mechanism remains to be seen[90].

In concluding this section the importance of the motor unit must again be stressed, since it is the all-or-none unit of striated muscle activity. It has been shown that motor units may vary widely in size and contractile performance, and that both of these characteristics are determined by the parent motoneurone. It would appear plausible to imagine that the development of all skeletal muscle proceeds along a uniform course until the arrival of the motor innervation. The larger diameter, and therefore faster growing, axons manage to gather a greater number of muscle fibres (thereby forming larger motor units). Subsequently the development of the contractile machinery depends upon the discharge characteristics of the motoneurones. If the motoneurone discharges only bursts of impulses the fibres it innervates manufacture one form of myosin and in due course develop into a mature fast-twitch motor unit. If the motoneurone (by virtue of its size and reflex connections) discharges regularly at low frequency the muscle fibres it innervates produce a different myosin and development proceeds towards a mature slow-twitch motor unit. Such a scheme is clearly an oversimplification. As pointed out above there exist, in each species, not two clearly distinct sets of motor units, but rather a wide spectrum having a number (possibly three?) of modal characteristics. It seems probable that only a limited number of different myosins may be produced in each species (? three) and that the type of myosin produced by the muscle fibres of a particular motor unit depends upon some characteristic of the motoneurone discharge. The spread in the characteristics of the motor units containing similar myosins must therefore depend upon the calcium transients which occur within the muscle fibres of these units. Again there seems little doubt that the behaviour of the sarcoplasmic reticulum is also determined by the motoneurone, but whether this influence is exercised by a 'fine control' of the discharge pattern, or by some independent (trophic?) neuronal process is not yet known.

7.7 THE WHOLE ANIMAL

The jump from the consideration of a single motor unit, or even a single anatomical muscle, to the consideration of the coordinated use of the total body musculature is a large one. The transition may be eased by asking a number of questions. First, why, in so many mammals, are there fast-twitch and slow-twitch skeletal muscles? A clue to the apparent answer has already been stated above. During the early years of this century Sherrington, assisted by other able physiologists at Oxford, clearly demonstrated that there existed in the mammal tonic reflexes concerned with the maintenance of a fixed posture against gravity, phasic reflexes, concerned with protective responses to nocuous stimuli, and (by inference) willed movements. It was also shown that slow-twitch muscle was primarily concerned with the maintenance of a fixed posture, and the fast-twitch muscles were used to bring about changes in this posture whether reflex or willed. It was inferred that slow-twitch muscle was the more efficient type of muscle to use for steady maintained contractions, but the validation of this hypothesis has only recently been achieved by the myothermic work of Gibbs and Gibson[67] and Wendt and Gibbs[68]. The advantages of using fast-twitch muscle to bring about changes of posture or willed movement are obvious, since it endows the animal with speed of action.

A second question may now be asked, why are the fast-twitch muscles of the rat faster than those of the cat, and again, why are the fast-twitch muscles of the mouse faster than those of the rat? If one assumes, as was done in the previous paragraph, that the function of the fast-twitch muscle is to endow the animal with speed of action, it must be appreciated that the physical strength of the materials making up the body (muscle, tendon, bone) set a limit to the accelerations that may be produced without causing damage. When a mammal, such as a horse, is at full gallop it has to oscillate each limb back and forth. If the fast-twitch muscles which are responsible for this reciprocating action had a higher maximum shortening velocity than they actually possess, the forces set up when maximally accelerating the limbs would exceed the tensile strength of the materials concerned, and a muscle, a tendon, or even a bone, would be damaged. It appears that dimensionally similar animals have the intrinsic speed of comparable fast-twitch limb muscles adjusted by nature so that they live just inside their own safety limits. One consequence of this arrangement is that such a series of animals (mouse, rat, cat, dog, horse) have very similar maximum linear speeds[91].

A third question might be, why are the slow-twitch muscles in any given species always some three to four times slower than the fast-twitch muscles, even though this means that the slow-twitch muscles of the mouse are of the same intrinsic speed as the fast-twitch muscles of the cat? It seems likely that a compromise has had to be reached between energetic efficiency and the speed with which a slow-twitch muscle can relax when the animal wishes to make a rapid movement. Since the speed of relaxation is related to the speed of shortening if a small animal developed very rapidly contracting fast-twitch muscles, but had slow-twitch muscles appropriate in speed to a much larger animal it would be hampered by the slow relaxation of its slow-twitch muscles when it wished to start running.

The study of the coordinated movements of an intact animal is a fascinating occupation, and there is no better introduction to it than that given by James Gray[92,93]. The ability of a mammal to exert a thrust against some structure in the outside world depends upon its ability to operate its bones as levers, but it must be recalled that a muscle cannot exert tension against its insertion without simultaneously exerting an equal and opposite force against its origin. What may, at first sight, appear a simple movement almost invariably turns out to involve the integration of a large part of the somatic musculature in coordinated activity. Only in this way are torsional and other strains avoided. Space precludes further treatment of this topic but the study of skeletal muscle must surely have as its ultimate goal the understanding of the total somatic musculature regarded as a single functional unit.

7.8 SUMMARY

The aim of this review has been to draw attention to the diversity of interests of 'muscle physiologists'. So often in this age of cellular biology the mention of 'muscle' immediately calls to mind a picture of the sliding of actin relative to myosin. It is by no means wrong that it should, since the sliding filament hypothesis represented one of the biological 'break-throughs' of this century. However, it would be a pity if, lost in admiration for the work of the molecular biologists, one also lost sight of the more integrative aspects of muscle research. At the present time it is not impossible to visualise the complete understanding of the molecular events of the contraction process. Considerable understanding has been achieved concerning the organisation of motor units within anatomical muscle. Our knowledge of the coordinated activity of muscle is minimal. Time must remedy this defect.

References

1. Hill, A. V. (1965). Trails and Trials in Physiology, (Edward Arnold)
2. Hill, A. V. (1950). *Biochem. Biophys. Acta*, **4**, 4–11
3. Gutmann, E. (1962). *The Denervated Muscle*, Chapter 1 (E. Gutmann, editor) (Czechoslovak Academy of Sciences)
4. Walton, J. (1973). *Disorders of Muscle*, 3rd ed. (London: J. and A. Churchill Ltd.) (in the press)
5. Carlsöö, S. (1972). *How Man Moves* (London: Heinemann)
6. Kuffler, S. W. and Vaughan Williams, E. M. (1953). *J. Physiol.*, **121**, 318
7. Hill, A. V. (1938). *Proc. Roy. Soc.B.*, **126**, 136–95
8. Bowman, W. (1840). *Phil. Trans.*, **130**, 457
9. Huxley, H. E. (1953). *Biochim. Biophys. Acta*, **12**, 387
10. Huxley, H. E. (1958). *Sci. Amer.*, **199**, 67
11. Huxley, A. F. and Niedergerke, R. (1954). *Nature (London)*, **173**, 971
12. Huxley, A. F. and Niedergerke, R. (1958). *J. Physiol.*, **144**, 403
13. Huxley, H. E. and Hanson, J. (1954). *Nature (London)*, **173**, 973
14. Fatt, P. and Katz, B. (1951). *J. Physiol.*, **115**, 320
15. Hill, A. V. (1948). *Proc. Roy. Soc.B.*, **135**, 446
16. Hill, A. V. (1949). *Proc. Roy. Soc.B.*, **136**, 399
17. Sten-Knudsen, O. (1954). *J. Physiol.*, **125**, 396
18. Porter, K. R. and Palade, G. E. (1957). *J. Biophys. Biochem. Cytol.*, **3**, 269
19. Porter, K. R. and Franzini-Armstrong, Clara (1965). *Sci. Amer.*, **212**, 72
20. Huxley, A. F. and Taylor, R. E. (1955). *Nature (London)*, **176**, 1068
21. Huxley, A. F. and Taylor, R. E. (1958). *J. Physiol.*, **144**, 426
22. Huxley, A. F. and Straub, R. W. (1958). *J. Physiol.*, **143**, 40P
23. Adrian, R. H. and Peachey, L. D. (1974). *J. Physiol.* (in the press)
24. Mines, G. R. (1913). *J. Physiol.*, **46**, 188
25. Ebashi, S. and Lipmann, F. (1962). *J. Cell. Biol.*, **14**, 389
26. Winegrad, S. (1968). *J. Gen. Physiol.*, **51**, 65
27. Ashley, C. C. and Ridgeway, E. B. (1970). *J. Physiol.*, **209**, 105
28. Huxley, A. F. and Peachey, L. D. (1961). *J. Physiol.*, **156**, 150
29. Gordon, A. M., Huxley, A. F. and Julian, F. J. (1966). *J. Physiol.*, **184**, 170
30. Lowey, H., Slayter, S., Weeds, A. G. and Baker, H. (1969). *J. Mol. Biol.*, **42**, 1
31. Tregear, R. T. and Miller, A. (1969). *Nature (London)*, **222**, 1184
32. Huxley, A. F. (1957). *Progress in Biophysics*, Vol. 7 (London: Pergamon Press)
33. Huxley, A. F. and Simmons, R. M. (1971). *Nature (London)*, **233**, 533
34. Huxley, A. F. (1973). *Proc. Roy. Soc.B.*, **183**, 83
35. Brown, G. L. (1937). *J. Physiol.*, **89**, 438
36. Ginetzinsky, A. G. and Shamarina, N. M. (1942). *Uspekhi Sovremennoi Biologii*, **15**, 289
37. Axelsson, J. and Thesleff, S. (1959). *J. Physiol.*, **147**, 178
38. Diamond, J. and Miledi, R. (1962). *J. Physiol.*, **162**, 393
39. Buller, A. J. (1966). *Brit. Med. Bull.*, **22**, 45
40. Bagust, J., Lewis, D. M. and Westerman, R. A. (1973). *J. Physiol.*, **229**, 241
41. Brown, M. C. and Matthews, P. B. C. (1960). *J. Physiol.*, **151**, 436
42. Harrison, R. G. (1910). *J. Exp. Zool.*, **9**, 787
43. Barker, D. and Ip, M. C. (1966). *Proc. Roy. Soc.B.*, **163**, 538
44. Jansen, J. K. S., Lomo, T., Nicolaysen, K. and Westgaard (1974). *Science* (in the press)
45. Goldspink, G. (1968). *J. Cell. Sci.*, **3**, 539
46. Williams, P. E. and Goldspink, G. (1971). *J. Cell. Sci.*, **9**, 751
47. Tabary, J. C., Tabary, C., Tardieu, C., Tardieu, G. and Goldspink, G. (1972). *J. Physiol.*, **224**, 231

48. Close, R. (1964). *J. Physiol.*, **173**, 74
49. Buller, A. J., Eccles, J. C. and Eccles, E. M. (1960). *J. Physiol.*, **150**, 399
50. Close, R. and Luff, A. R. (1974). *J. Physiol.*, (in the press)
51. McPhedran, A. M., Wuerker, R. B. and Henneman, E. (1965). *J. Neurophysiol.*, **28**, 71
52. Olson, C. B. and Swett, C. P. (1966). *J. Comp. Neurol.*, **128**, 475
53. Wuerker, R. B., McPhedran, A. M. and Henneman, E. (1965). *J. Neurophysiol.*, **28**, 85
54. Burke, R. E. (1967). *J Physiol.*, **193**, 141
55. Close, R. (1967). *J. Physiol.*, **193**, 45
56. Bagust, J., Knott, Sarah, Lewis, D. M., Luck, J. C. and Westerman, R. A. (1973). *J. Physiol.*, **231**, 87
57. Weeds, A. G. and Pope, B. (1971). *Nature (London)*, **234**, 85
58. Amako, T., Koga, J., Kobayashi, A., Tokunaga, J. and Urakado, S. (1962). *Kyushu J. Med. Sci.*, **13**, 205
59. Buller, A. J. (1974). The contractile behaviour of mammalian skeletal muscle. *Oxford Biology Readers* (Oxford University Press) (in the press)
60. Close, R. (1972). *Physiol. Rev.*, **52**, 129
61. Bagust, J. (1971). *Ph.D. thesis*, University of Bristol
62. Fenn, W. O. and Marsh, B. S. (1935). *J. Physiol.*, **85**, 277
63. Wilkie, D. R. (1950). *J. Physiol.*, **110**, 249
64. Al-Amood, W. S. and Pope, R. (1972). *J. Anat.*, **113**, 49
65. Buller, A. J., Kean, C. J. C. and Ranatunga, K. W. (1971). *J. Physiol.*, **213**, 66P
66. Woledge, R. C. (1968). *J. Physiol.*, **197**, 685
67. Gibbs, C. L. and Gibson, W. R. (1972). *Amer. J. Physiol.*, **223**, 864
68. Wendt, I. R. and Gibbs, C. L. (1974). *Amer. J. Physiol.* (in the press)
69. Eccles, J. C., Eccles, R. M. and Lundberg, A. (1958). *J. Physiol.*, **142**, 275
70. Buller, A. J., Eccles, J. C. and Eccles, R. M. (1960). *J. Physiol.*, **150**, 417
71. Close, R. (1965). *Nature (London)*, **206**, 831
72. Close, R. (1969). *J. Physiol.*, **204**, 331
73. Buller, A. J. and Kean, C. J. C. (1973). *J. Physiol.*, **233**, 24P
74. Bárány, M. (1967). *J. Gen. Physiol.*, **50**, Suppl. 2, 197
75. Bárány, M. and Close, R. (1971). *J. Physiol.*, **213**, 455
76. Samaha, F. J., Guth, L. and Albers, R. W. (1970). *Exp. Neurol.*, **27**, 276
77. Sreter, F. A. and Gergely, J. (1964). *Biochem. Biophys. Res. Commun.*, **16**, 438
78. Mommaerts, W. F. H. M., Buller, A. J. and Seraydarian, K. (1969). *Proc. Nat. Acad. Sci.*, **64**, 129
79. Close, R. (1965). *J. Physiol.*, **180**, 542
80. Hoh, J. F. Y. (1969). *Aust. J. Exp. Biol. Med. Sci.*, **47**, 17
81. Granit, R., Henatsch, H. D. and Steg, G. (1956). *Acta Physiol. Scand.*, **37**, 114
82. Kuno, M. (1959). *J. Physiol.*, **149**, 374
83. Liddell, E. G. T. and Sherrington, C. S. (1924). *Proc. Roy. Soc. B.*, **96**, 212
84. Denny-Brown (1929). *Proc. Roy. Soc. B.*, **104**, 252
85. Vrbová Gerta (1963). *J. Physiol.*, **166**, 241
86. Vrbová Gerta (1963). *J. Physiol.*, **169**, 513
87. Salmons, S. and Vrbová, Gerta (1969). *J. Physiol.*, **201**, 535
88. Sreter, F. A., Gergely, J., Salmons, S. and Romanul, F. (1973). *Nature New Biology*, **241**, 18
89. Al-Amood, W. S., Buller, A. J. and Pope, R. (1974). *Nature (London)* (in the press)
90. Guth, L. (1968). *Physiol. Rev.*, **48**, 645
91. Hill, A. V. (1950). *Sci. Prog. (London)*, **38**, 209
92. Gray, J. (1953). *How Animals Move* (London: Cambridge University Press)
93. Gray, J. (1956). *Brit. Med. Bull.*, **12**, 203
94. Needham, Dorothy (1971). *Machina Carnis* (Cambridge University Press)
95. Katz, B. (1966). *Nerve, Muscle and Synapse* (McGraw Hill Book Co.)
96. Huxley, H. E. (1969). *Science*, **164**, 1356

8
Neural Substrates of Somatic Sensation

J. J. G. BOIVIE
Karolinska Institute, Stockholm
and
E. R. PERL
University of North Carolina

8.1	INTRODUCTION	305
8.2	RECEPTIVE MECHANISMS	307
	8.2.1 *Transduction*	307
	8.2.2 *Stimulus location*	308
	8.2.3 *Receptors and stimulus quality*	309
	8.2.3.1 *Sensory receptor types*	311
	8.2.3.2 *Afferent fibre size*	317
	8.2.4 *Intensity*	318
	8.2.4.1 *Single receptors*	318
	8.2.4.2 *Population dynamics*	320
8.3	CENTRAL PROJECTIONS OF PRIMARY AFFERENT NEURONS	321
	8.3.1 *Morphological considerations*	321
	8.3.1.1 *Branching*	321
	8.3.1.2 *Termination loci*	322
	8.3.1.3 *The nature of synaptic termination*	323
	8.3.1.4 *Connections of primary afferent neurons*	324
	8.3.2 *Synaptic mechanisms*	325
	8.3.2.1 *Postsynaptic excitation*	325
	8.3.2.2 *Presynaptic inhibition*	327
	8.3.2.3 *Spinal 'gates'*	329
	8.3.2.4 *Postsynaptic inhibition*	329
8.4	METHODS AND APPROACHES	330
	8.4.1 *Anatomical methods*	330

8.4.1.1   *Light* versus *electron microscopy*   331
8.4.1.2   *Characterisation of cells*   331
8.4.1.3   *Pathway tracing*   332
          (a) *Orthograde degeneration*   333
          (b) *Retrograde methods*   333
8.4.1.4   *Techniques based upon transport of substances*   333
8.4.2   *Physiological methods*   334
8.4.2.1   *The single neuron*   334
8.4.2.2   *Evoked responses*   335
8.4.2.3   *Afferent input*   335
8.4.3   *Behavioural approaches*   335
8.4.3.1   *Deficits from lesions*   336
8.4.3.2   *Appropriateness of tests for sensory capacity*   336

8.5   ASCENDING SOMATOSENSORY SYSTEMS   337
8.5.1   *Pathways of the dorsal spinal cord*   338
8.5.1.1   *The dorsal column system*   338
          (a) *The dorsal columns*   338
          (b) *Dorsal column nuclei (DCN)*   341
          (c) *Physiology of the dorsal column nuclei*   342
          (d) *Projection from the dorsal column nuclei*   344
8.5.1.2   *Spinal pathway via nucleus Z*   345
          (a) *Nucleus Z*   345
8.5.1.3   *The spino-cervicothalamic pathway*   346
          (a) *The spinocervical tract*   346
          (b) *Lateral cervical nucleus*   348
          (c) *Cervicothalamic tract*   349
8.5.2   *Ascending tracts of the ventral quadrants*   349
8.5.2.1   *The spinothalamic projection*   349
          (a) *The spinothalamic tract*   349
          (b) *Cells of origin*   351
8.5.2.2   *Spinoreticular and related systems*   352
          (a) *Spinoreticular pathway*   353
          (b) *Nuclei of termination*   354
          (c) *Ascending projections*   356

8.6   SOMATOSENSORY PROJECTIONS TO DIENCEPHALIC NUCLEI   357
8.6.1   *Intimate thalamic anatomy*   358
8.6.1.1   *Cellular structure*   358
8.6.1.2   *Synaptic morphology*   359
8.6.2   *Ascending pathways*   359
8.6.2.1   *Projections from the dorsal column nuclei*   360
8.6.2.2   *Projections from the lateral cervical nucleus*
          (cervicothalamic)   360
8.6.2.3   *Spinothalamic projections*   361
8.6.2.4   *Projections from nucleus Z*   362
8.6.2.5   *Reticulothalamic connections*   363
8.6.3   *Physiological activation*   363

	8.6.3.1	*Ventroposterior region*	363
		(a) *Specificity of the input*	364
		(b) *Pain*	366
		(c) *Relation of function to afferent pathway*	367
		(d) *Spindling activity in the VPL*	369
		(e) *Synaptic mechanisms*	370
	8.6.3.2	*Posterior group*	371
	8.6.3.3	*Intralaminar nuclei*	372
8.6.4	*Lemniscal and non-lemniscal*		373

8.7	THE CEREBRAL CORTEX		374
8.7.1	*Morphological considerations*		375
	8.7.1.1	*Cellular and synaptic features*	375
	8.7.1.2	*Cytoarchitecture and its correlations*	376
8.7.2	*Somatotopy revisited*		377
8.7.3	*Thalamocortical and corticothalamic connections*		377
8.7.4	*Cortico–cortical connections*		378
8.7.5	*S-I: functional considerations*		379
	8.7.5.1	*Modality*	379
	8.7.5.2	*Directional properties*	380
	8.7.5.3	*Pathways to S-I*	381
8.7.6	*S-II: functional considerations*		381
	8.7.6.1	*Effective stimuli*	382
	8.7.6.2	*Pathways to S-II*	382
8.7.7	*Other cortical areas*		383

| 8.8 | SUMMARY DIAGRAMS | 383 |

8.9	FUNCTION AND PATHWAYS		385
8.9.1	*Traditional concepts*		385
8.9.2	*Dorsal columns and behaviour*		385
8.9.3	*The dorsolateral fasciculus and behaviour*		386
8.9.4	*Ventral spinal pathways and sensation*		387

| 8.10 | CONCLUDING COMMENTS | 387 |

8.1 INTRODUCTION

This account is an attempt to overview the present knowledge on structure and function of the neural apparatus subserving sensation derived from cutaneous and musculoskeletal tissue. We have limited our consideration to systems suspected to relate more or less directly to alterations of consciousness and recognition of the quality of stimuli. To make the account manageable, the afferent inflow from the head has not been specifically treated since it introduces a number of additional ramifications, although some of the discussion focuses on features applying to it as well. Moreover, clinical data suggest that by fixing upon consciousness, those systems terminating in the cerebellum may be left aside since removal of the cerebellum in man does not produce a major change in somatic sensation. Even with these restrictions, one must account for a remarkably diverse set of circumstances and mechanisms.

In setting things down on a complex subject, writers must make assumptions about readers. We planned this material for readers who have limited knowledge of part or much of the field. Consequently, the discussion of each facet begins with widely accepted facts or ideas and then explores newer developments. It turns out that in spite of our several limitations, it has proven impossible to cover all facets. Many discoveries or observations are at the moment left unconnected to things understood. We have chosen not to deal with certain of these; some that were left out undoubtedly will prove to be very important. In sum, what follows should be viewed as much as a recounting of our ignorance as of our knowledge.

Many situations changing the external or internal environment of the body are paralleled by distinguishable sensory reactions in man. It seems reasonable to believe that a frame of reference for somatosensory mechanisms can be derived from commonly shared conscious experience or a more rigorous counterpart, psychophysical analysis. Guidelines of this kind offer a rationale for attention to certain topics in the subsequent discussions. While sensation as we experience it cannot be proven to occur in animals, they discriminate between stimuli in ways which suggest processes similar to man's experiences. This is the justification for carrying over results obtained by necessity in animals to proposals for somatic, or in fact any, sensation in man.

As a start, consider the ability of mammals to locate the site of a stimulus. The capacity for the identification of place varies with the nature of the stimulus and the part of the body affected. Skin pressure can be more precisely located than skin warming; movement of an articulation of a digit can be better detected than movement of a proximal joint of the same limb. Our discussion of somatosensory mechanisms must consider neural arrangements of probable importance for determination of the body region involved.

Normal man recognises differences in the nature of events affecting his body. The contact between an external object and our skin can be detected and an idea gained about its movement. In the absence of disturbances of consciousness or injury to nervous pathways, we distinguish radiant skin warming from skin contact by a solid object, and circumstances deforming the skin alone from those producing disturbance of subcutaneous structures. A human being's ability to make these distinctions between stimuli and consciously to recognise their quality or modality seems to be paralleled by other mammals. Monkeys can be trained to indicate the size of a cutaneous stimulator and/or to differentiate between static and moving contact[1-3]. The ability to recognise reliably the characteristics of somatic stimuli must be explained at the level of both the transduction process itself, i.e. the sensory apparatus, and the subsequent operation of central systems.

The relation between stimulus intensity and perceptual intensity represents a major focus of psychophysics and, as such, has received systematic attention since the end of the last century. Changes in the magnitude of stimuli alter not only the intensity of a perceptual experience but, at certain levels, also cause a change in the nature of the sensation itself; mechanical pressure or skin warming may change to discomfort or pain at reasonably reproducible intensities. Animals must also have similar experiences with variations in intensity since they can be trained to respond differentially to variations of stimulus magnitude within the same ranges[4-6]. Intensity is not the only stimulus quality related to its quantitative characteristics; both duration and dynamic (rate of change or movement) features of the stimulus are appreciated by man to varying degrees.

So far, conscious perception and its implied differentiation between qualities of events have been mentioned; however, there are important responses to somatic stimuli of quite a different type. Under certain conditions, somatosensory input provokes a change in consciousness along the continuum from wakefulness to sleep. In these 'alerting' responses, somatic, visual and auditory stimuli may cause similar if not identical reactions; they seem to represent the antithesis of perceptual differentiation and discrimination. For these reasons effects upon the levels of consciousness must also be considered in an analysis of the neural activity attendant upon somatosensory events.

8.2 RECEPTIVE MECHANISMS

8.2.1 Transduction

A variety of receptive structures make up the peripheral portions of the somatic sensory apparatus. At the minimum each consists of

(1) a neuronal soma located within a dorsal root (or cranial nerve) ganglion,

(2) a peripheral process (primary or first order afferent fibre) extending through peripheral nerves to terminate in somatic tissue and

(3) a process ramifying within the central nervous system. Generally the peripheral terminations are considered the receptive portion, the locus of part of the transduction of physical events into neural activity. It has been recognised since the late 19th century that peripheral terminations of primary afferent neurons are often associated with special, non-neural elements. This combination of neural elements and other tissue makes up somatic sense organs varying in complexity from structures such as the muscle spindle to 'bare' nerve endings. The receptive terminals and their primary afferent fibres are often labelled a *receptor*.

There was a vogue among the microscopists around the turn of the century to ascribe every apparent variation in neural termination to a new and different type of sensory structure[7]. There has been changing sentiment over the years about the relation between histologically identifiable structures and functional characteristics. At the start there was enthusiasm for a match in functional specificity and morphological features; this was often based on highly circumstantial grounds[8]. Dictum on the functional significance of histological structures in some textbooks date from these early analyses. Subsequently, arguments favouring the lack of stimulus and/or morphological specialisation of the terminal[9,10] became prevalent. At present a solid and increasing body of evidence again favours a close correlation between functional characteristics and sensory nerve morphology[11-13].

Details of the transduction of physical or chemical conditions into neural activity and the way that non-neural tissue interacts with the neural terminal is beyond the scope of the present review. A few comments, however, are in keeping to summarise our present understanding and to point out some areas of uncertainty; interested readers should consult recent reviews by Fuortes[14], Loewenstein[15] and Flock[16].

A local depolarisation of the sensory nerve terminal, graded in amplitude according to the magnitude of the stimulus, has been shown to be a regular feature of the activation of mechanoreceptors. From the time of Katz's[17] description, this local potential has been presumed to be a critical step in the activation of sensory nerve fibres by their receptive terminals. While the existence of a generator or receptor potential has been reasonably established, the underlying molecular changes will remain a subject for speculation[18-20] until the structural features of biological membranes are further elucidated. However, the nerve terminal may not be the sole point for transduction in somatic mechanoreceptors. Synaptic activation of afferent terminals in somatic sense organs is still at issue; evidence in favour of it has been put forth for mechanoreceptors of the auditory and vestibular apparatus[16] and chemoreceptors[21] of the vascular system. One cutaneous sensory structure, the Pinkus haarschiebe[22,23], contains a specialised epithelial element, the Merkel cell, in close proximity to an expanded terminal from a sensory nerve fibre[24]. Iggo and Muir[23] have pointed out the possibility that the approximation of epithelial cells containing dense staining granules and nerve terminals represent a synapse in which a chemical agent stored in the non-neural element diffuses across the intercellular gap to act upon the sensory ending. A similar concept has existed for receptive structures important in pain; several investigators have postulated liberation of a substance by pain-producing stimuli which then act to excite nerve terminals (see review by Lim[25]).

In some primary sensory neurons, conducted action potentials ordinarily are not initiated in the same membrane region as that producing the generator potential; instead they are triggered at more centrally located points of the nerve fibre by electrotonic current flow produced by the generator potential[26,27]. These two transductions, one from stimulus to a graded and localised change at the sensory terminal, and the second by which the local change is converted to conducted impulses, impose important restrictions on the transfer of neural information about the stimulus and on subsequent manipulations of these data by central systems.

8.2.2 Stimulus location

The generally accepted route for sensory information from the body to the central nervous system is by way of the dorsal roots even though the idea of afferent fibres in the ventral roots has been revitalised. Coggeshall, Coulter and Willis[28] have shown that cat ventral roots contain unmyelinated fibres in considerable numbers which do not degenerate upon division of motor nerves, dorsal roots central to its ganglia or the sympathetic trunk. The conclusion is that the perikarya of unmyelinated fibres are in the dorsal root ganglia, and enter the spinal cord through the ventral root. A cell body in the dorsal root ganglion can be taken to imply a sensory function. In any case, the capacity for stimulus localisation begins with the innervation of a particular and restricted body part by a given spinal root fibre. To the degree that a receptive unit formed by a dorsal root neuron responds only to stimuli restricted to this vicinity, its impulses specify action of a stimulus there. Since the stimulus may cause effects elsewhere as well, the activity of a single afferent element is not sufficient to identify the locus. Prior to any central processing, essential data about the region and structures acted upon by a stimulus is provided by the ensemble of elements activated as well as those unaffected.

Place or locus is so clearly encoded by the fraction of the population of receptive elements activated that logic suggests use be made of the information for the process of sensory localisation. Nevertheless, some literature on somatosensory organisation prefers to emphasise the absence of place-coded effects in the projections from primary sensory neurons. Over the past three and one-half decades much effort has gone into establishing the existence of neural systems organised in a fashion reflecting the regional nature of input. The projection of primary afferent fibres from their segmental entrance to central neurons in these systems suggest that the segmental arrangement is restructured by a systematic convergence to make body region rather than segmental origin the important factor in excitation of particular neurons. This *somatotopic* arrangement is particularly apparent in systems projecting to the first somatosensory area (S-I) of the cerebral cortex. In somatotopically arranged pathways, the dermatome or the skin area (or equivalent deeper regions), representing the afferent innervation by one dorsal root, is replaced by a regional pattern; however, the segmental order is maintained[29]. *A priori* it would appear that those neural mechanisms in which excitation of a neuron is not dependent upon the location of the stimulus must be concerned with processes other than those that provide data for the decision on locus.

8.2.3 Receptors and stimulus quality

A signalling system dependent upon the intervals between impulses of primary afferent neurons could code features of stimuli in several ways. One possibility is a population of primary afferent units with a unimodal gradient of characteristics. In such a situation, different features or qualities of a somatic stimulus could be signalled by altering the frequency of activity in individual elements and/or altering the pattern of activity over the population of elements; this represents an extension of a postulate formulated by Erb[30] for the process leading to pain. Another conceivable means of signalling complex differences between stimuli by a single class of receptors would be to have a pattern of impulses other than a simple increase or decrease of impulse frequency represent quality. Any variations in discharge of individual elements could be extended by variations in the population, whether they were presumed to be uniform or continuously varying in some fashion; a pattern theory in the latter format was originally proposed by Nafe[31] and extended by Sinclair[9] and Weddell[32].

An alternate to frequency or pattern codes in one general class of receptive organs has been the concept that there are receptors with some specific responsiveness to particular kinds of stimuli. The latter is an outgrowth of the 'doctrine' of specific nerve energies set down by Müller[33]. In the minds of physiologists[34], the issues on the method by which stimulus type and modality are related seems to have been settled in favour of specificity at the beginning of the 20th century by psychophysical studies on cutaneous sense and von Frey's[35-37] resultant deductions on morphologically different receptors for touch, cold, warmth and pain. However, during the past sixty years the concept of specificity and von Frey's conclusion about receptor types have been repeatedly challenged (for a review see Sinclair[9]). Pain, with its ubiquitous receptive fields and the relative paucity of physiologically identified receptors with qualities appropriate for it, has been a particular rallying point for opponents of sense organ specificity. On the other side of the question, electrophysiological observations by a number of laboratories has generally concurred that individual dorsal root neurons have unique and differing responses to the gamut of stimuli which might affect the body surface and subcutaneous tissue. The functional features of somatic sense organs, their morphology and the available correlates to sensation are discussed in several current reviews[11-13,39]. The following summary is provided as a basis for consideration of central mechanisms.

As presently understood, somatosensory primary or first-order units (receptors) consist of a number of types or classes, each with unique features. A sensory receptor type in these terms really consists of a population of elements with a certain variation but with a group of common characteristics which serve to distinguish them from other populations. A given characteristic or feature may have quantitative overlap from one receptor type to another, but the composite of characteristics for each type is unique. When regarded from the point of view of somatic stimuli likely to exist during the evolutionary or natural history of mammals, overlap in functional features tends to be at the limits of the population[12,13]. Receptors were suggested to differ in this way in pioneering electrophysiological studies by Adrian[40,41]. Adrian and Zotterman[42], Matthews[43], and Zotterman[44]. These early works showed that different receptive units respond differently to given stimuli and that there was a consistent positive relation between the intensity of a particularly effective stimulus and the number of discharges produced by an afferent fibre. The two decades following World War II saw the responsive characteristics of muscle mechanoreceptors documented and correlated to morphology (see review by Matthews[45]), observations on articular receptors and a gradual enlightenment of the complex situation for the integument. Extension of these observations to the large afferent population with small diameter afferent fibres[96], and the resultant description of highly sensitive thermoreceptors were particularly important steps[46-49]. During this period, work on cutaneous mechanoreceptors strongly supported major differences between distinctive receptive units[50-52], reducing, but by no means eliminating, objections to the concept of specificity for sense organs of the skin[10]. Still a further advance in this direction came when the kind of functional and structural correlations made for muscle receptors was extended to those of the cutaneous realm with analyses on the Pacinian corpuscle and the tactile corpuscle[23,52-54].

The final bastion of non-specificity has also succumbed. Adrian[41,55] and his co-workers had noted the appearance of activity in an apparently special class of sensory elements to intense or damaging stimuli; however, confirmation and description of such elements was slow in coming. Zotterman[44,56] while agreeing with the idea that special sense organs were responsible for pain, provided ammunition to doubters when he pointed out that receptors with fibres of the small diameter implicated in pain or pain-like responses responded to gentle mechanical stimulation. The latter point was emphasised during the mid-1950s when Douglas and Ritchie[57] (see also Douglas, Ritchie and Straub[58]) showed, by colliding naturally evoked activity with compound action potentials, that a large fraction of cat C (unmyelinated) fibres could be effectively activated by gentle mechanical stimulation of the skin. Single unit studies of small diameter fibres had described certain elements with elevated thresholds for all forms of natural stimulation; however, the number studied were so few and their described features so inconsistent, that as late as 1965, Melzack and Wall[38] discarded the notion of a specific set of sense organs for pain. Since then, systematic study of the population of afferent units with slowly conducting (thin) fibres by Burgess and Perl[60], Perl[61], and Bessou and Perl[62] has demonstrated that a considerable fraction of primary afferent units have elevated thresholds for all kinds of stimuli as well as other unique features, a view an earlier critic, Wall[59], no longer disputes. High-threshold receptors appear to be the sole group of primary afferent fibres from the skin capable of reliably signalling the presence of noxious mechanical or thermal events and differentiating them from innocuous stimuli[61,62].

8.2.3.1 Sensory receptor types

The evolution of evidence just described identifies three major categories of somatosensory receptive elements: mechanoreceptors, thermoreceptors and nociceptors. Of the known sensory receptor types, aside from the special senses of the head, this list excludes those with a primary responsiveness to changes in chemical constituents of tissue, blood or luminal contents of hollow organs (i.e. carotid body receptors and pH-sensitive receptors). The latter are usually thought of as visceral receptors and have not been established to have a place in conscious experience.

As already pointed out, mechanoreceptors are a diverse population. Traditionally, mechanoreceptive sense organs have been classified by the tissue in which they are located and by the adaptation of their responses to a prolonged, constant mechanical displacement of tissues. Differences in the latter test led first Adrian and Zotterman[42] and successive generations of physiologists to speak of 'rapidly' and 'slowly' adapting receptors, even though early in this history it was clear that such tests defined many intermediate variations. In recent years, quantitative testing of receptors has uncovered dynamic features which in some cases uniquely specify an element's receptive characteristics. Defining mechanical stimuli by effects upon the

Table 8.1 Somatic mechanoreceptors

Tissue, receptor type and name	Effective stimuli/response	Terminal morphology/associated structures	Afferent fibre	References
A. Cutaneous				
1. Hairy regions				
a. Displacement and velocity responsive				
i. Type II	skin deformation/regular discharge	Ruffini end organs	myelinated A_β, 45–65 m sec^{-1} (cat)	63, 65–67
ii. Type I	indentation of dome/irregular discharge	dome (haarschiebe) with Merkel's cells	myelinated A_β, 50–70 m sec^{-1} (cat)	23, 63, 65, 67
b. Primarily velocity responsive				
i. G_2 hair—T hair	guard, tylotrich hair and skin movement, relatively slow to rapid	specialised termination in hair follicle	myelinated A_β, 35–65 m sec^{-1} (cat)	61, 63, 68, 69
ii. Field	skin indentation	unknown	myelinated A_β, 40–70 m sec^{-1} (cat)	61, 63
iii. D (delta) hair	down (fine)/guard hair skin deflection/slow to rapid	? specialised termination at hair base	myelinated A_δ, 16–27 m sec^{-1} (cat)	61, 63, 68, 69
iv. C Mechanoreceptors	slowly moving skin distortion	unknown, rare in distal portions of primate limbs	unmyelinated C, 0.7–1.1 m sec^{-1} (cat)	51, 70
c. Transient responsive				
i. Pacinian (P.C.) 'phasic', 'tap'	mechanical transients, vibration of 50–500 Hz	multilamellated corpuscles	myelinated $A_{\alpha\beta}$, 50–75 m sec^{-1} (cat)	52, 71, 72
ii. G_1 hair	high velocity guard and tylotrich hair or skin deflection	specialised terminations at base of hair follicles	myelinated A_α, 66–87 m sec^{-1} (cat)	63, 68, 69
2. Glabrous regions				
a. Displacement and velocity responsive				

313

i. SA ('slowly-adapting') probably two types	skin indentation	associated with Merkel's cells: ? second type with Ruffini organs	myelinated A_β, 40–70 m sec^{-1} (cat) 55–60 m sec^{-1} (monkey)	61, 72–76
b. Primarily velocity responsive i. RA ('rapidly-adapting')	skin indentation	? Meissner's corpuscles	myelinated $A_{\alpha\beta}$, 46–78 m sec^{-1} (cat)	72–75
c. Transient responsive Pacinian (P.C.) phasic, tap	see above (l.c.i.)			76
B. Muscle, tendon, fascia 1. Displacement and velocity i. Secondary spindle	muscle length	secondary coils and spray in muscle spindle	myelinated, Group II, (A_β) 30–66 m sec^{-1}	45, 77–79
ii. Primary spindle	muscle length	annulospiral and associated spray	myelinated, Group I$_a$ (A_α) 72–120 m sec^{-1}	43, 45, 78–80
iii. Tendon organs	fascia or muscle tension	Golgi spray	myelinated, Group I$_b$ (A_α) 72–110 m sec^{-1}	43, 78, 79, 81
iv. Pressure	pressure on belly, fascial distortion	unknown	myelinated, Group III, (A_δ) 12–40 m sec^{-1}	82, 83
2. Transient responsive i. P.C. type	taps, vibration (50–500 Hz)	lamellated capsule	myelinated, Group II, ($A_{\alpha\beta}$) 50–90 m sec^{-1}	52, 84
C. Articular tissue 1. Displacement and velocity i. S.A. type 1 (tendon organ)	joint position and movement	Golgi spray	myelinated, >10 μm	85–88
ii. S.A. type 2	joint bending	Ruffini-type	myelinated, 7–10 μm (A_β)	64, 86–88
2. Velocity signalling i. 'phasic'	joint movement (bend, twist)	unknown	myelinated, $A_{\alpha\beta}$, 50–80 m sec^{-1}	64
3. Transient signalling i. 'Tap'	mechanical transients in joint movements	? paciniform	myelinated, $A_{\alpha\beta}$ 50–80 m sec^{-1}	64, 86, 87

Table 8.2 Somatic thermoreceptors and nociceptors

Tissue, receptor type and name	Effective stimuli/ response	Terminal morphology/ associated structure	Afferent fibre	References
A. Cutaneous				
1. Thermal signalling				
a. cooling	temperature decrease >0.1°C from 35°C to 15°C	bulb-like terminals in basal epidermis	cat: unmyelinated, C, 0.7–1.2 m sec^{-1}; primate: myelinated, A$_\delta$, 5–15 m sec^{-1}	48, 49, 61, 89, 90
b. warming	temperature increase >0.1°C from 30°C to 43°C	unknown	unmyelinated, C, ∼/m sec^{-1}	48, 90
2. Noxious signalling				
a. High threshold mechanoreceptor	high shearing force	multiple, unknown structure	myelinated, A$_\delta$, 5–35 m sec^{-1}	49, 60, 61
b. Thermal-mechanical				

i. heat nociceptor	noxious heat (or mechanical)	unknown	myelinated, A_δ, 3–7 m sec^{-1}	91
ii. cold (sensitive)	noxious mechanical, prolonged cold	unknown	unmyelinated, C, 0.9–2.5 m sec^{-1}	62, 92
c. Polymodal nociceptor	noxious heat, mechanical, chemical	unknown	unmyelinated, C, 0.3–1.1 m sec^{-1}	62, 92
B. Subcutaneous 1. Noxious signalling a. Muscle				49, 82, 83
i. Pressure	high pressure, excessive muscle length	unknown	myelinated, Group III, 5–25 m sec^{-1}	
ii. Group IV (C) nociceptors	strong pressure, temperature extreme, anoxia	unknown (? free ending)	unmyelinated, Group IV, 0.4–1.6 m sec^{-1}	93, 94
b. Articular* i. Nociceptor	joint overextension	unknown	myelinated, A_δ, <30 m sec^{-1}	64

* Nothing is known of the function of receptors with C fibres in articular regions

position (p) or displacement of the sense organ in tissue, or derivatives of position relative to time [velocity (dp/dt), acceleration (d^2p/dt^2), jerk (d^3p/dt^3)] and examining receptor signals on this basis has led to a classification of mechanoreceptors in terms of displacement, velocity, etc., rather than simply slowly adapting or rapidly adapting[12]. While this latter classification undoubtedly will be the subject of debate and change, it does simplify and give meaning to an almost chaotic collection of observations. It points out that the bulk of mechanoreceptors, aside from those of skeletal muscle, are velocity detecting elements with each type best suited or 'tuned' to a part of the spectrum of movement speeds common in nature. The best examples of mammalian displacement or static detectors are the mechanoreceptors of skeletal muscle and their tendons (all displacement receptors show some sensitivity to velocity); displacement receptors make up a minor fraction of the receptors of skin and larger joints[63,64]. Detecting and signalling very high stimulus velocities, changing velocity (the higher derivatives — acceleration and jerk) or the transients which produce them are also the province of a relatively small fraction of the mechanoreceptor population. Table 8.1 lists mechanoreceptor types according to this scheme; additional references and rationale are given by Burgess and Perl[12]. It must be emphasised that designation of a receptor type is only partially dependent upon the most effective stimulus; ordinarily, a constellation of properties emerges as the distinguishing features of a given kind of primary sensory unit. These include the location and distribution of receptive field (receptive terminals), the associated specialised structures, the conduction velocity of the primary afferent fibre, and the pattern of transmitted discharge. The data in Table 8.1 point out that part of the apparent multiplicity of mechanoreceptor types derives from replication of units sensing similar parameters of mechanical changes in tissues forming the body surface, the skeletal motor apparatus and the supporting skeleton. For example, the displacement signalling elements of hairy skin (Type I and Type II) are paralleled by types with a similar balance of static and dynamic properties in glabrous skin (SA) and by receptive elements of skeletal muscle (the muscle spindle Group Ia and II ending). In another instance, while velocity-signalling receptors of cutaneous tissue apparently differ in maximal responsivity at different velocities, some overlap exists between types such as G_2 hair and the 'field' types; however, the G_2 receptor is related to an appendage of the skin, hairs, and the field receptor is associated with the skin proper.

Table 8.2 summarises primary sensory units classified as thermally sensitive or nociceptive. All receptors in Table 8.2 are characterised by higher thresholds ($1.0–10^3 \times$) for mechanical stimuli than those of the mechanoreceptors listed in Table 8.1 when thermally neutral stimuli are used. It is important to note that receptive units with A (myelinated) and with C (unmyelinated) fibres belong to three major categories: mechanoreceptors, thermoreceptors and nociceptors.

One view of functionally distinctive somatic sense organs would be analogous to von Frey's explicit 'specificity' concept: each receptor type could be conceived as the beginning of a different modality of conscious sensation (or the subconscious equivalent of modality) and the starting point of a private path to equally dedicated central regions. This sort of arrangement would demand eight to ten varieties of cutaneous sensation since there are at least that many receptor types. An alternate idea is that receptor special-isation serves the dual purposes of differentiation between classes of events by limiting the effective stimuli for each element and maintenance of maximal sensitivity to the wide variety of naturally occurring stimuli. In this alternate view of specificity, modalities of sensation result from activation of particular central regions by the projected activity from combinations of receptor types such as those specially responsive to velocity, or from the several kinds of nociceptors, or from thermoreceptors. Thus, in most cases, a given receptor would not be equivalent to a given sensation and there would be more receptor types than unique ascending pathways and sensations.

8.2.3.2 Afferent fibre size

Afferent fibres vary in cross-sectional diameter from about 0.4 μm to 20 μm. It has been known for many years that the frequency of occurrence of fibres as a function of cross-sectional diameter is multimodal, a fact which gained considerable importance when the distribution of fibre size was related to peaks in the compound action potential[95]. The grouping of fibre diameters around particular model values seems to be a reasonably regular character-istic of mammalian nerves, although there are systematic regional and species differences[96]. Unfortunately, several terminologies have been used for the modal peaks of fibre diameter and their close, parallel, components of the compound action potential. In a classification used since the mid-1930s[97], A fibres cover the full range of myelinated fibres (5–120 m sec^{-1}, 2–20 μm in cross-sectional diameter) and are both motor and sensory in function; B fibres are myelinated (10–15 m sec^{-1}, 1.5–4 μm) preganglionic motor fibres of the autonomic system (some shifts in B usage took place in the literature of the 1930s); the most slowly conducting (0.4–2.2 m sec^{-1}, 0.3–1.5 μm) or C group are unmyelinated. The first or A component of the compound action potential of a vertebrate mixed nerve contains several peaks designated as α, β, γ and δ. One source of difficulty has been the application to cutaneous nerves of a designation originally proposed for muscle afferent fibre groups: I (72–120 m sec^{-1}, 12–20 μm), II (24–66 m sec^{-1}, 5–11 μm), III (6–20 m sec^{-1}, 2–4 μm)[98,99]. In muscle nerve these groups have relatively little overlap and do have an established functional significance[100]. Un-fortunately, the spectra of velocities and diameters in cutaneous and muscle nerves are not comparable and, for this reason, it would seem best to restrict the group I–IV nomenclature to muscle afferent fibres.

Tables 8.1 and 8.2 also relate functional characteristics of afferent units and the cross-sectional diameter/conduction velocity of their peripheral nerve fibres. The data show that in spite of generalities in the classes of receptors served by each part of the spectrum of afferent fibres, no given diameter/conduction velocity uniquely specifies a receptor class. It is true that fibres conducting over 50 m sec^{-1} (>8 μm diameter) originate from mechanoreceptors and the various types of nociceptors are largely served by fibres conducting under 35 m sec^{-1} (<6 μm diameter). On the other hand, the tables document the diversity of afferent units with fibres conducting over 50 m sec^{-1} and the presence of other than nociceptive elements in the population conducting at $A\delta$ or C fibre velocities (<25 m sec^{-1}). In summary, from the functional standpoint any given size range of afferent fibres in most mammalian nerves represents a mixed input.

The term 'flexor reflex afferents' (FRA) has been used to describe the nature of afferent input impinging upon certain ascending sensory systems. The term originates from the relation established between components of the compound action potential and the polysynaptic spinal reflex to flexor motoneurons on the one hand, and suprasegmental control of interneurons on the other[99,194,195]. This nomenclature has appeal since it represents a shorthand for describing the parallelism between initiation of different neural mechanisms and reflex effect by afferent fibres of certain conduction velocity ranges. However, its use implies that the identical afferent fibres are responsible for the flexor reflex and the other mechanisms in question, something which usually has not been adequately tested. It is one of several instances in which all fibres making up peaks in the compound potential may be given a functional connotation of the basis of features possibly associated only with part of the population. This point is probably understood by many users of the term, but not necessarily by their audience. We do not mean to imply that ascending or other connections attributed to 'flexor reflex afferents' do not stem from elements with this reflex action, but rather that the designation is imprecise. It suggests an unproven common function for a mixed population of sensory elements and may do more to confound than to clarify issues.

8.2.4 Intensity

8.2.4.1 *Single receptors*

A sense organ's generator potential is closely linked to the production of conducted impulses, the number of impulses being a function of its amplitude, its duration and the characteristics of the process leading to the action potential. Demonstration of similar relationships in different phyla[17,101-103] suggest that the correlation represents enough of a general principle to make possible the use of conducted impulses as an indicator of the generation process. Both direct recording of generator potentials and/or analyses of the conducted impulses in primary afferent fibres indicate a reasonably rigorous relation between the magnitude of stimulus variables and receptor output for a given set of conditions. In the case of a mechanoreceptor signalling displacement, this relation exists between position, which is related to an intensity parameter (force), and the discharge frequency in the primary fibre. The representation of intensity by the frequency of discharge for displacement mechanoreceptors was recognised in pioneering studies of sense organ function by Adrian and Zotterman[42] and has been generally accepted since. The general rule is that the reciprocal of the interval between successive impulses (frequency for a regularly discharging receptor) increases with increasing intensity; more impulses per unit time are representative of increased intensity.

Classification of somatosensory receptors only as rapidly or slowly adapting makes it difficult to deal rationally with time variant features of quantitative relations between stimulus and receptor output; a number of differences of interpretation arise in part from this problem. The notion that mechanoreceptors have particular velocity or acceleration (vibration) sensitivities may help resolve some of the debate on the nature and meaning of input–output (transfer) functions for receptors. It should be obvious that a quantitative input–output description usually has functional meaning only when appropriate stimuli are used; in other words, this requires use of displacement to test a displacement receptor, velocity for a velocity receptor and acceleration for a receptor particularly sensitive to acceleration. Moreover, since mechanoreceptors or other kinds of somatic sense organs rarely, if ever, have sensitivities exactly fitting physical definitions, their responses will differ quantitatively according to the prominent features of the stimulus, i.e. movement from one position to another contains a transient component (velocity) as well as a static component (position). Thus, it must be recognised that while quantity may be signalled in part by individual receptors, the quantity is not necessarily amplitude alone.

There is disagreement on the relation between stimulus input and receptor response. Matthews[43,104,105] pointed out some time ago that the plot of discharge frequency of a 'slowly adapting' receptor as a function of the force provoking the displacement could be approximated by a logarithmic function (frequency of discharge $f = k + a \log S$, where k and a are constants and S is a measure of the stimulus magnitude). During the past decade considerable significance has been attached to the observation that a close fit between the frequency of discharge and stimulus amplitude often can be obtained by using a power function ($f = kS^n$), with an exponent less than or equal to one (the latter converting it to a linear function[67,68,106,107]. Mountcastle[108] has suggested that it is possible to infer features of the neural mechanisms operating on sensory information from input–output data on sense organs and equivalent measurements on central neural activity or perception. On careful examination of evoked first-order neural activity and human perception using identical stimuli, work in his laboratory found similar power functions to fit both sets of results[67,106,108,111]; this has led to the hypothesis that the central processing of intensity information consists of linear operations since non-linear intermediary steps would be expected drastically to alter the quantitative relationship[108,111]. Scepticism about the hypothesis has surfaced for several reasons[109,110]:

(1) input–output curves change with slight manipulation of stimulus conditions;

(2) the exponent of power function most closely descriptive of results varies for different experimental conditions;

(3) disparate conclusions have been reached on the curve-fitting results[106,112,113].

To make the situation more complicated, a number of receptors change their transfer functions with time, probably as a result of adaptation, saturation or fatigue[12,110]. The concept of linear operation by central neural mechanisms associated with discriminative sensation is interesting and provocative, but in view of the doubts which have been expressed, more support is necessary before it can be given credence.

Discharge frequency can vary in more than one fashion and patterns of discharge theoretically could be important in conveying information. A pattern theory for coding the nature of the stimulus has been mentioned; although still occasionally defended, no direct experimental support for it has been mustered. On the other hand, there is evidence that the pattern of discharge is an important part of the signalling process for certain specialised receptors. The Pacinian corpuscle is activated by high-frequency components of mechanical events and while it is very sensitive to these, even greatly suprathreshold stimuli may evoke only one impulse. Repeated discharges from Pacinian corpuscles indicate multiple transients rather than increases in the amplitude of the signal[54,71,76,114,115], a feature which appears in certain ascending pathways excited by these receptors[118,119]. A special pattern of activity also emerges in the response of cutaneous thermoreceptors; at temperatures evoking maximal responses, they show grouping of discharges at relatively high frequencies separated by considerably longer intervals between bursts. According to Iggo[90] the number of impulses in each burst and the interval between successive bursts for cooling receptors indicates direction of temperature change and other information, not specified by average frequency. Probably other instances will be found in which discharge frequency by individual sensory elements is not the sole indicator of intensity or in which it signals a parameter other than intensity.

8.2.4.2 Population dynamics

The behaviour of the whole sense organ population must be considered in analyses of intensity and other features of sensory signalling. Differences in sensitivity exist among individuals of one receptor type, in part owing to variations in the sense organ itself. This variation is enhanced by differences in the distance between stimulating point and the receptive terminals and in the structural characteristics of the tissue surrounding them. Elasticity of muscle varies considerably from the central to the polar region and even at a given level owing to variations in the proportion of contractile to connective tissue elements. Similarly, the physical characteristics of the skin are not uniform, even for adjacent areas; the relatively thin hairy skin is softer and more pliant that nearby glabrous skin of the palm. Stresses set up by force against the integument over a bony protrusion are much different from the same force applied to skin over the belly of a large muscle. Therefore, the physical transmission of stimulus properties will cause variation in the response of otherwise identical elements.

Operation of these considerations can be illustrated by an example. The very lightest pressure applied to hairy skin by a blunt small object, just threshold for an immediately subjacent Type II unit, would evoke impulses in it alone. If the pressure increases, it will progressively distort the skin farther and farther away from the point of application; since Type II units are sensitive to stretch, the stronger stimuli will recruit into activity progressively more and more elements. Thus, in the case of a uniformly sensitive population, coding of the intensity of effective stimuli will be a function of the number of elements excited as well as the degree of activity within each element[41]. With moderate to strong stimuli, one can envision a population of active afferent units wherein the highest frequency of discharge appears in those located at the place of the stimulus application with progressively lesser activity as distance from this site increases. The picture will be modified by factors introduced from a lack of uniformity in characteristics of the skin as well as differences in the threshold or responsiveness of the individual elements making up the population. The fact that the messages about somatic stimuli ordinarily are represented by the activity of more than one element has long been recognised. Nonetheless, attempts to describe quantitatively population dynamics for particular sense organs has only been done in a limited number of situations; from what has just been said such an analysis obviously involves consideration of the physical nature of tissue and its effect upon the transmission of the stimuli as well as the distribution of attributes among the sensory elements[120-122].

So far, receptors have been considered from the viewpoint of differentiating or distinguishing stimuli. Receptor types may have considerable importance in indicating the level and/or intensity of stimuli. For example, the response of cutaneous cold receptors for a 5 °C increase in temperature when the temperature of the skin is below 20 °C is a decreased average frequency and a decreased number of impulses per burst[13]. If the starting temperature, on the other hand, is 30 °C, and 5 °C warming occurs, not only will there be a decrease (probably cessation) in activity of cold receptors but some warm units will begin to discharge. Consideration of a 5 °C warming step starting at 40 °C adds another facet: more warm receptor activity will appear and, as the skin temperature exceeds 42–44 °C, discharges will appear in some polymodal nociceptors. We do not know the use made of these shifting patterns in activity, which can be expected for mechanical as well as thermal stimuli; it appears likely that the information the population behaviour contains is utilised in central mechanisms leading to discriminative behaviour and modality appreciation. In summary, the signalling of intensity by the first order neurons has at least three facets: modulation in the frequency of activity of individual sensory elements, variations in the active ensemble consisting of one receptor type and variations in the mixture of activity of different receptor types.

8.3 CENTRAL PROJECTIONS OF PRIMARY AFFERENT NEURONS

8.3.1 Morphological considerations

8.3.1.1 Branching

Most primary afferent neurons divide after entering the spinal cord or brainstem[124,125]. The division may take place at or near the segmental level of entry, some distance away, or at several different levels. Both morphological and physiological evidence suggests that branches are smaller in diameter than the parent fibres. It is common for a division into a number of branches to occur as the fibre approaches its place of synaptic contact[124]. The Pacinian corpuscle may differ and represent an exception in not having major branches at the segmental level; its lack of branching is deducible from the absence of change of conduction velocity of the Pacinian primary fibre in its central passage and fits with the paucity of spinal reflex effects associated with its excitation[126-131].

We have only fragmentary and indirect information on a primary afferent fibre's total branches, although it certainly differs from one species of receptive unit to another. Estimates for cat muscle spindle Ia fibres are available from analyses of monosynaptic reflex connections. A single Ia afferent fibre of medial gastrocnemius distributes at least one excitatory terminal to each of the approximately 300 medail gastrocnemius moto-neurons and to about one-half of the roughly 400 synergistic motoneurons (lateral gastrocnemius and soleus)[132]. Branches of the same fibre to inhibitory pathways (destined for motoneurons supplying antagonistic muscles) and divisions ending upon neurons of Clarke's column (forming part of the dorsal spinal cerebellar projection)[151,163] must be added to those upon motoneurons. Thus, a Ia spindle primary fibre has more than 500 terminal branches. Whether this is typical for primary afferent fibres is not known; techniques of dye injection or radioactive labelling have recently evolved which conceivably could permit direct estimation of the distribution of all central connections[133,134].

8.3.1.2 Termination loci

On morphological grounds, incoming fibres are known to have systematic differences in the distribution of endings to different parts of spinal and medullary cellular complexes[124,125,136,137]. Edinger[138] and later Ranson[139-141] noted dorsal root fibres formed two bundles, a medially coursing group of thick (myelinated) fibres which pass through the lateral part of the dorsal column and a lateral bundle of thinner ones entering the dorsal horn directly. Ramon y Cajal[124] pointed out that certain thick (therefore medially entering) fibres have a branch which runs directly to the spinal ventral horn and synapses with motoneurons while other fibres terminate more superficially in the dorsal horn. We know that the former are la primary afferent fibres of the muscle spindle[99]. A similar specificity of termination has emerged for myelinated fibres of cutaneous mechanoreceptors to cells of the spinal dorsal horn[144] and for fine fibres to the marginal cells of the dorsal horn[142,143].

In addition to terminations made in the immediate vicinity of their spinal entry, dorsal root fibres also connect to neurons several (2–6) segments rostrally or caudally in arrangements representing the first stage of ascending pathways and/or local reflexes. In Ramon y Cajal's[124] diffuse reflex a primary afferent fibre is shown terminating upon interneurons which in turn end upon motoneurons of several segments. Lloyd[99] showed that the latter arrangement is the probable substrate for the flexor reflex. Flexor and other polysynaptic spinal reflexes are initiated by a variety of stimuli which also excite ascending pathways, leading to the view that some primary afferent units are common to flexor reflex pathways and to ascending systems (see also Section

8.2.3.2)[34,99,145,146]. We lack evidence for an arrangement wherein a spinal interneuron could serve both a reflex pathway and an ascending projection, although this is a possibility which must be considered. In any case, without information on a neuron's connectivity, it must be remembered that evocation of a response by somatic afferent input does not classify cells as part of a sensory system, a point which seems to have escaped some authors.

On cytoarchitectural considerations, Rexed[147] divided the spinal cord grey substance into a series of laminae. Subsequently, the laminar identification has provided a valuable terminology for specifying the location of cellular elements. Various patterns of connectivity between primary afferent fibres and laminae I–VI have been suggested[142,148-150]. Rexed's cytoarchitectural analysis was carried out on the cat; however, other workers have extended laminar terminology to the primate without experimental justification. Morphological considerations suggest that Rexed's original dorsal to ventral lamination scheme may not be readily applicable without modification[125].

Dorsal root fibres contribute terminals to certain nuclei considerably rostral to the entrance segments. Of major concern to us are those myelinated dorsal root fibres entering via the medial division of the dorsal root which have a branch passing rostrally through the dorsal columns to the gracilis and cuneate nuclei at the spinal cord–medulla oblongata junction. On the basis of anatomical studies, Glees and Soler[152] estimate that only about one-fifth of the fibres which enter the dorsal columns continue to the dorsal column nuclei. Many primary fibres connecting to other ascending systems such as the spinocervical and the ventrolateral spinal tracts also pass through the dorsal columns for a number of segments before terminating in synapses with second-order neurons[172a-c].

8.3.1.3 The nature of synaptic termination

Rethelyi and Szentagothai[125] have surveyed morphological evidence on the nature of synaptic contacts within segmental and special regions of termination such as Clarke's column; their description illustrates the diversity of synaptic terminations made by dorsal root fibres. At the same time, there is a paucity of information on the type of synapses associated with the fibres from specific sensory elements. With the exception of the Ia junction to Clarke's column cells, functional attributes of a primary afferent neuron have not been correlated to the morphology of its synaptic connections.

Reference will be made to specific synaptic morphology in the detailed discussions of synaptic stations along ascending pathways. General discussions of the ultramicroscopic features of synapses and differences in the kinds of synaptic contacts appear in reviews by Gray and Guillery[154] and by Bodian[155]. Prior to the era of electron microscopy, identification of synaptic action as excitation or inhibition on morphological grounds was highly tenuous, even though morphologists had postulated differences in synaptic significance for contacts on different parts of a neuron, i.e. axodendritic versus axosomatic. Morphological study of synaptic regions[156] added a new dimension and gained greatly in significance after 1966. In that year, Bodian[157,157a] and Hirata[158] differentiated two kinds of presynaptic terminals on the basis of the structure of the microvesicles, a differentiation which presumably correlated with different chemically acting synaptic agents. Chemically different substances raised the issue of excitation versus inhibition. Recognition of increasing complexity of the subsynaptic situation as ultramicroscopic analyses became better controlled and more systematised has led to a progression of ideas; the present situation has been succinctly summarised by Bodian[155].

8.3.1.4 Connections of primary afferent neurons

It is not known whether any primary afferent fibres solely serve ascending projections without contributing to segmental or regional mechanisms. At the moment, the only candidate for this kind of dedicated function is the Pacinian corpuscle and the evidence on it is not complete (see Section 8.3.1.1). In most cases, several neural systems receive inputs from each primary fibre. Multiplicity of function would favour caution in emphasising an effect to the exclusion of other, possibly masked, processes depending upon the same sense organs.

Considering the substantial interest in presynaptic modulation of afferent activity, it is important to know whether one primary afferent fibre makes synaptic contact with another. Primary fibre to primary fibre contact has been suggested on the grounds of a short latency dorsal root reflex after an afferent volley in adjacent fibres[153]. Such evidence is indirect and needs confirmation, particularly since the cited data has a marginal latency for an unequivocal monosynaptic connection.

Afferent fibres join the central nervous system in segmental sequence which have topographical relations and this lays the foundation for topographical patterns within the dorsal horn[125,159]. Topographical (somatotopographical) features also appear in the functional organisation of ascending sensory systems beginning with the dorsal horn[160]. Within the dorsal columns an initial segmental layering of afferent fibres, in which the more rostral segments are represented most laterally, undergoes systematic reorganisation in the rostral passage of the fibres into a regional or somatopic pattern[161,162,192].

One consequence of branching of primary afferent fibres is the diffusion of effect, labelled divergence[34]. Divergence, simply stated, is the distribution of the processes of a given neuron, i.e. primary afferent element, to more than one other neuron. Divergence in distributions to sensory nuclei seem to be the rule; the receptive fields of neurons forming ascending projections show overlap consistent with an overlapping input from primary units[159,164,165]. Divergence also follows from the branching of primary fibres in the dorsal columns since they terminate in different regions—some near the segmental entrance and others a number of segments away. Convergence was the term Sherrington[34] used to describe synaptic endings on a cell from several presynaptic neurons. In recent years, considerable attention has been paid to 'convergent systems'. In evaluating the concepts and evidence related to the latter designation, it must be borne in mind that several kinds of convergence may exist:

(1) Input to a central neuron from more than one type of primary afferent neuron, i.e. Pacinian corpuscle, polymodal nociceptor, etc.

(2) One can consider primary units in broader terms according to general functional criteria such as those signalling mechanical displacement, or mechanical movement, or thermal or noxious conditions. In this light, convergence could take place from the several receptor types without necessarily imparting multimodal characteristics to the postsynaptic cell. This is an obvious but rarely considered interpretation of response patterns obtained from electrical excitation of peripheral nerves. For example, a neuron with an input from afferent elements with special responsiveness to moving mechanical distortion (velocity), could receive excitation from afferent fibres of the largest (Aa) through the smallest (C) diameter groups.

(3) True multimodal convergence would consist of inputs from receptors of obviously different responsiveness to natural stimulation such as mechanoreceptors, thermoreceptors and nociceptors. There are numerous reports of segmental and suprasegmental neurons excited by this variety of somatosensory stimuli. It seems self-evident that convergence from receptors with widely differing responsiveness has different significance from that from a single type or a class with common functional attributes. Care in defining input is necessary to distinguish between the kinds of convergence.

8.3.2 Synaptic mechanisms

8.3.2.1 Postsynaptic excitation

There are very limited data on synaptic transmission between primary afferent (first order) neurons and projecting cells of ascending sensory systems. It is possible only to surmise the possible situations from information obtained in studies of other mammalian synapses.

A first question concerns the means by which synaptic action is accomplished. One possibility is electrical coupling between presynaptic and postsynaptic elements, an arrangement which at one time was seriously considered as the process underlying synaptic excitation and inhibition[166,167]. Electrical coupling fell out of favour with the avalanche of evidence for chemically mediated transmission, only to be demonstrated for certain synapses in the past decade (see review by Bennett[168]); electrical linkage between pertinent primary afferent fibres and central neurons has become a possibility deserving of serious consideration as a consequence of Wylie's[169] observations in the rat suggestive of electrotonic coupling between vestibular nerve fibres and neurons of the vestibular nuclei. Special extracellular pathways for current flow necessary for electrotonic transmission apparently are present in the synapses of some vestibular nerve fibres with cells of the lateral vestibular nucleus[170,171]. The reader interested in details of the morphological and the physiological characteristics typical of electrical and chemical synapses should consult Bennett's review[168].

The majority of synaptic contacts between primary afferent fibres and central nervous system cells are not of the type which is associated with electrotonic coupling elsewhere. This leads to the presumption that transmission to second-order somatosensory neurons usually occurs by means of a chemical intermediary. Chemical transmission commonly, if not always, has a quantal basis. The chemical agent transmitting activity between presynaptic terminals and postsynaptic membranes is released in unit packets; release of a number of packets is synchronised by the invasion of the presynaptic terminal by an impulse[172]. Evidence for quantal synaptic events has been accumulated for several central nervous system synapses in the absence of knowledge of the putative agent. Candidate substances for excitatory synaptic transmission by vertebrate dorsal root fibres include the amino acid L-glutamate as well as related compounds[173,174a,174b] and a polypeptide similar or identical to hypothalamic substance 'P'[174]. At least two substances have been suggested as mediators for inhibition in the vertebrate nervous system, glycine and γ-aminobutyric acid (GABA)[173], but there is no evidence suggesting inhibition at a synapse between primary fibres and second order neurons. It must be emphasised that up to the present, arguments presented in favour of particular mediators for any mammalian central synapses are open to legitimate dispute and even tentative identification is lacking for junctions of the somatosensory systems.

Convergence from different presynaptic sources has major influence on synaptic action. The duration of an excitatory or inhibitory process will be influenced both by the length of time that a given synaptic process, electrical or chemical, acts and by the arrival of impulses over different fibres. In other words, staggering of the arrival of impulses travelling over different presynaptic terminals or repetitive impulses over a given terminal can prolong the duration of synaptic action provided that the duration of synaptic action is greater than the interval between action potentials. Hunt and Kuno[180] showed that many spinal interneurons (cells other than dorsal or ventral root neurons) fire repetitively at frequencies up to $700 \, \text{sec}^{-1}$ to a single dorsal root volley; the repetitive discharge reflected a sequence of bombardment of the postsynaptic cell by temporally dispersed arrival of afferent activity. Postsynaptic discharge, of course, is governed by postsynaptic factors as well. Typically, spinal interneurons have smaller post-impulse (or post-spike) hyperpolarisations than motor neurons[180]; a small hyperpolarisation after an impulse would be expected to enhance the ability of excitatory postsynaptic potentials to trigger an impulse and would be consonant with repetitive discharge during a prolonged excitatory action. While intracellular studies have been done on only a limited sampling of cells of somatosensory pathways, extracellular analyses of activity at every level of the major ascending pathway have noted the common occurrence of high frequency repetitive discharge[181-185]. Until additional information is available we are forced to presume that features associated with repetitive discharge of spinal interneurons apply to specific sensory system neurons with the same behaviour. Other postsynaptic factors such as interconnections between neurons of a nucleus or other nuclei and recurrent excitation of an element of the type proposed by Lorente de No[186] may also be factors in the tendency for sensory system neurons to discharge repetitively.

8.3.2.2 Presynaptic inhibition

For two decades there has been a major interest in inhibition manifested presynaptically. Schmidt[191] has provided an extensive survey of the question; we shall comment on only part of the issues involved and refer the reader to his article for additional information and more extensive citations of original literature. In presynaptic inhibition, suppression of synaptic transmission or its consequences, such as reflex action, occurs by agents acting on presynaptic terminals without involvement of the postsynaptic cell's excitability. Presynaptic effects were suggested in 1938 by Barron and Matthews[187] as a possible mechanism for the suppression of a dorsal root to ventral root reflex evoked by stimulation of an adjacent dorsal root. Subsequently, Renshaw[175a] found that components of a response recorded with microelectrodes from within the spinal grey matter attributed to presynaptic elements could be suppressed by stimulation of primary afferent fibres. The formal suggestion that inhibition can take place by blocking of activity in primary afferent fibres was made by Howland, Lettvin, McCulloch, Pitts and Wall in 1955[175]. The concept received a major impetus when Frank and Fuortes[176] described depression of a monosynaptically generated excitatory postsynaptic potential without an accompanying change of membrane conductance. The implications of the latter observation were grasped by Eccles and his associates, who provided much data on the subject. Eccles and Malcolm[177] had already postulated that block of conduction in primary afferent fibres could be produced by a depolarisation initiated in the synaptic region. Eccles and Krnjevic[178] showed that activity in one set of primary afferent fibres could evoke a depolarisation in the intraspinal portion of other primary fibres. This correlated well with Wall's[196] 1958 demonstration of increases in the excitability of primary afferent fibres with a time course parallel to a dorsal cord (positive) and dorsal root (negative) potentials. These observations were followed by a spate of publications correlating negative dorsal root potentials, changes in presynaptic excitability and inhibitory effect (see review by Eccles[197]). In essence the concept which has evolved argues that primary afferent fibres may be depolarised by means of axo–axonic synapses[179] near the fibre's termination upon a second-order cell. In a fibre so depolarised, conduction may be blocked (cathodal block); however, more likely, the terminal would still conduct an action potential of decreased amplitude. Recordings made close to presynaptic terminals confirm that the peak or reversal of the action potential takes place at nearly the same level regardless of the initial polarisation of the fibre and in depolarised fibres the overall amplitude of the conducted potential is smaller. In this concept of presynaptic modulation, transmitter release in a chemically mediated synaptic action from a primary afferent terminal is assumed to be positively correlated with the swing of the potential during an impulse. Eccles, Kostyuk and Schmidt[188] showed that polarisation of the spinal cord, modulating the terminal's transmembrane potential, produced the expected changes in excitatory synaptic action. More direct evidence on a presynaptically determined decrease in excitatory transmitter release has come from estimations of the quantal release of excitatory agents at the crayfish neuromuscular junction by Dudel and Kuffler[189] and at the mammalian motor neuron by Kuno[190]. In a number of instances in both vertebrate and invertebrate nervous systems, a reasonably convincing argument in favour of presynaptic inhibitory action has been gathered; however, the organisation of the presynaptic input and how it fits into integrated activity or the functional arrangements of the afferent systems remains an open issue.

Initially, presynaptic inhibition of transmission by primary fibres seemed ubiquitous. Cutaneous afferent input was reported to depress transmission from many types of cutaneous afferent fibres and widespread presynaptic effects were described on the input from muscle receptors by Ib fibres of the Golgi tendon organs. These results came from experiments in which afferent volleys in nerves or dorsal roots, generated by electrical stimulation, interacted with similarly evoked volleys from other nerves; even if volleys are restricted to a given size range of afferent fibres, they represent considerable mixing of receptor characteristics. Less diffuse effects emerged when physiological stimulation of receptors was substituted for electrically initiated volleys. It now appears that one pattern of presynaptic action on the termination of cutaneous receptors represents inhibition initiated by activation of similar receptors in nearby regions of the skin[131,198].

Many studies have used only dorsal root potentials to judge presynaptic interactions. Even when a more direct test, the excitability of primary afferent terminals, was employed the magnitude of the effect upon synaptic transmission was not ascertained. As Kellerth[199] has pointed out, indirect measurement of presynaptic inhibition makes comparison with powerful postsynaptically mediated actions difficult. Even greater difficulties are encountered when attempts are made to assess the place of presynaptic effects upon primary or other neurons of ascending sensory systems originating from higher centres[191]. While it is clear that presynaptic modulation of afferent transmission is important, insight on its organisational significance is also hampered by the heavy reliance on results obtained by electrical stimulation of afferent fibres or descending pathways.

Wall[200] and Schmidt[191] have suggested that the presynaptic effects on primary afferent fibres are part of mechanisms controlling sensory input to the central nervous system; Schmidt[191] proposes that presynaptic interactions are required by the tonic background discharge of afferent fibres which, when combined with specifically induced activity, might overload the transmission systems conveying information to rostral parts of the brain. This proposition, while seemingly reasonable, may be based upon a faulty assumption; in the absence of external stimuli there is remarkably little activity in much of the primary afferent spectrum. The notable exceptions are the Group Ia and II fibres from muscle spindles, the Type II cutaneous receptor and cutaneous thermal receptors. Observations made using natural stimuli suggest that presynaptic inhibitory effects are more finely focused than this global view implies and with the possible exception of the muscle spindle input, could act within populations of afferent neurons signalling common features of stimuli to discriminate against marginally excited elements. Only further experimentation will help decide between these proposals.

8.3.2.3 Spinal 'gates'

Presynaptic action may be tonic as well as phasic[191]. That is, a given set of primary terminals may be constantly bombarded by a depolarising input from other neurons. This could cause a persisting depression of the terminal's liberation of transmitter at the time of action potentials. If the neurons producing tonic presynaptic depolarisation are themselves depressed or inhibited, the membrane potential at the presynaptic terminal would increase, enhancing transmitter release with impulses, i.e. disinhibition. The concept of disinhibition came into prominence in association with Melzack and Wall's[38] theory about mechanisms operating in systems leading to pain. Melzack and Wall proposed a presynaptic control of afferent input by neurons of the substantia gelatinosa; the control of afferent activity was postulated to act as a switch or gate in the connection to projection neurons. The gate theory still has considerable popularity in spite of the fact that its crucial assumptions have been refuted. It was presumed that there were no primary afferent units responding in a particular way to pain-causing or noxious stimuli; there now is much evidence that such receptors do exist (Section 8.2.3.1 and Table 8.2). In the original construction, the gate mechanism was presumed to be dependent upon the balance of activity in large diameter and small diameter fibres, the former adapting rapidly and the latter slowly to maintained stimuli. This relation between afferent fibre diameter and adaptation rate has no basis in fact (Section 8.2.3.1). It was also assumed that small fibre activity, particularly from the unmyelinated fibres, would disinhibit or block presynaptic depolarisation of large-diameter afferent fibres. Suppression of tonic presynaptic inhibitory action should cause increases, in afferent fibre polarisation which should be manifest as a positive dorsal root potential. Positive dorsal root potentials do occur[201,202]. Mendell and Wall[203] reported positive root potentials to pure C fibre volleys, but their observation has been challenged by others on the basis of results with both electrically induced afferent volleys[204,205] and adequate (natural) stimulation of C fibres[206,408]. The weight of evidence now favours the view that volleys restricted to small diameter cutaneous afferent fibres primarily evoke presynaptic depolarisation of other afferent fibres. Gating or switching at the spinal level in sensory systems related to pain has retained favour in part owing to clinical evidence suggesting that selective stimulation of the dorsal columns or large diameter fibres in peripheral nerve can lead to amelioration of pathological pain[208,209]. Such stimulation, of course, could produce activity interacting at synaptic stations other than those at spinal levels and its value as a therapeutic measure needs the seasoning of time.

8.3.2.4 Postsynaptic inhibition

The mechanisms of postsynaptic inhibition have been ably reviewed by Eccles[197], Otsuka[173] and Schmidt[191]; the latter has given it special attention from the standpoint of the ascending somatosensory systems. In brief, the common features of postsynaptic inhibitory mechanisms are conductance changes in the postsynaptic neuron brought about by chemical synaptic mediators. These conductance changes hyperpolarise the cell or shunt excitatory synaptic potentials, decreasing the effectiveness of excitatory action.

Postsynaptically mediated inhibition is widespread in ascending sensory systems and probably represents a major means for controlling and modulating the subsequent effects of sensory input. Various patterns of inhibitory interaction exist at different synaptic stations; examples will be given when particular regions are discussed. It has the advantage over presynaptic inhibition at the primary afferent neuron level of acting after afferent messages have entered the central nervous system; in this situation the sensory impulses would be registered prior to being suppressed or extinguished in favour of activity generated by other inputs. At junctions between some first-order and second-order neurons, interactions take place between excitatory and inhibitory projections resulting in surround or adjacent area inhibition; the inhibitory actions are probably postsynaptic in part[191,228], although the organisation of presynaptic inhibition as presently understood at the sequential level could also favour development of a surround pattern. In essence, surround inhibition describes the arrangement in which afferent neurons with terminals in the centre of the receptive field are excitatory and those innervating tissues around the peripheral excitatory zone are inhibitory to a central neuron. The importance of inhibition of the surround type in somatosensory projections was called to attention by the work of Mountcastle and Powell[454].

8.4 METHODS AND APPROACHES

The variety of techniques which have been used to gain information on central portions of the somatosensory system make it appropriate to provide a brief critical commentary on methodology since an interpretation of an investigation and the impact of its conclusions depend upon them. Following tradition we have classified experimental procedures as anatomical, physiological and behavioural (the latter to include clinical data), although some of the earliest work combined approaches.

8.4.1 Anatomical methods

Important morphological features of somatosensory systems include
  (1) the constituent neuronal types and the arrangement of their processes;
  (2) the origin, arrangement and types of incoming fibres;
  (3) the synaptic organisation upon and between the neurons in question and
  (4) the destination of the efferent or projection fibres from a group of cells.
As might be expected, no one technique has been able to provide a complete picture of these factors.

8.4.1.1 *Light* versus *electron microscopy*

The electron microscope has proven a particularly powerful tool for the analysis of neural structures and the information it provides has revolutionised thinking on synaptic structures and organisation. Recently, it has also been of great value in tracing neural connectivity through its ability to indicate changes associated with degeneration. In the eyes of some observers, the power of the electron microscope has decreased the value of studies based upon light microscopy. This is an unrealistic judgement. The very advantage that electron microscopy gains, in terms of the high magnification, causes problems in terms of the extent of tissue which can be surveyed. It takes hundreds of serial sections at the thickness necessary for good electron microscopic resolution (fractions of a micron) to cover the extent of a single, medium-sized neuron. Effective use of the electron microscope frequently is a problem in sampling; survey of widely dispersed processes or terminations becomes nigh impossible unless there is firm guidance from lower power analyses using the light microscope. The ideal province of the electron microscope is the study of synaptic termination and ultrastructure of the neuron; it can help trace longer pathways provided that its high-power window is appropriately aimed. On the other hand, our present understanding of neural connectivity has such gaps that use of procedures based upon light microscopy still can be expected to provide major information.

8.4.1.2 *Characterisation of cells*

The classic way of examining neural tissue and characterising its cells is to stain the cell's surface or cytoplasmic inclusions with materials and dyes. The Golgi procedure and its variations have been primary tools in describing the cellular outline; in brief, the method impregnates neurons with silver salts so that cells stand out as more or less opaque structures. The importance of careful Golgi work is dramatically emphasised by the accomplishments of Ramon y Cajal[124] who, in about two decades ending in 1909, had assembled a body of knowledge about the structural arrangements of the vertebrate central nervous system which is being extended only gradually and painfully. A good Golgi preparation impregnates much, if not all, of a cell so that the extent of the neuronal processes, their general dimensions and orientation can be appreciated. A major failing of Golgi methods is that at the best they are capricious; not all cell types can be stained adequately, and not all processes of a cell may take up the metallic salts. In addition the procedure works best in immature animals and only lately has been employed successfully on adult nervous systems. The range of the Golgi method has recently been extended by combining it with electron microscopy[193,210,211,586].

Staining with aniline dyes is another traditional method for studying the distribution of different cell types — their size and, to some extent, the shape of cell bodies. Stains such as cresyl violet and thionin have the virtue of being reliable and easy to use, although in some preparations they do not permit ready differentiation of small neurons from glial cells.

Some newer techniques have considerable potential in terms of elucidating morphological particulars of chosen neurons. In one arrangement physiological measures are used for the intracellular localisation of the tip of a microelectrode from which the fluorescing dye, procion yellow, is iontophoretically passed. The dye then migrates or is transported throughout the cell, filling dendritic and axonic processes; when exposed to short-wavelength light, procion yellow fluoresces brilliantly and in thick sections or whole mounts provides striking pictures of a cell's geometry and extension. Procion brown, a non-fluorescing stain, may be used in light and electron microscopic studies in a similar fashion[212]. Intracellularly applied dyes have found their greatest success as morphological tools in invertebrate preparations, although the technique has been made to work for the mammalian motor neuron[133]. Fundamentally, the same approach may be used with radioactive compounds, particularly amino acids labelled with tritium (^{3}H) or ^{14}C. Localised or intracellular application (pressure injection or iontophoretic) of ^{3}H-labelled amino acids provides a radioactive substrate which is incorporated into protein (minutes to hours) and subsequently transported to processes of the cells by one of the several phases of intracellular flow[213,214]. The tissue is then handled in ordinary histological fashion and sections are coated with a photographic emulsion for autoradiography. Autoradiograms prepared in such a fashion can provide substantial information on the geometry of the cell and represents a powerful new tool for tracing connections (see Section 8.4.1.3). Autoradiograms may be examined by both light and electron microscopy; in the latter they can be used to identify specific synaptic architecture in normal tissue.

8.4.1.3 Pathway tracing

A number of questions may be asked about the more distant connections of neurons.

(1) Where do cells of a particular area project?

(2) Where does a particular pathway terminate?

(3) What are the sources of afferent input to a particular neuronal area?

(4) Where do the cell bodies of a particular fibre or fibre tract originate?

Either the Golgi or other staining of neurons can be helpful in identifying local connections. Silver staining of fibres in normal tissue (Cajal and Bielschowsky methods) were tools of the earlier anatomists. Analyses utilising maturation or myelination of tracts are not as important at the moment as at times in the past, although historically such approaches have provided valuable insights.

Two principles underlie the more important of the current methods for answering the above questions for longer pathways. In one case, the neuron's reaction to injury is used to identify either the cells of origin or the course of certain fibres. The second technique, the transport of substances along the processes of a cell, has already been alluded to.

(a) *Orthograde degeneration*—Until 1950 the Marchi method was the standard procedure for tracing a neural pathway by detecting orthograde degenerative changes in fibres separated from their parent soma. The Marchi procedure is based upon osmium staining of degenerating myelin and, therefore, is valid only for following myelinated fibres. The methods pioneered by Glees and Nauta employ silver solutions to impregnate degenerating axons and with variations can be used to distinguish terminals as well. In particular, Nauta-type methods have proven reliable and are more general than the Marchi since they also stain the axon cylinder so that both myelinated and unmyelinated tracts may be followed. Neuroanatomical data has blossomed as a consequence of the introduction of these silver staining methods (see review by Heimer[215]).

Electron microscopic views of degenerating nerve processes are distinctive and add another dimension to methods based upon light microscopy. Comparison of electron micrographs of normal terminals and terminals undergoing orthograde degeneration allow not only a reliable marker of a region of termination but also the location of synaptic site and the probable nature of synaptic contact.

(b) *Retrograde methods*—The traditional retrograde reaction is observed in Nissl preparations; in systems like spinal motor neurons or the geniculate-striate projections, retrograde changes provide relatively unambiguous information on the cells of origin of certain fibres. Unfortunately, retrograde changes are not readily recognised in all cells with Nissl staining, particularly those in which the cell bodies are small. In addition, neurons with projections to two quite different regions may not show the reaction to injury when only one is divided. In some cases, it may be possible that changes interpreted as retrograde in origin may have been orthograde and transynaptic[216]. Grant[217] showed that retrograde changes can also be demonstrated using Nauta preparations and that this method has potential use in tracing long dendritic as well as axon processes.

8.4.1.4 Techniques based upon transport of substances

Reference has already been made to the autoradiographic procedures based upon the incorporation of tritiated amino acids into the proteins of a cell. The power and advantages of this technique has recently been emphasised by Cowan *et al.*[218] and Barrett, Cook, Ledburg, Zucker and Whitlock[134]. Lesions used to produce degeneration reactions often interrupt fibres of passage or terminal fibres in addition to cells or processes under specific scrutiny, making interpretation of the results difficult. In contrast, the labelled amino acids are apparently picked up only by the cell in the immediate vicinity of its nucleus and not by extended processes such as axons. This means that accidental labelling of nearby fibres originating from other cells is minimal and the course of processes emanating from particular cell bodies may be analysed.

A new and interesting method is based upon the observation that a large particle such as horseradish peroxidase may be picked up by the terminals of an axon and antidromically transported back to the cell body[219,221-223]. LaVail and LaVail[220] demonstrated the potential of this method by histochemically staining the peroxidase which had been transported to the regions of cell bodies in visual pathways of chick embryos. Originally it was thought that the horseradish peroxidase was transported only retrogradely and had value as a unique antidromic marker; however, at least in some systems it may be moved both in the retrograde and orthograde direction[224,225].

8.4.2 Physiological methods

Investigations based upon functional attributes of neuronal systems also can provide information on the origin and destination of particular neurons or aggregates of neurons and fibre pathways they contribute to; however, in addition, they can reliably distinguish between the two major classes of neuronal effect, excitation and inhibition. Separation of the latter on the basis of morphological considerations has heretofore been debatable even under the best circumstances[155]. Physiological studies of neuronal activity can provide information on the possible functional significance of particular pathways in that the nature of stimuli necessary for activation can be correlated to those provoking particular sensations of behavioural reactions (see Section 8.4.3). Finally, electrophysiological procedures have a unique ability to trace pathways through several neurons in a chain and rapidly establish connectivity. Several kinds of question about somatosensory pathways may be answered by physiological methods:

(1) Does a process of a given neuron(s) extend between one point and another?

(2) Is the effect of a given presynaptic fibre upon a postsynaptic element excitatory or inhibitory?

(3) What kinds of stimuli or what kinds of sense organs activate the neurons or pathway under consideration?

(4) What kinds of transformations take place between peripheral input or prior neural activity and postsynaptic activity? In other words, how is the information being manipulated or coded?

8.4.2.1   The single neuron

Electrical recording of impulses in single neurons now has a history of approximately 50 years. Criteria for establishing electrical recordings of extracellular action potentials as coming from individual elements were set down in 1926 by Adrian and Zotterman's[42] pioneering work on impulses in peripheral fibres, and have been repeatedly confirmed since then by electrical recordings with microelectrodes from the central nervous system[183,226]. Electrical recordings can be used to establish that a given single cell has a process (or processes) between a point of excitation (usually single electric shocks) and the recording loci and has proven particularly useful for tracing projection of a neuron whose orthograde activation can also be analysed. Continuity of a single neuron is usually presumed if the element can respond to repetitive stimulation of several hundred times per second in a one to one fashion without the small variations in latency of response typical for transynaptic excitation.

8.4.2.2 Evoked responses

Early physiological analyses of the somatosensory systems employed gross recordings of evoked potentials. A peripheral stimulus such as natural activation of cutaneous sense organs was found by Marshall, Woolsey and Bard (see Bard[227]) to elicit an electrical transient recordable only from a limited portion of the cerebral cortical surface. Use of evoked potentials has provided a body of knowledge about major projections in the somato-sensory system; the extension of the evoked potential technique to recordings from single neurons ('units') has provided insight into not only excitatory but also inhibitory pathways. One problem with the evoked potential method is that without additional procedures or information it is impossible to be sure of the pathway by which the activity reaches the recording locus. In addition, evoked potential recordings may not be capable of indicating the complexity of the neuronal chain carrying activity from the place of stimu-lation to the point of recording, particularly for slowly conducting afferent systems.

8.4.2.3 Afferent input

The validity of information provided by electrophysiological recordings in sensory pathways is dependent not only upon the nature of the recording process but also on appropriateness of the initiating stimuli. This is an especially important consideration when electrical excitation is used to generate afferent activity from either peripheral nerves or central nervous system structures. Electrical excitation provides a precision of timing which may prove valuable in demonstrating a connection or in analysing features of synaptic function. At the same time it cannot be too strongly emphasised that electrical excitation of any neural tissue, including peripheral nerve, throws into activity an artificial combination of neural elements which may never occur under natural conditions. Since afferent input evokes inhibition as well as excitation, one possible pitfall in using electrical excitation is that a combination of excitatory and inhibitory activity could mask a response. Still another possible problem is that unnatural synchronous activation of neuronal elements may initiate activity of exaggerated proportions.

8.4.3 Behavioural approaches

Combining a behavioural observation with other measures or procedures has provided much of our knowledge on somatosensory function. It represents the only means for placing the functional significance of neuronal groups or mechanisms into perspective. We can classify as behaviourally based, the results obtained through human communication about sensation and in disease, in addition to experiments man performs on animals using learned or unlearned motor reactions as an indicator.

8.4.3.1   Deficits from lesions

No better justification for a technique can be given than its success in providing a major understanding. A beginning appreciation of specificity in neural pathways for somatic sensation came from Schiff's[229] testing of the effects of spinal injury by an animal's reaction to manipulation of its body below the level of the injury. Unfortunately, this historically established procedure has also been the source of misconceptions about the functional role of different structures and pathways in somesthesis. The difficulty is akin to that which would be encountered in trying to deduce operating principles of an internal combustion engine from observing the effects of removing parts while it was running. The point is that deficits show not the function of the injured (missing) part but the functional capabilities of the remaining apparatus. Moreover, the practical problems of either producing destruction of a single structure or pathway in animal investigations or finding well-defined injuries in the experiments nature performs upon man add to the difficulties. The result of even circumscribed and appropriate lesions may be related to the inevitable mixture of neuronal populations at particular loci as well as processes (fibres) only passing through.

Similar difficulties arise when artificial stimulation of nerves or brain are used in studies with behavioural endpoints as are found in those employing evoked potentials:

(1) the end result may be attributed to the wrong elements of a mixture;

(2) the effect may be related to processes in the vicinity rather than somata resident in the region stimulated;

(3) one effect may dominate or mask others important in more physiological functioning.

The plasticity of the vertebrate nervous system poses yet another problem. An endpoint requiring complex neural processing after the input may show change with time after lesions or other manipulations[230].

8.4.3.2   Appropriateness of tests for sensory capacity

Common sense suggests that a behavioural test must be closely attuned to normal function if it is to be a reliable measure of modifications in a system's operation. For instance, withdrawal of the hind quarters or flick of an animal's tail upon a mechanical contact or burning heat is a poor indicator of mechanisms for the sensation of pain, yet such tests are employed for this purpose. It should be obvious that somatic stimuli can produce reactions through linkages in the spinal cord or other lower centres without engagement of rostral parts of the brain more closely related to perception. In another instance, it may be appropriate to test for 'touch' sensation by contacting skin with the blunt end of a pencil, but this does not properly evaluate somesthetic capacities coming into play when size and movement are appreciated. Meaningful correlations between neural systems and their significance in sensation will appear only when the behavioural questions, methods of stimulation and manipulations of the neural apparatus are carefully chosen for suitability. However difficult this may be, it is possible and we shall cite studies which have employed ingenious methods for insuring that a behavioural response is closely related to a process akin to a human sensory experience. In other work behaviour dependent on quantitative distinctions of stimulus parameters has been and will continue to be crucial for ultimately linking neural structures and measures to somatic sensation.

8.5 ASCENDING SOMATOSENSORY SYSTEMS

Classification of a system of neurons as part of the somatosensory apparatus is not simple. Primary afferent neurons engage neurons whose function is other than conveying afferent information to rostral centres. How can one decide whether or not a given series of connections and the pathway they form represent an ascending projection system? At the present time there are no incisive guidelines. One is forced to fall back on multiple and occasionally vague criteria, a fact that undoubtedly contributes to confusion and controversy. It has been appreciated for many years that there are groups of neurons whose processes form well-defined central tracts which ascend from segmental levels to suprasegmental structures. Moreover, certain of these pathways contain inputs from afferent fibres of many segments and, therefore, major portions of the body. The tradition of labelling such projections as major ascending somatosensory projections appears reasonable. Excluding those destined for the cerebellum, an anatomical treatise of two decades ago would have listed two pathways of spinal origin as somatosensory, the dorsal column–medial lemniscal projection and the spinothalamic tract. These two pathways are still considered major routes for somatosensory information; they are sometimes referred to as oligosynaptic or 'direct', since some of their thalamic terminations are from second order cells, i.e. after a single synapse. 'Indirect' pathways are those considered to involve more neurons and more synapses. We know now that there are problems with implications of the direct–indirect concept. Some complex pathways actually are capable of conveying information from sense organs of both skin and deep somatic structures more rapidly to the forebrain than the 'direct' systems; moreover, portions of both 'direct' systems include connections to the diencephalon involving more than two neurons and one synapse.

We shall first take up ascending pathways passing rostrally in the dorsal half of the spinal cord, the dorsal column–medial lemniscal system and two more recently established routes, the spino–cervicothalamic and the spino–medullothalamic (via nucleus Z) pathways. The two known pathways of the ventrolateral portions of the spinal cord, the spinothalamic and the spino–reticulothalamic projections, will then be dealt with. Following this, the major thalamic regions and the cerebral cortical areas closely associated with somatosensory activity will be discussed. Consideration of the thalamic and cortical somatosensory receiving areas separate from discussion devoted to ascending systems was more than a dictate of convenience. Our enlarging understanding of the interrelations between thalamic and cortical regions suggests considerable functional interaction at these higher levels between inputs ascending via different pathways. This makes it unlikely that activities of particular thalamic or cortical regions are fully dedicated to afferent messages transmitted by any particular ascending chain of neurons.

A diagrammatic representation of the pathways to be discussed is given in Figure 8.2 (p. 384) and may prove helpful in following the text.

8.5.1   Pathways of the dorsal spinal cord

The dorsal column, spinocervical and nucleus Z pathways pass rostrally in the dorsal half of the spinal cord, have principally an ipsilateral input and have synaptic transfers close to the spinal cord's junction with the medulla lemniscus.

8.5.1.1 The dorsal column system

The traditional view of the dorsal column pathway was that it consisted of the ascending branches of primary afferent fibres which course rostrally to synapse on cells of the dorsal column nuclei; the latter's axons cross as the internal arcuate fibres to form the medial lemniscus. The only termination of the medial lemniscus in the classical picture was the ventral postero-lateral nucleus of the thalamus contralateral to the dorsal column fibres. As a corollary, the input to cells of the dorsal column nuclei forming the medial lemniscus was conceived to originate solely from myelinated fibres of dorsal root neurons. Dorsal column fibres derived from spinal cord cells[231] were believed to represent intraspinal (propriospinal) connections. We shall consider modifications that new observations impose on these traditional ideas on the dorsal column system and its projections.

(a) *The dorsal columns*—The primary afferent component of the dorsal column consists of some relatively fine myelinated fibres (under 25 m sec^{-1} in peripheral nerve), as well as the larger diameter fibres usually attributed to it[126]. The descending branch of primary afferent fibres in the dorsal column is often also not given due attention; it may contribute importantly to the input to second order cells of ascending pathways and its presence will be reflected in the dorsal column composition. As we have already mentioned and shall point out again, the dorsal columns include dorsal root fibres passing only to rostral spinal levels. In 1968 Uddenberg[234] added a new facet by reporting that a number of deeply located fibres of the cuneate tract as high as the first cervical segment differed from primary afferent fibres by (1) responding with repetitive discharge to a single peripheral afferent volley, (2) not responding in a one to one fashion at stimulation frequencies expected for primary fibres, and (3) responding to volleys in more than one peripheral nerve. These were all consistent with recordings from elements postsynaptic to the primary fibre. By using Uddenberg's criteria and in addition variations in latency of the evoked response, a number of postsynaptic fibres of the gracilis fasciculus were shown to reach the level of the dorsal column nuclei[235,236]. At the lower thoracic level about 10% of gracilis fibres were of postsynaptic origin and most could be antidromically excited from the first cervical segment by electrical stimulation of the dorsal column[236]. Evidence has been presented for an excitatory input to these postsynaptic fibres from both mechanoreceptors of low threshold and high threshold (nociceptive) receptors with unmyelinated afferent fibres[236]. Rustioni[237,238] has demonstrated that postsynaptic dorsal column fibres terminate synaptically on cells of the dorsal column nuclei by both light and electron microscopic degeneration techniques. These postsynaptic fibres possibly originate from cells of laminae III to VI [239]. Thus, the dorsal columns are composed not only of ascending and descending branches from large-diameter primary afferent fibres and propriospinal bundles but also contain a significant number of ascending branches from spinal cord cells.

Ascending fibres in the dorsal columns of dorsal root origin are arranged according to body region. The medial bundle (fasciculus gracilis) is composed of branches from dorsal root ganglion cells from segments below the mid thoracic region while the laterally located cuneate fasciculus contains fibres from upper thoracic and cervical segments. Studies based upon Marchi degeneration uncovered a segmental grouping of fibres within the dorsal columns with the most caudal segments being represented most medially and the most rostral segment lying lateral, closest to the root entrance zone[240a]. Kuhn's[242] electrophysiological analysis of recordings made from small groups of dorsal root fibres suggested that a laminar segmental arrangement was an oversimplification; he proposed that the organisation of the incoming primary fibres was regional in which the grouping of fibres was made on the basis of input from small overlapping regions rather than whole segmental dermatomes. Recently, results of extensive recordings from single elements of the dorsal column have offered data reconciling the morphological and electrophysiological evidence in demonstrating a systematically changing composition in the dorsal columns with progression rostrally from the root entrance; the change consists of a resorting of the segmental arrangement into a somatotopic pattern[161,243]. Along with the somatotopic resorting, the population of afferent fibres in the dorsal column also alters in the progression from the segmental root entrance to the level of the dorsal column nuclei. The most recent evidence for the latter comes from recordings of single fibres of either the dorsal columns or peripheral nerves with intact connections peripherally (the receptive terminals) and rostrally (upper cervical levels)[126,245] This method permits testing of both the receptive characteristics of the unit by various kinds of natural stimuli and the projection of its afferent fibre by electrical excitation of the dorsal columns[126,233]. Table 8.3, taken from Petit and Burgess[126], compares a population of afferent units recorded from the sural nerve of cats to the fraction found projecting to cervical levels of the dorsal columns. Note the relative dominance of receptors particularly responsive to moving stimuli — such as the G1 and G2, field, Pacinian corpuscle and tap — which reach the upper levels of the cord. Burgess and Clark[64] used the same technique to examine the projection of knee joint receptors in the dorsal column and found, in startling contrast to standard textbook descriptions, that very few joint receptors (10% or less of a particular

Table 8.3   Dorsal column projection of 828 sural receptors*

Receptor type	% of sural sample	% of peripherial primary afferent fibres found at cervical level
G₁ hair	12.8	96
G₂ hair	8.7	78
D hair	15.7	2
Type I	18.8	0
Type II	10.2	100
Field	12.4	79
Pacinian Corpuscle	4.1	100
Tap	1.9	67
High-threshold	13.0	0
Insensitive Hair	1.6	100
Subcutaneous	0.6	33

* Modified from Petit and Burgess[126]. Courtesy of the American Physiological Society

nerve) have a primary afferent fibre extending the full length of the dorsal column. Moreover, those joint receptors with long dorsal column fibres consisted exclusively of elements responsive to movement and not position, i.e. in traditional nomenclature, they were rapidly adapting. The predominance of cutaneous elements in the primary fibres of the dorsal column projection to the dorsal column nuclei is emphasised in another way for the monkey by Table 8.4, constructed from Whitsel, Petrucelli, Sapiro and Ha's[161] data; it illustrates the decrease in the proportion of dorsal column fibres excited by subcutaneous structure at rostral levels compared to the root entrance region, not differentiating between primary afferent and post-synaptic units. These newer observations are consistent with the pattern of projection of Group I afferent fibres of hindlimb muscles, the majority of which terminate by the midthoracic level[232]. A complete sampling of the dorsal root spectrum is yet to be done; nevertheless, the existing data are

Table 8.4*

Location of receptive field	Number of units studied		Proportion of 'skin'		Proportion 'deep' units	
	at L6	at Cl—C4	L6	Cl—C4	L6	Cl—C4
Tail	105	81	83%	100%	17%	0%
Leg	428	108	22%	94%	78%	6%
Ankle-foot	247	56	70%	98%	30%	2%

* Compiled from Whitsel, Petrucelli and Sapiro[192]

consistent with the concept that the rostral projections of the funiculus gracilis are dominated by a cutaneous input, particularly that associated with responses to movements or transients.

(b) *Dorsal column nuclei (DCN)*—One may consider the dorsal column nuclei as rostrally located spinal cord gray matter inasmuch as they receive synaptic terminals from dorsal root fibres. The medially-located gracilis (Goll) nucleus receives its principal input from lower thoracic and more caudally located segments while the laterally located cuneate (Burdach) nucleus receives its primary afferent input from more rostral levels. Experimental anatomical analyses have shown that incoming fibres to both the gracilis and cuneate nuclei are distributed in sagitally oriented laminae representing a systematic progression of body areas[240]. The older literature presumed that the ascending afferent input was strictly from primary afferent fibres. As pointed out above, postsynaptic dorsal column fibres terminate in the dorsal column nuclei[237]. In addition to a primary afferent and a non-primary afferent input via the dorsal columns, there is evidence that the dorsolateral funiculus also feeds synaptically terminating fibres to the DCN[237,238,246-249]. Most of the dorsal lateral fasciculus fibres terminate in the rostral portions of both the gracilis and cuneate nuclei[237,238,248]. The functional significance of the dorsolateral fasciculus and the non-primary input to the dorsal column is not yet clear; however, it suggests that previously accepted ideas on the place in sensation of the dorsal columns, the dorsal column nuclei and their projections must be reconsidered.

Information on cytoarchitectural details of the dorsal column nuclei largely comes from work on the cat, although there is enough confirmatory material from the primate to suggest a similar morphology. Kuypers and Tuerck[250] have provided the most complete picture of the DCN architecture by combining study of Golgi and Nissl material with results from degeneration experiments. They conclude that there are two main types of neurons in the dorsal column nuclei, a large round cell with a richly branching and bushy dendritic tree (cluster cells) and a medium-sized cell with varying shapes of somas characterised by long radiating dendrites (radiating cells). The first, or round cells, are present throughout the rostral–caudal extent of the nuclei but are most common in the middle dorsal portion where they appear in clusters. Radiating cells dominate in areas without clusters of round cells, although they are also found scattered between such clusters. Degeneration following dorsal root section was very heavy in patches among cell clusters and more diffusely spread in other areas. In addition, all cluster cells showed severe signs of retrograde degeneration after lesions of the medial lemniscus, while the radiating cells varied considerably in this regard; those of the rostral or ventral portions of the nucleus were largely unaffected. It should be noted that the absence of a retrograde degeneration reaction does not necessarily imply that a process in the medial lemniscus was not sectioned, since some cells do not show retrograde changes when only one of several branches of an axon are cut. Another piece of evidence consistent with the delineation between the cluster and radiating cells is the latter frequency in regions receiving input from non-primary fibres[237]. Although possible differences may exist between the gracilis and cuneate nuclei, other morphological studies have agreed with a rostral–caudal variation in the dorsal column distribution of round and of radiating cells[251-253]. It is possible that more than two types of cell are present in the primate DCN, with one being comparable with the round or cluster cells. The dorsal root input to the DCN in cat and monkey appear similar, although details of termination in the cluster areas might vary[254,255], possibly related to differences in the way the somatotopic organisation is reflected in the dorsal columns and in the ventroposterior nuclei of the thalamus. The spinal input terminates as both small and large boutons on the somatic and dendritic regions of neurons and as an axo–axonal connection to other spinal fibres[256-258]. Lesions of the somatosensory cerebral cortex produce degeneration principally of the small boutons making axo–dendritic connections[257].

(c) *Physiology of the dorsal column nuclei*—The patterns of convergence upon DCN cells have a number of facets. One feature concerns the distribution of receptive fields of the body exciting particular cells. The somatotopic organisation anticipated by the anatomically established laminae of first-order fibres[240 240a] was confirmed by Kruger, Siminoff and Witkovsky by the use of unitary recordings[259]. Superimposed upon somatotopy is another topographical arrangement in which neurons receiving input from receptors located distally on limbs have smaller peripheral receptive fields than those with a proximal limb or trunk input[228,259-261]. In addition to the relation to body region, receptive field size is related to the kind of primary afferent input[228]; cells receiving an input from only hair deflection receptors have considerably smaller receptive fields than those activated by slowly adapting mechanoreceptors of the skin proper. The excitatory hair receptor projection is associated with an inhibitory input from sense organs innervating a zone surrounding the excitatory receptive field[228]. The location of the cell within the rostral–caudal extent of the nuclei is a third factor in receptive field organisation; units with larger fields are the most common in the rostral regions[262-266].

Perl, Whitlock and Gentry[228] pointed out that the input of some DCN neurons is highly specific in terms of receptor type, observations generally confirmed and extended by Gordon and Jukes[264]. A number of feline gracilis cells are excited largely or exclusively by hair follicle receptors; another group receives excitatory input from contact receptors of the skin with little contribution from hair receptors; a third group's responses are dominated by vibration sensitive receptors of the Pacinian corpuscle type; and a limited number respond with a slowly adapting discharge to movement of the claws or distal digit joints. Each category gave indications of convergence from like receptors, but only the cells responding to contact of the skin clearly received an excitatory input from functionally different primary afferent units. Contact or touch cells respond not only to maintained skin pressure but also to heating, cooling, skin stretch and excitation of afferent fibres in deep nerves. Gracilis neurons driven by hair receptors have lateral or surround inhibition; it is conspicuously missing for neurons excited by skin contact. With information from subsequent work, some of the peculiarities of the response noted for the touch gracilis cells can be accounted for. The only cutaneous displacement mechanoreceptor whose axon runs the full length of the dorsal columns is the Type II (Table 8.4); some characteristics of the gracilis touch units can be attributed to an input from this type of element, including excitation by skin stretch and sudden cooling. The response to heating and the input from other than cutaneous elements could be related to excitatory terminations from the non-primary projections in the dorsal columns[236] or dorsolateral tract[267]. The information on functional attributes of the dorsal column nuclei has come from work on cat and rat; therefore, there is no physiological data which can be used to gain insight on the reported differences in the structure of the feline and primate nuclei.

In retrospect, the absence of elements specifically responsive to joint movement in the dorsal columns[458] is consistent with the paucity of prominent effects on dorsal column nuclear cells from proximal joint receptors noted by several authors[228,262,264,265]; however, in experiments reported by Kruger et al.[259] and by Winter[260], about 10% of cells sampled in the DCN were excited by joint movement. According to Winter[260], joint responsive elements are concentrated in the rostral portion of the gracilis. The latter represents another indication of a functional distinction between rostral and caudal portions of the nuclei. Rosen[268] concludes that a separate ventral portion of the cuneate nucleus receives an input from the largest diameter afferent fibres of muscle. The nucleus Z, rostral to the main portion of the gracilis nucleus, also receives a projection from the large diameter afferent fibres, its input coming from hindlimb muscles (see Section 8.5.1.2). In this context, one could argue that the rostral region of the gracilis nucleus together with nucleus Z and the ventral portion of the cuneate nucleus form a complex which is part of a system transmitting information centrally from subcutaneous position (deflection) receptors, e.g. slowly adapting muscle and joint sensory units.

The transmission of activity to a dorsal column nuclei cell is subject both to excitatory and inhibitory modulation by other afferent inputs. In addition, there are important descending connections to the dorsal column nuclei from rostral centres, particularly the somatosensory region of the cerebral cortex; detailed consideration of these descending modulatory effects can be found in reviews by Towe[269] and Schmidt[191].

Inhibitory interactions in the dorsal column nuclei have been the subject of a number of investigations since Amassian and DeVito[182] first demonstrated their existence. Substantial effort has gone into documenting the presence of presynaptic inhibition and differentiating it from postsynaptically mediated changes. Andersen and various colleagues[270-273] have made an extensive analysis of synaptic transmission in the cuneate nucleus, utilising a combination of techniques—gross potential recordings, excitability testing of presynaptic fibres by direct electrical stimulation, transmembrane recordings from presynaptic fibres and postsynaptic cells, and tests for antidromic activation from the medial lemniscus. This frontal attack corroborated modification of synaptic transmission in the cuneate nucleus similar to those established for some laminae of the spinal dorsal horn. Excitatory afferent input to cuneate cells generate large intra-cellularly recorded excitatory postsynaptic potentials (EPSPs) suggesting a high degree of synaptic security. As in many ascending sensory pathways, cuneate projection neurons tend to fire repetitively to single afferent volleys. On the inhibitory side, slow waves, similar to those seen at the dorsal surface of the spinal cord in association with the presynaptic depolarisation, can be recorded from the nucleus surface. Both peripheral afferent and cerebral cortical stimulation evoke a deflection attributable to presynaptic depolarisation, apparently mediated by internuncial neurons, which correlates in time with directly measured depolarisation of cuneate primary fibres and an enhanced excitability of their presynaptic terminals. Hyperpolarising potentials, indicative of postsynaptic inhibitory processes, can be induced in cuneate neurons projecting in the medial lemniscus by peripheral afferent stimulation. In spite of the powerful excitatory synaptic action, both peripheral afferent and cerebral cortical stimuli can effectively interfere with transmission through the nucleus.

The analyses by Andersen et al.[270-273] were based upon results obtained with electrical excitation of both peripheral afferent fibres and central structures and left unanswered questions on the functional organisation of the inhibitory processes. Andersen, Etholm and Gordon[277] have settled the issue of presynaptic action during normal excitation by showing that stimulation of the skin in a natural fashion can initiate both primary afferent depolarisation and postsynaptic inhibition. Nevertheless, major mysteries about the synaptic interactions and the convergent patterns within the dorsal column nuclei still remain. For example, Jabbur and Banna[282] have reported that electrical stimulation of the skin anywhere in the body provoke effects of the type associated with presynaptic inhibition, including reduced transmission through the nucleus.

(d) *Projection from the dorsal column nuclei*—The passage of axons from cells of the dorsal column nuclei as internal arcuate fibres to form the contralateral medial lemniscus is well established[278-280]. There is some overlap of cuneate and gracilis fibres in the medial lemniscus; Walker[278] suggests that gracilis fibres are located ventral in the medulla oblongata, ventrolateral in the pons and caudal midbrain to become the dorsal-most part of the lemniscus near the diencephalon. The principal target of the medial lemniscus is unquestionably the diencephalon; however, some fibres from the dorsal column nuclei terminate in the midbrain tectal region[250,281]. In addition, at least some fibres originating from the dorsal column nuclei end in the cerebellum. Cutaneously excited neurons located in the rostral part of the cuneate nucleus and intermingled with those projecting to the contralateral medial lemniscus are reported to project to the ipsilateral vermis[283,284]. The possibility has been raised that some cells of the most rostral portion of the gracilis nucleus also have terminations in the cerebellum[285].

Gordon and Jukes[264] found that 90% of the cells activated by hair follicle receptors and exhibiting afferent inhibition [see Section 8.5.1.1(c)] project in the contralateral medial lemniscus. In contrast, only one third of the gracilis neurons excited by receptors responding to direct skin contact (touch cells) could be shown to have fibres in the medial lemniscus. The largest proportion of projecting cells is found in the middle third of the gracilis nucleus, which correlates well with the fact that almost all of the cluster cells, predominating in this region, show retrograde changes following lesions of the contralateral medial lemniscus.

Andersen, Eccles, Schmidt and Yokota[271] found cuneate neurons which do not appear to project over the medial lemniscus and concluded that they were interneurons of the nucleus. The test for projection—antidromic invasion after medial lemniscus stimulation — cannot identify cells sending processes by other tracts and may be criticised in relation to its adequacy for all lemniscal cells; however, the classification of some cuneate neurons as inter-neurons is supported by other differences from cells with lemniscal axons. Stimulation of the somatosensory cortex is known to excite some DCN neurons[275,276]; the bulk of the non-projecting cuneate cells were excited by cortical stimulation while cuneate cells with lemniscal processes were not. Lemniscal cuneate cells were found in the middle portions of the nuclei, while non-projecting cells were concentrated rostal and ventral to them; the cortical excitation of non-projecting neurons is in keeping with anatomical observations that cortical fibres terminate in ventral parts of the dorsal column nuclei[250,274].

8.5.1.2 Spinal pathway via nucleus Z

The pathway to the thalamus involving nucleus Z has been discovered recently; the nucleus itself was recognised as a separate entity in 1957[286]. It shares features with the dorsal column system on one hand and the spino-cervicothalamic pathway on the other.

(a) *Nucleus Z*—Brodal and Pompeiano[286] described the nucleus they labelled 'Z' in the cat. It is located about 3 mm rostral to the obex and about the same distance lateral to the midline, just rostral to the nucleus gracilis. A similar nucleus has a corresponding location in man[287]. Originally, nucleus Z and the vestibular nuclei were thought to be related, but the absence of an input from vestibular afferent fibres and the lack of a projection to the cerebellum appears to rule this out[286,288,289].

Nucleus Z took on importance in 1971 following Landgren and Silf-venius's[290] demonstration of a projection of Group I afferent fibres in muscle nerve through it to the cerebral cortex. The principal or exclusive input to nucleus Z comes from regions caudal to forelimb spinal segments. Landgren and Silfvenius[290] concluded from experiments employing electrophysiological recordings and selective spinal lesions that the entire input to nucleus Z arrived over the dorsolateral fasciculus; however, Hand[251] found evidence for a small contribution from lumbar dorsal root fibres in the dorsal columns in a study utilising silver staining of degenerating fibres. Rustioni[237] con-firmed the contribution from both the dorsolateral fasciculus and from the dorsal columns to nucleus Z again by staining fibres caused to degenerate by selective lesions. Rustioni's cats were chronically deafferented by complete ipsilateral rhizotomy, indicating that the dorsal column fibres do not arise from dorsal root neurons. The integrity of nucleus Z is crucial for the trans-mission of activity from the largest diameter afferent fibres of hindlimb muscle to the cerebral cortex[290]. Hindlimb Group I activity evoking short latency cortical responses ascends in the dorsal column to about the third lumbar segment; the pathway then courses rostrally in the dorsolateral fasciculus, presumably after a synapse in the dorsal horn at that level. This arrangement is remarkably similar to that for the Group I input to Clarke's column (nucleus dorsalis) and the relay there to form the dorsal spinocere-bellar tract.

The physiology of nucleus Z has been evaluated so far solely on the basis of electrical excitation of peripheral nerves. Most of the Z-nucleus cells can be excited by stimulation of only one hindlimb muscle nerve, the major excitatory drive coming from Group I fibres. Some neurons also responded to volleys in cutaneous nerves and/or to a Group II input from muscle nerves. A few cells responded solely to stimulation of a hindlimb cutaneous nerve. The overall pattern is that of a relatively limited spatial convergence. Nucleus Z cells are capable of following high frequencies of afferent stimulation. Similarities between characteristics of the input to nucleus Z cells and features of the dorsal spinocerebellar pathway raises the possibility that the input to the nucleus may derive from collaterals of the Clarke's column projection.

The projection from nucleus Z crosses the midline at its level in a fashion similar to the internal arcuate fibres and then joins the medial edge of the medial lemniscus to stay well separated from the gracilis contribution throughout its course[291-293,295].

8.5.1.3   The spino–cervicothalamic pathway

A new centrally directed pathway for afferent activity of cutaneous origin was brought to light by a series of studies beginning with Morin's 1955 observation[296] that responses evoked in the cerebral cortex by cutaneous afferent stimulation are in part mediated by fibres of the spinal dorsolateral fasciculus. The spinal portion, which has come to be known as the spino-cervical tract, is fed by an input from the same side of the body like the other ascending pathways of the dorsal spinal cord. Its first synaptic junction is located in the dorsal horn with a second synaptic link in the lateral cervical nucleus at the upper end of the spinal cord. Fibres from the lateral cervical nucleus cross the midline in the anterior spinal commissure and pass rostrally with the medial lemniscus as far as the nucleus ventralis posterolateralis of the thalamus. The spinocervical system appears to be more prominent in the carnivore than in the primate, although its existence in the latter has been established. As will be mentioned, it may convey sensory information in addition to that arising from the skin.

(a) *The spinocervical tract*—The tract important for the spinocervical connection lies for the most part relatively superficially in the dorsolateral fasciculus just lateral to the dorsal root entrance zone. It is made up of fibres conducting between 17 and 103 m sec^{-1}, with a mean of 60 m sec^{-1}, an average conduction velocity considerably greater than the average for primary fibres in the dorsal column[297,298].

The location of the spinocervical tract corresponds with that of the dorsal spinocerebellar projection, and it has been argued that the input to the lateral cervical nucleus consists of collaterals of the spinocerebellar tract. Several observations suggest that these fibres are not the sole input. Firstly, electrical stimulation along the course of the dorsolateral fasciculus and in the spino-cerebellar tract above and below the level of the nucleus demonstrate the presence of fibres which leave the tract at the level of the nucleus[160,297,298]. Secondly, attempts to activate cells of the lateral cervical nucleus by cerebellar stimulation, which antidromically excites spinocerebellar fibres and presumably all of their branches, have been largely unsuccessful[299]. Thirdly, many neurons of the dorsolateral fasciculus, and particularly those reaching the lateral cervical nucleus, originate caudal to the origin of the dorsal spinocerebellar tract in Clarke's column[160,300]. Thus, the largest fraction of the ascending projection to the lateral cervical nucleus seems to stem from fibres other than those of the dorsal spinocerebellar system.

Originally, the spinocervical tract in the cat was reported to originate from neurons of lamina IV and V of the dorsal horn in the vicinity of segments contributing to the pathway[301,302]. More recent work by Bryan, Trevino, Coulter and Willis[160] has suggested a more extensive distribution of somata giving rise to its fibres. They reported electrophysiological evidence of antidromic excitation from rostral levels of the dorsolateral fasciculus for cells scattered from lamina III to the ventral horn, although most were located in laminae IV, V and VI[160]. Bryan et al.[160] also noted a somatotopic organisation in the distribution of spinocervical tract cells; medial skin areas were represented more rostrally than lateral ones and dorsal skin surfaces projected more laterally than ventral cutaneous areas. The number of fibres comprising the spinocervical tract (roughly approximated at 2000–3000 for the cat) is much smaller than the number of neurons in lamina IV to VI[160,303], so these dorsal horn layers contribute to other systems and mechanisms (see Section 8.2.3.2 and 8.5.2). In monkey, spinocervical tract neurons may have a less scattered distribution, lying principally in regions corresponding to lamina IV and V; they apparently are organised in the same somatopic pattern shown to exist in cat[305].

Rexed and Strom[304], in their original description of the lateral cervical nucleus, recognised its afferent inflow from cutaneous sense organs. Subsequent analyses based upon both intracellular and extracellular recordings have established that the spinocervical elements receive monosynaptic excitation from large-diameter afferent fibres of skin nerves and polysynaptic excitatory input from the small diameter, including C afferent fibres from muscle and skin[297,302,308]. Some of the fibres connecting to spinocervical tract neurons are branches of primary afferent fibres also projecting rostrally in the dorsal column[297].

Utilising carefully controlled natural stimulation of the skin, Brown and Franz[298] established several patterns of convergence from the response of spinocervical tract neurons. They found the specificity of the excitatory connections and related inhibitory patterns to vary according to the kinds of experimental preparation and the class of the unit. Many spinocervical elements are excited by both receptors responsive to hair movement and those requiring direct stimulation of the skin; some are excited by hair follicle receptors alone; in decerebrate animals, some units respond only to strong pressure and pinching of the skin[307]. Afferent inhibition to spinocervical tract cells apparently is not of the surround type and is at least partially mediated postsynaptically[298,302,306]. It is noteworthy that in two studies virtually all spinocervical units responded to noxious heating of body skin (a stimulus exciting the cat's C-fibre polymodal nociceptors); the degree of response to heat varied according to the preparation and other characteristics of the unit[267,298].

Identified spinocervical units are not excited by either the Type I or Type II cutaneous tactile receptors[298], in spite of verification of a Type I activation of numerous lamina IV and V cells[144]; this is additional information emphasising the contribution of these layers to other systems. A point still to be reconciled is Mendell's[308] attribution of a C-fibre input to only a small fraction of spinocervical fibres of the dorsolateral fasciculus, in contrast to the regularity of this finding in Brown and Franz's[298] analysis.

(b) *Lateral cervical nucleus*—The lateral cervical nucleus received little attention until Rexed and Brodal[309] described it in some detail and attributed it to a spinocerebellar linkage. The nucleus is most clearly developed in carnivores; in the cat, it lies just lateral and ventral to the dorsal horn from about the first to the third cervical segments. Each nucleus contains from about 3000 to 6000 cells in carnivores, depending upon the species[310-312]. In monkey the nucleus appears to be relatively smaller than it is in carnivore; in man, the cells appear to be scattered within what has beeen called the 're-ticular formation' of the spinal cord[281,313-315]. In some species neurons located along the dorsolateral fasciculus at many spinal cord levels could represent homologues of the cells forming the carnivore nucleus[316,317]. The feline lateral cervical nucleus appears to consist of two different cell types. Approxi-mately 90% of the neurons are relatively large (approximately 50 by 25 µm) with approximately 40% of the perikaryon covered by synaptic terminals from ipsilateral spinocervical tract fibres[318,319]. Some 10% of the neurons in the nucleus have considerably smaller cell bodies (maximum dimension of 20 µm) and receive only a few synaptic terminals on their soma, none attributable to the ipsilateral spinocervical tract[319,320]. Most (80%) of the nucleus' neurons undergo retrograde changes following lesions of the contra-lateral medial lemniscus in the midbrain[310,321]. It seems reasonable to believe that the large cells are projecting cells and that the smaller ones may be intranuclear interneurons.

In anesthetised carnivores, three-quarters of the lateral cervical nucleus cells can be excited by peripheral stimuli limited to movement of hairs[311,312,322,323]. Twenty per cent or less of single units recorded from the nucleus require skin contact to be driven; some elements are reported to require strong pressure or squeezing of the skin for excitation. In recordings made directly from the nucleus, no evidence of joint or muscle input has been demonstrated. The receptive fields of single units vary in a fashion similar to that noted for the dorsal column nuclei, with the most distally located fields being smaller than those situated on proximal portions of a limb. A clearcut somatotopic organisation has not been established, although Horrobin[299] suggests that units excited from the hindlimb tend to lie more medially and those driven by forelimb stimulation more laterally within the nucleus. Wall and Taub[324] report an input to the lateral cervical nucleus from the head and face region which has not been confirmed.

Afferent inhibition exists at the level of the lateral cervical nucleus as well as in the projection to it. The mass discharge of the contralateral medial lemniscus to stimulation of the dorsolateral fasciculus (after rostral section of the dorsal columns) can be profoundly depressed by volleys from a cutaneous nerve located in any of the four limbs[325]. These inhibitory effects are apparently mediated by pathways in the ventral half of the spinal cord.

Inhibitory postsynaptic potentials evoked by afferent volleys from skin nerves or by thinner afferent fibres of muscle have been demonstrated in lateral cervical nucleus neurons responding to brushing of body hair; typically, an inhibitory projection arises from the limb ipsilateral to the one from which excitation occurs. Presynaptic effects, in addition, are suggested by enhanced excitability of incoming spinocervical tract fibres after noxious mechanical stimulation of the forepaw skin[325].

(c) *Cervicothalamic tract*—The lateral cervical nucleus projects strictly contralaterally in both carnivores and monkeys[326-329] and sends no branches to the cerebellum[299,310,330,331]. The projection crosses at the upper cervical level and ascends superficially in the ventral funiculus to the level of the decussation of the pyramidal tract, where it moves slightly laterally in the medulla and passes the nucleus of the inferior olive. It was originally thought to send terminals to the nucleus of the inferior olive[326,328,332], but Boivie[281] (see also Mizuno[333]) was unable to establish terminal degeneration in the latter after lesions of the lateral cervical nucleus, even though some cervicothalamic fibres traverse the nucleus itself. The bulk of the cervicothalamic bundle runs ventrolateral to the nucleus of the inferior olive and rostral to this level from the lateral and dorsolateral portions of the medial lemniscus.

8.5.2 Ascending tracts of the ventral quadrants

The main ascending tracts of the ventral half of the spinal cord are largely (if not exclusively in some species) crossed and are postsynaptic to the primary afferent neurons. The spinothalamic and spinoreticular projections will be taken up separately, although it is not certain to what extent they represent different systems.

8.5.2.1 The spinothalamic projection

The concept of a sensory path in which fibres from neurons of the spinal dorsal horn form a tract reaching the contralateral diencephalon is usually attributed to Edinger[138,334]. The steps by which classical investigators correlated the tract Edinger located in the ventrolateral portion of the spinal cord to the sensation of pain, including Sherrington's[34] work on animals and the convincing clinical–pathological deductions of Spiller[335] and Petran[336], are eloquently recounted by Keele[337]. The interested reader can also gain historical perspective on morphological investigations of this pathway in Mehler, Feferman and Nauta's[338] article.

(a) *The spinothalamic tract*—Many treatises on neural function describe a lateral and ventral spinothalamic tract; the former is generally said to carry activity necessary for the perception of pain and temperature, whereas the ventral tract is linked to touch and pressure sensation. Much evidence cited as indicative of this division in the spinothalamic system is open to question or alternative interpretation, because it is based upon material in which the central course of cervicothalamic fibres may have been confused with the projection originating from the contralateral dorsal horn[138,334,340-343]. Kuru[339] deduced from analyses of retrograde chromatolytic changes after chordotomies that there were two distinct pathways in the ventrolateral portion of the human spinal cord. He concluded that more laterally situated fibres in the ventral quadrant stem from contralateral posteromarginal cells (pericornual); their retrograde involvement after chordotomy correlated well with the segmental distribution of the loss of pain and temperature sensation. His material also was interpreted as showing more ventrally situated spinal fibres to originate from contralateral cells of the centre of the dorsal horn (nucleus proprius) and to have a more medial course to the caudal midbrain than the lateral bundle of fibres. Spatial separation between spino-thalamic fibres important for pain and temperature and for other modalities of sensation, as Kuru[339] and many texts suggest, is but part of the argument regarding two spinothalamic pathways. Segregation of function within the spinal cord is often confounded with another question, namely a difference in the central distribution of spinothalamic fibres into lateral and medial regions of the brainstem. Mehler[344,425] concluded from comparative studies that, in subprimates, some fibres passing through the ventrolateral portion of the spinal cord have a medial course through the brainstem; these medially-located fibres were labelled by Herrick and Bishop[425a,425b] because they were thought to be phylogenetically older than the latter or neo-spinothalamic components. Furthermore, the former have been assumed to terminate in the intralaminar thalamic region and the latter in the ventroposterior thalamic nucleus. Other ventral quadrant fibres of subprimates and all those of primates at the midbrain and above pass laterally along with the medial lemniscus. Some commentators have linked pain or temperature to the medial or paleospinothalamic distribution, based on the view that such sensations are phylogenetically old and less discriminative; this latter contains an antomical construction quite the opposite to what Kuru[339] has suggested. At the present, definitive evidence on whether or not there are two functionally, possibly phylogenetically, different parts of this pathway is lacking and we believe it best to leave the issue open.

For the purposes of the discussion which follows, Boivie's[427] definition of the spinothalamic tract as fibres to the diencephalon from spinal cord cells, other than those from the lateral cervical nucleus, will be used. As usually envisioned and applying to much of the pathway in primates, cells of the dorsal horn have an axon which crosses (probably in the ventral commissure) within a few segments and turns rostrally in the ventral quadrant to terminate in several diencephalic nuclei. In the spinal cord spinothalamic fibres accompany those of two other pathways, the spinoreticular projection and the ventral spinocerebellar tract.

Degeneration after section of the ventrolateral tracts demonstrates a segmental lamination[241,345-348]. Fibres ascending from the most caudal levels are located most laterally with progressively more rostral segments arranged sequentially on the medial side. The segmental lamination arrangement was established by the use of Marchi-stained material and as such reflects solely the arrangement of the myelinated fibres. The lamination is apparently retained, at least in part, as the tract continues rostrally through suprasegmental levels[241,348,349]. In all species the number of fibres, as judged from degeneration following ventrolateral spinal lesions, decreases as the pathway passes cephalad owing to termination of elements at medullary, pontine and midbrain levels. Fibres ending caudal to the diencephalon will be discussed separately (Section 8.5.2.2.).

(b) *Cells of origin*—There has been uncertainty about the neurons from which spinothalamic fibres arise from the time of Edinger's original description. Part of the doubt derives from the other ascending fibres in the ventral spinal quadrants. While morphological studies may not have provided definitive answers to the problem, they have offered consistent and important clues. Prior to Kuru's[339] work and its conclusions, Foerster and Gagel[345] also had suggested both the posteromarginal cells of the dorsal horn and larger cells of the centre of the dorsal horn (nucleus proprius) as the source of the spinothalamic projection on the basis of retrogade changes following human chordotomy. Moreover, Morin, Schwartz and O'Leary's[348] analysis of experimental chordotomy in cats and monkeys similarly had pointed at the posteromarginal cells and large cells of the nucleus proprius, a conclusion largely overlooked. The latter work also noted retrograde chromatolytic changes in cells of the ventral horn scattered among the motor neurons and at its lateral border. The overall picture has left most authors of anatomical treatises undecided, perhaps because of suspected vagaries in the identification of retrograde changes or because of conflicting reports. Pearson[350] added cells of the substantia gelantinosa to the list while other observers have deduced that no cells of the feline dorsal horn contributed to crossed pathways[351]. Considerable clarification has taken place during the past four years as a consequence of combined physiological and morphological analyses. A first step occurred when Christensen and Perl[142] showed in the cat, by use of controlled afferent input and dye deposition from recording electrodes, that cells located at the border of the dorsal horn, the posteromarginal neurons forming Rexed's lamina I, receive a specific input from cutaneous nociceptors and thermoreceptors. Subsequently, lamina I neurons of the monkey dorsal horn were found to receive similar nociceptive and thermoreceptive projection; antidromic testing from the contralateral cervical cord established that some of these marginal cells give rise to a long ascending pathway[143]. These results presented a functional framework for the earlier chordotomy evidence. Recent studies using antidromic excitation of the spinothalamic projection to search for antidromically excited spinal neurons have provided results of great value for reconciliation of the various ideas on the tract's origins. Dilly, Wall and Webster[353], in the cat, placed one of 56 units antidromically excitable from the midbrain in lamina I and all the others in laminae V and VI of the spinal dorsal horn. Again, in the cat, Trevino, Maunz, Bryan and Willis's[354] systematic search located 85% of units antidromically excited from the caudal border of the diencephalon in laminae VII and VIII of the lumbar ventral horn, with 15% in laminae V and VI or the dorsal grey matter. At almost the same time, Levante and Albe-Fessard[355] could only find evidence of neurons antidromically excitable from the diencephalon in the cat's ventral horn (laminae VII and VIII). Using the same techniques, Trevino, Coulter and Willis[356, 433b] obtained a quite different pattern in the monkey; cell bodies of fibres projecting to the diencephalon were distributed from the posterior horn margin, lamina I, across the spinal grey matter to the region equivalent to lamina VIII in the medial part of the ventral horn. In the monkey, the predominant contribution comes from laminae IV and V. The difference in location of antidromically excitable spinothalamic cells between the carnivore and the primate has been confirmed by Levante, Lamour and Albe-Fessard[433a]. Thus, most predictions of the earlier anatomical studies and their disparity can be supported. There appears to be a systematic difference between the studies using the cat such as those by Szentagothai[351] and those based upon primate material, including man. In the cat the bulk of the spinothalamic projection arises from cells situated at the base of the dorsal horn or in the ventral grey matter, while in the primate the projection arises principally from dorsal horn neurons, including those of the most superficial layers.

In the cat the conduction velocity of spinothalamic fibres calculated from the latency of antidromic impulses varies from 9 to nearly 100 m sec^{-1} with a median of 33 m sec^{-1} [354]. In the monkey a systematic difference was found according to the location of the cell, with the more slowly projecting fibres originating from laminae I, VI–VIII and rapidly conducting fibres arising from neurons of the centre of the dorsal horn (laminae IV and V)[356]. Trevino et al.[356] found the natural stimulation most effective for exciting projecting cells to correlate with the neuron's location. Cells in lamina I could be activated only by mechanical stimuli of noxious intensity; however, other elements responsive only to strong mechanical stimuli were also found in laminae, IV, V and VI. Their most commonly recorded spinothalamic unit was excited by gentle mechanical stimulation of hair or skin and was located laterally in laminae IV and V. All cells in laminae VII and VIII (ventral horn) appeared to be excitable by subcutaneous receptors. A number of the terminations on cells of origin of the spinothalamic system are likely to come directly from primary afferent fibres. A possibility which must be explored, however, is that some spinothalamic neurons, particularly in more ventral laminae, receive their afferent input exclusively from other spinal cells more dorsally located.

In summary, the spinothalamic tract originates from a variety of cell layers located in different regions of the spinal cord. In the cat, most of the cells giving rise to fibres projecting to the level of the diencephalon are located ventrally. Combining the evidence gathered from morphological and electrophysiological studies in primates, including man, posteromarginal neurons (lamina I) and cells in the middle of the dorsal horn are the principal sources of spinothalamic fibres. In the monkey some fibres reaching the contralateral thalamus also originate from more deeply located cells; they appear to be associated with an input from subcutaneous receptors. The only source suggested by anatomical studies which has not been borne out is the lateral border of the ventral horn; its implication by experimental chordotomy studies probably is attributable to lesions of the ventral spinocerebellar tract in that material[207].

8.5.2.2 Spinoreticular and related systems

The groups of neurons lying within the core of the medulla oblongata, pons and mesencephalon, surrounded and interlaced by a network of fibres, are generally referred to as the reticular formation. The diversity and extent of this region makes the term spinoreticular pathway very broad. We shall reserve it for pathways terminating in nuclear regions of the reticular core of the brainstem: the gigantocellular nucleus of the medulla, the pontine reticular and the mesencephalic reticular nuclei. This excludes spinal projections to structures such as the inferior olivary and the vestibular nuclei as well as the medullary nuclei contributing to the medial lemniscus (dorsal column and Z). Even so, it is difficult to develop a coherent picture of the nature and significance of the ascending projection to the complex network of cells and fibres making up these regions. The inherent problems of dealing with such a variegated area have been added to by a number of circumstances associated with work on the question. To start with, the terminology applied to constituents of the reticular formation is diverse, making comparisons between different experimental results difficult. For example, Brodal[137,358] and Mehler[344] have used similar, though not identical, terminology with the former based upon the Meessen and Olszewski's[359] usage for the rabbit and the latter upon Olszewski and Baxter's[360] nomenclature for the human brainstem; confusion has arisen from the mixing of these terminologies for given structures. A lack of precision in both morphological and functional studies in describing or contemplating the significance of lesions has compounded this difficulty. In addition, physiological approaches have often drawn unwarranted conclusions about the nature of excitation produced by electrical stimulation of peripheral nerve or central neural tissue. As has been stated previously, the patterns of activity, the magnitude of projections and the complexity of interactions made with electrically initiated activity may not reflect functional arrangements existing under the more selective conditions usually imposed by nature.

The diverse anatomy amalgamated as the reticular formation accompanies its association with a large range of function. The reticular formation includes cell groups concerned with motor integration in general and in particular that related to afferent and efferent cranial nerve neurons (skeletal, respiratory cardiovascular). A place in states of consciousness and the cycle of sleep and wakefulness is another role attributed to reticular formation structures. Finally, modulatory actions upon somatosensory activity mediated by reticular formation neurons must be considered. The latter are pertinent to our topic but on present information it is hard to sort out organisation or effects referable to the latter from other activities. In what follows, we shall only touch upon the mass of literature on the reticular formation and its features of possible significance of somatic sensation. The reader desiring an extensive bibliography and commentary should consult the detailed overview by Pompeiano[361].

(a) *Spinoreticular pathway*—Fibres of spinal origin ending in the brain stem caudal to the thalamus ascend in the ventral quadrants of the spinal cord[338,344,362,363,364,365]. Rossi and Brodal[362] believed that the bulk of these fibres are located in the ventral half of the lateral funiculus since they found nearly maximal terminal degeneration in Nauta material after lesions restricted to this area. However, Kerr[366] has a current report describing degeneration in a number of reticular nuclei in primate following lesions restricted to the ventral spinal funiculus. Thus, in part, reticular-directed components occupy similar if not identical spinal locations as fibres destined for the diencephalon. The morphological studies based upon degeneration suggest that in their passage through the medulla to the level of the caudal midbrain, two groups of fibres can be distinguished: a lateral group which lies close to the brainstem surface and a medial bundle which is centred between the midline and the lateral surface. The input to the gigantocellular, caudal pontine reticular, subcoeruleus and mesencephalic reticular nuclei comes from the medial fascicle, while other areas are supplied by the lateral branch[338,344,362]. Some earlier work had suggested that the spinoreticular fibres were branches of those forming spinothalamic projections. Estimations of the size of the tract and phylogenetic comparisons make this seem unlikely[338,344,362], although at best the arguments are indirect. Support for independence of the two pathways is provided by the recent observation that in cat, only three of 22 spinal cells antidromically excited from the medial bulbar reticular region could also be antidromically driven from the thalamus[355]; however, the sample size limits generalisation of the observations. A final decision on the extent to which branches of a fibre represents both a spinoreticular and a spinothalamic projection will probably have to await studies based upon some of the newer ways of labelling all of the processes of a given neuron.

There is limited information available on the cells of origin of the spinoreticular projection. The coexistence or proximity of spinothalamic and spinoreticular fibres in the ventral quadrant of the spinal cord and at accessible points in the brainstem prevents studies based upon retrograde changes from distinguishing their somata of origin. Limited data comes from Levante and Albe-Fessard's[355] recording from neurons antidromically excited by electrical stimulation of the cat 'bulbar reticular' formation (probably the gigantocellular nucleus); all of their 22 units were located in the ventral horn-some in Rexed's lamina VII, the majority lying in lamina VIII.

The degree to which the spinoreticular projection is ipsilateral to primary afferent neurons and/or the recrossing which may occur within the brainstem is uncertain. After dorsal horn lesions in the cat, Rossi and Brodal[362] found orthograde degeneration to be largely contralateral. Lesions of one ventral quadrant in primate are reported to cause mostly ipsilateral degeneration in reticular structures[344] with signs of bilateral termination appearing principally in the gigantocellular and subcoeruleus nuclei[338]. In lower forms, electrophysiological recordings in the reticular region coupled with acute lesions of the spinal cord have suggested a bilateral pathway through one ventral quadrant to the gigantocellular nucleus[363,364] and, more rostrally, to the periaquaductal grey of the midbrain[365].

(b) *Nuclei of termination*—The following nuclei of the reticular formation or related areas may have some place in somatosensory function and, on the basis of morphological studies, receive direct projections from fibres of spinal cells which course in the ventrolateral funiculus:

(1) Brodal's ventral reticular nucleus in the caudal medulla oblongata;
(2) the gigantocellular nucleus in the medulla;
(3) the caudal pontine reticular nucleus;
(4) the nucleus subcoeruleus in the pons;
(5) the lateral tegmental process of the pontine grey matter;
(6) the midbrain reticular formation (mesencephalic tegmentum);

(7) parts of the mesencephalic periaquaductal grey region; and

(8) Olszewski and Baxter's intercollicular nucleus.

Little is known about the nature and function of the spinal connection to several of these structures. Most of the ascending spinal connections are with medially located nuclei containing large cells in the bulbar and caudal pontine reticular areas, to the laterally located nucleus subcoeruleus and the nearby lateral pontine tegmental nuclei, and to parts of the mesencephalic reticular formation[344,362,366-368]. In the medulla the area of maximal termination roughly corresponds to the outline of the gigantocellular nucleus.

We have only sketchy information on the intimate anatomy of the reticular formation nuclei and know even less about how this relates to function. Two types of neuron have been recognised in the ventral reticular (nucleus reticularis ventralis), the gigantocellular nuclei of the medulla and the nucleus of the posterior commissure. One kind of cell has five to six long straight main dendrites with spines on the somata and proximal dendrites (polydendritic cells). The polydendritic cell is the most common element of the gigantocellular nucleus. Another type (oligodendritic cell), which has only one or two primary dendrites and does not have spines in the soma-dendritic region, is particularly common in the nucleus reticular ventralis. Electron microscopic analyses indicate the existence of only a few degenerating synaptic boutons after ventrolateral spinal lesions, even in the giganto-cellular nucleus, a structure reportedly receiving a heavy input from this pathway[319,369-371].

The presence of convergence from different afferent sources has been a commonly emphasised feature in the reports of physiological studies on the reticular formation. Unfortunately, some investigations have either not reported or have not controlled the precise loci of recording, making inter-pretation and comparison of limited value. In addition, the afferent pathway or the synaptic linkage to the cells of this region seems to be peculiarly sensitive to the state of the preparation, including the type and level of anaesthesia. The latter fact has served to complicate the issue and to make analogies with other parts of the somatosensory system difficult. Studies on the ventral reticular nucleus of the medulla, the gigantocellular nucleus and the mesencephalic reticular formation agree that a large proportion of the cells have convergence not only from different somatic regions but also from other sensory systems, such as auditory, visual and vestibular[363,364,372-377]. It is also generally reported that cells in these areas cease responding after only a few rapidly repeated stimuli to a somatic structure. The somatic input to the gigantocellular region stems principally from afferent fibres of the Aδ conduction velocity (10–30 m sec^{-1}), while the ventral reticular nucleus of the medulla is reported to receive a C fibre input, as well as one from more rapidly conducting primary elements[364,377]. The kinds of natural somatic stimuli described as effective for exciting individual neurons of particular nuclei have varied according to the experimental conditions. For instance, it has been reported in one study on chloralose-anaesthesized cats that cells of the gigantocellular nucleus respond to innocuous mechanical stimuli[363], and in another on decerebrate cats that most are activated only by noxious stimuli[364]. Similar differences appear in descriptions of unitary responses from the nucleus reticularis ventralis[373,375,376].

The periaquaductal grey substance and the mesencephalic reticular region have often been lumped together in work descriptions of physiological results. Liebeskind and Mayer's[365] attention to the periaquaductal region of the rat is an exception; they reported that periaquaductal neurons respond to non-noxious stimuli but show increased activity when graded electrical stimulation of the skin is increased to the noxious level. Units in the mesencephalic reticular formation and the periaquaductal grey of decorticate cats are reported to respond specifically to non-noxious or to noxious cutaneous stimulation, the latter type being the most common[378]. Unmyelinated (C) primary afferent fibres have been shown to have a special projection to the mesencephalic reticular region[379]. These various studies have been interpreted by a number of authors as indicative of a significant relation between nuclei of the reticular formation and the periaquaductal grey region to the sensation of pain. This may be the case for some cell groups but it is hard to square with the poorly localised and multisensory activation commonly described; normally, pain is produced by only certain stimuli and it can often be reliably localised to the area affected. In evaluating such proposals, the effects produced by noxious stimulation other than pain must be taken into account; autonomic reactions such as increased blood pressure and heart rate, increased respiration and increased alertness are all common results of pain-causing stimuli. It seems more appropriate to think of regions which receive polysensory inputs as related to reflex and other subconscious reactions, rather than to perception. In this view, sensation would be affected by peripheral afferent inputs to such portions of the brain only indirectly through whatever effect they may have on the state of consciousness.

The situation for the periaquaductal grey region and possibly parts of the mesencephalic reticular formation may be different. Stimulation of parts of the periaquaductal grey of the mesencephalon in both rats and cats has been stated to reduce responsiveness to noxious stimuli, even to the extent of anaesthesia[381]. Before attributing meaning to these observations it will be necessary to reconcile specific activation of some periaquaductal neurons by noxious stimulation[365] with analgesia-like effects evoked from the same general, although possibly not identical, vicinity. Some of the periaquaductal stimulation experiments have equated effects on spinal reflexes, such as the heat-induced tail flick of the rat, to pain[382]; these have been supplemented by confirmatory results using observations on the modification of behaviour by rats and cats which may be more closely akin to perceptually related reactions[380]. Periaquaductal stimulation has now been shown to inhibit neurons of spinal laminae IV and V of the cat[383]. Unfortunately for the logic relating these effects to pain, in cat these laminae apparently are not the source of the ventrolateral pathways[354,355] important for the behaviour taken as indicative of pain[34].

(c) *Ascending projections*—Regions of the reticular formation of the medulla, pons and midbrain have been suggested to act as relays for somatic afferent activity destined for the forebrain. In part, the concept is based upon recordings of potentials in rostral structures, such as the nucleus of the posterior commissure, the mesencephalic reticular formation or the thalamic centrum medianum evoked by electrical stimulation of regions identified as to location only by stereotaxic coordinates[363,372,384]. These conclusions do have a measure of support from anatomical studies. Retrograde degenerative changes in perikarya and silver impregnation of orthograde degeneration after lesions suggest that some cells of the medial two-thirds of the reticular formation of the medulla and pons project rostrally as far as the medial nuclei of the thalamus. In the case of the gigantocellular nucleus in the medulla, the long ascending connections arise from smaller cells rather than the large neurons. On the same grounds, the caudal part of the nucleus reticularis pontis is thought to send fibres to the mesencephalic reticular formation, the periaquaductal grey and the hypothalamus[385-387]. Fibres from the ventral portion of the periaquaductal region have been shown to terminate in the midline and intralaminar nuclei of the thalamus and in the subthalamus[579]. Furthermore, the dorsal and possibly the ventral parts of the periaquaductal grey substance are reported to send fibres to the hypothalamus[579,580]. The connections from both the medullary and pontine reticular regions and from the periaquaductal structures to the intralaminar nuclei of the thalamus are interesting, since this portion of the thalamus receives direct spinothalamic projections as well. The fact that several of these regions and the intralaminar nuclei (see Section 8.6.7) contain neurons responding in a special way to noxious stimulation may indicate participation in some common mechanism.

8.6 SOMATOSENSORY PROJECTIONS TO DIENCEPHALIC NUCLEI

The preceding material has followed major ascending pathways of spinal origin to the level of the diencephalon. The material in this section will take up their termination in the diencephalon and their functional characteristics. Connections from the cerebral cortex to thalamic nuclei will only be mentioned as they shed light on other features and will be discussed briefly again in Section 8.7. Furthermore, even though somatosensory input to the hypothalamus may have an important place in the regulation of the latter's control of autonomic and skeletal motor function, these projections will not be considered.

Terminology and species differences pose special problems for the reviewer of structure, afferent connections and function of thalamic nuclei. The thalamus, with its relatively large and non-homogeneous collection of nerve cells, has been divided into nuclei of varying boundaries on the grounds of several criteria. In addition, the advent and popularity of the stereotaxic approach spawned a number of atlases of the forebrain reproducing sections cut according to planes of fixation of the instrument to the animal's skull. The orientation of the brain varies considerably with the points of reference used for different species, changing the appearance of the thalamus in histological cross sections and adding another factor which results in different names for identical or homologous nuclei. We shall use terminology based upon atlases by Olszewski[388] for the macaque monkey and Jasper and Ajmone–Marsan[389] for the cat. Correlations between this nomenclature and that applied to the human thalamus have been made by Hassler[390] and Carpenter[391].

The ascending spinal pathways project to three general regions of the mammalian thalamus — the ventral, the intralaminar and the posterior nuclei. In the ventral thalamus, our major concern will be with the nuclei ventralis posterior lateralis (which with the ventralis posterior medialis constitutes Rose and Mountcastle's[392] ventrobasal complex), ventralis posterior inferior and a transitional zone between the rostral portion of the ventralis posterior lateralis and ventralis lateralis (recently labelled by Mehler[393] as ventralis intermedius after Hassler[390]). From a broad viewpoint, the intralaminar group consists of nuclei centralis lateralis, paracentralis, parafascicularis and centrum medianum.

Rose and Woolsey[394] proposed the posterior nuclear group as anatomical entity less than two decades ago; its status has been reviewed recently by Jones and Powell[395]. The posterior group has been most thoroughly studied in the cat where it lies between the small-celled portion of the medial geniculate body, the nucleus lateralis posterior-pulvinar and the ventral thalamic nuclei; it is considered to include parts of the magnocellular medial geniculate and the suprageniculate nuclei. Primate homologies of the carnivore posterior group are not settled; if the monkey posterior group is defined as that region caudal to the ventral posterior nuclei which receives an input from ascending spinal pathways, it would also contain portions of the suprageniculate and magnocellular medial geniculate nuclei.

8.6.1 Intimate thalamic anatomy

8.6.1.1 Cellular structure

Most of our limited knowledge on the details of neuronal structure in thalamic nuclei comes from studies of the nucleus ventralis posterior lateralis (VPL). The VPL is classified as an extrinsic nucleus[396]; its input is principally from extrathalamic neurons and its large cells project outside the thalamus. The majority (75%) of VPL neurons are relatively large with somata measuring about 25–30 μm in diameter[397]. These large cells degenerate following ablation of the cortical somatosensory areas and have a limited number of primary dendrites which branch to form an extensive dendritic arbor[398,399] extending about 300–400 μm[400]. It has been estimated that 20–25% of cortically projecting neurons of the VPL have recurrent collaterals from their relatively thick axons. Axons of most projecting VPL cells also give off collaterals as they pass through the thalamic reticular nucleus[398].

Two additional kinds of cells have been recognised in the VPL. One is a Golgi Type II element, a relatively small cell with a soma 12–18 μm in diameter. The dendritic tree of Golgi Type II neurons is about the same size as that of the larger projecting cells, but the axon does not course further than twice the range of the dendritic spread. Both projecting cells and the intrinsic neurons show protrusions from the dendrites in Golgi material, usually taken as an indication of a synaptic site; the protrusions on the non-projecting cells appear relatively more distally on the dendritic tree than those on the larger neurons[399,400]. In addition to the Golgi type II neurons, a small cell with a soma 3–6 μm across and a dendritic spread of some 40 μm has been noted in the ventral and intralaminar nuclei[401]. These small cells are thought to lack an axon, but their general appearance is that of neurons and they are considered as axonless neurons.

8.6.1.2 Synaptic morphology

Golgi-impregnated material has consistently shown a very dense terminal arborisation throughout the VPL from a system of ascending, relatively thick fibres[124,298,402]. In the monkey, each such incoming fibre distributes terminals to an area large enough to contain around 50 thalamic nerve cell bodies. The fibres making this kind of termination have been assumed to stem from the dorsal column nuclei, since they are the source of the only projections which are homogeneously and densely distributed through the VPL. However, it is now uncertain whether or not each ascending input to the VPL has a characteristic method of ending because differences in the arrangements were usually described in newborn animals and tend to become less clear with maturation[398-400]. In contrast to the ascending termination, descending connections from the cerebral cortex consist of relatively thin fibres giving rise to a limited number of short branches along a relatively long trajectory across the VPL[402].

Terminal boutons in the VPL have been classified in different ways[397,405,406]. Ralston and Herman[397] listed three types according to size with about 10% being over 3 μm, 16% between 2 and 3 μm and over 70% under 2 μm in diameter. Almost all of the large boutons degenerate after lesions of the dorsal column nuclei[404], while a substantial proportion of the small ('dark') boutons stem from cerebral cortical neurons[406]. The medium-sized ('pale') boutons are reported by Ralston and Herman[397] to contain both round and flattened vesicles, in contrast to the large and small boutons which have only round vesicles. According to some morphologists[157,157a,407], the flattened vesicles contain inhibitory transmitter and the round vesicles excitatory agent, an unusual combination in one terminal. A majority of synaptic junctions in the VPL are of the axo–dendritic type. Axo–axonal synapses are rare and have never been seen with the postsynaptic element as a large bouton. Differences of opinion are expressed about the existence and frequency of localised collections of synaptic contacts within lamellar glial sheaths, an arrangement labelled synaptic glomeruli in other sensory nuclei[397,398,402,403,405,410]. It is clear that our understanding of the cellular and subcellular structure of the thalamus is still in its infancy.

8.6.2 Ascending pathways

The most convincing evidence for afferent projections to thalamic nuclei from a particular source has come from morphological evidence, although important clues about a termination often have been provided by electro-physiological studies. The following comments are largely based upon anatomical evidence and emphasise recent analyses, even though some of the conclusions have been anticipated by classical work[137,411].

8.6.2.1 Projections from the dorsal column nuclei

Fibres originating from the dorsal column nuclei end in the VPL, the medial part of the posterior group and the zona incerta[280,412,413,416]. As earlier work based upon Marchi[278] or electrophysiological mapping[414,415] had suggested, the input to the VPL is topographically organised with the gracilis projection lateral and that from the cuneate more medially located[280,416]. Fibres from the dorsal column nuclei are densely and evenly distributed over the entire VPL[280,413,416].

It appears likely that the projection from the dorsal column nuclei to the posterior nuclear region is similar in cats and primates, although the terminology used for the regions in the two species is not identical. In the monkey the area includes the magnocellular medial geniculate nucleus and the ventrolateral portion of the suprageniculate nucleus[280,413]. In the cat the termination is in the PO$_m$ (medial part of posterior group) of Jones and Powell[395]. The morphological organisation of the DCN input to the posterior nuclear group differs from that to the VPL in at least two features. The distribution of DCN fibres to the posterior group are scattered and never as dense as in the VPL. In addition, there is no evidence for somatotopic organisation since the gracilis and the cuneate nuclei have overlapping areas of termination[280]. The projection to the zona incerta is also scattered and has no signs of a somatotopic organisation[280].

8.6.2.2 Projections from the lateral cervical nucleus (cervico-thalamic)

The termination of the cervicothalamic portion of the medial lemniscus in the cat, the only animal so far studied in detail, has both similarities to and differences from those of the dorsal column nuclei[327]. Cervicothalamic fibres are distributed to both the VPL and the posterior group. The endings in the VPL avoid the central part of the nucleus to concentrate on the dorsal, lateral and ventral rims, differing notably from those from the dorsal column nuclei. These anatomical observations are consistent with Landgren, Nordwall and Wengstrom's[417] earlier findings that stimulation of the spinal dorsolateral fasciculus evokes activity in outer portions of the contralateral VPL. Projections to the VPL from rostral and caudal parts of the lateral cervical nucleus show no obvious differences[327]. Fibres from the lateral cervical nucleus do not have a substantial projection to the dorsomedial or medial portions of the VPL, the region found by Andersen, Andersson and Landgren[418] to be excited by the large diameter afferent fibres of forelimb muscles. The morphology of the cervicothalamic terminals seems to be similar to that of endings derived from DCN fibres[419,420].

The lateral cervical nucleus, as the dorsal column nuclei, has a sparser projection to the posterior group than to the VPL. There are suggestions of a denser cervicothalamic termination in the medial part of the magnocellular medial geniculate nucleus than from the DCN[327,427].

8.6.2.3 Spinothalamic projections

Fibres from the spinal ventral quadrants terminate in the ventral, the intra-laminar and the posterior nuclei of the thalamus. The bulk of the direct evidence demonstrating this distribution is again morphological; although Whitlock and Perl's[421-423] electrophysiological studies on animals with sectioned dorsal tracts first called attention to a somatosensory input to the posterior group.

A projection to the ventral thalamic nuclei of man and other primates from spinal cells has been appreciated for a long time[278,345,424]. The studies of recent years have added details, including contributions of the fine calibre fibres through the use of the Nauta method and its modifications. In the monkey, the spinothalamic input is disbursed throughout the VPL in a unique pattern; in silver staining of degenerating fibres, patches or clusters of dense spinothalamic terminal fields are scattered in regions with fewer and more uniformly distributed terminals[338,344,413,416,426]. The clustering of endings from the spinothalamic pathway contrast sharply with uniform distribution of the medial lemniscus projection to the same nucleus. Another dimension surfaced in Boivie's studies on the somatosensory projection to the cat thalamus. Lesions which distinguished between the spinothalamic and cervicothalamic projections showed the spinothalamic projection to be rostral to that of the dorsal column nuclei[280,327,427]. Preliminary observations in monkey indicate that, even though the spinothalamic and dorsal column nuclear projections overlap considerably, there is a tendency for spino-thalamic projections also to external rostral to terminations of cuneate and gracile fibres[416]. The termination of the dorsal column nuclear fibres in the feline VPL[280] compares closely with Rinvik's cytoarchitectonic defi-nition of this nucleus; in Rinvik's classification the extent of the VPL which matches the corticothalamic projection from the first and second somato-sensory regions[428,471] is smaller than that defined in Jasper and Ajmone–Marsan's[389] atlas. In this more restricted definition of cat VPL, the spino-thalamic projection lies outside that nucleus in a transitional zone between the region having the cytoarchitecture of the VPL and that typical for the more rostrally located nucleus ventralis lateralis. The topographical location of the transitional zone is similar to that of Hassler's[390] nucleus ventralis intermedium (V. im.) and seems partially to overlap the termination region for fibres from nucleus Z[292].

There are other interesting features of the transitional zone between the VPL and nucleus ventralis lateralis. Mehler[425] suggested a zone of overlap between spinal and cerebellar projections in the general vicinity of the region of ventralis intermedius (V. im.). Hassler[390] had earlier predicted that nucleus ventralis intermedius would project to the cortical area 3a, a cortical area dominated by an input from receptors of muscle. This prediction has been borne out by Strick[429], who found that the transitional zone in the cat equiva-lent to V. im. does in fact project to the cortical area receiving afferent input from large afferent fibres of muscle; its cortical termination is distinct from the area receiving fibres from the more caudally located VPL. In summary, this new view of the VPL arising from Rinvik's[428] and Boivie's[280,327,427] analyses raises the possibility that the several somatosensory pathways actually terminate on different cells of the ventral thalamic nuclei even when their projection fields overlap within the same nucleus. In attempting to assess the significance of such independence of termination, it is well to keep in mind the mounting evidence for functionally distinctive groups, populations (or columns) of cells in major sensory nuclei.

The more recent investigators of the spinothalamic pathway have described a bundle of fibres ending medially as well as laterally in the diencephalon[338,344,367,413,427]. According to Mehler[425], the medial termination lies within a continuous zone of the intralaminar region containing darkly-staining, medium-sized cells; he identifies the region as part of nucleus centralis lateralis. In the monkey, Olszewski's[388] classification would have placed this zone as partially within the nuclei parafascicularis and medialis dorsalis.

Morphological analyses generally agree that fibres of the spinal ventral quadrants send terminals to the posterior nuclear group[338,395,413,416,427]. In the monkey, these endings are distributed to the magnocellular medial geniculate and the supergeniculate nuclei[338,413,416,425]. Most of the spinothalamic contributions to the feline posterior nuclear group are to the medial portion of the magnocellular medial geniculate nucleus[427], i.e. ventromedially in the PO_m of Jones and Powell[395].

Several investigators have reported terminal degeneration in the ipsilateral subthalamus after lesions of the ventrolateral spinal quadrant[367,386,427]. Boivie[427] localised the subthalamic endings in the zona incerta; this could have a relation to the reported descending connections from the zona incerta to the periventricular grey region of the mesencephalon[411] and the latter's proposed involvement in pain (see Section 8.5.2.2). In cat, a few spinothalamic fibres have been reported to end in the nucleus centralis medialis of the midline thalamic nuclei[427].

Anatomical data do not indicate a somatotopical organisation in the spinothalamic projection other than to the VPL[425]. Even in the VPL somatotopy has been denied[426,427], although studies based upon histology probably could not detect differences in termination unless they were to relatively widely separated portions of the nucleus. Judgements about somatotopy from the usual morphological material can be dangerous; even with fairly diffuse patterns of termination individual cells may be dominated by input from a particular body region owing to the nature or concentration of synaptic contact.

8.6.2.4 Projections from nucleus Z

The projection of nucleus Z of the medulla has already been mentioned in considering the spinothalamic contribution to the VPL region. Grant, Boivie and Silfvenius[292] determined that a lesion restricted to nucleus Z of cat caused terminal degeneration dorsolateral and rostral to the dorsal column nuclei's projection to the ventroposterior region. Most terminations of fibres from nucleus Z are in the transitional zone of nucleus ventralis lateralis (V. im.), although there may be some overlap with the gracilis projection in VPL. Thus, in the only species so far studied, the projecton of nucleus Z to the ventroposterior thalamus in part overlaps topographically that of the spinothalamic tract and that from the dorsal column nuclei.

8.6.2.5 Reticulothalamic connections

The thalamic connections of those reticular nuclei which receive somato-sensory projections has been previously touched upon (Section 8.5.2.2). In general, certain neurons of the medullary, pontine and mesencephalic reticular formation and portions of the periaquaductal grey — the regions with input from spinal ventral quadrants — send processes mainly to the interlaminar nuclei[137,361].

8.6.3 Physiological activation

There is considerable controversy about the way thalamic neurons respond to various somatosensory stimuli and the functional significance of their responses. A good deal of the reported differences in results and conclusions have arisen due to variations in experimental conditions. Anaesthesia is one such factor and its influence will be mentioned in the course of the discussion. Another problem arises from the nature of afferent input; activation of sense organs is not equivalent to electrically initiated volleys in peripheral nerves or central tracts. When considering higher levels of the nervous system it is necessary to examine the presumption that increasing the strength of electrical shock to a nerve bundle or tract increases the magnitude of input. This may be true to the extent that fibres converging upon a central cell have actions of the same type, but often a uniform or common effect is not a feature of the underlying organisation. Fibres with inhibitory projections to a neuron may be recruited in varying proportions relative to those producing excitation at different stimulus intensities. Another possibility is that relatively sparse (weak) convergence which, under natural situations is functionally subthreshold and/or depressed by inhibition, may be converted to supra-threshold levels through synchronous activation of many elements normally not simultaneously active owing to spatial separation of their receptive terminals.

8.6.3.1 Ventroposterior region

A conceptual framework for the functional organisation of the somatosensory projection to the ventroposterior nuclei was set down by a series of electro-physiological investigations by Mountcastle and his collaborators. They obtained three dimensional 'maps' of the relation between the body surface and the ventral thalamic nuclei by recording neural activity evoked by natural stimulation of cutaneous sense organs in anaesthetised animals. Systematic exploration using stereotaxic coordinates with careful histological reconstruction of the electrode penetrations and comparisons to cytoarchi-tectural details demonstrated a somatotopic, tactile projection to the ventroposterior nuclei (ventralis posterolateralis – VPL — and ventralis posteromedialis – VPM) in cat, rabbit and monkey[392,414,415,430,431]. The thalamic representation of cutaneous receptors uncovered by these studies bears a considerable resemblance to that established in the pioneer topographic analyses of somatosensory activation of the cerebral cortex by Marshall, Woolsey and Bard[432]; diagrams showing how the body surface is related to the thalamic structures are caricatures of the contralateral half of the animal with feet ventrally located and facing toward the midline so that the back is dorsal, the head medial, the tail lateral and the forelimb medial to the hindlimb. The volume of thalamic tissue devoted to input from the face areas and distal portions of the limb is disproportionately large, mimicking the situation on the cerebral cortex. The somatotopic arrangements have been confirmed by other investigators[434,435] and basically similar patterns have been shown to exist in man[436-439] and other species[440].

(a) *Specificity of the input*—The somatotopic pattern was established with electrical recordings of activity from populations of thalamic neurons; however, determination of the modalities of stimulation effective for the projection needed the finer focus provided by recordings from single cells. In the intact, anaesthetised or unanaesthetised animal, a large proportion of ventroposterior units can be excited by innocuous mechanical stimuli[431,435,441,442]. Both in unanaesthetised monkeys[431] and awake man[443], about 50% of excitable units are driven by mechanical stimulation of the skin with the remainder responding to activation of subcutaneous receptors associated with joints or muscles. For elements responding to cutaneous stimuli, distinctions have been made between those activated from hair follicle receptors and those requiring 'touch' of the skin[430,431,435,441,442]. Neurons of the VPL are reported to be stimulus specific, responding to hair movement, direct skin stimulation, joint movement or mainpulation of the limb; only a limited number are fired by more than one of this spectrum of stimuli[435,442]. For example, Nakahama et al.[441] reported cells which were excited by direct skin contact from receptive fields consisting of from one to five discrete spots separated by less than 5 mm; these are features suggestive of a relatively pure, dominant projection from either Type I or Type II cutaneous receptors. Unfortunately, even the most recent analyses have not taken full advantage of stimuli which might distinguish between peripheral receptor types. Moreover, important dynamic parameters of mechanical stimuli (velocity, direction, etc.) are just coming into use in the study of central systems. For these reasons, a number of questions on the degree of convergence from different kinds of primary afferent units to neurons of the VPL or other somatosensory nuclei cannot be answered.

Within the ventroposterior region the class of stimuli effective in exciting an element is correlated with the latter's location; cells excited by subcutaneous receptors are concentrated in the dorsal and rostral portions of the nucleus while hair and 'touch' units are ventrally located[431,435,442]. Similarly, stimulation of Group I afferent fibres in muscle nerves is found to evoke responses at the rostral pole of the feline VPL, dorsomedially from the forelimb and dorsolaterally from the hindlimb[293,418,444,445]. Parenthetically, the last mentioned results are inconsistent with Poggio and Mountcastle's[431] conclusion that the 'deep' category of cells making up most of their VPL population receive their excitation from joint and fascia receptors; few joint and fascia sense organs have Group I afferent fibres. The conclusion from animal studies that receptor representation in the ventroposterior nuclei is segregated, elements activated by joint movement or muscle contraction being situated rostral and dorsal to cells excited by tactile stimuli, is supported by like observations in recordings made during human brain surgery[436-439,448,449].

New evidence on the nature of sensory receptors of the knee joint poses another problem for the interpretation of responses by thalamic neurons to joint movement. The myelinated fibre receptors making up the bulk of those found in Burgess and Clark's survey[64] have quite different properties from those Mountcastle, Poggio and Werner[452] used for comparing activity in sense organs and thalamic neurons. A population of VPL neurons was described which had a steady-state discharge frequency approximated by a power function transformation of joint angle (position)[452]. Mountcastle *et al.*[452] presumed that the thalamic cell discharges related to joint position were initiated by sense organs in joint tissue; however, in nerves to the knee joint of cat (and one species of monkey), there are few if any first-order neurons producing steady-state discharges with maxima at intermediate joint angles in the fashion described for thalamic units[64]; the only slowly adapting joint sense organs found gave a maximal discharge at the limits of joint position. It is possible that the thalamic unitary activity represents a synthesis of the input from such receptors. Alternatively, the thalamic and the similar responses observed at the cerebral cortical level[453,454] are related to the projection from sense organs of muscle previously mentioned. This issue can only be resolved by additional experiments with careful identification of the sensory structures being stimulated.

An interesting point was made by Andersen *et al.*[418] in their study of thalamic activity evoked from muscle nerves. They located a narrow lamina of cells which responded to activation of slowly conducting myelinated afferent fibres from muscle and had a longer latency response to excitation of cutaneous nerves than more ventral and caudal VPL units. This lamina lay dorsal to the thalamic zone receiving the Group I mucle projection. These observations on a thin afferent fibre projection are reminiscent of Poggio and Mountcastle's[431] report of thalamic units in an apparently similar location responding solely to strong stimulation of widely distributed deep tissues.

A limited number of VPL units are said to have convergence from hair follicle and skin contact receptors[435,441]. Field or D hair receptors are relevant to this kind of apparent covergence; both are movement-sensitive elements and input from them along with that from other velocity detection receptors does not carry the same implication as would convergence from movement and position receptors. Burton *et al.*[450] mentioned that a substantial number of VPL cells responsive to tactile stimuli increase their firing rate during fairly marked cooling, while none respond to warming. Type II receptors, D hair receptors and some field receptors respond to sudden, relatively marked cooling, so an apparent convergent response could reflect solely primary afferent characteristics. One obviously needs to know more than the fact that a central cell responds to mechanical and to thermal stimuli to decide on the mixture or purity of the primary afferent projection.

The situation is different for Martin and Manning's[451] observation that sudden heating excites a small proportion of VPL cells also responsive to gentle mechanical stimuli; this combination of effective stimuli cannot be explained on the basis of a single kind of primary afferent unit and indicates true multi-modal convergence. Responses to heat and innocuous tactile stimuli could reflect an input from nonprimary dorsal column and/or spinocervical fibres, since they exhibit these features (Sections 8.5.1.1; 8.5.1.3); this possibility needs examination inasmuch as the destination of these spinal fibres is a mystery.

(b) *Pain*—The question of a specialised input to the ventral thalamus important for pain has taken on a new significance with the establishment of a special linkage from nociceptors to particular spinal cells. Gaze and Gordon[459] noted that a few neurons of the ventroposterior region in cat and monkey required activity in Aδ myelinated fibres for excitation and responded only to intense mechanical stimuli; this contrasted with the activation of over 80% of their 64 units by hair movement and rapidly conducting primary fibres. In animals with sectioned dorsal spinal tracts, Perl and Whitlock[145] also reported observations on neurons in the ventroposterior region of cat and monkey that were excited only by noxious (mechanical and/or heat) stimuli applied to small receptive fields. Other studies of unitary responses from the ventroposterior nuclei have not described nociceptive units in intact preparations and their existence has been doubted or explained as products of other deafferentation or deep anaesthesia[455,455a]. A source for a specific nociceptive input to the ventral thalamus has now been uncovered by the demonstration of laminae I and IV–V neurons excited only by noxious stimuli which project rostrally, some as far as the thalamus[143,352,356]. The number of ventroposterior thalamic cells with specific nociceptive function may be small, and their presence normally masked by the much larger population of elements responding to innocuous stimuli. Support for the existence of a set of neurons with a special significance for localised pain, possibly in a particular thalamic locus, is provided by observation made during stereotactic procedures on man attempting to relieve chronic pain or symptoms of Parkinsonism. Hassler[456] reported 15 years ago that stimulation caudal and inferior to the main body of the VPL evokes reports of severe pain in conscious patients. Moreover, lesions of the region, labelled by Hassler[456] as nucleus ventralis posterior inferior, are said to be successful in alleviating certain painful states. Hassler's argument for a region in this locality with significance for pain sensation is supported by Halliday and Logue[457], who describe evocation of unpleasant paresthesias, identified or defined by conscious patients as burning or sharp pain; they also place this region caudal and inferior to that responding to innocuous stimulation of the contralateral body. In Halliday and Logue's subjects, similar electrical stimulation small distances from the region where the painful paresthesia was produced evoked tingling without a painful quality.

(c) *Relation of function to afferent pathway*—While anatomical evidence agrees in indicating that all major ascending somatosensory pathways send terminals to the ventroposterior region, the nature of the activity carried by each system is a matter of considerable disagreement. Several possibilities exist including:

(1) convergence of excitatory activity from different pathways upon a given thalamic cell;

(2) primary excitation from one route and modulatory impulses over another to act on a given neuron; and/or

(3) quite separate neuronal populations within the region, each concerned with the peripheral afferent traffic conveyed to them over a separate route.

Contrary to impressions given by much of the literature and many textbooks, a good deal of the traditional view on functional attributes of the dorsal column–medial lemniscus contribution to the thalamus is based upon inference from complex clinical situations. As we have pointed out earlier (see Section 8.6.2.4), direct experimental evidence favours the idea that Group I muscle receptor activity reaches the rostral VPL region via the contralateral medial lemniscus after synapses in the ventral portion of the cuneate nucleus (forelimb)[268,445-447,460] or in the dorsal horn and nucleus Z (hindlimb)[290,293,295]. Direct physiological observations supported by behavioural studies also suggest that in animals a major fraction of the velocity- and vibration-sensitive cutaneous receptors synapse in the dorsal column nuclei and are part of the medial lemniscus projection to the VPL [Section 8.2.3, 8.5.1.1(a)]. In addition, afferent fibres from Type II cutaneous receptors link with projecting cells of the dorsal column nuclei; this input presumably contributes to the displacement (and sudden cooling) component of cutaneously evoked responses in the VPL [Section 8.6.3.1(a)]. Thus, some 'hair' and 'touch' units of the VPL proper appear to receive at least part of their excitation over the dorsal column–dorsal column nuclei–medial lemniscus system; these tactile projections are both stimulus-specific (hair and vibration) and stimulus-mixed (touch), but overall still have characteristics consistent with the kinds of modality segregation reported for VPL neurons. It must be noted, though, that observations indicating the nature of the VPL response to afferent input over the dorsal column–medial lemniscus in isolation are lacking. Wall[461] reports the startling finding that behavioural responses cannot be evoked by stimulation of body regions below a level at which all of the spinal cord is transected except the dorsal columns.

Although some investigators have contended that the excitatory input to the VPL arises strictly from the contralateral body half[430,432,462], there are accounts of VPL neurons being activated by ipsilateral somatic stimulation[463]. Jabbur, Baker and Towe[463] describe excitation of cat VPL neurons by electrical stimulation of the ipsilateral dorsal columns under conditions eliminating physical spread; the VPL responses to the dorsal column stimuli mimicked those evoked by electrical stimulation of the skin of an ipsilateral limb. McLeod's[463a] observation that VPL neurons which are readily driven by light tactile stimulation of contralateral receptive fields respond to electrical excitation of the ipsilateral splanchnic nerve also conflicts with the idea that functional excitation of this nucleus is limited to a contralateral input. Chloralose anaesthesia is a common feature in studies demonstrating ipsilateral excitation of the VPL and could represent a critical variable, since the concept of a strictly crossed projection to this nucleus is founded on observations in barbiturate or unanaesthetised preparations. It appears unlikely that chloralose anaesthesia can create ipsilateral neuronal connections. On the other hand, an agent with selective effects upon the excitability of different neurons conceivably could modify inhibitory interactions so as to allow observation of excitatory connections suppressed under certain forms of anaesthesia or in the unanaesthetised brain.

There is even less information on the kinds of adequate stimulation and the receptor population which contribute to activation of VPL cells via the dorsolateral spinal fasciculus than exists for the dorsal column system. Two sets of experiments have attempted to differentiate between pathways of the dorsolateral spinal cord and the spinal dorsal columns in activation of thalamic cells[417,418]. By electrical stimulation of the dorsolateral fasciculus or the dorsal columns, isolated from the rest of the spinal cord, the dorsolateral fasciculus was shown to excite a shell of neurons around the central core of the VPL. This outer zone corresponds closely to the region of degenerating terminals produced by lesions of the lateral cervical nucleus[327]. With rare exceptions, neurons in the core surrounded by the shell respond to dorsal column excitation but not to spinocervical input. In the shell, most of the neurons receive an input from both the spinocervical pathway and the dorsal column; one third respond only to the dorsolateral fasciculus and 10% only to the dorsal column input. Unfortunately, testing of the adequate forms of stimulation are not possible in such experiments. Demonstration of this kind of convergence from the two dorsal spinal pathways upon some ventroposterior neurons and their independent excitation of others in carefully done experiments must be accounted for in any conceptual proposal.

Perl and Whitlock[145] approached the question of the spinothalamic input by recording thalamic activity in barbiturate anaesthetised cats and monkeys after transection of the dorsal columns and the contralateral dorsolateral fasciculus. This approach has inherent limitations due to possible modification of responses by removal of background or contributory effects. Nevertheless, it does give information of the functional capabilities of the residual pathways and turns out to fit with some other observations. In these animals with dorsal cord transections, evoked activity was regularly seen in the VPL region but many spontaneously active units were encountered which could be driven neither by electrical stimulation of intact nerves nor natural stimulation of the body. Two-thirds of some 70 verified ventroposterior units in preparations could be driven by hair movement or transient contact with the skin and another 15% by direct pressure on the skin, confirming Gaze and Gordon's[464] discovery of a tactile projection to the thalamus in the absence of the dorsal columns. Unexpectedly, a few cells, including some in both species, were excitable by joint movement under conditions in which inadvertent activation of cutaneous sense organs and the receptors of contractile parts of muscle had been minimized. Eight of 70 neurons, some in each species, responded only to noxious cutaneous pinching or heat, and were driven by nerve volleys only when slowly conducting myelinated components were included. Recently, Bowsher[465] split crossing fibres in the cat's upper cervical spinal cord and lower medulla to eliminate dorsal column and lateral cervical nucleus contributions and also found VPL cells to respond to peripheral stimulation. Approximately one-third of Bowsher's units were excited by electrical stimuli applied to the skin of one limb alone with the remainder responding to stimulation of the skin of several limbs. Thus, physiological data demonstrates that the projection from tracts in the ventral quadrants of the spinal cord to the ventroposterior nuclei in both carnivore and primate is partially excitatory and in part shows stimulus- and place-specific qualities.

Connections and interactions between ventroposterior nuclei of opposite sides have been the subject of a series of studies by Bava, Fadiga and Manzoni[466-459]. Their work has not only indicated the nature of effects one nucleus may produce on the other, but also describe remarkable but systematic variations associated with different preparations. Studies summarised by Fadiga and Manzoni[470] indicate that almost all VPL cells in unanesthetised acutely decorticated cats, (1) had inputs limited to the contralateral body side from restricted receptive fields and (2) showed limited stimulus modality convergence. Interestingly, only the few 'non-specific' elements encountered in such preparations could be excited by stimulation of the contralateral VPL. In contrast, in similar experiments in cats anaesthetised by chloralose, approximately one-third of the units did not show the specificity typical of VPL core cells and these same elements responded to stimulation of the opposite VPL. With chronic decortication, projecting VPL cells undergo retrograde degeneration; in such preparations again about one-third of the unitary elements encountered were 'non-specific' while the remainder were typical of the modality specific type. Over 50% of all the cells in chronically decorticate animals could be excited by electrical stimulation of the opposite VPL. Inhibitory interactions suggestive of a presynaptic locus of action were also noted from one VPL nucleus to its contralateral homologue[469]. The crossed excitatory interactions were dependent upon the integrity of the posterior commissure, while the inhibitory ones disappeared following lesions in the region of the massa intermedia.

(d) *Spindling activity in the VPL*—Both the first (S-I) and second (S-II) somatosensory cortical areas have somatotopically arranged descending connections to the VPL[405,406,428,471,473,474]. The pattern of interconnections between the thalamus and the cortex appear reciprocal in that somatotopically equivalent regions each project to the other; e.g. the forelimb portion of the thalamus sends fibres to the forelimb area of the cortex and receives fibres back from the same cortical region.

The reciprocity between thalamus and cortex seems to be correlated with spindling activity or rhythmic discharges seen both in the VPL and in the cerebral cortex during sleep and deep barbiturate anaesthesia. In the cat, thalamic spindles consist of about 10 sec^{-1} bursts of activity lasting several seconds and separated by intervals of relative quiescence. Spindles may occur in the absence of specific afferent input or may be evoked by afferent stimulation, although the two types differ in their onset characteristics. The following comments are based largely upon Andersen and Andersson's[475] extensive monograph on the topic and the reader is referred to it for further details. Spindling is encountered in the ventral, lateral, intralaminar and medial thalamic nuclei as well as in the cerebral cortex, but it is not seen in structures such as the caudate, the hypothalamus or the mesencephalic reticular formation[476]. There is a degree of synchronisation between spindle activity in the thalamus and in the cerebral cortex with a particularly close linkage between somatotopically equivalent portions of the VPL and the somatosensory cortex. By contrast, different portions of the somatosensory cortex and different portions of the VPL do not show synchronisation of spindles so that cells 100 μm apart may be participating in spindling bursts with different timing[477]. Andersen, Andersson and Lomo[478] demonstrated the dependence of spindling in S-I upon the VPL by showing that destructions of the thalamic nucleus abolished spindling in S-I. At the same time, lesions of the medial thalamic nuclei had relatively little effect upon cortical spindling.

Intracellular recordings made during spindling cycles reveal that each cycle or wave of the spindle has its reflection in individual elements as an initial depolarisation during which the cell may produce a burst of discharges and then a subsequent prolonged hyperpolarisation. Andersen et al.[483] argued that the hyperpolarisation was an inhibitory potential caused by interneurons with widely distributed effects; the interneurons were presumed to be activated through recurrent collaterals of the thalamocortical neurons. The recurrent collateral concept was based upon the observation that similar inhibitory postsynaptic potentials could be evoked both by ascending afferent input and by antidromic excitation of thalamocortical fibres. Different mechanisms have been proposed for the initial depolarisation, including an internally generated effect due to a rebound from prolonged inhibition[475] or excitatory synaptic bombardment from other sources[478a].

During spontaneous spindling, the thalamic response to afferent input varies according to the phase of spindle activity; in general, the evoked response is markedly depressed immediately after and for a considerable fraction of the interspindle period[482]. Evoked thalamic activity, particularly that arriving by way of the spino–cervicothalamic path, can be markedly depressed by stimulation of the equivalent somatotopic portion of the S-I cortex; this observation may have a relation to the inhibitory postsynaptic potential associated with the interspindle interval[418].

(e) *Synaptic mechanisms*—Excitatory synaptic activation of VPL cells appears to follow rules established for other parts of the nervous system. Excitatory postsynaptic potentials of relatively large size are evoked upon stimulation of medial lemniscus fibres, triggering repetitive impulses[478a]. Smaller depolarising postsynaptic potentials which may occur in seemingly random patterns or in rhythmical bursts are also a common feature. When the latter 'spontaneous' potentials summate, an impulse is generated[478a]. Excitatory postsynaptic potentials evoked by afferent nerve volleys are consistently followed by large postsynaptic hyperpolarisations lasting about 100 msec; the latter are powerful enough to prevent the cell from being discharged during much of their time course. During the latter part of inhibitory postsynaptic potentials, VPL cells appear to have a lowered threshold for impulse generation[478a]. At this writing, nothing is known about the nature of either the excitatory or the inhibitory mediators in the VPL.

Inhibition and associated inhibitory postsynaptic potentials may be evoked in thalamic neurons by afferent input. Interneurons of the VPL, i.e. neurons which cannot be antidromically activated from the cerebral cortex, have been suggested as the mediators of postsynaptic inhibition[479,483]. The question of presynaptic inhibition within the VPL is controversial; some authors have reported weak effects of this type upon fibres from the dorsal column nuclei[483], but others have denied its existence[480]. While there have been a number of accounts of inhibitory interactions due to ascending input to the VPL, the generality of the effect is disputed. VPL neurons typically discharge in the absence of specific stimulation in unanaesthetised preparations; inhibition of the spontaneous discharge has been reported for only a small fraction of VPL units[431,435]. On the other hand, when inhibition is tested against an evoked response, a much larger fraction of VPL units is found to have inhibitory receptive fields, often of the surround type[441]. Inhibitory effects on VPL neurons are suppressed much more by barbiturate than by chloralose anaesthesia[481].

8.6.3.2 Posterior group

Poggio and Mountcastle[430] identified the posterior group as a cytoarchitectural entity much larger than the region which receives a direct input from ascending sensory pathways (see Section 8.6.1). They reported that in cats lightly anaesthetised with barbiturate, most cells within this larger area respond only to noxious manipulation of bilateral and widely distributed deep body structures. The remainder of their posterior region elements were excited by brusque, but innocuous mechanical stimulation of large regions of the integument. Characteristics of posterior group units contrasted sharply with those of typical VPL neurons, the latter in Poggio and Mountcastle's view reflecting on afferent input largely from the dorsal column–medial lemniscus system. This logic led to the deduction that the posterior group was excited via the spinothalamic tract. In addition, the intense stimulation necessary to excite the majority of posterior group neurons led to the postulate that the region was important in pain mechanisms.

Subsequent work has not confirmed domination of the posterior nuclear region either by nociceptive activity or by a spinothalamic input. In intact, although apparently deeply anaesthetised cats, Curry[485] found that all but 3% of posterior group neurons responded to innocuous mechanical stimulation of the skin, particularly hair movement. This agrees with the predominantly mechanoreceptive cutaneous input described earlier in both cat and monkey with divided dorsal columns and dorsolateral tracts[145]. The differences between Poggio and Mountcastle's results and those of other investigators may be attributable to the former's use of more lightly anaesthetised preparations and recordings from regions other than those receiving direct somatosensory projections. Nevertheless, it must be explained why nociceptive characteristics have not appeared for neurons located in the portion of the posterior group directly receiving terminations from somatosensory pathways under conditions permitting their observation elsewhere[145,365].

All investigators agree that the receptive fields of posterior nuclear group neurons are large and often involve three or four limbs. Thus, spatial convergence is unquestioned. A clear somatotopic organisation is absent, although a tendency for neurons having most effective excitation from one body region to be located in particular regions has been noted[484]. Posterior group units with bilateral receptive fields usually respond more vigorously to contralateral than to ipsilateral stimuli and when electrical shocks to nerves or the skin are used, the response latency is shortest for contralateral stimulation[145,422,485]. No major differences have been observed between posterior nucleus responses between the cat and monkey[145,434].

A considerable fraction of posterior group neurons show afferent inhibition with the inhibitory receptive field varying in size and location relative to the excitatory area. Gentle movement of body hair inhibits the spontaneous discharge of many elements[485]. Stimulation of the somatosensory cortical areas also inhibit a number of posterior group cells[486,487] and a good proportion of cortically inhibited cells also can be facilitated from cortical loci[487]. On the basis of antidromically evoked responses, a small fraction of posterior group cells have a fibre reaching the S-I cortical area and a somewhat larger proportion have one extending to S-II; one instance was reported of antidromic driving from both cortical areas[487].

Both physiological and anatomical evidence indicates that the dorsal column nuclei–medial lemniscus pathway, the cervicothalamic tract and the spinothalamic tract terminate within restricted portions of the posterior nuclear region. When electrical stimuli are limited by lesions and dissection of fascicles either to the dorsal columns, or the dorsolateral fasciculus or the ventral quadrants of the spinal cord, Curry and Gordon[484] found the dorsal columns to evoke the most prominent activity in the posterior nuclear region. Evaluated in this fashion, the contralateral dorsolateral fasciculus was the next most powerful projecting system while fibres of the ventral quadrants were the least effective.

Not only the role of the posterior group in pain mechanisms, but also its overall functional significance remains in doubt. It is an area receiving a convergent somatosensory input and at least some of its neurons are also excited by auditory activity[431,485]. The posterior group has been postulated to be a source of thalamic projection to S-II of the cerebral cortex[430,488] as well as to other areas[489,490]. The overall evidence is sufficiently conflicting to raise doubts about the posterior group functioning as a relay region comparable with the ventroposterior nuclei[487].

8.6.3.3 Intralaminar nuclei

Both the direct spinothalamic and spinoreticular–thalamic pathways terminate within part of the intralaminar complex of the thalamus (see Sections 8.6.3.3 and 8.6.3.4); work done to date does not distinguish between functional activity arriving over one or the other. Physiological observations first pointed out the existence of a somatosensory projection to thalamic structures located medial to the ventrobasal nuclei[491-493]. Kruger and Albe-Fessard[433,494] noted that single afferent volleys evoke a double response of neurons in the centrum medianum–parafasicular complex. The shortest response latency in the intralaminar region to somatosensory volleys is nearly twice that of responses evoked in the ventroposterior thalamus by identical stimuli. Dorsal column and dorsolateral tract fibres apparently do not contribute an excitatory input to the intralaminar region[363,495]. Adequate stimulation of intralaminar neurons in chloralose- or barbiturate-anaesthetised cat and monkey is usually described as brusque tapping, pinching or squeezing of the skin over large receptive fields[145,433,434,496-498]. However, Casey[499] points out that the kind of response obtained is a function of anaesthetic level; noxious stimuli are effective in awake and deeply anaesthetised animals, while both noxious and innocuous stimuli are effective in very lightly anaesthetised preparations. Intralaminar neurons responding to ascending afferent input can be deeply inhibited by stimulation of the caudate nucleus[500], cortical S-II and the inferior temporal region of the ipsilateral cerebral cortex[501]. In addition, Albe-Fessard and Gillett[501] and Dila[502] describe excitatory effects on centrum medianum neurons from stimulation of the mesencephalic reticular formation. It has been suggested that the centrum medianum region is a relay to 'association' regions of the cerebrum[493]; supporting evidence for direct corticopetal fibres from the centrum medianum–parafasicular region to these cortical areas has not appeared[503].

8.6.4 Lemniscal and non-lemniscal

The term 'lemniscal' and its antonym, 'non-lemniscal', have achieved some currency over the past decade, contributing a semantic problem to concepts about the somatosensory system. This nomenclature's present usage derives from differences in the behaviour of elements recorded from the thalamic ventroposterior nuclei and the posterior group. Poggio and Mountcastle[431,432] reported that most VPL neurons, presumably thalamocortical relay cells, had the following properties:

(a) they were activated by mechanical stimulation of a restricted part of the contralateral half of the body;

(b) they were excited only by a limited class of mechanical stimuli (a characteristic termed modality specificity); and

(c) they displayed a high degree of synaptic security expressed as an ability to follow repeated stimulation at frequencies in excess of 10 or 20 sec^{-1}.

VPL neurons with these features (and neurons in other locations with similar properties) were labelled 'lemniscal' based upon the assumption that the afferent input responsible for the characteristics arrived over the medial lemniscus (via the dorsal column–dorsal column nuclei linkage). In contrast, posterior group elements excited from large receptive fields, receiving projections from both sides of the body, having convergence from obviously different types of sensory receptors, were classified as 'non-lemniscal' under the assumption that the somatosensory input came from the spinothalamic projection[431,432]. The term 'lemniscal' was equated with discriminative and linked to Head's[504,506] concept of epicritic sensation; a similar correspondence was suggested for 'non-lemniscal' and protopathic sense. These equivalencies were abetted by Poggio and Mountcastle's concept of pain as a largely non-discriminative sensation and their finding of diffuse nociceptive responses by posterior region neurons — responses they assumed were derived from a non-lemniscal input, the spinothalamic projection. These terms and associated arguments gave Head's notion of a duality in sensation the morphological organisation and thalamic home he had hypothesised but which he and others had been unable to demonstrate[505].

The terminology represents simple designations for certain attributes of neurons in the somatosensory system and have become widely disseminated in the literature. A variety of anatomical and physiological observations conflicts with the implications and assumptions associated with the terms lemniscal and non-lemniscal. To begin with there is the well-established contribution of spinothalamic tracts to the ventroposterior nuclei of the primate and the demonstration of 'lemniscal-like' characteristics for part of that projection. The fact that medial lemniscal elements make up a major part of the input to the posterior group, the very region which spawned the non-lemniscal idea is probably even a more compelling consideration. In addition, there is the difficulty that some medial lemniscal elements have the type of receptor and spatial convergence attributed to 'non-lemniscal' systems. The misleading anatomical connotations are only some of the considerations for arguing against continued use of lemniscal and non-lemniscal. As the material in this article shows, the notion that there are just two kinds of organisational arrangements within the somatosensory system does not fit the facts. The concept associated with lemniscal derives to a considerable extent from observations on the projections of mechanical movement detectors. The ability to follow rapid changes in excitation by mechanical events is certainly appropriate for a discriminative system but it is not any more discerning than the ability to detect the difference between warm and burning hot. Therefore, we feel that the notion of the qualities defined as lemniscal as being those characteristic of a discriminative system also should be dispelled.

It will be difficult to abandon a widely used but inappropriate nomenclature. We admit the convenience of labelling groups of characteristics for ease of discussion but hope words can be chosen implying neither incorrect morphological attributes nor dubious psychophysical–philosophical ones. A possible alternative to lemniscal could be 'specified' since we often know much about part of an arrangement making up the constellation of characteristics now labelled lemniscal. A substitute for 'non-lemniscal' could be 'unspecified', which at times simply would be an admission of ignorance. We believe these terms to be superior to the terminology 'convergent' and 'non-convergent' utilised by Albe-Fessard and Besson[503], since almost every kind of ascending projection has at least convergence of input from like elements in its organisation.

8.7 THE CEREBRAL CORTEX

The existence of cortical regions with special importance for somatic sensation is an old idea; it gained great impetus from the development of the evoked potential technique which permitted direct demonstration of the projection from peripheral sense organs to the cerebral mantle[227, 432, 507]. With use and refinement of cortical surface recordings, several different cortical areas with reproducible boundaries were demonstrated to receive excitation from somatic sensory receptors. Our attention will be principally directed at two of these, labelled by Adrian[507] as first (S-I) and second (S-II) to signify their chronological discovery, not — as the terms primary and secondary might imply — relative importance[508]. In addition to S-I and S-II, S-III[509], a suprasylvian fringe area[510], an area on the orbital cortex, and portions of the motor areas have been associated with somatosensory projections. Anatomical features[508], physiological considerations[159] and descending effects[269] of cortical somatosensory regions have recently been thoroughly reviewed. For these reasons, we shall limit our comments to general considerations and changes in point of view.

8.7.1 Morphological considerations

In primates, S-I begins anteriorly at the depth of the central sulcus and extends posteriorly as part of the parietal cortex; from anterior to posterior it is comprised of cytoarchitectonic areas 3a, 3b, 2 and 1. The anterior border of the feline S-I begins just in front of the postcruciate dimple, which forms part of the borderline between the homologues of areas 3a and 3b. In both primates and carnivore, S-I begins on the medial surface of the cortex and extends laterally to the junction with S-II. Cortical sensory areas are characterised by a large number of small, mostly stellate, neurons (Golgi Type II) which give it a granular appearance. In the terminology of cyto-architecture, the S-I cortical area is koniocortex, differing from the prokonio-cortex of S-II. In the monkey, S-II lies on the anterior bank of the lateral (Sylvian) fissure, while in the cat it is located largely in the anterior ectosylvian gyrus. In the cat, the suprasylvian fringe area lies immediately rostral and dorsal to the first auditory area, while S-III lies posterior to S-I in the anterior suprasylvian gyrus. The orbito-insular region of the cat lies in the orbital gyrus ventral to the orbital sulcus.

8.7.1.1 Cellular and synaptic features

The predominant neurons of the cerebral cortex are pyramidal and stellate (or granule) cells. Pyramidal neurons have an apical dendrite as well as a number of thick basal dendrites; all have many spines. The apical dendrite ascends to layer I and branches there. Pyramidal cell axons descend to the cortical white matter, some giving off recurrent collaterals before they leave the cellular areas. Axons of stellate cells are short and stay within the cortical mantle; their dendrites are thick and have many branches but few spines. Lorente de No[409] made note of the fact that cortical cells are arranged in cylinders approximately perpendicular to the surface; this observation provides an anatomical substrate for the concept advanced by Mountcastle[511], and Powell and Mountcastle[512] that a column of cortical cells represents a functional unit (see Section 8.7.1.2). Afferent fibres to S-I from the thalamus appear to be distributed so that each branch ascends within one column of cells, although its effects may not be confined to the cells of the column. Commissural fibres to S-I also run perpendicular to the surface apparently within the confines of one column[508]. According to Jones and Powell[508], the afferent terminations in S-II seem less strictly oriented toward the perpen-dicular cell cylinders and take a more oblique course through the cortical layers. Thalamocortical fibres make synaptic contact principally on dendritic spines throughout the layer IV of the cortex, in adjacent parts of layers III

and V, and in the deep portion of layer I[513]. The general belief is that thalamocortical fibres synapse on pyramidal cells; however, the actual evidence from
electronmicroscopic studies can only specify with certainty a connection to
dendritic spines. Since the dendrites of both pyramidal and stellate cells have
spines, the possibility remains that the dendritic contact is to stellate cells.
Fibres to S-I from S-II and from the opposite hemisphere terminate most
heavily at the same levels as the thalamocortical projections.

8.7.1.2 Cytoarchitecture and its correlations

The figures detailing somatotopic projections to the cerebral cortex are
familiar in many textbooks of neuroanatomy, physiology and neurology. The
remarkable fit between the boundaries of carefully made maps of S-I and
structurally determined cytoarchitectonic details is probably not as generally
appreciated as is the presence of somatotopic representation. The correlation
to cytoarchitecture becomes especially clear when the particulars of a pattern
of evoked activity are compared directly with histological delineation of
cortical structure in the fashion pioneered by Powell and Mountcastle[512, 533].
As a result there has been a rekindled interest in cortical cytoarchitectonics
and the latter adds an important dimension to current studies of cerebral
function[508, 514, 515]. Mountcastle's[511] proposal of functional columns, while at
times challenged or misunderstood, now is supported by a solid body of
data for S-I[159, 508]. Stated simply, it argues that a column of neurons arranged
perpendicular to the surface of a particular part of the cortex contains
elements which are similar in their peripheral receptive fields and in the
stimuli necessary to activate them. In practical terms, this means that when
an S-I neuron is excited by light mechanical stimulation of a leg skin area,
the receptive fields of other cells in the same column respond to the
same general class of stimulus to overlapping but not necessarily coextensive
skin areas. One millimetre away, a different column of cells may be related
to joint movement or other deep tissue distortion, from the region of the
lower leg. These conclusions are drawn from studies in which discharges
have been recorded from single neurons or small groups of neurons with
microelectrodes inserted progressively through layers of the cerebral cortex.
Most recordings have been made from depths equivalent to layers III and
IV, but they have been coupled with enough observations both deeper and
more superficially so as to lend credence to the columnar organisation concept
The finding that tangential or angled penetrations, in contrast to those made
carefully perpendicular to the true cortical surface, usually encounter sudden
discontinuities or jumps in the functional characteristics of one small group
of cells to the next is advanced as consistent with the columnar scheme. The
latter observation has served as a principle in experimental design used to
make correlations and comparisons between different areas or for examining
changes imposed by experimental conditions[29, 162, 516-520]. While columnar
organisation seems to be a reality in the functional architecture of the
visual[516, 517, 581], auditory[582, 583], and motor cerebral cortical regions[584], it may
not be equally well developed in all areas. The latter factor, the experimental
approach used, and the nature of associated morphological analyses — all

probably contribute to reported differences in the observations on vertically organised arrangements within the cortex.

8.7.2 Somatotopy revisited

The original evoked potential maps showed the cortical representation of the body surface to be grossly distorted with much larger portions devoted to the face, hand and foot than to proximal portions of the body. When examined using adequate stimulation of peripheral receptors, individual S-I neurons, with rare exceptions, are excited from the opposite side of the body. Receptive fields of single S-I units are smallest when they are distally located on the extremities and largest in size proximally on the body[162, 454, 511].

The early somatotopic maps corresponded reasonably well with the area thought to be somatosensory on other grounds. Systematic examination of the receptive fields and kinds of stimuli exciting single neurons presented a new degree of complexity; the representation of body surface, the basic feature of the earlier somatotopic maps, was supplemented by data on projections activated by specific modes of stimulation — subcutaneous as well as cutaneous. Increased detail in the somatotopic map also emerged. Imagine turning the cortex of a macaque monkey into a flat sheet without convolutions by unfolding it. Neurons of S-I in such a sheet would have receptive fields successively arranged in a sequence reflecting the segmental dermatomes as one moves along a line from the medial to the lateral border close to the junction between areas 3b and 1[29, 162, 243, 518-520, 522, 523]. On the other hand, the pattern of the receptive fields of single cells from the anterior to the posterior border of S-I would change in a sequence at right angles to segmental levels and in some places these would follow a circular course around a body part. There are differences of opinion on whether to call the observed sequence and its pattern 'dermatomal' or 'somatotopic'; however, the basic observations are not disputed[440, 523].

8.7.3 Thalamocortical and corticothalamic connections

Morphological studies have established that both S-I and S-II receive terminals directly from neurons of the ventroposterior nuclei in a topically organised fashion. No anatomical evidence exists for direct projections from the ventroposterior nuclei to any other cortical area. The region of cat S-III (cortical area 5) receives fibres from the nucleus lateralis posterior of the thalamus as well as from the ipsilateral S-I[524, 525]. Finally, the somatosensory activation of the cat orbital cortex can be blocked by manipulations in the ventroposterior region, but not from a number of other thalamic structures[526]; the apparent lack of direct connections between the ventroposterior nuclei and cortical regions other than S-I and S-II suggests that pathways to the former through VPL are multisynaptic.

Reciprocal, topographically organised connections between many cortical areas and the thalamic nuclei from which they receive ascending input has been mentioned earlier. Both S-I and S-II project back to the ventroposterior nuclei in a detailed place to place arrangement and are the only cortical regions to do so[508]. Jones and Powell[508] call attention to the possibility that the thalamic neuron projecting to a certain group of S-I or S-II cortical cells may in turn receive a set of terminals from them. An arrangement of this type could represent either a negative feedback or a feedforward mechanism depending upon whether the reciprocal corticothalamic contact is excitatory or inhibitory. By and large, the effects which have been seen are inhibitory[272], although Iwamura, Gardner and Spencer[479] express the view that conditions for positive feedback also may exist. The posterior nuclear group may be a possible exception to the general principle of reciprocity. The medial part of the posterior group region, PO_m[395], is a somatosensory input region which Heath and Jones[490] argue does not project to either S-I or S-II in the cat, but receives fibres from both areas; they believe that PO_m sends fibres only to the suprasylvian fringe cortex. On the other hand, some investigators propose projections from PO_m to S–II proper[425,489]. The main source of cortical fibres to the intralaminar nuclei are the motor and premotor cortical areas of the frontal lobe[472,472a,527]. Area 3a of S-I may have connections to the caudal portions of nuclei centralis lateralis and centrum medianum[528].

An interesting and new interpretation of the interrelations between cortex and thalamus is proposed by Jones and Powell[395]. They argue that the sensory systems — somatic, auditory and visual — all have relations with three major regions of the thalamus: the specific sensory nuclei, the posterior and intralaminar groups, and the reticular nucleus. They postulate that the posterior group and the intralaminar nuclei are different portions of the same entity. Part of this hypothesis is based upon the composite of the afferent input to the posterior group and the intralaminar nuclei as well as their descending cortical connections. Some of the possible contradictions and mysteries of the connectivity in the somatosensory region may be explicable in terms of this hypothesis; however, it needs more investigation both at the level of morphological interconnections and related physiological features.

8.7.4 Cortico–cortical connections

Different cortical areas related to the somatosensory system have an intricate series of interconnections, both within one hemisphere and between areas of the two hemispheres. Some of these, depicting material summarised by Jones and Powell[508], are shown in Figure 8.1. There are interconnections which tie together rather large somatotopic subsections of S-I, such as the hand area. Different major somatotopic regions, for example the hand as opposed to the face area, are not so linked. S-I is connected to the motor cortex, to S-II, to area 5 ipsilaterally and to S-II and S-I contralaterally. In turn, S-II projects ipsilaterally to S-I, to the motor region as well as to the contralateral S-II. Intrinsic association fibres connecting different subdivisions of S-I or (S-II) together appear to run within the grey matter and thus cross a large number of cortical columns; they could make connections in their passage between various columns. Connections between S-I and another major area, such as S-II, pass subcortically.

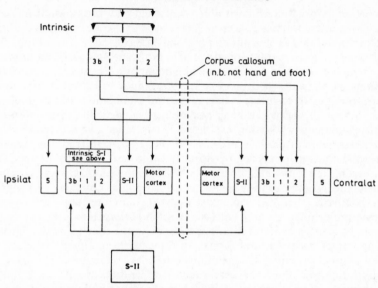

Figure 8.1 Intrinsic, hemispheric and intrahemispheric connections of somatosensory cortical regions. The beginning of a connection is shown as a short vertical line and its distribution by the horizontal lines; termination points are indicated by the vertical lines with arrows. The blocks labelled as 5, 3b, 1 and 2 are Brodmann's cytoarchitectonic designations of cortical areas. S-I and S-II refer to the first and second somatosensory regions.

8.7.5 S-I: functional considerations

8.7.5.1 Modality

Few studies of S-I have used stimuli appropriate for identifying the particular cutaneous or subcutaneous sense organs responsible for activating individual neurons, but even so they have been able to demonstrate a clear modality specificity. Most neuronal units recorded with microelectrodes from S-I respond only to a limited kind of stimulation and usually can be excited by stimulation of receptors located in one kind of tissue. Many S-I neurons in cat and monkey are vigorously excited by hair movement alone; another large fraction respond best to direct stimulation of the skin — some adapting rapidly and some slowly to a maintained skin deformation. Under similar conditions other S-I neurons are driven by joint movements or deep tissue manipulation and are not excited by skin stimulation[162, 455, 511, 512]. General surveys of responses in the feline or simian S-I report few cells preferentially excited by thermal or noxious stimuli, although such elements have been seen[454, 529]. Experiments specifically directed at a search for cortical thermoreceptive units have demonstrated a projection from cold receptors of the tongue to S-I[531] and the activation of cortical cells in both S-I and S-II by transient, non-noxious warming[531]. Activity can be evoked in the cat S-I by volleys in small-diameter myelinated and C fibres of peripheral nerves after conduction in larger myelinated fibres is blocked[532]; a projection from slowly conducting afferent fibres conceivably is related to the thermoreceptive input. Another possibility is that the C fibre and induced heat input results from projections of postsynaptic dorsal column and some spinocervical units.

Convincing evidence for the functional importance of cytoarchitectonic divisions of cortical somatosensory regions comes from the distribution of cells responding to particular kinds of natural stimulation. For example, the input to area 3b appears to be principally cutaneous with a high proportion of cells giving slowly adapting responses to maintained skin pressure[515, 533, 534]. In contrast, more posteriorly, area 2 is dominated by cells receiving excitation from subcutaneous receptors, particularly those associated with joints, their surrounding tendons and fascia[453, 515, 533]. The situation in area 3a, buried deep in the primate central sulcus, is an especially compelling case for a correspondence between somatosensory cytoarchitecture and specific afferent projections. Experiments based upon surface recordings of evoked potentials in anaesthetised cats at one time led to the conclusion that Group I muscle afferent fibres do not project to the cerebral cortex[521, 560]. However, under different experimental conditions it has been unequivocally shown that Group I impulses do activate cerebral cortical neurons in both cat and monkey through straightforward pathways[535-542]. When units in areas 3a, 3b and 1 of the primate were systematically surveyed, only those in area 3a were excited by impulses from Group I fibres and brief rapid stretches of a single muscle[542]. Group I fibres also excited a focus in the motor cortex (area 4γ), in area 2 and the S-II suprasylvian fringe region[539-541]. The evidence taken as a whole is convincing that the muscle afferent projection derives from the Group Ia fibre of the muscle spindle[538, 540-542, 544]. In cat's area 3a, there is an input from cutaneous afferent fibres to cells receiving Group I excitation[537]; however, in primate, gentle cutaneous stimulation does not activate neurons responding to Group I input and muscle stretch[542].

To summarise, in primate S-I consists of an anterior border area (3a) with a predominantly muscle afferent input, a central core (area 3b and the anterior portion of area 1) dominated by a cutaneous afferent projection and a posterior border (the posterior part of area 1 and area 2) with predominantly, although not exclusively, subcutaneous input[515].

8.7.5.2 Directional properties

Observations on directional discrimination provide a clue to transformations of the sensory information in the process of projection to S-I neurons. Whitsel, Roppolo and Werner[520] found that approximately one out of five S-I cells gave much more vigorous responses when a stimulating object was moved across the skin in certain directions than in others. Directional discriminatory units were concentrated in layer III of the cortex, a lamina that also contains cells with less spontaneous discharge than was seen with cells either of more superficial or deeper levels. Directionality is an important feature of visual cortical responses[516] and appears to be a part of the visual system's pattern recognition arrangement. The same possibility may apply to the somatosensory system. The time, position and movement dependent transformations important for shape and texture recognition would seem to be reasonable tasks for the kind of projection operated on by S-I neurons; the functional role of the S-I cortex may be associated with cutaneous and cutaneous–subcutaneous pattern recognition. In any case, generation of a direction-sensitive response from receptors not having such a characteristic implicates a systematic set of interactions more complex than those applicable to simple excitatory and inhibitory receptive fields.

8.7.5.3   Pathways to S-I

In the cat, afferent fibres of large diameter project to the S-I region through both the dorsal columns and the dorsolateral fasciculus[546-548]. The latter represents the route for the Group I projection from the hindlimbs[290, 540]. Overall the dorsolateral fasciculus pathway appears to be more rapidly conducting even though at least one additional synapse is intercalated (Section 8.5.1.2). Large numbers of S-I neurons lose their excitatory input if both the dorsal columns and the dorsolateral fasciculus are cut[455, 455a, 549]. Activation of S-I via the spinal dorsolateral fasciculus is more important in carnivores than in primates[550]. In a careful comparison of the effects produced by division of the dorsal columns, the dorsolateral fasciculus or the ventral quadrant, Dreyer, Schneider, Metz and Whitsel[515] uncovered a differential distribution of the several ascending pathways to monkey S-I. Cells specifically excited by rapidly adapting mechanoreceptors of the skin (velocity type) receive their input over the dorsal columns, a fact consistent with the latter's makeup (Section 8.5.1.1). These cutaneously excited neurons were principally located in area 3b and the anterior portion of area 1. Cells in the posterior portion of S-I, which are excited by subcutaneous stimulation of proximal body parts, receive their spinal input via dorsolateral fasciculus pathways. Ventral quadrant pathways influence the projection to the distal limb representation in the posterior portion of S-I and to area 3a in the rostral portion of S-I. After spinal lesions or following peripheral denervation, units with unusual characteristics appear in the primate S-I; altered features include the emergence of a number of recordings from cells with large, discontinuous and/or ipsilateral receptive fields and units responding only to massive strong stimulation[515, 534, 551].

8.7.6   S-II: functional considerations

Surface recordings of evoked potentials in the S-II region reveal two prominent differences from S-I. The somatotopic projection to S-II is less obviously detailed than that in S-I and there is a conspicuous input to S-II from the ipsilateral body surface[552, 553]. Recordings from individual S-II cells also demonstrate bilateral activation[518, 554, 555]. The projection from the ipsilateral side of the body is particularly sensitive to anaesthesia[557]. It also seems probable that there are differences between the feline and primate S-II[518, 555]. Both large and small receptive fields have been observed for individual neurons of S-II. Like those of S-I, the smallest receptive fields are related to inputs from distal portions of the body while cells with the largest fields receive their input from proximal locations[518,555]. Some discussions of S-II imply that receptive fields of S-II neurons are all large; however, in the unanaesthetised monkey, receptive fields of individual elements frequently are small but bilaterally symmetrical[518]. Activation from the contralateral body side is more effective for S-II cells with bilateral receptive fields[518,555].

8.7.6.1   Effective stimuli

Most of the input to the rostral two-thirds of S-II apparently stems from cutaneous receptors; the same kinds of stimuli are effective from both sides of the body. Some differentiation exists between elements excited by hair movement alone and those requiring direct stimulation of the skin; the sum of the two types represents approximately 90% of the elements encountered[518,555,558] Gentle joint movement is not an effective stimulus for S-II cells[554,555,558,559]. The rostral and caudal portions of S-II differ; the caudal region contains a number of cells with multisensory convergence such as auditory and somatic as well as a prominent fraction of neurons with very large receptive fields. Some of the latter are excited only by intense (noxious) stimuli[518,554,555].

Many neurons of S-II are excited through connections not having the overall security of synaptic transfer typical for neurons of S-I[518,554]. This is evidenced by the inability to follow even moderate frequencies of repetitive stimulation. Vibration and direct stimulation of Pacinian corpuscles or their afferent fibres are striking exceptions. The vibration-Pacinian corpuscle projection shows more consistent response in S-II than S-I[543,560].

8.7.6.2   Pathways to S-II

All three major ascending pathways of the spinal cord contribute an input to S-II. Andersson[559] investigated the contribution of ascending spinal cord tracts by recording from S-II cells in cats in which lesions left various combinations of pathways intact. S-II cells with the smallest receptive fields were activated through the dorsal column system and afferent inhibition could be identified for about one-third of these. Receptive fields from units receiving excitation through the dorsolateral fasciculus were occasionally small, but never as small as those dependent upon the integrity of the dorsal columns. The dorsally located tracts carry projections from receptors responsive to innocuous mechanical stimulation of the skin and/or deep structures. When the ventral pathways alone were left intact, the receptive fields of feline S-II neurons were large and intense mechanical stimulation was typically required to evoke discharge. The latter observation may be related to a projection from the smaller-diameter myelinated fibres of subcutaneous nerves to cells of S-II[521,561,562]. Some S-II units are activated by gentle mechanical stimulation of large areas of the body after interruption of the ventral quadrants, indicating that afferent input through them is not the sole source contributing to the synthesis of large receptive fields.

The latency of responses evoked in S-II in the intact animal are comparable with those in S-I, the most rapidly conducted activity reaching S-II via the dorsolateral fasciculus as it does in S-I. S-II responses in preparations having only the ventral tracts intact have a considerably longer in latency than when the spinal cord is intact[559].

8.7.7 Other cortical areas

Somatosensory excitation of cortical areas of the parietal region (areas 5 and 7 or the equivalent in the cat) and the premotor region of the frontal cortex exhibits extensive spatial and modality convergence, poor responses to rapidly repeated stimuli and long latencies to electrical stimulation of skin or nerves[563, 564]. Units recorded from these areas have very large and bilateral receptive fields. The ipsilateral projection to the orbital cortex is mediated through the contralateral cerebral hemisphere in contrast to S-II, where hemidecortication does not interfere with ipsilateral projections[526, 563]. Cells of the orbital cortex in the cat can be excited only by brusque taps, pinching of the skin, noxious pressure on muscles and noxious cutaneous heat. Orbital cortex neurons also receive an input from visceral structures (mesentry). The reader is referred to Albe-Fessard and Besson[503] for further comment on such 'non-primary' cortical areas and the possible significance of somatic input to them.

8.8 SUMMARY DIAGRAMS

Figure 8.2 summarises trajectories and synaptic stations for the principal ascending somatosensory systems. The schematic diagrams illustrate major features of each system but do not attempt to account for areas of controversy or less fully understood arrangements, such as possible bilateral representation within the spinal cord. Figure 8.2a schematises the system associated with the dorsal column nuclei (DCN). Its spinal input arrives over both the dorsal columns (DC) and the dorsolateral fasciculus (DLF); the muscle afferent pathway through nucleus Z is included with the projection from the DCN. As indicated, the dorsal column nuclei and nucleus Z receive an ipsilateral excitatory input and project to the contralateral thalamus via the medial lemniscus (ML). Figure 8.2b outlines the spino–cervicothalamic system. Its first synaptic junction is in the spinal cord grey matter near to the segment of primary afferent entry and a second synapse occurs in the lateral cervical nucleus (LCN) of the upper cervical segments. The spinocervical pathway also projects via the medial lemniscus to the contralateral thalamus; it is ipsilateral until fibres from the lateral cervical nucleus cross in the upper portions of the cervical spinal cord. Figure 8.2c outlines the pathways with fibres passing through the ventral spinal quadrants, the spinoreticular (SRP) and the spinothalamic (STT) projections. The ventral spinal pathways have a synapse in the segment of dorsal root entry or nearby and are mostly crossed shortly thereafter. The ventral quadrant pathways terminate at different levels in the brainstem reticular formation and in thalamic nuclei. Note that the dorsal column–dorsal column nucleus–medial lemniscus, the spinocervical system and the spinothalamic projection all contribute terminations to the posterior group and to the ventroposterior region of the thalamus. Moreover, all three systems have projections to both the first (S-I) and the second (S-II) somatosensory regions of the cerebral cortex. Only the spinoreticular and spinothalamic pathways of the ventral spinal quadrants have established connections directly to the brainstem reticular formation and the intralaminar nuclei (ILN) of the thalamus.

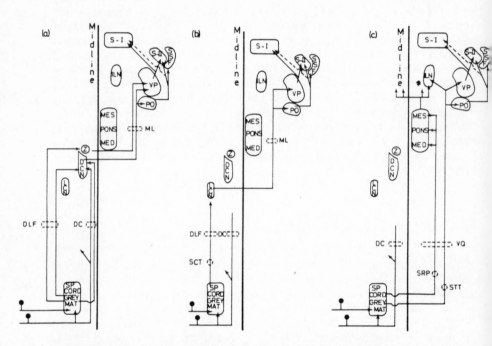

Figure 8.2 Schematic representations of major ascending sensory pathways. Connections without synapses are shown as continuous lines. Enclosed labelled structures represent nuclear regions. A connection (fibre pathway) starts with the beginning of a line and ends at the nuclear region pointed to by an arrow where a synaptic transfer takes place. The midline is marked by the long, heavy vertical line for each drawing. (a) Dorsal column nucleus–medial lemniscus system. (b) Lateral cervical nucleus–medial lemniscus system (spino–cervicothalamic pathway). (c) Spinoreticular and spinothalamic systems.

DC, dorsal columns; DCN, dorsal column nuclei (gracilis and cuneatus); DLF, dorsolateral fasciculus; ILN, intralaminar nuclei of the thalamus; LCN, lateral cervical nucleus; MAT, matter; MED, medulla oblongata; MES, mesencephalon; ML, medial lemniscus; PO, posterior group of the thalamus; PONS, pons; S-I, first somatosensory area of the cerebral cortex; S-II, second somatosensory area of the cerebral cortex; SCT, spinocervical tract; SP, spinal; SRP, spinoreticular pathway; SSF, suprasylvian fringe area of the cerebral cortex; STT, spinothalamic tract; VP, ventroposterior nucleus (ventralis posterior lateralis, ventralis intermedius) of the thalamus; VQ, ventral quadrant of the spinal cord; Z, nucleus Z of Brodal and Pompeiano.

8.9 FUNCTION AND PATHWAYS

8.9.1 Traditional concepts

Stereotyped points of view pervade many textbook descriptions of the somatosensory system. In these, the projections passing through the dorsal columns are described as being necessary for perception of joint position and other kinesthetic sense, for perception of vibration, for accurate localisation of cutaneous stimuli and for the kind of tactile appreciation tested by two-point discrimination. The spinothalamic tract is ordinarily described as the pathway important for pain and temperature sensation and for 'crude touch'. Even if sense organ projections through the two pathways were appropriate, the interactions at every level of somatosensory organisation and in particular, at thalamic and cortical levels, argue against so simple a concept. Some of the necessary sense organs do not contribute afferent information to the spinal tract as these dicta propose. As evidence inconsistent with the traditional concepts has accumulated, the most vigorous attacks have been aimed at suppositions about the dorsal column–medial lemniscus pathway. A recent critical appraisal by Wall[461] speculated that the dorsal column pathway has only an indirect part in conscious sensation. Instead he proposes that its function lies primarily in controlling analyses of information arriving over other pathways and in mechanisms initiating the motor exploration (i.e. palpation) necessary for identification of objects. This seemingly outrageous proposal drew support from the literature, such as the reports that surgical interruption of the dorsal columns in man produces almost no permanent deficit in tactile or proprioceptive sense other than a possible loss of vibration detection[566, 567]. Part of the evidence for Wall's proposal was his own observations on rats in which the spinal cord at the lower thoracic level had been transected with the exception of the dorsal columns; these animals ignored somatic stimulation at segmental levels below the lesion for some days, although potentials could still be evoked at the cerebral cortex from the affected regions[461]. Originally, the idea that the dorsal columns are important for tactile and proprioceptive sense derived from clinical observations, particularly on cases of tabes dorsalis; the degeneration of dorsal column fibres seen in this disease was often associated with a combination of tactile and position sense deficits. We have already pointed out that lesions of the dorsal column are not equivalent to lesions of the dorsal column nucleus–medial lemniscus pathway. Furthermore, the pathology of tabes dorsalis also involves the dorsal root ganglia.

8.9.2 Dorsal columns and behaviour

The best information on the importance of the various spinal pathways for sensory-related behaviour comes from analyses of deficits produced by controlled experimental lesions. These data suffer from the problem already mentioned; the results only indicate the residual capacity of the uninjured pathways. Vierck[3], in a series of well-documented experiments on monkeys, describes prolonged deficits in tactile size discrimination on the side below the level of a dorsal column lesion; a gradual recovery to preoperative competence takes place. Addition of a dorsolateral fasciculus transection after recovery from the effects of dorsal column section causes return of a major difficulty in size recognition for many months. In other work Vierck[585] observed a persisting inability to detect the direction of a moving stimulus in monkeys following dorsal column lesions; the loss of direction detection did not result from a lack of capacity to differentiate between a moving and stationary object. High cervical lesions of the dorsal columns impair a monkey's ability to place his limbs accurately and to pick up small objects[568]. Results with carnivores are essentially similar to those obtained for primates. After dorsal column transection cats can still approximately localise and appropriately respond to a tactile stimulus, although threshold may slightly increase[548,570]. Interruption of almost all the fibres in the dorsal columns impair roughness discrimination in cats for considerable periods of time[545]. These results imply that the dorsal columns do carry important tactile discriminatory information, but that the capacity for some aspects of this function is not unique to that pathway. They further emphasise the multiple facets of mammalian somatic sense and the necessity for more accurate and appropriate tests for proper insight into the contributions by various neural systems.

Several investigations have stressed important deficits in movements following lesions of the dorsal columns. Gilman and Denny-Brown[569] found that interruption of the monkey's dorsal column impairs fine palpatory exploration of objects within arm's reach. Subsequent studies have also noted the absence of the common exploratory movements of the hand or foot after division of the dorsal column; the paucity of movements is postulated to result from absence of an appropriate input or feedback[571,572]. Controlled experiments have been consistent in showing that division of the dorsal columns in monkeys produces only transient deficits of knee joint position sense[573] and weight discrimination[575,576].

8.9.3 The dorsolateral fasciculus and behaviour

Dorsolateral fasciculus lesions alone cause no evident impairment of localisation or roughness discrimination in carnivores, although permanent deficits in these functions appear when the dorsolateral fasciculus lesion is combined with division of the dorsal column[545,548,549,570]. Combined transections of the dorsal columns and the dorsolateral fasciculus produce a permanent impairment in the ability of monkeys to recognise the size of gaps, two-point discrimination and persisting impairments of joint position sense[3,573,574].

Vierck, Hamilton and Thornby[6] have made interesting observations on the response of monkeys to noxious stimulation after lesions of the dorsal quadrants. Ipsilateral dorsal column lesions increase the latency and decrease the intensity of a monkey's response to noxious shocks, while leaving threshold unaffected. In contrast, ipsilateral lesions of the dorsolateral tract produced significant reductions in the latency and increases in the force of responses to the same kind of noxious stimulation without altering threshold. These results again bring to mind the fact that noxious stimulation contributes to the response of some dorsolateral tract neurons and of postsynaptic fibres in the dorsal columns.

8.9.4 Ventral spinal pathways and sensation

Tracts of the ventral spinal quadrants have been known to be important for pain and reactions typical of it since the classic reports by Spiller[335], Sherrington[34] and Petren[336]. The therapeutic sections of the ventral spinal quadrants have provided many opportunities for clinical observations[230, 339, 345]. The general concensus of this experience is that section of the ventrolateral spinal tracts in man causes enduring, but not necessarily permanent, loss of pain appreciation beginning a few segments below the level of the lesion. Pinprick recognition and the ability to discriminate between objects of different temperatures is lost for considerable periods of time. Chordotomy in human beings is often reported to have only a temporary effect in ameliorating chronic pain, and there is a high percentage of recurrence of discomfort in patients whose basic disease allows them long survival. Considerable evidence also exists for close correlation between lesions of the spinothalamic tract, particularly rostral to the spinal cord, and the development of pathological pain of a type different than that originally experienced by the subject[577].

The clinical evidence, while extensive, leaves much to be desired in terms of the care with which sensory testing was done and/or the correlations with morbid anatomy. There are few careful experimental analyses of the effects of ventral spinal quadrant deficits upon somesthetic function of animals. Intensity of electrical stimulation and mechanical pinch to the contralateral body surface of a monkey necessary to evoke reactions interpreted as indicating a disagreeable experience increases below the level of a ventral quadrant transection [6, 578]. However, Christiansen[578] did not find a change in the reaction to noxious heat following ventral quadrant lesions. Furthermore, neither joint position sense nor two point discrimination have been shown to change following ventral quadrant lesions[573, 574]. The combination of a dorsal quadrant lesion on one side and a ventral quadrant lesion on the other side produced total and permanent loss of both position sense and tactile two-point differentiation on the side of the dorsal column lesion.

8.10 CONCLUDING COMMENTS

If nothing else, this survey should illustrate that our information on somatosensory mechanisms is still fragmentary in spite of much work. We do know that there is considerable diversity in the neural systems contributing to somatic sensation. This diversity is manifest at the very first stage in the sense organs themselves. It continues in the rostral projection over the several pathways and within parts of pathways traditionally considered to have some units of function. Finally, the rostral terminations are also multiple and while largely mysterious, clearly different. In this context, the notions of duality of function as proposed by Head[504] seem strangely out of place. Similarly, the modern extension of duality implying that somatic sensation is explicable in terms of two major organisational features — lemniscal and non-lemniscal (or convergent and non-convergent) — appear inappropriate. It would seem both realistic and prudent to refrain from dogmatic labelling until we have better qualitative information on the overall functional organisation of the sensory systems dealing with the body. At this point we do not know the place in function of the apparent redundancy between the different afferent pathways and we have only conflicting information on the part played by such important way stations in the ascending pathways as the reticular regions of the lower brainstem, the thalamic posterior group and the thalamic intra-laminar nuclei. Much of the existing data can be criticised because of the lack of careful control of the stimulus, the site of lesions or the site of recordings. Some quantitative information has begun to emerge but one should wonder about its significance. Rigid control of one parameter without carefully antici-pating the influence of other factors may result in misleading results. It would seem that the time for major insights from quantitative studies of neuronal discharge probably still lies in the future.

ACKNOWLEDGEMENTS

We are grateful for the efforts of Ms. L. Sedivec in preparation of the biblio-graphy and the manuscript.

Preparation of this review was supported by USPHS research grant NS 10321.

The final stages of the effort were aided by Swedish Medical Research Grant 12X-3391.

References

1. Vierck, C. J. Jr. and Jones, M. B. (1970). Influences of low and high frequency oscil-lation upon spatio-tactile resolution. *Physiol. Behav.*, **5**, 1431
2. Mountcastle, V. B., LaMotte, R. H. and Carli, G. (1972). Detection thresholds for stimuli in humans and monkeys: comparison with threshold events in mechano-receptive afferent nerve fibres innervating the monkey hand. *J. Neurophysiol.*, **35**, 122
3. Vierck, C. J. Jr. (1973). Alterations of spatio-tactile discrimination after lesions of primate spinal cord. *Brain Res.*, **58**, 69
4. Cragg, B. G. and Downer, J. de C. (1967). Behavioural evidence for cortical involve-ment in manual temperature discrimination in the monkey. *Exp. Neurol.*, **19**, 433
5. Schwartzman, R. J. and Semmes, J. (1971). The sensory cortex and tactile sensitivity. *Exp. Neurol.*, **33**, 147
6. Vierck, C. J., Hamilton, D. M. and Thornby, J. I. (1971). Pain reactivity of monkeys after lesions to the dorsal and lateral columns of the spinal cord. *Exp. Brain Res.*, **13**, 140
7. Ruffini, A. (1905). Sur les expansions nerveuses de la peau, chez l'homme et quelques autres mammifères. *Rev. Gén. Histol.*, **1**, 419
8. Von Frey, M. (1910). Physiologie der Sinnesorgane der Menschlichen Haut. *Ergebnisse Physiol.*, **9**, 351
9. Sinclair, D. C. (1955). Cutaneous sensation and the doctrine of specific energy. *Brain*, **78**, 584
10. Melzack, R. and Wall, P. D. (1962). On the nature of cutaneous sensory mechanisms. *Brain*, **85**, 331

11. Andres, K. H. and Von Düring, M. (1973). Morphology of Cutaneous Receptors. In: *Handbook of Sensory Physiology*, Vol. **2**, 1 (A. Iggo, editor) (Berlin: Springer-Verlag)
12. Burgess, P. R. and Perl, E. R. (1973). Cutaneous Mechanoreceptors and Nociceptors. In: *Handbook of Sensory Physiology*, Vol. 2, 29 (A. Iggo, editor) (Berlin: Springer-Verlag)
13. Hensel, H. H. (1973). Cutaneous Thermoreceptors. In: *Handbook of Sensory Physiology*, Vol. 2, 79 (A. Iggo, editor) (Berlin: Springer-Verlag)
14. Fuortes, M. G. F. (1971). Generation of Responses in Receptor. In: *Handbook of Sensory Physiology*, Vol. 1, 243 (W. R. Loewenstein, editor) (Berlin: Springer-Verlag)
15. Loewenstein, W. R. (1971). Mechano-electric Transduction in the Pacinian Corpuscle. Initiation of Sensory Impulses in Mechanoreceptors. In: *Handbook of Sensory Physiology*, Vol. 1, 269 (W. R. Loewenstein, editor) (Berlin: Springer-Verlag)
16. Flock, A. (1971). Sensory Transduction in Hair Cells. In: *Handbook of Sensory Physiology*, Vol. 1, 396 (W. R. Loewenstein, editor) (Berlin: Springer-Verlag)
17. Katz, B. (1949). The efferent regulation of the muscle spindle in the frog. *J. Exp. Biol.*, **26**, 201
18. Loewenstein, W. R. (1959). The generation of electric activity in a nerve ending. *Ann. New York Acad Sci.*, **81**, 367
19. Loewenstein, W. R. (1961). Excitation and inactivation in a receptor membrane. *Ann. New York Acad Sci.*, **94**, 510
20. Teorell, T. (1971). A Biophysical Analysis of Mechano-electrical Transduction. In: *Handbook of Sensory Physiology*, Vol. 1, (W. R. Loewenstein, editor) (Berlin: Springer-Verlag)
21. Eyzaguirre, C., Nishi, K. and Fidone, S. (1972). Chemoreceptor synapses in the carotid body. *Fed. Proc.*, **31**, 1385
22. Pinkus, F. (1902). Über einen bisher unbekannten Nebenapparat am Haarsystem des Menschen: Haarscheiben. *Derm. Z.*, **9**, 465
23. Iggo, A. and Muir, A. R. (1969). The structure and function of a slowly adapting touch corpuscle in hairy skin. *J. Physiol. (London)*, **200**, 763
25. Lim, R. J. S. (1970). Pain. *Ann. Rev. Physiol.*, **32**, 269
26. Diamond, J., Gray, J. A. B. and Sato, M. (1956). The site of initiation of impulses in Pacinian corpuscles. *J. Physiol. (London)*, **133**, 54
27. Edwards, C. and Ottoson, D. (1958). The site of impulse initiation in a nerve cell of a crustacean stretch receptor. *J. Physiol. (London)*, **143**, 138
28. Coggeshall, R. E., Coulter, J. D. and Willis, W. D. Jr. (1973). Unmyelinated fibers in the ventral root. *Brain Res.*, **57**, 229
29. Werner, G. and Whitsel, B. L. (1968). Topology of the body representation in somatosensory area I of primates. *J. Neurophysiol.*, **31**, 856
30. Erb, Z. (1939). Krankheiten der peripherischen cerebrospinalen Nerven. 1874. As cited in: K. M. Dallenbach, (1939). Pain: History and Present, *J. Psychol.*, **52**, 336
31. Nafe, J. P. (1929). A qauntitative theory of feeling. *J. Gen. Psychol.*, **2**, 199
32. Weddell, G. (1955). Somesthesis and the chemical senses. *Ann. Rev. Psychol.*, **6**, 119
33. Müller, J. (1840). *Handbuch der Physiologie des Menschen*, **2**, 249
34. Sherrington, C. S. (1906). *The Integrative Action of the Nervous System* (New Haven: Yale Univ. Press)
35. Von Frey, M. (1895). Beiträge zur Sinnesphysiologie der Haut. *Ber. über die Verhandlungen der Königl. Säch.*, **47**, 166
36. Von Frey, M. (1896). Untersuchungen über die Sinnesfunctionen der Menschlichen Haut: Druckempfindung und Schmerz. *Abhandlungen der mathematisch-physischen Classe der Königl. Sächsischen Gesellschaft der Wissenschaften*, **23**, 175
37. Von Frey, M. (1897). Beiträge zur Sinnesphysiologie der Haut. *Ber. über die Verhandlungen der Königl. Säch.*, **49**, 462
38. Melzack, R. and Wall, P. D. (1965). Pain mechanisms: a new theory. *Science*, **150**, 971
39. Skoglund, S. (1973). Joint Receptors and Kinaesthesis. In: *Handbook of Sensory Physiology*, Vol. 2, 111 (A. Iggo, editor) (Berlin: Springer-Verlag)
40. Adrian, E. D. (1926). The impulses produced by sensory nerve endings. Part IV. Impulses from pain receptors. *J. Physiol.*, **62**, 33
41. Adrian, E. D. (1931). The messages in sensory nerve fibres and their interpretation. *Proc. Roy. Soc B*, **109**, 1

42. Adrian, E. D. and Zotterman, Y. (1926). The impulses produced by sensory nerve-endings. Part II. The response of a single end-organ. *J. Physiol. (London)*, **61**, 151
43. Matthews, B. H. C. (1933). Nerve endings in mammalian muscle. *J. Physiol. (London)*, **78**, 1
44. Zotterman, Y. (1939). Touch, pain and tickling: an electrophysiological investigation on cutaneous sensory nerves. *J. Physiol. (London)*, **95**, 1
45. Matthews, P. B. C. (1964). Muscle spindles and their motor control. *Physiol. Rev.*, **44**, 219
46. Hensel, H. and Zotterman, Y. (1951). Quantitative relation between the discharge from single cold fibers and temperature. *Acta Physiol. Scand.*, **23**, 291
47. Hensel, H. H. (1952). Physiologie der Thermoreception. *Erge. Physiol.*, **47**, 166
48. Hensel, H. H., Iggo, A. and Witt, I. (1960). A quantitative study of sensitive cutaneous thermoreceptors with C afferent fibres. *J. Physiol. (London)*, **153**, 113
49. Iriuchijima, J. and Zotterman, Y. (1960). The specificity of afferent cutaneous C fibres in mammals. *Acta Physiol. Scand.*, **49**, 267
50. Maruhashi, J., Mizuguchi, K. and Tasaki, I. (1952). Action currents in single afferent nerve fibres elicited by stimulation of the skin of the toad and the cat. *J. Physiol. (London)*, **117**, 129
51. Iggo, A. (1960). Cutaneous mechanoreceptors with afferent C fibres. *J. Physiol. (London)*, **152**, 337
52. Hunt, C. C. and McIntyre, A. K. (1960). An analysis of fibre diameter and receptor characteristics of myelinated cutaneous afferent fibres in cat. *J. Physiol. (London)*, **153**, 99
53. Gray, J. A. B. and Matthews, P. B. C. (1951). A comparison of the adaptation of the Pacinian corpuscle with accommodation of its own axon. *J. Physiol. (London)*, **114**, 454
54. Sato, M. (1961). Response of Pacinian corpuscles to sinusoidal vibration. *J. Physiol. (London)*, **159**, 391
55. Adrian, E. D. (1930). Impulses in sympathetic fibres and in slow afferent fibres. *J. Physiol. (London)*, **70**, xx
56. Zotterman, Y. (1936). Specific action potentials in the lingual nerve of cat. *Skand-arch.*, **75**, 105
57. Douglas, W. W. and Ritchie, J. M. (1957). A technique for recording functional activity in specific groups of medullated and non-medullated fibres in whole nerve trunks. *J. Physiol. (London)*, **138**, 19
58. Douglas, W. W., Ritchie, J. M. and Straub, R. W. (1960). The role of non-myelinated fibres in signalling cooling of the skin. *J. Physiol. (London)*, **150**, 266
59. Wall, P. D. (1973). Dorsal Horn Electrophysiology. *Handbook of Sensory Physiology*, Vol. 2, 253 (A. Iggo, editor) (Berlin: Springer-Verlag)
60. Burgess, P. R. and Perl, E. R. (1967). Myelinated afferent fibres responding specifically to noxious stimulation of the skin. *J. Physiol. (London)*, **190**, 541
61. Perl, E. R. (1968). Myelinated afferent fibres innervating the primate skin and their response to noxious stimuli. *J. Physiol. (London)*, **197**, 593
62. Bessou, P. and Perl, E. R. (1969). Response of cutaneous sensory units with unmyelinated fibers to noxious stimuli. *J. Neurophysiol.*, **32**, 1025
63. Burgess, P. R., Petit, D. and Warren, R. M. (1968). Receptor types in cat hairy skin supplied by myelinated fibers. *J. Neurophysiol.*, **31**, 833
64. Burgess, P. R. and Clark, F. J. (1969). Characteristics of knee joint receptors in the cat. *J. Physiol. (London)*, **203**, 317
65. Chambers, M. and Iggo, A. (1967). Slowly-adapting cutaneous mechanoreceptors. *J. Physiol. (London)*, **192**, 26P
66. Chambers, M., Andres, K. H., Von Düring, M. and Iggo, A. (1972). The structure and function of the slowly adapting Type II mechanoreceptor in hairy skin. *Quart. J. Exp. Physiol.*, **57**, 417
67. Harrington, E. and Merzenich, M. M. (1970). Neural coding in the sense of touch; human sensations of skin indentation compared with the responses of slowly adapting mechanoreceptive afferents innervating the hairy skin of monkeys. *Exp. Brain Res.*, **10**, 251
68. Brown, A. G. and Iggo, A. (1967). A quantitative study of cutaneous receptors and afferent fibres in the cat and rabbit. *J. Physiol. (London)*, **193**, 707
69. Merzenich, M. M. and Harrington, T. H. (1969). The sense of flutter-vibration evoked

by stimulation of the hairy skin of primates: comparison of human sensory capacity with the responses of mechanoreceptive afferents innervating the hairy skin of the monkeys. *Exp. Brain Res.*, **9**, 236

70. Bessou, P., Burgess, P. R., Perl, E. R. and Taylor, C. B. (1971). Dynamic properties of mechanoreceptors with unmyelinated (C) fibers. *J. Neurophysiol.*, **34**, 116

71. Hunt, C. C. (1961). On the nature of vibration receptors in the hind limb of the cat. *J. Physiol. (London)*, **155**, 175

72. Jänig, W., Schmidt, R. F. and Zimmermann, M. (1968). Single unit responses and the total afferent outflow from the cat's foot pad upon mechanical stimulation. *Exp. Brain Res.*, **6**, 100

73. Iggo, A. (1963). New specific sensory structures in hairy skin. *Acta Neurovegetativa*, **24**, 1

74. Jänig, W. (1971). Morphology of rapidly and slowly adapting mechanoreceptors in the hairless skin of the cat's hind foot. *Brain Res.*, **28**, 217

75. Knibestöl, M. and Vallbo, A. B. (1970). Single unit analysis of mechanoreceptor activity from the human glabrous skin. *Acta Physiol. Scand.*, **80**, 178

76. Talbot, W. H., Darian-Smith, I., Kornhuber, H. H. and Mountcastle, V. B. (1968). The sense of flutter-vibration: comparison of the human capacity with response patterns of mechanoreceptive afferents from the monkey hand. *J. Neurophysiol.*, **31**, 301

77. Appelberg, B., Bessou, P. and Laporte, Y. (1966). Action of static and dynamic fusimotor fibres on secondary endings of cat's spindles. *J. Physiol. (London)*, **185**, 160

78. Barker, D. (1962). The structure and distribution of muscle receptors. *Symposium on Muscle Receptors*, 227 (1962: Hong Kong)

79. Boyd, I. A. (1962). The structure and innervation of the nuclear bag muscle fibre system and the nuclear chain muscle fibre system in mammalian muscle spindles. *Phil. Trans. Roy. Soc. London B*, **245**, 81

80. Bessou, P., Laporte, Y. and Pages, B. (1968). Frequency grams of spindle primary endings elicited by stimulation of static and dynamic fusimotor fibres. *J. Physiol. (London)*, **196**, 47

81. Houk, J. and Henneman, E. (1967). Responses of Golgi tendon organs to active contractions of the soleus muscle of the cat. *J. Neurophysiol.*, **30**, 466

82. Bessou, P. and Laporte, Y. (1961). Étude des récepteurs musculaires innervés par les fibres afférentes du groupe III (Fibres myelinisées fines), chez le chat. *Arch. Ital. Biol.*, **99**, 293

83. Paintal, A. S. (1960). Functional analysis of group III afferent fibres of mammalian muscles. *J. Physiol. (London)*, **152**, 250

84. Zimmermann, M. (1972). Personal communication

85. Andrew, B. L. (1954). The sensory innervation of the medial ligament of the knee joint. *J. Physiol. (London)*, **123**, 241

86. Boyd, I. A. (1954). The histological structure of the receptors in the knee-joint of the cat correlated with their physiological response. *J. Physiol. (London)*, **124**, 476

87. Boyd, I. A. and Roberts, T. D. M. (1953). Proprioceptive discharges from stretch receptors in the knee-joint of the cat. *J. Physiol. (London)*, **122**, 38

88. Skoglund, S. (1956). Anatomical and physiological studies of knee joint innervation in the cat. *Acta Physiol. Scand.*, **36**, 1

89. Andres, K. H. (1971). Structure of cutaneous receptors. *Proc. Int. Union Physiol. Sci.*, **8**, 136

90. Iggo, A. (1969). Cutaneous thermoreceptors in primates and sub-primates. *J. Physiol. (London)*, **200**, 403

91. Iggo, A. and Ogawa, H. (1971). Primate cutaneous thermal nociceptors. *J. Physiol. (London)*, **216**, 77P

92. Iggo, A. (1959). Cutaneous heat and cold receptors with slowly conducting (C) afferent fibres. *Quart. J. Exp. Physiol.*, **44**, 362

93. Iggo, A. (1961). Non-myelinated afferent fibres from mammalian skeletal muscles. *J. Physiol. (London)*, **155**, 52P

94. Bessou, P. and Laporte, Y. (1958). Activation des fibres afférentes amyéliniques d'origine musculaire. *C. R. Soc. Biol. (Paris)*, **152**, 1587

95. Gasser, H. S. and Erlanger, J. (1927). The role played by the sizes of the constituent

fibers of a nerve trunk in determining the form of its action potential wave. *Amer. J. Physiol.*, **80**, 522

96. Ranson, S. W., Droegemueller, W. H., Davenport, H. K. and Fisher, C. (1935). Number, size and myelination of the sensory fibers in the cerebrospinal nerves. *Proc. A.R.N.M.D.*, **15** (Sensation, Its Mechanisms and Distribution.), 3

97. Erlanger, J. and Gasser, H. (1937). *Electrical Signs of Nervous Activity.* (Philadelphia: University Pennsylvania Press)

98. Lloyd, D. P. C. and Chang, H. T. (1948). Afferent fibers in muscle nerves. *J. Neurophysiol.*, **11**, 199

99. Lloyd, D. P. C. (1943). Neuron patterns controlling transmission of ipsilateral hind limb reflexes in cat. *J. Neurophysiol.*, **6**, 293

100. Hunt, C. C. and Perl, E. R. (1960). Spinal reflex mechanisms concerned with skeletal muscle. *Physiol. Rev.*, **40**, 538

101. Hartline, H. K., Wagner, H. G. and MacNichol, E. F. (1952). The peripheral origin of nervous activity in the visual system. *Cold Spring Harbor Symposia on Quantitative Biology*, **17**, 125

102. Eyzaguirre, C. C. and Kuffler, S. W. (1955). Processes of excitation in the dendrites and in the soma of single isolated sensory nerve cells of the lobster and crayfish. *J. Gen. Physiol.*, **39**, 87

103. Fuortes, M. G. F. (1971). Generation of responses in receptor. In: *Handbook of Sensory Physiology*, Vol. **1**, 243 (W. R. Loewenstein, editor) (Berlin: Springer Verlag)

104. Matthews, B. H. C. (1931). The response of a single end organ. *J. Physiol. (London)*, **71**, 64

105. Matthews, B. H. C. (1931). The response of a muscle spindle during active contraction of a muscle. *J. Physiol. (London)*, **72**, 153

106. Werner, G. and Mountcastle, V. B. (1965). Neural activity in mechanoreceptive cutaneous afferents: stimulus-response relations, Weber functions, and information transmission. *J. Neurophysiol.*, **28**, 359

107. Mountcastle, V. B., Talbot, W. H. and Kornhuber, H. H. (1966). The neural transformation of mechanical stimuli delivered to the monkey's hand. In: *Touch, Heat and Pain*, Ciba Foundation Symp. (A. V. S. DeRueck and J. Knight, editors) (Boston: Little, Brown), 325

108. Mountcastle, V. B. (1967). The problem of sensing and the neural code of sensory events. In: *The Neurosciences* (G. C. Quarton, T. Melnechuk, and F. O. Schmitt, editors) (New York: Rockefeller University Press), 393

109. Kenton, B. and Kruger, L. (1971). Information transmission in slowly adapting mechanoreceptor fibers. *Exp. Neurol.*, **31**, 114

110. Kruger, L. and Kenton, B. (1973). Quantitative neural and psychophysical data for cutaneous mechanoreceptor function. *Brain Res.*, **49**, 1

111. Werner, G. and Mountcastle, V. B. (1968). Quantitative relations between mechanical stimuli to the skin and neural responses evoked by them. In: *The Skin Senses* (D. R. Kenshalo, editor) (Springfield: C. C. Thomas), 112

112. Tapper, D. N. (1964). Cutaneous slowly adapting mechanoreceptors in the cat. *Science* **143**, 53

113. Kenton, B., Kruger, L. and Woo, M. (1971). Two classes of slowly adapting mechanoreceptor fibres in reptile cutaneous nerve. *J. Physiol. (London)*, **212**, 21

114. Gray, J. A. B. and Matthews, P. B. C. A comparison of the adaptation of the Pacinian corpuscle with the accommodation of its own axon. *J. Physiol. (London)*, **114**, 454

115. Gray, J. A. B. and Sato, M. (1953). Properties of the receptor potential in Pacinian corpuscles. *J. Physiol. (London)*, **122**, 610

118. Perl, E. R. (1964). Études sur la sensibilité tactile et sur la sensibilité vibratoire. *Actualités Neurophysiologiques*, **5**, 91

119. Mountcastle, V. B., Talbot, W. H., Sakata, H. and Hyvarinen, Y. (1969). Cortical neuronal mechanisms in flutter-vibration studied in unanesthetized monkeys. Neuronal periodicity and frequency discrimination. *J. Neurophysiol.*, **32**, 452

120. Armett, C. J. and Hunsperger, R. W. (1961). Excitation of receptors in the pad of the cat by single and double mechanical pulses. *J. Physiol. (London)*, **158**, 15

121. Armett, C. J., Gray, J. A. B., Hunsperger, R. W. and Lal, S. (1962). The transmission of information in primary receptor neurones and second order neurones of a phasic system. *J. Physiol. (London)*, **164**, 395

122. Johnson, K. O. (1974). Reconstruction of population response to a vibratory stimulus in quickly adapting mechanoreceptive afferent fiber population innervating glabrous skin of the monkey. *J. Neurophysiol.*, **37,** 48

124. Cajal, Ramon y, S. (1909). *Histologie du Système Nerveux de l'Homme et des Vertèbrès.* (Paris: Maloine)

125. Rethelyi, M. and Szentagothai, J. (1973). Distribution and connections of afferent fibres in the spinal cord. In: *Handbook of Sensory Physiology,* Vol. **2,** 207 (A. Iggo, editor) (Berlin: Springer-Verlag)

126. Petit, D. and Burgess, P. R. (1968). Dorsal column projection of receptors in cat hairy skin supplied by myelinated fibers. *J. Neurophysiol.*, **31,** 849

127. Widen, L. (1955). Cerebellar representation of high threshold afferents from splanchnic nerve. *Acta Physiol. Scand.*, **117,** 1

128. Downman, C. B. B. (1955). Skeletal muscle reflexes of splanchnic and intercostal nerve origins in acute spinal and decerebrate cats. *J. Neurophysiol.*, **18,** 217

129. Franz, D. N., Evans, M. H. and Perl, E. R. (1966). Characteristics of viscerosympathetic reflexes in the spinal cat. *Amer. J. Physiol.*, **211,** 1292

130. Pomeranz, B., Wall, P. D. and Weber, W. V. (1968). Cord cells responding to fine myelinated afferents from viscera, muscle and skin. *J. Physiol. (London)*, **199,** 511

131. Whitehorn, D. and Burgess, P. R. (1973). Changes in polarization of central branches of myelinated mechanoreceptor and nociceptor fibers during noxious and innocuous stimulation of the skin. *J. Neurophysiol.*, **36,** 226

132. Mendell, L. M. and Henneman, E. (1971). Terminals of single Ia fibers: location, density and distribution within a pool of 300 homonymous motor neurons. *J. Neurophysiol.*, **34,** 171

133. Barrett, J. N. and Crill, W. E. (1971). Specific membrane resistivity of dye-injected cat motoneurons. *Brain Res.*, **28,** 556

134. Barrett, J., Cook, M., Ledbury, P., Zucker, R. and Whitlock, D. (1973). Axoplasmic transport from rat dorsal root ganglia. *Anat. Rec.*, **175,** 269

136. Ranson, S. W. (1943). *The Anatomy of the Nervous System.* (Philadelphia: W. B. Saunders)

137. Brodal, A. (1969). *Neurological Anatomy.* (Oxford: Oxford University Press)

138. Edinger, L. (1889). Vergleichend-entwicklungsgeschichtliche und anatomische studien im bereiche des zentralnervensystems. *Anat. Anz.*, **4,** 121

139. Ranson, S. W. (1911). Non-medullated nerve-fibers in the spinal nerves. *Amer. J. Anat.*, **12,** 67

140. Ranson, S. W. (1912). The structure of the spinal ganglia and of the spinal nerves. *J. Comp. Neurol. Physiol.*, **22,** 159

141. Ranson, S. W. (1913). The course within the spinal cord of the non-medullated fibres of the dorsal roots: a study of Lissauer's tract in the cat. *J. Comp. Neurol. Physiol.*, **23,** 259

142. Christensen, B. N. and Perl, E. R. (1970). Spinal neurons specifically excited by noxious or thermal stimuli: marginal zone of the dorsal horn. *J. Neurophysiol.*, **33,** 293

143. Kumazawa, T., Perl, E. R., Burgess, P. R. and Whitehorn, D. (1971). Excitation of posteromarginal cells (Lamina I) in monkey and their projection in lateral spinal tracts. *Proc. Int. Union Physiol. Sci.*, **9,** 328

144. Tapper, D. N., Brown, P. B. and Moraff, H. (1973). Functional organization of the cat's dorsal horn: connectivity of myelinated fiber systems of hairy skin. *J. Neurophysiol.*, **36,** 817

145. Perl, E. R. and Whitlock, D. G. Somatic stimuli exciting spinothalamic projections to thalamic neurons in cat and monkey. *Exp. Neurol.*, **3,** 256

146. Oscarsson, O. and Lundberg, A. (1962). Two ascending spinal pathways in the ventral part of the cord. *Acta Physiol. Scand.*, **54,** 270

147. Rexed, B. (1952). The cytoarchitectonic organization of the spinal cord of cat. *J. Comp. Neurol.*, **96,** 415

148. Ralston, H. J. III (1965). The organization of the substantia gelatinosa rolandi in the cat lumbosacral spinal cord. *Z. Zellforsch*, **67,** 1

149. Wall, P. D. (1967). The laminar organisation of dorsal horns and effects of descending impulses. *J. Physiol. (London)*, **188,** 403

150. Selzer, M. and Spencer, W. A. (1969). Convergence of visceral and cutaneous afferent pathways in the lumbar spinal cord. *Brain Res.*, **14,** 331

151. Oscarsson, O. (1973). Functional organization of spinocerebellar paths. In: *Handbook of Sensory Physiology*, Vol. 2, 339 (A. Iggo, editor) (Berlin: Springer-Verlag)

152. Glees, P. and Soler, J. (1951). Fibre content of the posterior column and synaptic connections of nucleus gracilis. *Z. Zellforsch*, **36**, 381

153. Van Harreveld, A. and Niechaj, A. (1967). A monosynaptic content of the dorsal root reflex in the cat. *Fed. Proc.*, **26**, 433

154. Gray, E. G. and Guillery, R. W. (1966). Synaptic morphology in the normal and degenerating nervous system. *Int. Rev. Cytol.*, **19**, 111

155. Bodian, D. (1972). Synaptic diversity and characterization by electron microscopy. In: *Structure and Function of Synapses* (G. D. Pappas and D. P. Purpura) (New York: Raven Press), 45

156. Gray, E. G. (1959). Axo-somatic and axo-dendritic synapses of the cerebral cortex: an electron microscope study. *J. Anat.*, **93**, 420

157. Bodian, D. (1966). Electron microscopy: two major synaptic types on spinal moto-neurons. *Science*, **151**, 1093

157a. Bodian, D. (1966). Synaptic types on spinal motoneurons: an electron microscopic study. *Bull. Johns Hopkins Hosp.*, **119**, 16

158. Hirata, Y. (1966). Occurrence of cylindrical synaptic vesicles in the central nervous system perfused with buffered formalin solution prior to OsO₄ fixation. *Arch. Histol. Japan*, **26**, 269

159. Werner, G. and Whitsel, B. L. (1973). Functional organization of the somatosensory cortex. In: *Handbook of Sensory Physiology*, Vol. 2, 621 (A. Iggo, editor) (Berlin: Springer-Verlag)

160. Bryan, R. N., Trevino, D. L., Coulter, J. D. and Willis, W. D. (1973). Location and somatotopic organization of the cells of origin of the spinocervical tract. *Exp. Brain Res.*, **17**, 177

161. Whitsel, B. L., Petrucelli, L. M., Sapiro, G. and Ha, A. (1970). Fiber sorting in the fasciculus gracilis of squirrel monkeys. *Exp. Neurol.*, **29**, 227

162. Whitsel, B. L., Petrucelli, L. M., Ha, H. and Dreyer, D. A. (1972). The resorting of spinal afferents as antecedent to the body representation in the postcentral gyrus. *Brain, Behavior and Evolution*, **5**, 303

163. Kuno, M. and Miyahara, J. T. (1968). Factors responsible for multiple discharge of neurons in Clarke's column. *J. Neurophysiol.*, **31**, 624

164. Brown, A. G. (1973). Ascending and long spinal pathways: dorsal columns, spino-cervical tract and spinothalamic tract. In: *Handbook of Sensory Physiology*, Vol. 2, 315 (A. Iggo, editor) (Berlin: Springer-Verlag)

165. Gordon, G. (1973). The concept of relay nuclei. In: *Handbook of Sensory Physiology*, Vol. 2, 137 (A. Iggo, editor) (Berlin: Springer-Verlag)

166. Eccles, J. C. (1945). Electrical hypothesis of synaptic and neuromuscular transmission. *Nature (London)*, **156**, 680

167. Brooks, C. McC. and Eccles, J. C. (1947). An electrical hypothesis of central inhibition. *Nature (London)*, **159**, 760

168. Bennett, M. V. L. (1972). A comparison of electrically and chemically mediated synaptic transmission. In: *Structure and Function of Synapses*, 221 (G. D. Pappas and D. P. Purpura, editors) (New York: Raven Press)

169. Wylie, R. M. (1973). Evidence of electrotonic transmission in the vestibular nuclei of the rat. *Brain Res.*, **50**, 179

170. Korn, H., Crepel, F. and Sotelo, C. (1972). Couplage électronique entre les neurones géants du noyau vestibulaire latéral chez le Rat. *C.R. Acad. Sci. (Paris) D*, **274**, 1365

171. Sotelo, C. and Palay, S. L. (1970). The fine structure of the lateral vestibular nucleus in the rat. *Brain Res.*, **18**, 93

172. Kuno, M. (1971). Quantum aspects of central and ganglionic synaptic transmission in vertebrates. *Physiol. Rev.*, **51**, 647

172a. Sprague, J. M. and Ha, H. (1964). The terminal fields of dorsal root fibers in the lumbosacral spinal cord of the cat, and the dendritic organization of the motor nuclei. In: *Progress in Brain Research: Organization of the Spinal Cord*, Vol. 11, 120 (J. C. Eccles and J. P. Schade, editors) (Amsterdam: Elsevier)

172b. Sterling, P. and Kuypers, H. G. J. M. (1967). Anatomical organization of the brachial spinal cord of the cat. I. The distribution of dorsal root fibers. *Brain Res.*, **4**, 1

172c. Imai, Y. and Kusama, T. (1969). Distribution of the dorsal root fibers in the cat. An experimental study with the nauta method. *Brain Res.*, **13**, 338

173. Otsuka, M. (1972). γ-Aminobutyric acid in the nervous system. In: *The Structure and Function of Nervous Tissue*, Vol. IV, 249 (G. H. Bourne, editor) (N.Y.: Academic Press)

174. Otsuka, M., Konishi, S. and Takahashi, T. (1972). A further study of the moto-neuron-depolarizing peptide extracted from dorsal roots of bovine spinal nerves. *Proc. Jap. Acad.*, **48**, 747

174a. Curtis, D. R., Phillis, J. W. and Watkins, J. C. (1959). The depression of spinal neurones by γ-amino-n-butyric acid and β-alanine. *J. Physiol. (London)*, **146**, 185

174b. Van Harreveld, A. (1959). Compounds in brain extracts causing spreading depression of cerebral cortical activity and contraction of crustacean muscle. *J. Neurochem.*, **3**, 300

175. Howland, B., Lettvin, J. Y., McCulloch, W. S., Pitts, W. H. and Wall, P. D. (1955). Reflex inhibition by dorsal root interaction. *J. Neurophysiol.*, **18**, 1

175a. Renshaw, B. (1946). Observations on interaction of nerve impulses in the gray matter and on the nature of central inhibition. *Amer. J. Physiol.*, **146**, 443

176. Frank, K. and Fuortes, M. G. F. (1957). Presynaptic and postsynaptic inhibition of monosynaptic reflexes. *Fed. Proc.*, **16**, 39

177. Eccles, J. C. and Malcolm, J. L. (1946). Dorsal root potentials of the spinal cord. *J. Neurophysiol.*, **9**, 139

178. Eccles, J. C. and Krnjevíc, K. (1959). Presynaptic changes associated with post-tetanic potentiation in the spinal cord. *J. Physiol. (London)*, **149**, 274

179. Gray, E. G. (1962). A morphological basis for pre-synaptic inhibition? *Nature (London)*, **193**, 82

180. Hunt, C. C. and Kuno, M. (1959). Background discharge and evoked responses of spinal interneurones. *J. Physiol. (London)*, **147**, 364

181. Amassian, V. E. and DeVito, J. L. (1954). Time characteristics of single unit activity in cuneate nucleus. *Fed. Proc.*, **13**, 3

182. Amassian, V. E. and DeVito, J. L. (1957). La transmission dans le noyau de Burdach (Nucleus cuneatus). Etude analytique par unités isolées d'un relais somato-sensoriel primaire. *Colloq. Int. Cent. Nat. Rech. Sci.*, **67**, 355

183. Mountcastle, V. B. and Rose, J. E. (1954). Activity of single neurons in the tactile thalamic region of the cat in response to a transient peripheral stimulus. *Bull. Johns Hopkins Hosp.*, **94**, 238

184. Mountcastle, V. B., Davies, P. W. and Berman, A. L. (1957). Response properties of neurons of cat's sensory cortex to peripheral stimuli. *J. Neurophysiol.*, **20**, 374

185. Amassian, V. E. (1953). Evoked single cortical unit activity in the somatic sensory areas. *Electroenceph. Clin. Neurophysiol.*, **5**, 415

186. Lorente de No, R. (1938). Limits of variation of the synaptic delay of motoneurons. *J. Neurophysiol.*, **1**, 187

187. Barron, D. H. and Matthews, B. H. C. (1938). The interpretation of potential changes in the spinal cord. *J. Physiol. (London)*, **92**, 276

188. Eccles, J. C., Kostyuk, P. G. and Schmidt, R. F. (1962). The effect of electric polariza-tion of the spinal cord on central afferent fibres and on their excitatory synaptic action. *J. Physiol. (London)*, **162**, 138

189. Dudel, J. and Kuffler, S. W. (1961). Presynaptic inhibition at the crayfish neuro-muscular junction. *J. Physiol. (London)*, **155**, 543

190. Kuno, M. (1964). Mechanism of facilitation and depression of the excitatory synaptic potential in spinal motoneurons. *J. Physiol. (London)*, **175**, 100

191. Schmidt, R. F. (1973). Control of the access of afferent activity to somatosensory pathways. In: *Handbook of Sensory Physiology*, Vol. **2**, 151 (A. Iggo, editor) (Berlin: Springer-Verlag)

192. Whitsel, B. L., Petrucelli, L. M. and Sapiro, G. (1969). Modality representation in the lumbar and cervical fasciculus gracilis of squirrel monkey. *Brain Res.*, **15**, 67

193. Blackstad, T. W. (1965). Mapping of experimental axon degeneration by electron microscopy of Golgi preparations. *Z. Zellforsch.*, **67**, 819

194. Oscarsson, O. (1958). Further observations on ascending spinal tracts activated by muscle, joint and skin nerves. *Arch. Ital. Biol.*, **96**, 199

195. Holmquist, B., Lundberg, A. and Oscarsson, O. (1960). Supraspinal inhibitory control of transmission to three ascending spinal pathways influenced by the flexion reflex afferents. *Arch. Ital. Biol.*, **98**, 60

196. Wall, P. D. (1958). Excitability changes in afferent fibre terminations and their relation to slow potentials. *J. Physiol. (London)*, **142**, 1
197. Eccles, J. C. (1964). *The Physiology of Synapses*. (Berlin: Springer)
198. Jänig, W., Schmidt, R. F. and Zimmerman, M. (1968). Single unit responses and the total afferent outflow from the cat's foot pad upon mechanical stimulation. *Exp. Brain Res.*, **6**, 100
199. Kellerth, J.-O. (1968). Aspects on the relative significance of pre- and postsynaptic inhibition in the spinal cord. In: *Structure and Functions of Inhibitory Neuronal Mechanisms*. (C. Von Euler, S. Skoglund and U. Söderberg, editors) (Oxford: Pergamon Press), 197
200. Wall, P. D. (1964). Presynaptic control of impulses at the first central synapse in the cutaneous pathway. In: *Progress in Brain Research*, Vol. **12**, 92 (J. C. Eccles and J. P. Schadé, editors) (Amsterdam: Elsevier Publishing Company)
201. Lloyd, D. P. C. and McIntyre, A. K. (1949). On the origin of dorsal root potentials. *J. Gen. Physiol.*, **32**, 409
202. Mendell, L. M. (1970). Positive dorsal root potentials produced by stimulation of small diameter muscle afferents. *Brain Res.*, **18**, 375
203. Mendell, L. M. and Wall, P. D. (1964). Presynaptic hyperpolarization: a role for fine afferent fibres. *J. Physiol. (London)*, **172**, 274
204. Zimmermann, M. (1968). Dorsal root potentials after C-fiber stimulation. *Science*, **160**, 896
205. Jänig, W. and Zimmermann, M. (1971). Presynaptic depolarization of myelinated afferent fibres evoked by stimulation of cutaneous C fibres. *J. Physiol. (London)*, **214**, 29
206. Vyklicky, L., Rudomin, P., Zajac, F. E. III and Burke, R. E. (1969). Primary afferent depolarization evoked by a painful stimulus. *Science*, **165**, 184
207. Burke, R., Lundberg, A. and Weight, F. (1971). Spinal border cell origin of the ventral spinocerebellar tract. *Exp. Brain Res.*, **12**, 283
208. Wall, P. D. and Sweet, W. H. (1967). Temporary abolition of pain in man. *Science*, **155**, 108
209. Shealy, C. N., Mortimer, J. T., Hagfors, N. R. (1970). Dorsal column electroanalgesia. *J. Neurosurg.*, **32**, 560
210. Stell, W. K. (1965). Correlation of retinal cytoarchitecture and ultrastructure in Golgi preparations. *Anat. Rec.*, **153**, 389
211. Rethelyi, M. (1968). The Golgi architecture of Clarke's column. *Acta Morph. Acad. Sci. Hung.*, **16**, 311
212. Christensen, B. N. (1973). Procion brown: an intracellular dye for light and electron microscopy. *Science*, **182**, 1255
213. Globus, A., Lux, H. D. and Schubert, P. (1968). Somadendritic spread of intracellularly injected tritiated glycine in cat spinal motoneurons. *Brain Res.*, **11**, 440
214. Schubert, P., Lux, H. D. and Kreutzberg, G. W. (1971). Single cell isotope injection technique, a tool for studying axonal and dendritic transport. *Acta neuropath. (Berl.) Suppl.*, **5**, 179
215. Heimer, L. (1970). Selective silver-impregnation of degenerating axoplasm. In: *Contemporary Research Methods in Neuroanatomy*. (W. J. H. Nauta, S. O. E. Ebbesson editors) (Berlin: Springer Verlag), 106
216. Cowan, W. M. (1970). Anterograde and retrograde transneuronal degeneration in the central and peripheral nervous system. In: *Contemporary Research Methods in Neuroanatomy*. (W. J. H. Nauta, S. O. E. Ebbesson, editors) (Berlin: Springer-Verlag), 217
217. Grant, G. (1968). Silver impregnation of degenerating dendrites, cells and axons central to axonal transection. II. A Nauta study on spinal motor neurons in kittens. *Exp. Brain Res.*, **6**, 284
218. Cowan, W. M., Gottlieb, D. I., Hendrickson, A. E., Price, J. L. and Woolsey, T. A. (1972). The autoradiographic demonstration of axonal connections in the central nervous system. *Brain Res.*, **37**, 21
219. Kristensson, K. and Olsson, Y. (1971). Retrograde axonal transport of protein. *Brain Res.*, **29**, 363
220. LaVail, J. H. and LaVail, M. M. (1972). Retrograde axonal transport in the central nervous system. *Science*, **176**, 1416
221. Ralston, J. H. and Sharp, P. V. (1973). The identification of thalamocortical relay

cells in the adult cat by means of retrograde axonal transport of horseradish peroxidase *Brain Res.*, **62**, 272

222. Litchy, W. J. (1973). Uptake and retrograde transport of horseradish peroxidase in frog sartorius nerve in vitro. *Brain Res.*, **56**, 377

223. Krishnan, N. and Singer, M. (1973). Penetration of peroxidase into peripheral nerve fibers. *Amer. J. Anat.*, **136**, 1

224. Lynch, G., Smith, R. L., Mensah, P. and Cotman, C. (1973). Tracing the dentate gyrus mossy fiber system with horseradish peroxidase histochemistry. *Exp. Neurol.*, **40**, 516

225. Lynch, G., Gall, C., Mensah, P. and Cotman, C. W. (1974). Horseradish peroxidase histochemistry: a new method for tracing efferent projections in the central nervous system. *Brain Res.*, **65**, 373

226. Renshaw, B. (1941). Influence of discharge of motoneurons upon excitation of neighboring motoneurons. *J. Neurophysiol.*, **4**, 167

227. Bard, P. (1938). Studies on the cortical representation of somatic sensibility. *Harv. Lect.*, **33**, 143

228. Perl, E. R., Whitlock, D. G. and Gentry, J. R. (1962). Cutaneous projection to second order neurons of the dorsal column system. *J. Neurophysiol.*, **25**, 337

229. Schiff, J. M. (1858). Lehrbuch der Physiologie des Menschen. *Cyclus Organische Verbund. Lehrbuch Sämmtl. Med. Wissensch.*, **1**, 234

230. White, J. C. and Sweet, W. H. (1955). *Pain: Its Mechanisms and Surgical Control.* (Springfield: C. C. Thomas)

231. Bok, S. T. (1928). Das Rückenmark, *Handbuch der mikroskopischen Anatomie des Menschen*, **4**, 478 (W. v. Möllendorf, editor) (Berlin: Springer)

232. Lloyd, D. P. C. and McIntyre, A. K. (1950). Dorsal column conduction of Group I muscle afferent impulses and their relay through Clarke's column. *J. Neurophysiol.*, **13**, 39

233. Whitehorn, D., Cornwall, C. C. and Burgess, P. R. (1971). Central course of identified cutaneous afferents from cat hindlimb. *Fed. Proc.*, **30**, 433

234. Uddenberg, N. (1968). Functional organization of long, second-order afferents in the dorsal funiculus. *Exp. Brain Res.*, **4**, 377

235. Petit, D., Lackner, D. and Burgess, P. R. (1969). Mise en évidence de fibres à áctivité postsynaptique au niveau des colomnes dorsales chez le Chat. *J. Physiol. (Paris)*, **61**, 372

236. Petit, D. (1972). Postsynaptic fibres in the dorsal columns and their relay in the nucleus gracilis. *Brain Res.*, **48**, 380

237. Rustioni, A. (1973). Non-primary afferents to the nucleus gracilis from the lumbar cord of the cat. *Brain Res.*, **51**, 81

238. Rustioni, A. (1974). Non-primary afferents to the cuneate nucleus in the brachial dorsal funiculus of the cat. *Brain Res.*, in press

239. Rustioni, A. (1974). Non-primary afferents to the dorsal column nuclei of cat distribution pattern and cells of origin. *Anat. Rec.*, **178**, 454

240. Ferraro, A. and Barrera, S. E. (1935). The nuclei of the posterior funiculi in *Macacus rhesus*. An anatomic and experimental investigation. *Arch. Neurol. Psychiat. (Chic.)*, **33**, 262

240a. Ferraro, A. and Barrera, S. E. (1935). Posterior column fibers and their termination in *Macacus rhesus*. *J. Comp. Neurol.*, **62**, 507

241. Weaver, T. A. Jr. and Walker, A. E. (1941). Topical arrangement within the spino-thalamic tract of the monkey. *Arch. Neurol. Psychiat.*, *(Chic)*, **46**, 877

242. Kuhn, R. A. (1953). Organisation of tactile dermatomes in cat and monkey. *J. Neurophysiol.*, **16**, 169

243. Werner, G. and Whitsel, B. L. (1967). The topology of dermatomal projection in the medial lemniscal system. *J. Physiol. (London)*, **192**, 123

245. Brown, A. G. (1968). Cutaneous afferent fibre collaterals in the dorsal columns of the cat. *Exp. Brain Res.*, **5**, 293

246. Dart, A. M. and Gordon, G. (1970). Excitatory and inhibitory afferent inputs to the dorsal column nuclei not involving the dorsal column. *J. Physiol. (London)*, **211**, 36P

247. Dart, A. M. and Gordon, G. (1973). Some properties of spinal connections of the cat's dorsal column nuclei which do not involve the dorsal columns. *Brain Res.*, **58**, 61

248. Gordon, G. and Grant, G. (1972). Afferents to the dorsal column nuclei from the dorsolateral funiculus of the spinal cord. *Acta Physiol. Scand.*, **84**, 30A

249. Hazlett, J. C., Dom, R. and Martin, G. F. (1972). Spino-bulbar, spino-thalamic and

medial lemniscal connections in the American opossum, *Didelphis* and *Marsupialis virginiana*. *J. Comp. Neurol.*, **146**, 95

250. Kuypers, H. G. J. M. and Tuerck, J. D. (1964). The distribution of the cortical fibres within the nuclei cuneatus and gracilis in the cat. *J. Anat.* (*London*), **98**, 143

251. Hand, P. J. (1966). Lumbosacral dorsal root terminations in the nucleus gracilis of the cat. Some observations on terminal degeneration in other medullary sensory nuclei. *J. Comp. Neurol.*, **126**, 137

252. Rustioni, A. and Macchi, G. (1968). Distribution of dorsal root fibers in the medulla oblongata of the cat. *J. Comp. Neurol.*, **134**, 113

253. Keller, J. H. and Hand, P. J. (1970). Dorsal root projections to nucleus cuneatus of the cat. *Brain Res.*, **20**, 1

254. Shriver, J. E., Stein, B. M. and Carpenter, M. B. (1968). Central projections of spina dorsal roots in the monkey. I. Cervical and upper thoracic dorsal roots. *Amer. J. Anat.*, **123**, 27

255. Carpenter, M. B., Stein, B. M. and Shriver, J. E. (1968). Central projections of spinal dorsal roots in the monkey. II. Lower thoracic, lumbosacral and coccygeal dorsal roots. *Amer. J. Anat.*, **123**, 75

256. Walberg, F. (1965). Axoaxonic contacts in the cuneate nucleus, probable basis for presynaptic depolarization. *Exp. Neurol.*, **13**, 218

257. Walberg, F. (1966). The fine structure of the cuneate nucleus in normal cats and following interruption of afferent fibers. An electron microscopical study with particular reference to findings made in Glees and Nauta sections. *Exp. Brain Res.*, **2**, 107

258. Blomquist, A. and Westman, J. (1971). An electron microscopical study of the gracile nucleus in the cat. *Acta Soc. Med. Upsal.*, **75**, 241

259. Kruger, L., Siminoff, R. and Witkovsky, P. (1961). Single neuron analysis of dorsal column nuclei and spinal nucleus of trigeminal in cat. *J. Neurophysiol.*, **24**, 333

260. Winter, D. L. (1965). N. gracilis of cat. Functional organization and corticofugal effects. *J. Neurophysiol.*, **28**, 48

261. Woudenberg, R. A. (1970). Projections of mechanoreceptive fields to cuneate-gracile and spinal trigeminal nuclear regions in sheep. *Brain Res.*, **17**, 417

262. Gordon, G. and Paine, C. H. (1960). Functional organization in nucleus gracilis of the cat. *J. Physiol.* (*London*), **153**, 331

263. Gordon, G. and Seed, W. A. (1961). An investigation of nucleus gracilis of the cat by antidromic stimulation. *J. Physiol.* (*London*), **155**, 589

264. Gordon, G. and Jukes, M. G. M. (1964). Dual organization of the exteroceptive components of the cat's gracile nucleus. *J. Physiol.* (*London*), **173**, 263

265. Gordon, G. and Jukes, M. G. M. (1964). Descending influences on the exteroceptive organizations of the cat's gracile nucleus. *J. Physiol.* (*London*), **173**, 291

266. McComas, A. J. (1963). Responses of the rat dorsal column system to mechanical stimulation of the hind paw. *J. Physiol.* (*London*), **166**, 435

267. Burgess, P. R. (1965). A study of the transmission of sensory information in the cat spinal cord. Ph.D. Dissertation, (New York: The Rockefeller University)

268. Rosén, I. (1969). Afferent connexions to group I activated cells in the main cuneate nucleus of the cat. *J. Physiol.* (*London*), **205**, 209

269. Towe, A. L. (1973). Somatosensory Cortex: Descending influences in ascending systems. In: *Handbook of Sensory Physiology*, Vol. 2 (A. Iggo, editor) (Berlin: Springer Verlag), 701

270. Andersen, P., Eccles, J. C., Oshima, T. and Schmidt, R. F. (1964). Mechanisms of synaptic transmission in the cuneate nucleus. *J. Neurophysiol.*, **27**, 1096

271. Andersen, P., Eccles, J. C., Schmidt, R. F. and Yokota, T. (1964). Slow potential waves produced in the cuneate nucleus by cutaneous volleys and by cortical stimulation. *J. Neurophysiol.*, **27**, 78

272. Andersen, P., Eccles, J. C., Schmidt, R. F. and Yokota, T. (1964). Depolarization of presynaptic fibers in the cuneate nucleus. *J. Neurophysiol.*, **27**, 92

273. Andersen, P., Eccles, J. C., Schmidt, R. F. and Yokota, T. (1964). Identification of relay cells and interneurons in the cuneate nucleus. *J. Neurophysiol.*, **27**, 1080

274. Walberg, F. (1957). Corticofugal fibres to the nuclei of the dorsal columns. An experimental study in the cat. *Brain*, **80**, 273

275. Jabbur, S. J. and Towe, A. L. (1959). Blocking and excitation of cuneate neurons by sensori-motor cortical stimulation in the cat. *Fed. Proc.*, **18**, 73

276. Jabbur, S. J. and Towe, A. L. (1960). Effect of pyramidal tract activity on dorsal column nuclei. *Science*, **132**, 547
277. Andersen, P., Etholm, B. and Gordon, G. (1970). Presynaptic and postsynaptic inhibition elicited in the cat's dorsal column nuclei by mechanical stimulation of skin. *J. Physiol. (London)*, **210**, 433
278. Walker, A. E. (1938). *The Primate Thalamus.* (Chicago: University of Chicago Press)
279. Matzke, H. A. (1951). The course of the fibers arising from the nucleus gracilis and cuneatus of the cat. *J. Comp. Neurol.*, **94**, 439
280. Boivie, J. (1971). The termination in the thalamus and the zona incerta of fibres from the dorsal column nuclei (DCN) in the cat. An experimental study with silver impregnation methods. *Brain Res.*, **28**, 459
281. Boivie, J. Unpublished work
282. Jabbur, S. J. and Banna, N. R. (1970). Widespread cutaneous inhibition in dorsal column nuclei. *J. Neurophysiol.*, **33**, 616
283. Cooke, J. D., Larson, B., Oscarsson, O. and Sjölund, B. (1971). Origin and termination of cuneocerebellar tract. *Exp. Brain Res.*, **13**, 339
284. Cooke, J. D., Larson, B., Oscarsson, O. and Sjölund, B. (1971). Organization of afferent connections to cuneocerebellar tract. *Exp. Brain Res.*, **13**, 359
285. Gordon, G. and Horrobin, D. F. (1967). Antidromic and synaptic responses in the cat's gracile nucleus to cerebellar stimulation. *Brain Res.*, **5**, 419
286. Brodal, A. and Pompeiano, O. (1957). The vestibular nuclei in the cat. *J. Anat. (Lond.)*, **91**, 438
287. Sadjadpour, K. and Brodal, A. (1968). The vestibular nuclei in man. A morphological study in the light of experimental findings in the cat. *J. Hirnforsch.*, **10**, 299
288. Walberg, F., Bowsher, D. and Brodal, A. (1958). The termination of primary vestibular fibres in the vestibular nuclei in the cat. An experimental study with silver methods. *J. Comp. Neurol.*, **110**, 391
289. Brodal, A. and Torvik, A. (1957). Über den Ursprung der sekundären vestibulocerebellaren Faseen bei der Katze. Eine experimentall-anatomische Studie. *Arch. Psychiat. Nervenkr.*, **195**, 550
290. Landgren, S. and Silfvenius, H. (1971). Nucleus Z, the medullary relay in the projection path to the cerebral cortex of group I muscle afferents from the cat's hind limb. *J. Physiol. (London)*, **218**, 551
291. Boivie, J., Grant, G. and Silfvenius, H. (1970). A projection from nucleus Z to the ventral nuclear complex of the thalamus in the cat. *Acta Physiol. Scand.*, **80**, 11A
292. Grant, G., Boivie, J. and Silfvenius, H. (1973). Course and termination of fibres from the nucleus Z of the medulla oblongata. An experimental light microscopical study in the cat. *Brain Res.*, **55**, 55
293. Landgren, S. and Silfvenius, H. (1970). The projection of group I muscle afferents from the hindlimb to the contralateral thalamus of the cat. *Acta Physiol. Scand.*, **80**, 10A
295. Silfvenius, H. (1972). Properties of cortical group I neurones located in the lower bank of the naterior suprasylvian sulcus of the cat. *Acta Physiol. Scand.*, **84**, 555
296. Morin, F. (1955). A new spinal pathway for cutaneous impulses. *Amer. J. Physiol.*, **183**, 245
297. Taub, A. and Bishop, P. O. (1965). The spinocervical tract: dorsal column linkage, conduction velocity, primary afferent spectrum. *Exp. Neurol.*, **13**, 1
298. Brown, A. G. and Franz, D. N. (1969). Responses of spinocervical tract neurones to natural stimulation of identified cutaneous receptors. *Exp. Brain. Res*, **7**, 231
299. Horrobin, D. F. (1966). The lateral cervical nucleus of the cat: an electrophysiological study. *Quart. J. Exp. Physiol.*, **51**, 351
300. Brodal, A. and Rexed, B. (1953). Spinal afferents to the lateral cervical nucleus in cat. An experimental study. *J. Comp. Neurol.*, **98**, 179
301. Eccles, J. C., Eccles, R. M. and Lundberg, A. (1960). Types of neurones in and around the intermediate nucleus of the lumbosacral cord. *J. Physiol. (London)*, **154**, 89
302. Hongo, T., Jankowska, E. and Lundberg, A. (1968). Postsynaptic excitation and inhibition evoked from primary afferents in neurones of the spinocervical tract. *J. Physiol. (London)*, **199**, 569
303. Van Beusekom, G. T. (1955). Fibre analysis of the anterior and lateral funiculi of the cord in the cat. Ph.D. Thesis, (Leiden: E. Ijdo, N.V.)

304. Rexed, B. and Strom, G. (1952). Afferent nervous connections of the lateral cervical nucleus. *Acta Physiol. Scand.*, **24**, 219

305. Willis, W. D., personal communication.

306. Taub, A. (1964). Local, segmental and supraspinal interaction with a dorsolateral spinal cutaneous afferent system. *Exp. Neurol.*, **10**, 357

307. Brown, A. G. (1970). Descending control of the spinocervical tract in decerebrate cats. *Brain Res.*, **17**, 152

308. Mendell, L. M. (1966). Physiological properties of unmyelinated fiber projection to the spinal cord. *Exp. Neurol.*, **16**, 316

309. Rexed, B. and Brodal, P. (1951). The nucleus cervicalis lateralis. A spino-cerebellar relay nucleus. *J. Neurophysiol.*, **14**, 399

310. Morin, F. and Catalano, J. (1955). Central connections of a cervical nucleus (nucleus cervicalis lateralis of the cat). *J. Comp. Neurol.*, **103**, 17

311. Ha, H., Kitai, S. and Morin, F. (1965). The lateral cervical nucleus of the Raccoon. *Exp. Neurol.*, **11**, 441

312. Kitai, S. T., Ha, H. and Morin, F. (1965). Lateral cervical nucleus of the dog: anatomical and microelectrode studies. *Amer. J. Physiol.*, **209**, 307

313. Mizumo, N., Nakano, K., Imaizumi, M. and Okamoto, M. (1967). The lateral cervical nucleus of the Japanese monkey (Macaca fuscata). *J. Comp. Neurol.*, **129**, 375

314. Kircher, C. and Ha, H. (1968). The nucleus cervicalis lateralis in primates, including the human. *Anat. Rec.*, **160**, 376

315. Truex, R., Taylor, M. and Smythe, J. (1968). The lateral cervical nucleus of the human spinal cord. *Anat. Rec.*, **160**, 443

316. Gwyn, D. G. and Waldron, H. A. (1968). A nucleus in the dorsolateral funiculus of the spinal cord of the rat. *Brain Res.*, **10**, 342

317. Waldron, H. A. (1969). The morphology of the lateral cervical nucleus in the hedgehog *Brain Res.*, **16**, 301

318. Westman, J. (1968). The lateral cervical nucleus in the cat. II. An electron microscopical study of the normal structure. *Brain Res.*, **11**, 107

319. Westman, J. (1971). The lateral cervical nucleus in the cat. V. A. quantitative evaluation on the bouton- and glia-covered surface area of different LCN-neurons. *Z. Zellforsch Mikrosk Anat.*, **115**, 377

320. Westman, J. (1969). The lateral cervical nucleus. III. An electron microscopical study after transection of spinal afferents. *Exp. Brain Res.*, **7**, 32

320a. Biedenbach, M. A. (1972). Cell density and regional distribution of cell types in the cuneate nucleus of the rhesus monkey. *Brain Res.*, **45**, 1

321. Grant, G. and Westman, J. (1969). The lateral cervical nucleus in the cat. IV. A light and electron microscopical study after midbrain lesions with demonstration of indirect Wallerian degeneration at the ultrastructural level. *Exp. Brain Res.*, **7**, 51

322. Morin, F., Kitai, S. T., Portnoy, H. and Demirjian, C. (1963). Afferent projections to the lateral cervical nucleus: a microelectrode study. *Amer. J. Physiol.*, **204**, 667

323. Oswaldo-Cruz, E. and Kidd, C. (1964). Functional properties of neurons in the lateral cervical nucleus of the cat. *J. Neurophysiol.*, **27**, 1

324. Wall, P. D. and Taub, A. (1962). Four aspects of the trigeminal nucleus and a paradox. *J. Neurophysiol.*, **25**, 110

325. Fedina, L., Gordon, G. and Lundberg, A. (1968). The source and mechanisms of inhibition in the lateral cervical nucleus of the cat. *Brain Res.*, **11**, 694

326. Busch, H. F. M. (1961). An anatomical analysis of the white matter in the brain stem of the cat. Thesis, 116 (Assen: van Gorcum)

327. Boivie, J. (1970). The termination of the cervicothalamic tract in the cat. An experimental study with silver impregnation methods. *Brain Res.*, **19**, 333

328. Hagg, S. and Ha, H. (1970). Cervicothalamic tract in the dog. *J. Comp. Neurol.*, **139**, 357

329. Ha, H. (1971). Cervicothalamic tract in the rhesus monkey. *Exp. Neurol.*, **33**, 205

330. Morin, F. and Thomas, L. M. (1955). Spinothalamic fibers and tactile pathways in cat. *Anat. Rec.*, **121**, 344

331. Grant, G., Boivie, J. and Brodal, A. (1968). The question of a cerebellar projection from the lateral cervical nucleus re-examined. *Brain Res.*, **9**, 95

332. DiBiagio, F. and Grundfest, H. (1955). Afferent relations of the inferior olivary

nucleus. II. Site of relay of the hind limb afferents into the dorsal spino-olivary tract in cat. *J. Neurophysiol.*, **18**, 299

333. Mizuno, N. (1966). An experimental study of the spino-olivary fibers in the rabbit and the cat. *J. Comp. Neurol.*, **127**, 267

334. Edinger, L. (1890). Eineges vom verlauf der gefuehlsbahnen im centralen nervensysteme. *Deutsche Medizinische Wochenschrift*, **16**, 421

335. Spiller, W. G. (1905). The occasional clinical resemblance between caries of the vertebrae and lumbothoracic syringomyelia, and the location within the spinal cord of the fibres for the sensations of pain and temperature. *Univ. Pennsyl. Med. Bull.*, **18**, 147

336. Petrén, K. (1910). Ueber die Bahnen der Sensibilität im Rückemarke, besonders nach den Fällen von Stichverletzung studiert. *Arch. psychiat.*, **47**, 495

337. Keele, K. D. (1957). *Anatomies of Pain.* (Oxford: Blackwell Scientific Publishers)

338. Mehler, W. R., Feferman, M. E., Nauta, W. J. H. (1960). Ascending axon degeneration following anterolateral cordotomy. An experimental study in the monkey. *Brain*, **83**, 718

339. Kuru, M. (1949). *Sensory Paths in the Spinal Cord and Brain Stem of Man.* (Tokyo: Sogensya)

340. Probst, M. (1900). Experimental untersuchungen über die schleifenendingugn, die haubenbahnen des dorsalen längsbundeln und die hinter commisur. *Arch. F. Psychiat. U. Nervenkr.*, **33**, 1

341. Rothmann, M. (1903). Zur anatomie und physiologie des vorderstranges. *Neurol. Centralbl.*, **22**, 744

342. Rothmann, M. (1904). Über die Leitungsbahnen des Berührungsreflexes unter Berücksichtigung der Hautreflexe des Menschen. *Arch. F. Anatomie und Entwiklungsgech S.*, 256

343. Rothmann, M. (1906). Ueber die leitung der sensibilität im Rückenmark *Berlin. Klin. Wochenschrift*, **43**, 76

344. Mehler, W. R. (1969). Some neurological species differences — a posteriori. *Ann. N.Y. Acad. Sci.*, **167**, 424

345. Foerster, O. and Gagel, O. (1931). Die Vorderseitenstrangdurchschneidung beim Menschen. Eine klinisch-pathophysiologisch-anatomische Studie. *Z. Ges. Neurol. Psychiat.*, **138**, 1

346. Hyndman, O. R. and Van Epps, C. (1939). Possibility of differential section of the spinothalamic tract: A clinical and histological study. *Arch. Surg.*, **38**, 1036

347. Gardner, E. and Cuneo, H. M. (1945). Lateral spinothalamic tract and associated tracts in man. *Arch. Neurol. Psychiat. (Chic.)*, **53**, 423

348. Morin, F., Schwartz, H. G. and O'Leary, J. L. (1951). Experimental study of the spinothalamic and related tracts. *Acta Psychiat. Neurol. Scand.*, **26**, 371

349. Walker, A. E. (1942). Somatotopic localization of spinothalamic and sensory trigeminal tracts in mesencephalon. *Arch. Neurol. Psychiat. (Chic.)*, **48**, 885

350. Pearson, A. A. (1952). Role of gelatinous substance of spinal cord in conduction of pain. *Arch. Neurol. Psychiat. (Chic.)*, **68**, 515

351. Szentagothai, J. (1964). Propriospinal pathways and their synapses. In: *Progress in Brain Research*, Vol. II, (J. C. Eccles and J. P. Schadé, editors) (Amsterdam: Elsevier Publishing Company), 155

352. Kumazawa, T. and Perl, E. R., Burgess, P. R. and Whitehorn, D. (1974). Ascending projections from marginal zone (Lamina I) neurons of the spinal dorsal horn. *J. Comp. Neurol.*, in press

353. Dilly, P. N., Wall, P. D. and Webster, K. E. (1968). Cells of origin of the spinothalamic tract in cat and rat. *Exp. Neurol.*, **21**, 550

354. Trevino, D. L., Maunz, R. A., Bryan, R. N. and Willis, W. D. (1972). Location of cells of origin of the spinothalamic tract in the lumbar enlargement of cat. *Exp. Neurol.*, **34**, 64

355. Levante, A. and Albe-Fessard, D. (1972). Localisation dans les couches VII et VIII de Rexed des cellules d'origine d'un faisceau spino-réticulaire croisé. *C.R. Acad. Sci. (Paris)*, **274**, 3007

356. Trevino, D. L., Coulter, J. D. and Willis, W. D. (1973). Location of cells of origin of spinothalamic tract in lumbar enlargement of the monkey. *J. Neurophysiol.*, **36**, 750

357. Bryan, R. N., Trevino, D. L., Coulter, J. D. and Willis, W. D. (1973). Location and

somatotopic organization of the cells of origin of the spino-cervical tract. *Exp. Brain Res.*, **17**, 177

358. Brodal, A. (1957). *The Reticular Formation of the Brain Stem. Anatomical Aspects and Functional Correlations.* (Edinburgh: Oliver and Boyd)

359. Meessen, H. and Olszewski, J. (1949). *A Cytoarchitectonic Atlas of the Rhombencephalon of the Rabbit.* (Basel: Karger)

360. Olszewski, J. and Baxter, D. (1954). *Cytoarchitecture of the Human Brain Stem.* (Basel: Karger)

361. Pompeiano, O. (1973). Reticular formation. In: *Handbook of Sensory Physiology*, Vol. 2 (A. Iggo, editors) (Berlin: Springer-Verlag), 381

362. Rossi, G. F. and Brodal, A. (1957). Terminal distribution of spino-reticular fibers in the cat. *Arch. Neurol. Psychiat.*, **78**, 439

363. Bowsher, D., Mallart, A., Petit, D. and Albe-Fessard, D. (1968). A bulbar relay to the centre median. *J. Neurophysiol.*, **31**, 288

364. Casey, K. L. (1969). Somatic stimuli, spinal pathways, and size of cutaneous fibers influencing unit activity in the medial medullary reticular formation. *Exp. Neurol.*, **25**, 35

365. Liebeskind, J. C. and Mayer, D. J. (1971). Somatosensory evoked responses in the mesencephalic central gray matter of the rat. *Brain Res.*, **27**, 133

366. Kerr, F. W. L. (1974). The ascending tracts of the ventral funiculus of the spinal cord with special reference to a spinothalamic system. *Anat. Rec.*, **178**, 389

367. Anderson, F. D. and Berry, C. M. (1959). Degeneration studies of long ascending fiber systems in the cat brain stem. *J. Comp. Neurol.*, **111**, 195

368. Bowsher, D. (1962). The topographical projection of fibres from the anterolateral quadrant of the spinal cord to the sub-diencephalic brain stem in man. *Mschr. Psychiat. Neurol.*, **143**, 75

369. Bowsher, D. and Westman, J. (1970). The gigantocellular reticular region and its spinal afferents: a light and electron microscope study in the cat. *J. Anat. (London)*, **106**, 23

370. Bowsher, D. and Westman, J. (1971). Ultrastructural characteristics of the caudal and rostral brain stem reticular formation. *Brain Res.*, **28**, 443

371. Westman, J. and Bowsher, D. (1971). Ultrastructural observations on the degeneration of spinal afferents to the nucleus medullae oblongata centralis (pars caudalis) of the cat. *Brain Res.*, **26**, 395

372. Bowsher, D. and Petit, D. (1970). Place and modality analysis in nucleus of the posterior commissure. *J. Physiol. (London)*, **206**, 663

373. Bowsher, D. (1970). Place and modality analysis in caudal reticular formation. *J. Physiol. (London)*, **209**, 473

374. Peterson, B. W. and Felpel, L. P. (1971). Excitation and inhibition of reticulospinal neurons by vestibular, cortical and cutaneous stimulation. *Brain Res.*, **27**, 373

375. Burton, H. (1968). Somatic sensory properties of caudal bulbar reticular neurons in the cat (Felis Domestica). *Brain Res.*, **11**, 357

376. Benjamin, R. M. (1970). Single neurons in the rat medulla responsive to nociceptive stimulation. *Brain Res.*, **24**, 525

377. Collins, W. F. and Randt, C. T. (1958). Evoked central nervous sytsem activity relating to peripheral unmyelinated or 'C' fibers in cat. *J. Neurophysiol.*, **21**, 345

378. Becker, D. P., Gluck, H., Nulsen, F. E. and Jane, J. A. (1969). An inquiry into the neurophysiological basis for pain. *J. Neurosurg.*, **30**, 1

379. Collins, W. F. and Randt, C. T. (1960). Midbrain evoked response relating to peripheral unmyelinated or 'C' fibers in cat. *J. Neurophysiol.*, **23**, 47

380. Liebeskind, J. C., Mayer, D. J. and Akil, H. (1974). Central mechanisms of pain inhibition: studies of analgesia from focal brain stimulation. In: *Advances in Neurology*, Vol. 4 (J. J. Bonica, editor) (New York: Raven Press), 1

381. Mayer, D. J., Wolfle, T. L., Akil, H., Carder, B. and Liebeskind, J. C. (1971). Analgesia from electrical stimulation in the brain stem of the rat. *Science*, **174**, 1351

382. Mayer, D. J. (1971). Analgesia produced by focal brain stimulation in the rat. Ph.D. Dissertation (University of California, Los Angeles)

383. Liebeskind, J. C., Guilbaud, G., Besson, J.-M. and Oliveras, J.-L. (1973). Analgesia from electrical stimulation of the periaqueductal grey matter in the cat: behavioural observations and inhibitory effects on spinal cord interneurons. *Brain Res.*, **50**, 441

384. Mancia, M., Grantyn, A., Broggi, G. and Margnelli, M. (1971). Synaptic linkage between mesencephalic and bulbo-pontine reticular structures as revealed by intracellular recording. *Brain Res.*, **33**, 491

385. Brodal, A. and Rossi, G. F. (1955). Ascending fibers in brain stem reticular formation of cat. *Arch. Neurol. Psychiat. (Chic.)*, **74**, 68

386. Nauta, W. J. H. and Kuypers, H. G. J. M. (1958). Some ascending pathways in the brain stem reticular formation. In: *Reticular Formation of the Brain.* (H. H. Jasper and L. D. Proctor, editors) (Boston: Little, Brown and Company), 3

387. Bowsher, D. (1957). Termination of the central pain pathway in man: the conscious appreciation of pain. *Brain*, **80**, 606

388. Olszewski, J. (1952). The Thalamus of *Macaca Mulatta* (New York: Karger)

389. Jasper, H. H. and Ajmone-Marsan, C. (1954). *A Stereotaxic Atlas of the Diencephalon of the Cat.* (Toronto: University of Toronto Press)

390. Hassler, R. (1959). Die zentralen systeme des Schmerzes. *Acta Neurochisurgica*, **8**, 353

391. Carpenter, M. (1967). Ventral tier thalamic nuclei. In: *Modern Trends in Neurology*, Vol. **4**, 1

392. Rose, J. and Mountcastle, V. (1952). The thalamic tactile region in rabbit and cat. *J. Comp. Neurol.*, **97**, 441

393. Mehler, W. R. (1971). Idea of a new anatomy of the thalamus. *J. Psychiat. Res.*, **8**, 203

394. Rose, J. E. and Woolsey, C. N. (1958). Cortical connections and functional organization of the thalamic auditory system of the cat. In: *Biological and Biochemical Bases of Behavior.* (H. F. Harlow and C. N. Woolsey, editors) (Madison: University of Wisconsin Press), 127

395. Jones, E. G. and Powell, T. P. S. (1971). An analysis of the posterior group of thalamic nuclei on the basis of its afferent connections. *J. Comp. Neurol.*, **143**, 185

396. Rose, J. E. and Woolsey, C. N. (1949). Organization of the mammalian thalamus and its relationships to the cerebral cortex. *EEG and Clin. Neurophysiol.*, **1**, 391

397. Ralston, H. J. and Herman, M. M. (1969). The fine structure of neurons and synapses in the ventrobasal thalamus of the cat. *Brain Res.*, **14**, 77

398. Scheibel, M. E. and Scheibel, A. B. (1966). Patterns of organization in specific and non-specific thalamic fields. In: *The Thalamus* (D. P. Purpura and M. D. Yahr, editors) (New York: Columbia University Press), 13

399. Tömböl, T. (1969). Terminal arborization in specific afferents in the specific thalamic nuclei. *Acta Morph. Acad. Sci. Hung.*, **17**, 273

400. Tömböl, T. (1969). Two types of short axon (Golgi 2nd) interneurons in the specific thalamic nuclei. *Acta Morph. Acad. Sci. Hung.*, **17**, 285

401. Scheibel, M. E., Davies, T. L. and Scheibel, A. B. (1972). An unusual axonless cell in the thalamus of the adult cat. *Exp. Neurol.*, **36**, 512

402. Tömböl, T. (1967). Short neurons and their synaptic relations in the specific thalamic nuclei. *Brain Res.*, **3**, 307

403. Scheibel, M. E. and Scheibel, A. B. (1972). Input–output relations of the thalamic nonspecific system. *Brain Behav. Evol.*, **6**, 332

404. Ralston, H. J. (1969). The synaptic organization of lemniscal projections to the ventrobasal thalamus of the cat. *Brain Res.*, **14**, 99

405. Jones, E. G. and Powell, T. P. S. (1969). An electron microscopic study of the mode of termination of cortico-thalamic fibres within the sensory relay nuclei of the thalamus. *Proc. Roy. Soc. B*, **172**, 173

406. Jones, E. G. and Powell, T. P. S. (1969). The cortical projection of the ventroposterior nucleus of the thalamus in the cat. *Brain Res.*, **13**, 298

407. Uchizono, K. (1965). Characteristics of excitatory and inhibitory synapses in the central nervous system of the cat. *Nature (London)*, **207**, 642

408. Franz, D. N. and Iggo, A. (1968). Dorsal root potentials and ventral root reflexes evoked by non-myelinated fibers. *Science*, **162**, 1140

409. Lorente de Nó, R. (1943). Cerebral Cortex: Architecture, Intracortical connections, Motor Projections. In: *Physiology of the Nervous System* (J. F. Fulton, editor), Chapt. XV, 274, (New York: Oxford University Press), 274

410. Forbes, D. (1972). Synaptic organization of somatosensory afferent projections to the squirrel monkey thalamus. *Soc. Neurosci.*, Second Annual Meeting, Houston, 146

411. Crosby, E. C., Humphrey, T. and Lauer, E. W. (1962). *Correlative Anatomy of the Nervous System.* (New York: Macmillan Company)

412. Hand, P. and Liu, C. N. (1966). Efferent projections of the nucleus gracilis. *Anat. Rec.*, **154**, 353
413. Bowsher, D. (1961). The termination of secondary somatosensory nuerons within the thalamus of *Macaca mulatta:* an experimental degeneration study. *J. Comp. Neurol.*, **117**, 213
414. Mountcastle, V. and Henneman, E. (1949). Pattern of tactile representation in thalamus of cat. *J. Neurophysiol.*, **12**, 85
415. Mountcastle, V. B. and Henneman, E. (1952). The representation of tactile sensibility in the thalamus of the monkey. *J. Comp. Neurol.*, **97**, 409
416. Boivie, J. (1974). Thalamic termination of fibres from the dorsal column nuclei and the spinal cord in the macaque. *Anat. Rec.*, **178**, 313
417. Landgren, S., Nordwall, A. and Wengstrom, C. (1965). The location of the thalamic relay in the spino–cervico–lemniscal path. *Acta Physiol. Scand.*, **65**, 164
418. Andersen, P., Andersson, S. and Landgren, S. (1966). Some properties of the thalamic relay cells in the spino–cervico–lemniscal path. *Acta Physiol. Scand.*, **68**, 72
419. Boivie, J. and Westman, J. (1968). Electron microscopy of medial lemniscal terminal degeneration in the ventral posterolateral thalamic nucleus of the cat. *Experientia (Basel)*, **24**, 159
420. Ralston, H. J. III (1973). Somatosensory projections to the thalamus of the cat. *Anat. Rec.*, **175**, 419
421. Whitlock, D. G. and Perl, E. R. (1957). Central projections of the 'spinothalamic' system in cats. *Anat. Rec.*, **127**, 388
422. Whitlock, D. G. and Perl, E. R. (1959). Afferent projections through ventrolateral funiculi to thalamus of cat. *J. Neurophysiol.*, **22**, 133
423. Whitlock, D. G. and Perl, E. R. (1961). Thalamic projections of spinothalamic pathways in monkey. *Exp. Neurol.*, **3**, 240
424. Collier, J. and Buzzard, E. F. (1903). The degeneration resulting from lesions of posterior nerve roots and from transverse lesions of the spinal cord in man. A study of twenty cases. *Brain*, **26**, 559
425. Mehler, W. R. (1966). Some observations on secondary afferent systems in the central nervous system. In: *Pain*. (R. S. Knighton and P. R. Dumke, editors) (Boston: Little Brown Company), 11
425a. Bishop, G. H. (1959). The relation between nerve fiber size and sensory modality, phylogenetic implications of the afferent innervation of cortex. *J. Nerv. Ment. Dis.*, **128**, 89
425b. Herrick, C. J. and Bishop, G. H. (1958). A comparative survey of the spinal lemniscus systems. In: *Reticular Formation of the Brain*. (H. H. Jasper and L. D. Proctor, editors) (Boston: Little Brown Company), 353
426. Kerr, F. W. L. and Lippman, H. (1973). Ascending degeneration following antero-lateral cordotomy and midline myelotomy in the primate. *Anat. Rec.*, **175**, 356
427. Boivie, J. (1971). The termination of the spinothalamic tract in the cat. An experimental study with silver impregnation methods. *Exp. Brain Res.*, **12**, 331
428. Rinvik, E. (1968). The corticothalamic projection from the second somatosensory cortical area in the cat. An experimental study with silver impregnation methods. *Exp. Brain Res.*, **5**, 153
429. Strick, P. L. (1973). Light microscopic analysis of the cortical projection of the thalamic ventrolateral nucleus in the cat. *Brain Res.*, **55**, 1
430. Poggio, G. F. and Mountcastle, V. B. (1960). A study of the functional contributions of the lemniscal and spinothalamic systems to somatic sensibility. *Bull. Johns Hopkins Hosp.*, **106**, 266
431. Poggio, G. F. and Mountcastle, V. B. (1963). The functional properties of ventrobasal thalamic neurons studied in unanaesthetized monkeys. *J. Neurophysiol.*, **26**, 775
432. Marshall, W. H., Woolsey, C. N. and Bard, P. (1941). Observations on cortical somatic sensory mechanisms of cat and monkey. *J. Neurophysiol.*, **4**, 1
433. Kruger, L. and Albe-Fessard, D. (1960). Distribution of responses to somatic afferent stimuli in the diencephalon of the cat under chloralose anesthesia. *Exp. Neurol.*, **2**, 442
433a. Levante, A., Lamour, Y. and Albe-Fessard, D. (1973). Localisation dans la couche V de Rexed de cellules d'origine d'un faisceau spinothalamique croise chez le Macaque. *C. R. Acad. Sci. (Paris)*, **276**, 1589

433b. Trevino, D. L., Coulter, J. D. and Willis, W. D. (1972). Excitation of cells of origin of the spinothalamic tract in the monkey. *Fed. Proc.*, **31**, 385

434. Albe-Fessard, D. and Bowsher, D. (1965). Responses of monkey thalamus to somatic stimuli under chloralose anaesthesia. *Electroenceph. Clin. Neurophysiol.*, **19**, 1

435. Baker, M. A. (1971). Spontaneous and evoked activity of neurons in the somatosensory thalamus of the waking cat. *J. Physiol. (London)*, **217**, 359

436. Albe-Fessard, D., Guiot, G., Lamarre, Y. and Arfel, G. (1966). Activation of thalamocortical projections related to tremorogenic processes. In *The Thalamus*. (D. P. Purpura and M. D. Yahr, editors) (New York: Columbia University Press), 237

437. Albe-Fessard, D., Arfel, G., Guiot, G., Derome, P. and Guilbaud, G. (1967). Thalamic unit activity in man. In: *Recent Advances in Clinical Neurophysiology*, (L. Widen, editor) (Amsterdam: Elsevier), 132

438. Jasper, H. and Bertrand, G. (1966). Thalamic units involved in somatic sensation and voluntary and involuntary movements in man. In: *The Thalamus* (D. P. Purpura and M. D. Yahr, editors) (New York: Columbia University Press), 365

439. Bertrand, G., Jasper, H. and Wong, A. (1967). Microelectrode study of the human thalamus: functional organization in the ventro-basal complex. *Confin. neurol. (Basel)*, **29**, 81

440. Welker, W. I. (1973). Principles of organization of the ventrobasal complex in mammals. *Brain. Behav. Evol.*, **7**, 253

441. Nakahama, H., Nishioka, S. and Otsuka, T. (1966). Excitation and inhibition in ventrobasal thalamic neurons before and after cutaneous input deprivation. In: *Progress in Brain Research*, **21A**, (T. Tokizane and J. P. Shadé, editors) (Amsterdam: Elsevier), 180

442. Harris, F. A. (1970). Population analysis of somatosensory thalamus in the cat. *Nature*, **225**, 559

443. Bates, J. A. V. (1973). Electrical recording from the thalamus in human subjects. In: *Handbook of Sensory Physiology*, Vol. 2 (A. Iggo, editor) (Berlin: Springer-Verlag), 561

444. Mallart, A. (1961). Données sur les types de fibres conduisant les afférences somatiques au noyau centre médian du thalamus. *J. Physiol. (Paris)*, **53**, 422

445. Mallart, A. (1968). Thalamic projection of muscle nerve afferents in the cat. *J. Physiol. (London)*, **194**, 337

446. Rosén, I. (1969). Excitation of the group I activated thalamocortical relay neurons in the cat. *J. Physiol. (London)*, **205**, 237

447. Rosén, I. (1969). Localization in caudal brain stem and cervical spinal cord of neurones activated from forelimb group I afferents in the cat. *Brain Res.*, **16**, 55

448. Albe-Fessard, D., Arfel, G., Guiot, G., Hardy, J., Vourc'h, G., Hertzog, E., Aleonard, P., Derome, P. (1962). Dérivations d'activités spontanées et évoquées dans les structures cérébrales profondes de l'homme. *Rev. Neurol.*, **106**, 89

448a. Albe-Fessard, D., Arfel, G., Guiot, G., Derome, P., Hertzog, E., Vourc'h, G., Brown, H., Aleonard, P., de la Herran, J. and Trigo, J. C. (1966). Electrophysiological studies of some deep cerebral structures in man. *J. Neurol. Sci.*, **3**, 37

449. Goto, A., Kosaka, K., Kubota, K., Nakamura, R. and Narabayashi, H. (1968). Thalamic potentials from muscle afferents in the human. *Arch. Neurol.*, **19**, 302

450. Burton, H., Forbes, D. J. and Benjamin, R. M. (1970). Thalamic neurons responsive to temperature changes of glabrous hand and foot skin in squirrel monkey. *Brain Res.*, **24**, 179

451. Martin, H. F. and Manning, J. W. (1971). Thalamic 'warming' and 'cooling' units responding to cutaneous stimulation. *Brain Res.*, **27**, 377

452. Mountcastle, V. B., Poggio, G. F. and Werner, G. (1963). The relation of thalamic cell response to peripheral stimuli varied over an intensive continuum. *J. Neurophysiol.*, **26**, 807

453. Mountcastle, V. B. and Powell, T. P. S. (1959). Central nervous mechanisms subserving position sense and kinesthesis. *Bull. Johns Hopkins Hosp.*, **105**, 173

454. Mountcastle, V. B. and Powell, T. P. S. (1959). Neural mechanisms subserving cutaneous sensibility, with special reference to the role of afferent inhibition in sensory perception and discrimination. *Bull. Johns Hopkins Hosp.*, **105**, 201

455. Levitt, J. and Levitt, M. (1968). Sensory hind-limb representation in SmL cortex of the cat. A unit analysis. *Exp. Neurol.*, **22**, 259

455a. Levitt, M. and Levitt, J. (1968). Sensory hind-limb representation in the SmL cortex of the cat after spinal tractotomies. *Exp. Neurol.*, **22**, 276

456. Hassler, R. (1959). Anatomy of the thalamus. In: *Introduction to Stereotaxis with an Atlas of the Human Brain.* (G. Schaltenbrand and P. Bailey, editors) (Stuttgart: Georg Thieme Verlag), Vol. 1 ,230

457. Halliday, A. M. and Logue. (1970). Personal communication.

458. Burgess, P. R. and Clark, F. J. (1969). Dorsal column projection of fibres from the cat knee joint. *J. Physiol. (London)*, **203**, 301

459. Gaze, R. M. and Gordon, G. (1954). The representation of cutaneous sense in the thalamus of the cat and monkey. *Quart. J. Exp. Physiol.*, **39**, 279

460. Andersson, S. A., Landgren, S. and Wolsk, D. (1966). The thalamic relay and cortical projection of group I muscle afferents from the forelimb to the cat. *J. Physiol. (London)*, **183**, 576

461. Wall, P. D. (1970). The sensory and motor role of impulses travelling in the dorsal column towards cerebral cortex. *Brain*, **93**, 505

462. Mountcastle, V. B. (1961). Some functional properties of the somatic afferent system. In: *Sensory Communication.* (W. A. Rosenblith, editor) (Cambridge, Mass.: M.I.T. Press), 403

463. Jabbur, S. H., Baker, M. A. and Towe, A. L. (1972). Wide-field neurons in thalamic nucleus ventralis posterolateralis of the cat. *Exp. Neurol.*, **36**, 213

463a. McLeod, J. G. (1958). The representation of splanchnic afferent pathways in the thalamus of the cat. *J. Physiol. (London)*, **140**, 462

464. Gaze, R. M. and Gordon, G. (1955). Some observations on the central pathway for cutaneous impulses in the cat. *Quart. J. Exp. Physiol.*, **40**, 187

465. Bowsher, D. (1971). Properties of ventrobasal thalamic neurons in cat following interruption of specific afferent pathways. *Arch. Ital. Biol.*, **109**, 59

466. Bava, A., Fadiga, E. and Manzoni, T. (1966). Interactive potentialities between thalamic relay-nuclei through subcortical commissural pathways. *Arch. Sci. Biol.*, **50**, 101

467. Bava, A., Fadiga, E. and Manzoni, T. (1967). Functional analysis of subcortical interactions between thalamic somatosensory relay-nuclei. *Arch. Sci. Biol. (Bologne)*, **51**, 263

468. Bava, A., Fadiga, E. and Manzoni, T. (1968). Extralemniscal reactivity and commissural linkages in the VPL nucleus of cats with chronic cortical lesions. *Arch. Ital. Biol.*, **106**, 204

469. Bava, A., Fadiga, E., Manzoni, T. and Maricchiolo, M. (1970). Inhibitory interactions between thalamic VPL nuclei of the two sides. *Arch. Ital. Biol.*, **108**, 462

470. Fadiga, E. and Manzoni, T. (1969). Relationships between the somatosensory thalamic relay nuclei of the two sides. *Arch. Ital. Biol.*, **107**, 604

471. Rinvik, E. (1968). A re-evaluation of the cytoarchitecture of the ventral nuclear complex of the cat's thalamus on the basis of corticothalamic connections. *Brain Res.*, **8**, 237

472. Rinvik, E. (1968). The corticothalamic projection from the gyrus proreus and the medial wall of the rostral hemisphere in the cat. An experimental study with silver impregnation methods. *Exp. Brain Res.*, **5**, 129

472a. Rinvik, E. (1968). The corticothalamic projection from the pericruciate and coronal gyri in the cat. An experimental study with silver-impregnation methods. *Brain Res.*, **10**, 79

473. Kawana, E. (1969). Projections of the anterior ectosylvian gyrus to the thalamus, the dorsal column nuclei, the trigeminal nuclei and the spinal cord in cats. *Brain Res.*, **14**, 117

474. Kawana, E. and Kusama, T. (1964). Projection of the sensory motor cortex to the thalamus, the dorsal column nucleus, the trigeminal nucleus and the spinal cord in the cat. *Folia Psychiat. Neurol. Jap.*, **18**, 337

475. Andersen, P. and Andersson, S. A. (1968). *Physiological Basis of the Alpha Rhythm.* (New York: Appleton-Century-Crofts), 235

476. Junge, K. and Sveen, O. (1968). Exclusive thalamic location of subcortical spontaneous barbiturate spindles. *Acta Physiol. Scand.*, **73**, 22

477. Verzeano, M. and Negishi, K. (1960). Neuronal activity in cortical and thalamic networks. A study with multiple microelectrodes. *J. Gen. Physiol.*, **43**, 177

478. Andersen, P., Andersson, S. A. and Lomo, T. (1967). Some factors involved in the thalamic control of spontaneous barbiturate spindles. *J. Physiol. (London)*, **192**, 257

478a. Maekawa, K. and Purpura, D. P. (1967). Properties of spontaneous and evoked synaptic activities of thalamic ventrobasal neurons. *J. Neurophysiol.*, **30**, 360

479. Iwamura, Y., Gardner, E. P. and Spencer, W. A. (1972). Geometry of the ventrobasal complex: functional significance in skin sensation. *Brain. Behav. Evol.*, **6**, 185

480. Dagnino, N., Favale, E., Loeb, C., Manfredi, M. and Seitun, A. (1969). Presynaptic and postsynaptic changes in specific thalamic nuclei during deep sleep. *Arch. Ital. Biol.*, **107**, 668

481. Gordon, G. and Manson, J. R. (1967). Cutaneous receptive fields of single nerve cells in the thalamus of the cat. *Nature*, **215**, 597

482. Andersen, P., Andersson, S. A. and Lomo, T. (1967). Nature of thalamocortical relations during spontaneous barbiturate spindle activity. *J. Physiol.* (*London*), **192**, 283

483. Andersen, P., Eccles, J. C. and Sears, T. A. (1964). The ventro-basal complex of the thalamus: types of cells, their responses and their functional organization. *J. Physiol.* (*London*), **174**, 370

484. Curry, M. J. and Gordon, G. (1972). The spinal input to the posterior group in the cat. An electrophysiological investigation. *Brain Res.*, **44**, 417

485. Curry, M. J. (1972). The exteroceptive properties of neurones in the somatic part of the posterior group (PO). *Brain Res.*, **44**, 439

486. Calma, I. (1965). Thalamo–cortical relations in the sensory nuclei of the cat. *Nature* (*London*), **205**, 394

487. Curry, M. J. (1972). The effects of stimulating the somatic sensory cortex on single neurones in the posterior group (PO) of the cat. *Brain Res.*, **44**, 463

488. Knighton, R. S. (1950). Thalamic relay nucleus for the second somatic sensory receiving area in the cerebral cortex of the cat. *J. Comp. Neurol.*, **92**, 183

489. Morrison, A. R., Hand, P. J. and Donoghue, J. (1970). Contrasting projections from the posterior and ventrobasal thalamic nuclear complexes to the anterior ectosylvian gyrus of the cat. *Brain Res.*, **21**, 115

490. Heath, C. H. and Jones, E. G. (1971). An experimental study of ascending connections from the posterior group of thalamic nuclei in the cat. *J. Comp. Neurol.*, **141**, 397

491. Magoun, H. W. and McKinley, W. A. (1942). The termination of ascending trigeminal and spinal tracts in the thalamus of the cat. *Amer. J. Physiol.*, **137**, 409

492. French, J. D., Verzeano, M. and Magoun, H. W. (1953). An extralemniscal sensory system in the brain. *Arch. Neurol. Psychiat.*, **69**, 505

493. Albe-Fessard, D. and Rougeul, A. (1958). Activités d'origine somesthésique évoquées sur le cortex non-spécifique du chat anesthésié au chloralose: rôle du centre médian du thalamus. *EEG and Clin. Neurophysiol.*, **10**, 131

494. Kruger, L. and Albe-Fessard, D. (1959). Dualité des réponses observées dans le centre médian lors de stimulations somatiques. Types d'afférences et voies spinales. *J. Physiol.* (*Paris*), **51**, 501

495. Petit, D. and Mallart, A. (1964). Voies spinales afférentes vers le noyau centre médian du thalamus chez le chat. *J. Physiol.* (*Paris*), **56**, 423

496. Albe-Fessard, D. and Kruger, L. (1962). Duality of unit discharges from cat centrum medianum in response to natural and electrical stimulation. *J. Neurophysiol.*, **25**, 4

497. Urabe, M., Tsubokawa, T., Watanabe, Y. and Kadoya, S. (1965). Driven and spontaneous activities of single neuron in the nucleus centrum medianum following stimulation of the peripheral nerve. *Brain and Nerve*, **18**, 25

498. Urabe, M., Tsubokawa, T. and Watanabe, Y. (1966). Alteration of activity of single neurons in the nucleus centrum medianum following stimulation of the peripheral nerve and application of noxious stimuli. *Jap. J. Physiol.*, **16**, 421

499. Casey, K. L. (1966). Unit analysis of nociceptive mechanisms in the thalamus of the awake squirrel monkey. *J. Neurophysiol.*, **29**, 727

500. Feltz, P., Krauthamer, G. and Albe-Fessard, D. (1967). Neurons of the medial diencephalon. I. Somatosensory responses and caudate inhibition. *J. Neurophysiol.*, **30**, 55

501. Albe-Fessard, D. and Gillet, E. (1961). Convergences d'afférences d'origines corticale et peripherique vers le centre médian du chat anesthésié ou eveille. *Electroenceph. Clin. Neurophysiol.*, **13**, 257

502. Dila, C. J. (1971). A midbrain projection to the centre median nucleus of the thalamus. A neurophysiological study. *Brain Res.*, **25**, 63

503. Albe-Fessard, D. and Besson, J. M. (1973). Convergent thalamic and cortical projections — the non-specific system. In: *Handbook of Sensory Physiology*, Vol. 2 (A. Iggo, editor) (Berlin: Springer Verlag), 489
504. Head, H. (1920). *Studies in Neurology*, Vol. 1 (Londres).
505. Walshe, F. M. R. (1942). The anatomy and physiology of cutaneous sensibility: a critical review. *Brain*, **85**, 48
506. Head, H., Rivers, W. H. R. and Sherren, J. (1905). The afferent nervous system from a new aspect. *Brain*, **28**, 99
507. Adrian, E. D. (1941). Afferent discharges to the cerebral cortex from peripheral sense organs. *J. Physiol. (London)*, **100**, 159
508. Jones, E. G. and Powell, T. P. S. (1973). Anatomical organization of the somatosensory cortex. In: *Handbook of Sensory Physiology*, Vol. 2 (A. Iggo, editor) (Berlin: Springer Verlag), 579
509. Darian-Smith, I. (1964). Cortical projections of thalamic neurones excited by mechanical stimulation of the face of the cat. *J. Physiol. (London)*, **171**, 339
510. Woolsey, C. N. (1961). Organization of cortical auditory systems: a review and a synthesis. In: *Neuronal Mechanisms of the Auditory and Vestibular Systems*. (G. L. Rasmussen and W. F. Windle, editors) (Springfield: C. C. Thomas), 165
511. Mountcastle, V. B. (1957). Modality and topographic properties of single neurons of cat's somatic sensory cortex. *J. Neurophysiol.*, **20**, 408
512. Powell, T. P. S. and Mountcastle, V. B. (1959). The cytoarchitecture of the postcentral gyrus of the monkey *Macaca mulatta*. *Bull. Johns Hopkins Hosp.*, **105**, 108
513. Jones, E. G. and Powell, T. P. S. (1970). An electron microscopic study of the laminar pattern and mode of termination of extrinsic afferent fibres in the somatic sensory cortex of the cat. *Phil. Trans.* B, **257**, 45
514. Hubel, D. H. and Wiesel, T. N. (1968). Receptive fields and functional architecture of monkey striate cortex. *J. Physiol. (London)*, **195**, 215
515. Dreyer, D. A., Schneider, R. J., Metz, C. B. and Whitsel, B. L. (1974). Differential contributions of spinal pathways to body representation in postcentral gyrus of *Macaca mulatta*. *J. Neurophysiol.*, **37**, 119
516. Hubel, D. H. and Wiesel, T. N. (1962). Receptive fields, binocular interaction and functional architecture in the cat's visual cortex. *J. Physiol. (London)*, **160**, 106
517. Blakemore, C. (1970). The representation of three-dimensional visual space in the cat's striate cortex. *J. Physiol. (London)*, **209**, 155
518. Whitsel, B. L., Petrucelli, L. M. and Werner, G. (1969). Symmetry and connectivity in the map of the body surface in somatosensory area II of primates. *J. Neurophysiol.* **32**, 170
519. Whitsel, B. L., Dreyer, D. A., Roppolo, J. R. (1971). Determinants of the body representation in the postcentral gyrus of macaques. *J. Neurophysiol.*, **34**, 1018
520. Whitsel, B. L., Roppolo, J. R. and Werner, G. (1972). Cortical information processing of stimulus motion on primate skin. *J. Neurophysiol.*, **35**, 691
521. Mountcastle, V. B., Covian, M. and Harrison, C. R. (1952). The central representation of some forms of deep sensibility. *Res. Publ. Ass. Nerv. Ment. Dis.*, **30**, 339
522. Pubols, B. H. and Pubols, L. M. (1969). Forelimb, hindlimb, and tail dermatomes in the spider monkey (Ateles). *Brain. Behav. Evol.*, **2**, 132
523. Pubols, B. H. and Pubols, L. M. (1971). Somatotopic organization of spider monkey somatic sensory cerebral cortex. *J. Comp. Neurol.*, **141**, 63
524. Jones, E. G. and Powell, T. P. S. (1968). The projection of the somatic sensory cortex upon the thalamus in the cat. *Brain Res.*, **10**, 369
525. Jones, E. G. and Powell, T. P. S. (1969). Connexions of the somatic sensory cortex of the rhesus monkey. I. Ipsilateral cortical connexions. *Brain*, **92**, 477
526. Korn, H. N., Wendt, R. and Albe-Fessard, D. (1966). Somatic projection to the orbital cortex of the cat. *Electroenceph. and Clin. Neurophysiol.*, **21**, 209
527. Petras, J. M. (1965). Fiber degeneration in the basal ganglia and diencephalon following lesions in the precentral and postcentral cortex of the monkey (Macaca mulatta) with additional observations in the chimpanzee. In: *Abstracts of the Eighth International Anatomical Congress*. (Wiesbaden)
528. Jones, E. G. and Powell, T. P. S. (1970). Connexions of the somatic sensory cortex of the rhesus monkey. III. Thalamic connexions. *Brain*, **93**, 37

529. Morse, R. W., Adkins, R. J. and Towe, A. L. (1965). Population and modality characteristics of neurons in the coronal region of somatosensory area I of the cat. *Exp. Neurol.*, **11**, 419

530. Landgren, S. (1957). Cortical reception of cold impulses from the tongue of the cat. *Acta Physiol. Scand.*, **40**, 202

531. Martin, H. F. III and Manning, J. W. (1969). Peripheral nerve and cortical responses to radiant thermal stimulation of skin fields. *Fed. Proc.*, **28**, 458

532. Handwerker, H. O. and Zimmerman, M. (1972). Cortical evoked responses upon selective stimulation of cutaneous group III fibers and the mediating spinal pathways. *Brain Res.*, **36**, 437

533. Powell, T. P. S. and Mountcastle, V. B. (1959). Some aspects of the functional organization of the cortex of the postcentral gyrus of the monkey: a correlation of findings obtained in a single unit analysis with cytoarchitecture. *Bull. Johns Hopkins Hosp.*, **105**, 133

534. Paul, R. L., Goodman, H. and Merzenich, M. (1972). Alterations in mechanoreceptor input to Brodmann's areas 1 and 3 of the postcentral hand area of *Macaca mulatta* after nerve section and regeneration. *Brain Res.*, **39**, 1

535. Amassian, V. E. and Berlin, L. (1958). Early projection of large muscle afferents from forelimb of cat to somatosensory cortex. *Fed. Proc.*, **17**, 3

536. Amassian, V. E. and Berlin, L. (1958). Early cortical projection of group I afferents in the forelimb muscle nerves of cat. *J. Physiol. (London)*, **143**, 61P

537. Oscarsson, O., Rosén, I. and Sulg, I. (1966). Organization of neurones in the cat cerebral cortex that are influenced from Group I muscle afferents. *J. Physiol. (London)*, **183**, 189

538. Oscarsson, O. and Rosén, I. (1963). Projection to cerebral cortex of large muscle spindle afferents in forelimb nerves of the cat. *J. Physiol. (London)*, **169**, 924

539. Oscarsson, O. and Rosén, I. (1966). Short-latency projections to the cat's cerebral cortex from skin and muscle afferents in the contralateral forelimb. *J. Physiol. (London)* **182**, 164

540. Landgren, S. and Silfvenius, H. (1969). Projection to cerebral cortex of group I muscle afferents from the cat's hind limb. *J. Physiol. (London)*, **200**, 353

541. Silfvenius, H. (1970). Projections to the cerebral cortex from afferents of the interosseos nerves of the cat. *Acta Physiol. Scand.*, **80**, 196

542. Phillips, C. G., Powell, T. P. S. and Wiesendanger, M. (1971). Projection from low-threshold muscle afferents of hand and forearm to area 3a of baboon's cortex. *J. Physiol. (London)*, **217**, 419

543. McIntyre, A. K., Holman, M. E. and Veale, J. L. (1967). Cortical responses to impulses from single Pacinian corpuscles in the cat's hind limb. *Exp. Brain Res.*, **4**, 243

544. Silfvenius, H. (1972). Properties of cortical group I neurones located in the lower bank of the anterior suprasylvian sulcus of the cat. *Acta Physiol. Scand.*, **84**, 555

545. Dobry, P. J. K. and Casey, K. L. (1972). Roughness discrimination in cats with dorsal column lesions. *Brain Res.*, **44**, 385

546. Norrsell, U. and Voorhoeve, P. (1962). Tactile pathways from the hindlimb to the cerebral cortex in cat. *Acta Physiol. Scand.*, **54**, 9

547. Norrsell, U. and Wolpow, E. R. (1966). An evoked potential study of different pathways from the hindlimb to the somatosensory areas in the cat. *Acta Physiol. Scand.*, **66**, 19

548. Norrsell, U. (1966). The spinal afferent pathways of conditioned reflexes to cutaneous stimuli in the dog. *Exp. Brain Res.*, **2**, 269

549. Dobry, P. J. K. and Casey, K. L. (1972). Coronal somatosensory unit responses in cats with dorsal column lesions. *Brain Res.*, **44**, 399

550. Andersson, S. A., Norrsell, K. and Norrsell, U. (1972). Spinal pathways projecting to the cerebral first somatosensory area in the monkey. *J. Physiol. (London)*, **225**, 589

551. Paul, R. L., Merzenich, M. and Goodman, H. (1972). Representation of slowly and rapidly adapting cutaneous mechanoreceptors of the hand in Brodman's areas 3 and 1 of Macaca mulatta. *Brain Res.*, **36**, 229

552. Woolsey, C. N. (1952). Patterns of localization in sensory and motor areas of the cerebral cortex. In: *The Biology of Mental Health and Disease*. (New York: Hoeber), 193

553. Benjamin, R. M. and Welker, W. I. (1957). Somatic receiving areas of cerebral cortex of squirrel monkey (*Saimiri sciureus*). *J. Neurophysiol.*, **20**, 286

554. Carreras, M. and Andersson, S. A. (1963). Functional properties of neurons of the anterior ectosylvian gyrus of the cat. *J. Neurophysiol.*, **26**, 100

555. Haight, J. R. (1972). The general organization of somatotopic projections to SII cerebral neocortex in the cat. *Brain Res.*, **44**, 483

557. Woolsey, C. N. and Wang, G. H. (1945). Somatic sensory areas I and II of the cerebral cortex of the rabbit. *Fed. Proc.*, **4**, 79

558. Morse, R. W. and Vargo, R. A. (1970). Functional neuronal subsets in the forepaw focus of somatosensory area II of the cat. *Exp. Neurol.*, **27**, 125

559. Andersson, S. A. (1962). Projection of different spinal pathways to the second somatic sensory area in cat. *Acta Physiol. Scand.*, **56**, 1

560. McIntyre, A. K. (1962). Cortical projection of impulses in the interosseus nerve of the cat's hind limb. *J. Physiol. (London)*, **163**, 46

561. Landgren, S., Silfvenius, H. and Wolsk, D. (1967). Somato-sensory paths to the second cortical projection area of the group I muscle afferents. *J. Physiol. (London)*, **191**, 543

562. Landgren, S., Silfvenius, H. and Wolsk, D. (1967). Vestibular, cochlear and trigeminal projections to the cortex in the anterior suprasylvian sulcus of the cat, *J. Physiol. (London)*, **191**, 561

563. Amassian, V. E. (1954). Studies on organization of a somesthetic association area, including a single unit analysis. *J. Neurophysiol.*, **17**, 39

564. Bignall, K. E. and Imbert, M. (1969). Polysensory and cortico-cortical projections to frontal lobe of squirrel and rhesus monkeys. *Electroenceph. Clin. Neurophysiol.*, **26**, 206

566. Rabiner, A. M. and Browder, J. (1948). Concerning the conduction of touch and deep sensibilities through the spinal cord. *Trans. Amer. Neurol. Assoc.*, **73**, 137

567. Cook, A. W. and Browder, E. J. (1965). Function of posterior columns in man. *Arch. Neurol.*, **12**, 72

568. Ferraro, A. and Barrera, S. E. (1934). Effects of experimental lesions of the posterior columns in *Macacus Rhesus* monkeys. *Brain*, **57**, 307

569. Gilman, S. and Denny-Brown, D. (1966). Disorders of movement and behaviour following dorsal column lesions. *Brain*, **89**, 397

570. Chambers, W. W. (1972). Role of cervicothalamic tract and dorsal column on tactile localization in cats. *Anat. Rec.*, **172**, 287

571. Melzack, R. and Bridges, J. A. (1971). Dorsal column contributions to motor behaviour. *Exp. Neurol.*, **33**, 53

572. Dubrovsky, B., Davelaar, E., Garcia-Rill, E. (1971). The role of dorsal columns in serial order acts. *Exp. Neurol.*, **33**, 93

573. Vierck, C. J. (1966). Spinal pathways mediating limb position sense. *Anat. Rec.*, **154**, 437

574. Levitt, M. and Schwartzman, R. (1966). Spinal sensory tracts and two-point tactile sensibility. *Anat. Rec.*, **154**, 377

575. DeVito, J. L. (1954). Study of sensory pathways in monkeys. Ph.D. Thesis (University of Washington)

576. DeVito, J. L., Ruch, T. C. and Patton, H. D. (1964). Analysis of residual weight discriminatory ability and evoked potentials following section of dorsal column in monkeys. *Indian J. Physiol. Pharmacol.*, **8**, 117

577. Cassanari, V. and Pagni, C. A. (1969). *Central Pain: A neurosurgical survey*. (Cambridge: Howard University Press)

578. Christiansen, J. (1966). Neurological observations of macaques with spinal cord lesions. *Anat. Rec.*, **154**, 330

579. Hamilton, B. L. and Skultety, F. M. (1970). Efferent connections of the periaqueductal grey matter in the cat. *J. Comp. Neurol.*, **138**, 105

580. Chi, C. C. (1970). An experimental silver study of the ascending projections of the central gray substance and adjacent tegmentum in the rat with observations in the cat. *J. Comp. Neurol.*, **139**, 259

581. Hubel, D. H. and Wiesel, T. N. (1969). Anatomical demonstration of columns in the monkey striate cortex. *Nature (London)*, **221**, 747

582. Hind, J. E. (1960). Unit activity in the auditory cortex. In: *Neural Mechanisms of*

the Auditory and Vestibular Systems (G. L. Rasmussen and W. F. Windle, editors) (Springfield: C. C. Thomas), 201

583. Abeles, M. and Goldstein, M. H. (1970). Functional architecture in cat primary auditory cortex: columnar organization and organization according to depth. *J. Neurophysiol.*, **33**, 172

584. Sakata, H. and Miyamoto, J. (1968). Topographic relationship between the receptive fields of neurons in the motor cortex and the movements elicited by focal stimulation in freely moving cats. *Jap. J. Physiol.*, **18**, 489

585. Vierck, C. J. (1972). Tactile deficits resulting from dorsal column lesions in monkeys. *Proc. Soc. Neurosci.*, **2**, 135

586. Ramon-Moliner, E. and Ferrari, J. (1972). Electron microscopy of previously identified cells and processes within the central nervous system. *J. Neurocytol.*, **1**, 85

Index

Abducens motoneurones
  response to rotation, 118
Acceleration
  otolith receptor stimulation by, 100
  semicircular canal stimulus by, 100
Acetylcholine
  as synaptic transmitter, 58
  skeletal muscle sensitivity to, 287
Actin
  muscle control by, 285
Adenosine diphosphate
  effect on sodium pump, 247, 249
Adenosine triphosphate
  hydrolysis, coupling of ion transport to, 247
Afferent fibres
  size, 317, 318
Afferent systems
  in movement performance, 170–175
Animals
  cells, sodium pump in, 236, 237
Aplysia
  axons, sodium influxes for, 234,
  behaviour, sensitisation, 14
  gill withdrawal response, habituation, 32–35
  identifiable neurone, 5
  Parabolic Burster in, 8
Arousal
  neural systems mediating, 36, 37
Autonomic functions
  vestibular effects on, 135, 136

Barium
  cations, transmitter release from nerve terminals and, 68
Behaviour
  dorsal column and, in somatosensory system 385, 386
  dorsolateral fasciculus and, in somatosensory system, 386, 387
  in somatosensory system examination, 335–337

Behaviour
  invertebrates, 10–16
  identifiable neurones and, 1–51
Branching
  of central projections of primary afferent neurones, 321, 322

Calcium
  ions, flux in resting nerves, 234
  in muscle contraction, 284
  transmitter release from nerve terminals and, 67–69
Cardiac ganglia
  neural system, mediating, 22–24
Cats
  collicular cell activity and eye movement in, 215
  cortico–collicular pathway in, properties, 209–212
  cupula motion during rotation of, 83
  optic nerve projection in, 189
  superior colliculus, electrical stimulation of, 216, 217
  function of various inputs to, 212, 213
  lesions in, effect of, 219, 220
  pattern discrimination, 221
  receptive fields of cells in deep layers of, 203–206
  receptive fields of neurones in superficial layers of, 195–200
Cebus monkey
  receptive fields of cells in deep layers of superior colliculus of, 207
  receptive fields of neurones in superficial layers of superior colliculus in, 203
Cells
  excitable, membrane properties, 54–56
  in somatosensory systems, characterisation of, 331, 332
Central programmes
  neural system mediating, 21–28
  sensory modulation of, 28–31
  vertebrate behaviour, 12
Cerebellar–vestibular projection, 125–127

413

Cerebellum
  effect on vestibulo–ocular reflex, 120, 121
  neuronal discharge recording, 169
Cerebral cortex
  somatosensory system and, 374–383
Chlorides
  flux in resting nerves, 234
Cholinesterase
  post-synaptic receptor density and, 74,
    75
Cockroaches
  nervous system development in, 38
Command elements
  invertebrate behaviour, 12, 13
Conditioning
  invertebrate behaviour, 14
Conductance
  decreases, post-synaptic action of trans-
    mitters and, 72
  excitatory changes, post-synaptic action
    of transmitters and, 70–72
Cortical stimulation
  effect on spinal motoneurones, 158–160
Cortico–collicular pathway
  cats, properties, 209–213
  mammals, 213
Cortico–cortical connections, 378, 379
Corticomotoneuronal synapses
  properties, 168
Corticospinal actions
  individual motoneurones and, 160–162
Corticospinal pathways
  destruction, effect on motoneurones, 164
Corticothalamic connections, 377, 378
Crabs
  identifiable neurones in, 6
Crayfish
  neuromuscular junction, synaptic trans-
    mission and, 60
  neurone somata in, 6
  tail flip, habituation, 31–32
    neural system mediating, 18–21
Crickets
  nervous system, development in, 38
  genetics of, 40
Crossed extensor reflex
  characteristics, 155, 156
Cross-reinnervation
  skeletal muscles, 295
Cupula motion
  during cat rotation, 83

Daphnia magna
  neuronal morphology, 9
Dendritic spikes
  in vestibular neurones, 100
Depolarisation
  transmitter release from nerve terminals
    and, 69

Development
  invertebrate nervous systems, 38, 39
Diencephalic nuclei
  somatosensory projections to, 357–374
Dorsal column
  nuclei, physiology, 342–344
    projection from, 344, 345, 360
    somatosensory system and, 341, 342
  somatosensory system in 338–345
    behaviour and, 385, 386
Dorsallateral fasciculus
  somatosensory system, behaviour and,
    386, 387
Dorsal spinocerebellar tracts
  recording of neurones in, 166
Doryteuthis plei
  axons, sodium influxes for, 234
Dosidicus gigas
  axons, sodium influxes for, 234
Drosophila
  nervous system genetics, 41

Efferent innervation
  vestibular receptors, 93–97
Electricity
  semicircular canals response to, 101
  superior colliculus stimulation by, 215–
    219
Electrogenic pumping
  effect on steady state resting potential
    of nerves, 257, 258
  sodium pump and, 250–262
Electromechanical coupling
  in skeletal muscle, 284
Electron microscopy
  somatosensory systems, 331
Evolution
  neural behaviour of mechanisms and, 37
Excitation
  chemical, in synaptic transmission, 58–60
  of cells, membrane potential and, 55, 56
Excitatory junctions
  synaptic transmission and, 58, 59
Extensor thrust reflex
  characteristics, 155, 156
Eye movement
  superior collicular cell activity and, 213–
    215
  superior collicular lesions and, 222, 223

Feeding
  conditioned response in Pleurobranchea
    californica, 15
  sensory modulation, 28
Fixed action patterns
  invertebrate behaviour and, 11, 12
Flexor reflex
  characteristics, 155, 156

Flight
  sensory modulation, 28

Genetics
  invertebrate nervous systems and, 39–42
Glycolysis
  in nerve, metabolism and, 262–266
Golden hamsters
  superior colliculus lesions pattern discrim-
      ination, 221
Ground squirrel
  cortico–collicular pathway in, 213
  optic nerve projection in, 189
  superior colliculus, receptive fields in, 208,
      209

Habituation
  invertebrates, 10
    behaviour, 14
    plasticity, 31–35
Hamsters
  superior colliculus lesions in effect of, 220
Heart—see Cardiac
Heat
  production by skeletal muscle, 282
  semicircular canals response to, 101
Helix aspersa
  axons, sodium influxes for, 234
Higher-order control
  invertebrate behaviour, 13, 14
Histochemistry
  invertebrate neurones, 6
Homarus americanus
  axons, sodium influxes for, 234
Horseradish peroxidase
  transport by somatosensory systems, 333
Hunt-and-poke approach
  neural identity, 4
Hydrogen
  ions, flux in resting nerves, 234

Inhibition
  chemical, in synaptic transmission, 58–
      60
  post-synaptic conductance changes and,
      72
Inhibitory junctions
  synaptic transmission and, 59, 60
Insects
  arousal, neural systems mediating, 36
  flight, 11
Intralaminar nuclei
  physiological activity, 372, 373
Invertebrates
  behaviour, 10–16
    identifiable neurones and, 1–51
  identifiable neurones of, 5–10

Ionic gradients
  in nerves, dissipation of, 233–235
Ions
  effect on sodium pump, 240–247
  movement in nerves during stimulation,
      235
  transport by sodium pump, 236–250
Iontophoresis, 255
Isometric recording
  skeletal muscle, 291
Isotonic recording
  skeletal muscle, 291

Kinocilium
  sensory cell polarisation and, 83

Labyrinthine input
  to vestibular nuclei, 97–115
Labyrinthine receptors
  convergence, vestibular neurones and,
      110, 111
Lagena organ
  morphology, 83
  physiology, 92
Lanthanum
  cations, transmitter release from nerve
      terminals and, 68
Lateral cervical nucleus
  projections from, 360, 361
  somatosensory system and, 348, 349
Leeches
  motoneurone in, 7
  nervous system development in, 39
  neuronal morphology, 10
  neurone somata of, 5
  reflex shortening, neural systems media-
      ting, 16–18
Lemniscal
  terminology, 373, 374
Lengthening reaction
  characteristics, 155, 156
Lesions
  somatosensory system analysis and, 336
  superior colliculus, effects of, 219–223
Lobsters
  neuronal geometry, 9
  neurone somata of, 5
Location
  of stimulus, 308, 309
Locomotion
  arthropod, command elements and, 13
  sensory modulation, 30
  vestibulo–spinal relations and, 131
Locusts
  arousal, neural systems mediating, 37
  flight, 12
    neural system mediating, 21
    sensory modulation, 28

Locusts *continued*
identifiable neurones in, 7
Loligo forbesi
axons, sodium influxes for, 234
Loligo pealei
axons, sodium influxes for, 234

Magnesium
ions, effect on sodium pump, 243
flux in resting nerves, 234
transmitter release from nerve terminals and, 68
Mammals
receptive fields in superior colliculus, 207–
209
Manganese
cations, transmitter release from nerve
terminals and, 68
Mechanoreceptors
somatic, 311–313
Membrane potential
effect on sodium pump, 258–261
of resting nerve, effect of sodium pump
on, 255–258
Membranes
excitable cells, properties, 54–56
nerve cell, density of pumping sites on,
237
post-synaptic, 58
presynaptic, 58
resting, excitable cells, 54, 55
Metabolism
effect on sodium pump, 249, 250
nervous activity and, 262–266
Microscopy
somatosensory systems, 331
Monkeys (*see also* Cebus monkey; Rhesus
monkey; Squirrel monkey)
optic nerve projection in, 188, 189
superior colliculus lesions in, effect of,
220, 221
pattern discrimination, 221, 222
Motion sickness, 136
Motoneurones, 152–164
corticospinal actions on individual, 160–
162
destruction of pathways influencing,
162–164
discharge pattern, 297–299
reflex activation of, 154–157
spinal, cortical stimulation and, 158–160
supraspinal activity and, 157, 158
Motor-unit, 287–289
Movement
neurone response in superficial layer of
cat superior colliculus and, 196
neurophysiology, 151–183
performance, afferent systems in, 170–
175

Movement *continued*
recording from neuronal elements during,
164–170
Muscle afferents
movement performance and, 172
Muscles
fast-twitch, 289–295
skeletal, motor-unit, 287–289
physiology, 279–302
slow-twitch, 289–295
speed, neural control of, 295–297
spindles, recording from, during movement, 165
Myosin
filaments, structure, 285

Nerves
recovery processes, 231–278
resting, effect of sodium pump on
membrane potential of, 255–258
Nerve terminals
transmitter release from, 60–70
Nervous activity
effect on metabolism, 262–266
Nervous tissue
electrogenic pumping in, 251, 252
Neural control
of muscle speed, 295–297
Neural substrates
of somatic sensation, 303–410
Neurones
biochemical characteristics, 7
of cerebral cortex, 375
contralateral excitation of single, 112
contralateral inhibition of single, 113
geometry, 8
identifiable, invertebrates, 5–10
limitations, 8–10
neural identity and, 4, 5
identity, hunt-and-poke approach, 4
identifiable neurone approach, 4, 5
population approach, 3, 4
injection of sodium ions into, hyperpolarisation and, 255
invertebrate behaviour and, 1–51
oscillating, 4
prefontal, recording from, 168
primary, vestibular receptors and, 82–93
primary afferent, central projections of,
321–330
connections of, 324, 325
receptive fields, in superficial layers of
superior colliculus, 195–203
recording from, movement and, 164–170
single, in somatosensory systems, 334, 335
thalamic, physiological activation, 363–
373
vestibular, intracellular studies, 100
receptor convergence on, 110, 111

Neurophysiology
  movement performance, 151–183
Nociceptors
  somatic, 314–317
Nucleus Z
  projections from, 362, 363
  spinal pathway via, 345, 346

Optic nerve projection
  in superior colliculus, 188–190
Oscillatory motor outputs
  neural mechanisms, 4
Otolith organs
  primary neurones in, 92, 93
  stimulation of, 107–110
Otolith receptors
  response to acceleration, 100
Oxygen
  consumption in nerve cells, 235, 236
    activity and, 262

Pain
  ventral thalamus and, 366
Parabolic Burster
  description, 8
Paramecium
  nervous system genetics in, 40
Pathway tracing
  in somatosensory systems, 332, 333
Pattern discrimination
  superior colliculus lesions and, 221, 222
Phosphates
  effect on sodium pump, 243
Physiology
  vestibular receptors, 86–88
Plasticity
  invertebrate, behaviour, 14–16
    habituation, 31–35
Population approach
  neural identity, 3, 4
Post-synaptic effects
  of transmitters, 70–75
Post-synaptic excitation
  primary afferent neurons, 325–327
Post-synaptic inhibition
  primary afferent neurons, 329, 330
Post-synaptic receptors
  at vertebrate end-plates, 74, 75
Potassium
  conductance, 262
  flux, coupling with sodium flux, 243–247
  ions, effect on sodium pump, 240–243
    flux in resting nerve, 234
Pressure
  semicircular canals response to, 101
Presynaptic inhibition
  primary afferent neurons, 327–329
  synaptic transmission and, 60

Primates
  superior colliculus, electrical stimulation
    of, 217–219

Rabbits
  cortico–collicular pathway in, 213
  superior colliculus, electrical stimulation
    of, 217
  receptive fields in, 208
Rats
  optic nerve projection in, 189
  superior colliculus lesions in, effect of,
    220
Receptive fields
  auditory, in deep layers of cat superior
    colliculus, 204–206
  of cells in deep layers of superior colli-
    culus, 203–207
  in lower mammals superior colliculus,
    207–209
  neurones, in superficial layers of superior
    colliculus, 195–203
  somatic, in deep cells of cat superior
    colliculus, 206
  superior colliculus, elaboration, 209–213
  visual, in deep layers of cat superior
    colliculus cells, 204
Receptive mechanisms
  of somatic sensation, 307–321
Receptors
  sensory, types, 311–317
  somatic, intensity, 318–320
  somatosensory, population dynamics,
    320, 321
  stimulus quality and, 309–318
Recording
  from neuronal elements during move-
    ment, 164–170
Recovery processes
  in nerve, 231–278
Reflexes
  motoneurone activation by, 154–157
  neural systems mediated in, 16–21
Respiration
  vestibular stimulation and, 136
Reticulospinal pathways
  destruction, effect on motoneurones, 164
  recording from neuronal units in, 166
  spinal motoneurones following electrical
    stimulation of, 157, 158
Reticulothalamic connections, 363
Rhesus monkey
  collicular cell activity and eye movement
    in, 213–215
  receptive fields of cells in deep layers of
    superior colliculus of, 206, 207
  receptive fields of neurones in superficial
    layers of superior colliculus in,
    201–203

Rubrospinal pathways
    destruction, effect on motoneurones, 164
    recording from neuronal units in, 166
    spinal motoneurones following electrical stimulation of, 157, 158

Sacculus organ
    morphology, 83
    physiology, 92
Self-reinnervation
    skeletal muscles, 295
Semicircular canals
    in mammals, morphology, 83
    primary vestibular neurones of, 88–92
    response to acceleration, 100
    response to stimulation of, 101–107
Sensation
    ventral spinal pathway and, somatosensory system, 387
Sensitisation
    invertebrate behaviour, 14
Sepia officinalis
    axons, sodium influxes for, 234
Simple reflexes
    invertebrate behaviour and, 11
Sliding filament hypothesis
    skeletal muscle, 283
Snails
    feeding, sensory modulation, 29
Sodium
    flux, coupling with potassium flux, 243–247
    ions, effect on sodium pump, 240–243
    flux in resting nerves, 234, 235
Sodium pump
    effect, of ADP on, 247–249
        of ions on, 240–247
        of membrane potential on, 258–261
        of metabolism on, 249–250
        on membrane potential of resting nerve, 255–258
    electrogenic operation of, 250–262
        physiological role of, 261, 262
    energy source for, 237–240
    ion transport by, 236–250
    kinetics, 238, 239, 241–243
    post-tetanic hyperpolarisation, 252–255
    stoichiometry, 243–247
Somatic sensation
    neural substances, 303–410
Somatosensory system
    ascending, 337–357
    function and pathway, 385–387
    lesions, study and, 336
    methods and approaches, 330–337
    projections to diencephalic nuclei, 357–374

Somatotopy, 377
Spinal chord
    dorsal, somatosensory system in, 338–349
    ventral quadrants, ascending tracts of, 349–357
Spinal gates
    in primary afferent neurons, 329
Spinal reflexes
    segmental, characteristics, 155, 156
Spinocervical tract
    somatosensory system and, 346–348
Spino–cervicothalamic pathway
    somatosensory system and, 346–349
Spinoreticular systems
    somatosensory system and, 352–357
Spinothalamic projections
    to diencephalic nuclei, 361, 362
    somatosensory system and, 349–352
Spinothalamic tract
    somatosensory system and, 349–351
Squirrel monkey
    cortico–collicular pathway in, 213
    receptive fields of neurones in superficial layers of superior colliculus in, 203
Stereocilia
    sensory cell polarisation and, 83
Stimulation
    natural, vestibular system response to, 100–110
    of nerves, ion movement during, 235
Stimulus
    location, 308, 309
    quality, receptors and, 309–318
Stomatogastric ganglion
    gastric mill cycle, neural systems mediating, 25–28
    pyloric cycle, neural system mediating, 24, 25
Stretch reflex
    characteristics, 155, 156
    recording from neuronal elements during, 165
Stridulation
    sensory modulation, 28
Strontium
    ions, transmitter release from nerve terminals and, 68
Subcorticospinal pathways
    destruction, effect on motoneurones, 164
Superior colliculus, 185–229
    anatomy, 188–195
    ascending efferents, 194
    cell activity, eye movement and, 213–215
    deep layers, receptive fields of cells in, 203–207
    descending efferents, 194, 195
    electrical stimulation of, 215–219

Superior colliculus *continued*
  lesions, effects of, 219–223 .
  non-visual inputs, 193, 194
  receptive fields, elaboration, 209–213
  receptive fields of neurones in super-
    ficial layers of, 195–203
  synaptic organisation, 192, 193
  topographic organisation, 190, 191
Supraspinal activity
  effect on spinal motoneurones, 157, 158
Synapses
  chemical, 57, 58
  corticomotoneuronal, properties, 162
  electrical, 57, 58
Synaptic cleft, 57
Synaptic mechanisms
  of primary afferent neurons, 325–330
Synaptic transmission, 53–79
Synaptic vesicles, 58

Tectospinal pathways
  spinal motoneurones following electrical
    stimulation of, 157, 158
Temperature
  effect on resting potential of nerves, 256,
    257
Termination
  of central projections of primary afferent
    neurons, 322, 323
Thalamocortical connections, 377, 378
Thalamus
  anatomy, 358, 359
  nucleus ventralis lateralis, recording
    from neurones in, 169
  neurones, physiological activation, 363–
    373
Thermoreceptors
  somatic, 314–316
Transduction
  receptive mechanisms and somatic sensa-
    tion, 307, 308
Transmitters
  post-synaptic action of, 70–75
  release from nerve terminals, 60–70
Transport
  in somatosensory system examination,
    333, 334
Tree shrew
  superior colliculus lesions in, effect of, 220
Tritonia
  fixed action pattern of, 12
Tropomyosin
  in skeletal muscle, protein binding to, 285

Utriculus organ
  morphology, 83
  physiology, 92

Ventilation
  sensory modulation, 28
Ventralis posterior lateralis
  neuronal structure in, 358
Ventral spinal pathway
  sensation and, somatosensory system
    and, 387
Ventroposterior region
  somatosensory projection to, 363–371
Vesicles
  transmitters in, 69, 70
Vestibular ganglion
  primary neurones in, 85
Vestibular nerve
  in amphibia, 86
Vestibular nuclei
  functional organisation of labyrinthine
    input, 97–115
Vestibular nystagmus
  vestibular–ocular relations and, 121–124
Vestibular organ
  morphology, 82
Vestibular receptors
  efferent innervation, 93–97
  physiology, 86–88
  primary neurones and, 82–93
Vestibular system, 81–149
Vestibulo–cerebellar interaction, 124–127
Vestibulo–cortical projection, 133–135
Vestibulo–occular reflex
  cerebellar influence on, 120, 121
  synaptology, 115–118
Vestibulo–occular relations, 115–124
  natural stimulation, 118–120
  vestibular nystagmus and, 121–124
Vestibulo–reticular interaction, 132, 133
Vestibulo–spinal interaction, 127–132
Vestibulo–spinal pathways
  destruction, effect on motoneurones, 164
  recording from neuronal units in, 166
  spinal motoneurones following electrical
    stimulation of, 157, 158
Vestibulo–spinal projection, 129–132
Visual cortical areas
  projection from, 190

Walking
  sensory modulation, 28